Benign diseases of the vulva and vagina

Benign diseases of the vulva and vagina

Herman L. Gardner, M.D.

Clinical Professor, Department of Obstetrics and Gynecology, Baylor College of Medicine, Houston, Texas; Chief of Obstetrics and Gynecology, St. Luke's Episcopal Hospital, Houston, Texas

Raymond H. Kaufman, M.D.

Acting Chairman, Department of Obstetrics and Gynecology; Associate Professor, Department of Pathology, Baylor College of Medicine, Houston, Texas

With 406 illustrations, including 2 color plates

The C. V. Mosby Company

Saint Louis   1969

Copyright © 1969 by
The C. V. Mosby Company

All rights reserved. No part of this book may be
reproduced in any manner without written
permission of the publisher.

Printed in the United States of America

Standard Book Number 8016-1726-X

Library of Congress Catalog Card
Number 74-78433

Distributed in Great Britain by Henry Kimpton,
London

Preface

The chief impetus for writing this book was the realization that benign diseases of the vulva and vagina, although constituting a large percentage of all gynecologic disease, are only sketchily covered in most of the general gynecologic texts. We believe that a single comprehensive volume devoted especially to the clinical and pathologic features of these diseases will prove useful to the physician whose practice, in whole or in part, consists of gynecology.

Many of the affections discussed come first to the attention of the dermatologist or urologist, a fact pointing up the overlapping interests of these specialties with gynecology. We hope that the subjects are presented in such a manner as to be of interest also to the dermatologist, urologist, and perhaps the pathologist.

We have endeavored to include all benign diseases involving the vulva and vagina that are likely to be encountered by clinicians practicing in the temperate zones of the world. Some lesions only rarely observed in the United States are included, with the thought that a ready reference source might preclude their complete disregard in differential diagnosis should they be presented unexpectedly. Several conditions are discussed that should have been omitted, while others have been omitted that probably should have been included. In view of the many voluminous treatises on the subject of invasive malignant lesions, these have been purposely omitted. Intraepithelial carcinoma of the vulva is included, however, because of its position between benign disease and invasive cancer. Such lesions as fistulas and relaxations, although intimately related to the vulva and vagina, do not fall within the scope of the planned text. The length of the discussions of most lesions is somewhat in keeping with their incidence and importance, although the length of the discussion of others is, perhaps, in accord with our own special interests. If the space allotted to histopathologic descriptions seems excessive in comparison to that in most nonpathology textbooks, it is because of our conviction that a knowledge of pathology is necessary for a thorough understanding of disease processes and for the optimal care of patients.

Despite every effort to give proper credit for significant contributions, such an accomplishment may have proved unattainable. Any failure in this regard is far from intentional. We are indebted to the many authors whose ideas have been incorporated. Some of the opinions expressed may be in conflict with published reports; in every such instance, however, we have attempted to weigh personal experiences with these opinions. In no instance has a contradictory opinion been advanced solely for the purpose of disagreement.

Most of the illustrations are from our personal files, the majority of those of gross lesions having been made from colored slides. Many authors and friends have graciously contributed other illustrations that seemed particularly instructive. A glossary of selected terms frequently used by the pathologist and the dermatologist is included for the use of students and clinicians to whom they may not be entirely familiar.

We were fortunate in being able to persuade Doctor Arnold A. Zimmermann to write the chapter on embryology. His many years of intimate contact with the subject as Professor of Anatomy at Baylor College of Medicine make him eminently qualified for the task. Doctors Robert R. Franklin and L. Russell Malinak, Department of Obstetrics and Gynecology at Baylor College of Medicine, because of their special knowledge and interest, were asked to contribute the chapter on developmental anomalies.

We wish to acknowledge gratefully the invaluable help and advice of our many colleagues and friends of the Houston medical community. These include Doctors John M. Knox, Marvin E. Chernosky, Elizabeth W. Rauschkolb, Joseph M. Glicksman, and Robert G. Freeman, all of the Department of Dermatology, Baylor College of Medicine; Doctor Willson J. Fahlberg, of the Department of Microbiology, Baylor College of Medicine; Doctor C. Dean Dukes, of the University of Arizona at Tuscon; and Mr. Reuben D. Wende, Director of Laboratories for the Department of Public Health for the City of Houston.

We wish to thank also Mrs. Allene Jefferson for her extensive editorial counsel, Miss Mary Smith for accumulating the bibliographic data and for editorial work, Miss Juanita Wells, M.T., for her many years of laboratory assistance and data processing, and Miss Joyce Lessard for her secretarial help. Particular indebtedness is expressed to Mrs. Velma Heiser, a long-time employee, for her dedicated efforts in every phase of the preparation and typing of the manuscript. The visual education departments of Baylor College of Medicine and the Methodist Hospital have been most cooperative in the preparation of the illustrations.

Finally, we wish to express apologies to our wives, LeNan and Patricia, for the deprivations that they experienced while this work was in progress, as well as appreciation of their tolerance of our occasional altered moods, which we only too willingly attributed to the undertaking.

Herman L. Gardner, M.D.
Raymond H. Kaufman, M.D.

Contents

1 Anatomy of the vulva and vagina, 1

2 Embryology, 12
Arnold A. Zimmermann, Ph.D.

3 Developmental anomalies of the vulva and vagina, 24
Robert R. Franklin, M.D., and L. Russell Malinak, M.D.

4 Solid tumors, 42

5 Cystic tumors, 70

6 Endometriosis, 98

7 Adenosis, 107

8 Dermatoses of the vulva, 111

9 Vulvar dystrophies, 121

10 Intraepithelial carcinoma of the vulva, 139

11 Candidiasis (moniliasis), 149

12 Trichomoniasis, 168

13 Haemophilus vaginalis vaginitis, 191

14 Nonvenereal bacterial vulvovaginitides, 208

15 Atrophic vulvovaginitis, 216

16 Viral infections, 230

17 Miscellaneous vulvovaginitides, 253

18 Miscellaneous mycoses, 269

19 Pediatric vulvovaginitis, 276

20 Contact vulvovaginitis—primary irritant and allergic reactions, 287

21 Pyodermas of the vulva, 298

22 Venereal diseases, 305

23 Traumatic lesions of the vulva and vagina, 328

24 Miscellaneous conditions, 336

Glossary, 345

Color plates

Plate 1 Vulvar manifestations of acute candidiasis, 154

Plate 2 Acute trichomoniasis, 176

Benign diseases of the vulva and vagina

Chapter 1

Anatomy of the vulva and vagina

THE VULVA

The vulva (Fig. 1-1) is that part of the female anatomy between the genitocrural folds laterally, the mons pubis anteriorly, and the anus posteriorly. It is composed of the labia majora, labia minora, mons pubis, clitoris, vestibule, urinary meatus, vaginal orifice, hymen, Bartholin's glands, Skene's ducts, and the vestibulovaginal bulbs.

Labia majora
Gross anatomy

The lateral boundaries of the vulva are formed by the labia majora, which consist of two large folds of adipose and fibrous tissue. Anteriorly, the labia majora fuse into the mons pubis; posteriorly, they become narrower and flatter and terminate 3 to 4 cm. anterior to the anus, where they are united by the posterior commissure or fourchette. The lateral aspects of the labia majora are covered by a considerable amount of coarse hair, and the inner aspects by little or no hair. Prior to puberty, the labia majora are inconspicuous and the labia minora protrude between them in a conspicuous fashion. At puberty, the labia majora develop as one of the secondary sexual characteristics, with their lateral aspects and the mons becoming covered by coarse hairs. In most women, the upper border of this hair is sharply defined. The skin of the labia majora is usually somewhat darker than the adjacent skin.

Histology

The labia majora are covered by skin composed of an outer lining of stratified squamous epithelium (Fig. 1-2) consisting of a basal layer of cells, the stratum malpighii, a thin granular layer (occasionally absent),

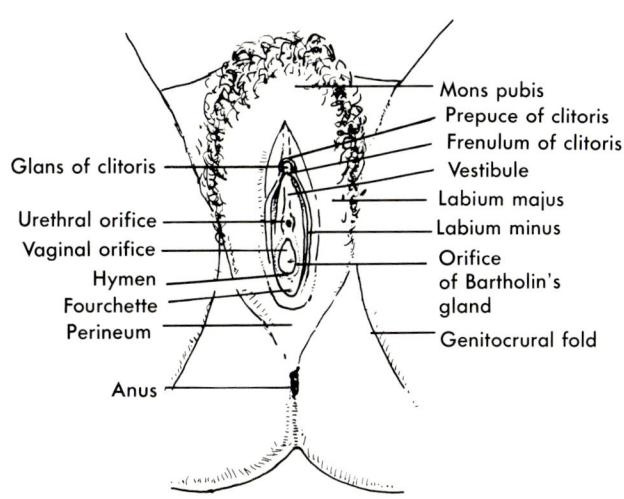

Fig. 1-1. Diagram of the vulva, showing its principal parts.

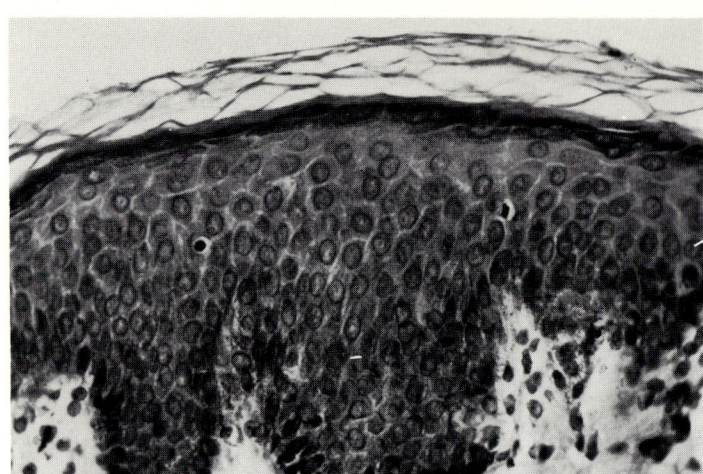

Fig. 1-2. Labium majus. Squamous epithelium; a thin granular layer and a slight degree of keratinization. (H & E × 495)

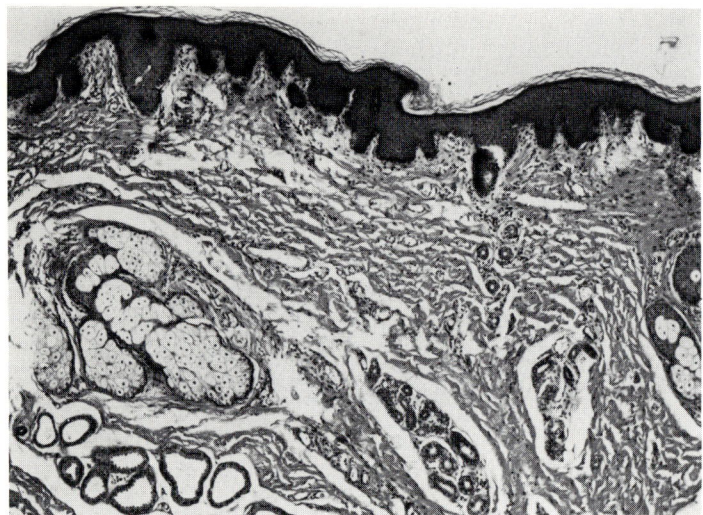

Fig. 1-3. Labium majus. Within the dermis are eccrine, apocrine, and sebaceous glands. (H & E × 77)

and a horny layer. These different layers represent the different stages of the conversion of the basal cells into cornified cells. (Odland, Selby, and Zellickson have published excellent works on the electron microscopy of the human skin to which the interested reader is referred.) Within the dermis of the skin are numerous hair follicles and sebaceous, sweat, and apocrine glands (Fig. 1-3).

The *sweat* or *eccrine glands* (Fig. 1-4) are tubular structures whose cells secrete and change only slightly in size and shape during this process. The sweat glands lead directly into the epidermis and are composed of three segments: a secretory portion, intradermal sweat duct, and intraepidermal sweat duct. The secretory portion of the gland has one distinct layer, consisting of secretory cells that contain a clear, slightly basophilic cytoplasm and abundant glycogen that disappears on sweating. Small myoepithelial cells are scattered between the bases

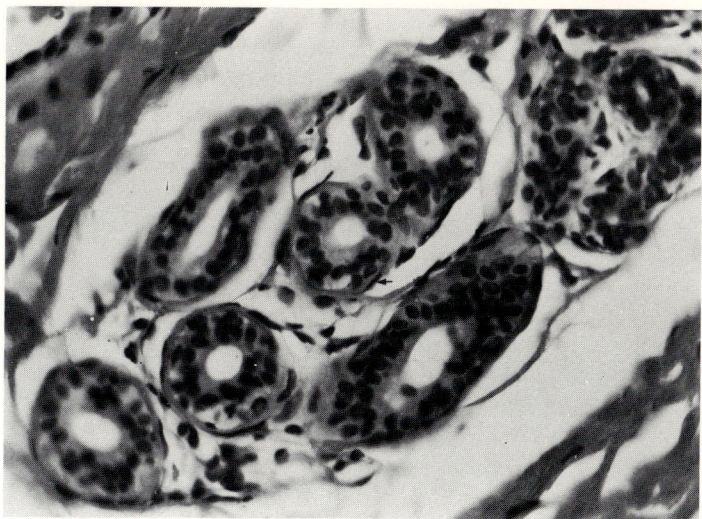

Fig. 1-4. Labium majus. Eccrine sweat glands and ducts. Arrow points to a myoepithelial cell. (H & E × 495)

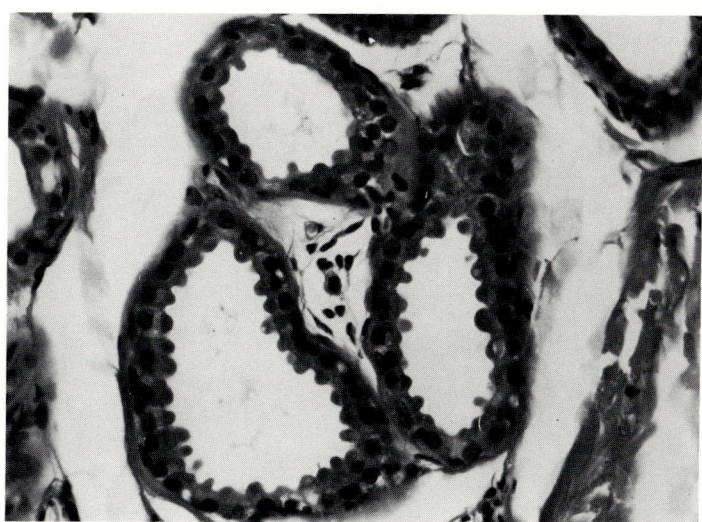

Fig. 1-5. Labium majus. Apocrine glands. Note variations in height of the secretory cells. The lumina of the glands are large as compared to those of the eccrine sweat glands. (H & E × 495)

of the secretory cells; contraction of the myoepithelial cells forces out the secretion of the latter. The intradermal portion of the sweat duct is composed of two layers of cuboidal, deeply basophilic cells. The intraepidermal duct consists of a single layer of cuboidal cells surrounded by a sheath of epidermal cells.

The *sebaceous glands* are alveolar, holocrine glands that have no lumen. Their secretion, which is formed by decomposition of the cells, is evacuated through the sebaceous ducts into pilosebaceous follicles. These follicles may or may not contain hair. Each gland is composed of several lobules, and at the periphery of each lobule one layer of deeply basophilic cuboidal cells, referred to as the *generative cells*, is present. The cells within the central portion of each lobule have a cytoplasm arranged in a delicate network and are filled by fat.

The *apocrine glands* (Fig. 1-5) of the

labia majora are identical to those found in the axilla, breasts, and perianal regions. Sometimes referred to as the scent glands, the apocrine glands are tubular structures whose cells pass through a full cycle of secretory stages. At the beginning of the cycle the cells are of a low cuboidal type. Gradually, they increase in height until they protrude into the lumen; then, upon releasing their secretion, they again become low cuboidal. Recent studies by Montes, Baker, and Curtis suggest that, contrary to prior opinion, the lining cells in these glands do not release part of their cytoplasm into the lumen during secretion. The secretory portion of the apocrine gland is lined by a distinct layer of epithelial cells that varies in height, depending upon the stage of the secretory cycle. The duct is lined by two layers of cuboidal epithelial cells.

Labia minora
Gross anatomy

The labia minora lie between the labia majora and consist of two flat folds of connective tissue that contain little or no adipose tissue. They are covered by skin on their lateral aspects, and partially so on their medial aspects. As a rule, the labia minora are 4 to 5 cm. in length and approximately 0.5 cm. in thickness, although in some females they are more elongated and protrude between the labia majora. Anteriorly, each divides into two parts, one passing over the clitoris to form the prepuce, or foreskin, and the other passing behind the clitoris to form the frenulum. Posteriorly, they tend to become smaller and blend with the medial surfaces of the labia majora or to unite anterior to the posterior commissure to form the fourchette. The cleft between the two labia minora is referred to as the *vestibule*, and into this vestibule open the vagina, the urethra, Skene's ducts, and Bartholin's gland ducts. Between the posterior fourchette and hymeneal ring is a depression, the *fossa navicularis*. As already mentioned, the labia minora are relatively more prominent in children, since the labia majora are not well-developed at this time. In the postmenopausal woman the labia majora tend to atrophy, and the labia minora again become relatively prominent. Occasionally, the labia minora may atrophy almost to the point of disappearance.

Histology

As the hymen is approached, the skin on the medial aspects of the labia minora changes into what many morphologists call a mucous membrane type of epithelium, although whether this covering is skin or mucous membrane is debatable (Fig. 1-6). Mucus is not secreted from the labia minora; however, these tissues often are bathed in the mucous secretion that comes from Bartholin's

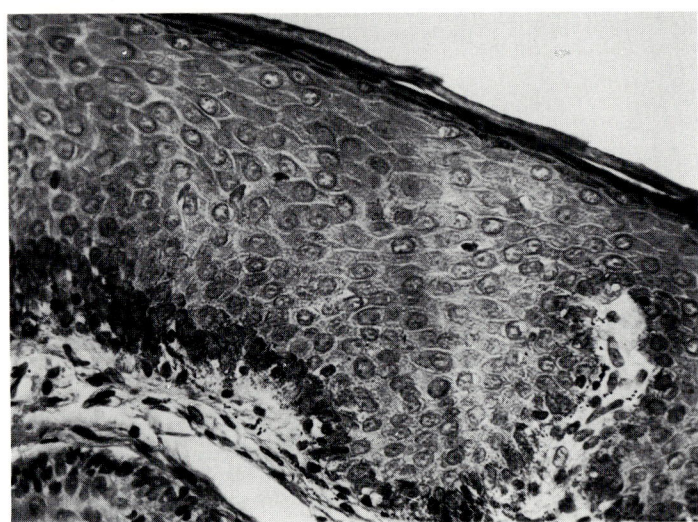

Fig. 1-6. Outer labium minus. The lining epithelium contains little keratin, and the granular layer is indistinct. (H & E × 495)

Anatomy of the vulva and vagina

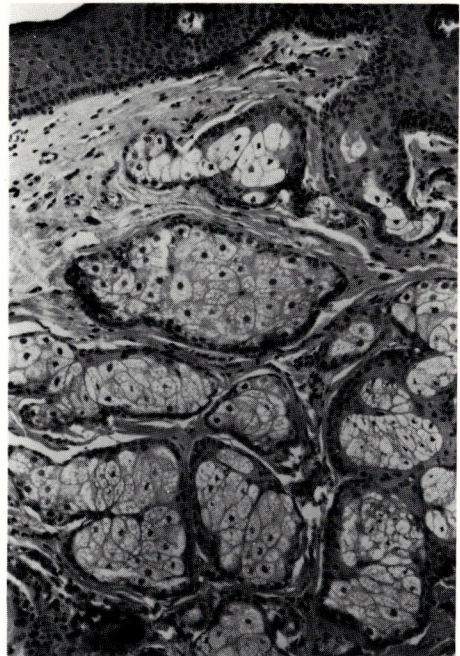

Fig. 1-7. Labium minus. Numerous sebaceous glands are apparent in the dermis. (H & E × 100)

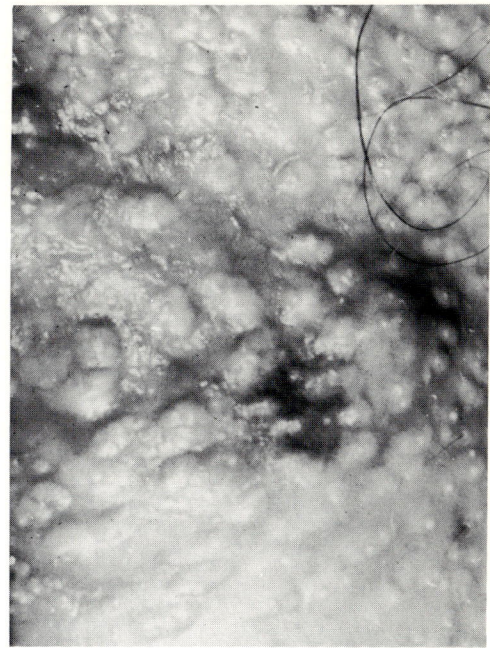

Fig. 1-8. Labium minus. Prominent sebaceous glands within the dermis may result in the presence of pinpoint papular structures.

glands and the cervix. The epithelial covering is much less cornified than true skin; it has a scant or no granular layer, and the dermis contains no hair follicles. The skin and mucosa of the labia minora are extremely rich in sebaceous glands (Figs. 1-7 and 1-8). These glands enter directly into the skin through tunnels in the epithelium. Sweat glands are sparse or completely absent.

The deeper tissues are composed of dense connective tissue containing many veins and some smooth muscle elements. Numerous bundles of elastic tissue are mixed within the connective tissue, and a minimal amount of fatty tissue is present. During sexual excitement, the labia minora frequently become swollen and congested and take on the appearance of erectile tissue.

The clitoris
Gross anatomy

The clitoris is the homologue of the penis. It consists of two cylindrical erectile bodies, called the *corpora cavernosa*, that terminate in the vestibule as the glans. The body of the

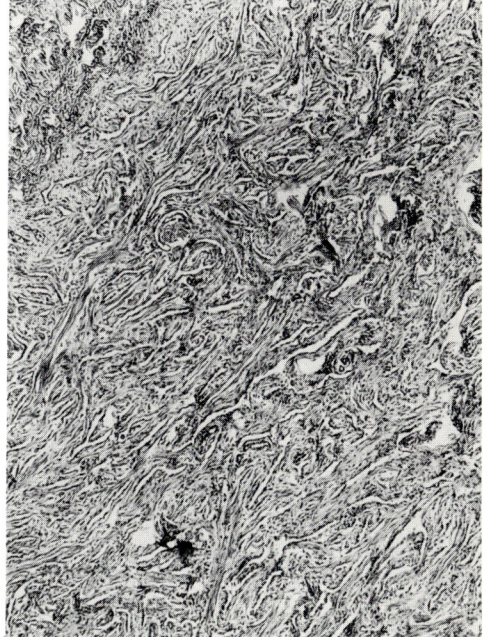

Fig. 1-9. Section through clitoris of 2-year-old child showing erectile tissue composed of numerous thin-walled vascular channels and nerve fibers. (H & E × 65)

6 Benign diseases of the vulva and vagina

clitoris, which is formed by fusion of the two corpora cavernosa, extends from the pubic arch anteriorly to the glans posteriorly and is approximately 2 cm. in length. At the inferior border of the pubic arch, the two corpora cavernosa separate and follow the inferior border of the inferior rami of the pubic bones, to which they are attached. These are the crura of the clitoris. They are covered by the ischiocavernosus muscles which, by contraction, trap blood within the corpora cavernosa to cause erection of the clitoris.

Histology

The glans clitoris is covered by a mucous membrane containing many specialized nerve end-organs. It is composed of erectile tissue (Fig. 1-9) with many large and small venous channels surrounded by large amounts of smooth muscle tissue. This erectile tissue is arranged into the corpora cavernosa.

The vestibule

The vestibule is the portion of the vulva extending from the clitoris to the fourchette that is visible on separation of the labia minora. It is the remains of the urogenital sinus of the embryo. The vagina, ducts of Bartholin's glands, Skene's ducts, and urethra open into the vestibule. The vestibule is covered by a mucosa lined by stratified squamous epithelium.

The hymen

The hymen is a thin membrane of connective tissue over the entrance of the vagina into the vestibule. It has a central

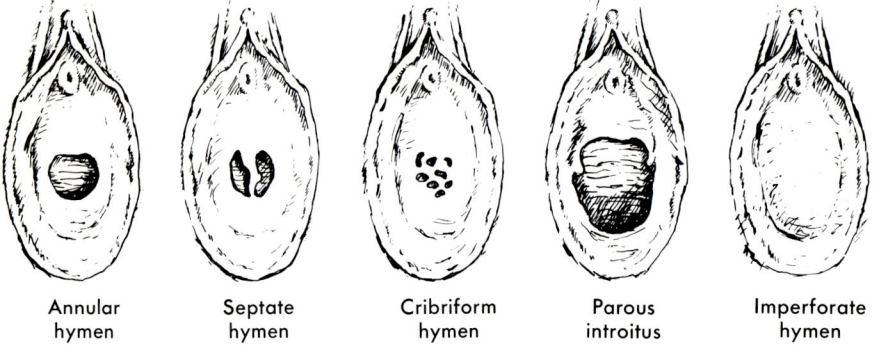

Fig. 1-10. Diagram of various types of hymens described in text.

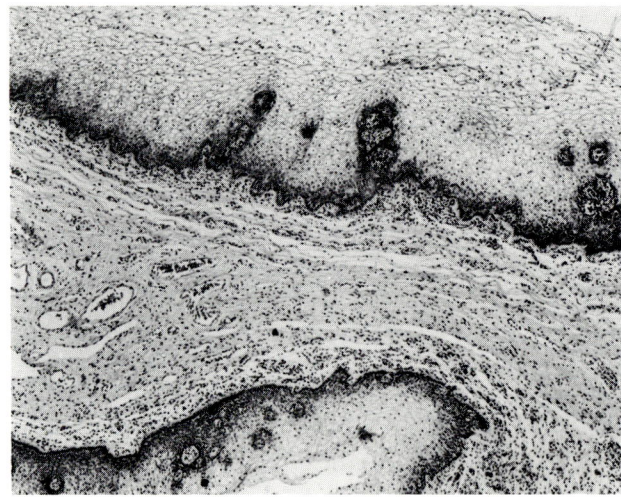

Fig. 1-11. Section through hymen. A lining of squamous epithelium on both inner and outer surfaces is separated by a relatively thin layer of connective tissue. (H & E × 52)

Anatomy of the vulva and vagina

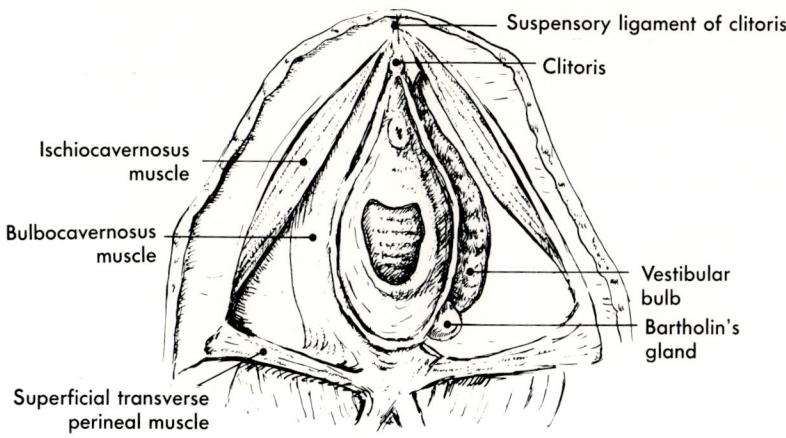

Fig. 1-12. Diagram of deeper structures of vulva, showing the location of Bartholin's glands and vestibular bulb.

opening that is usually round or concentric. In some hymens, a thin mucosal septa may create two or more openings; or the hymen may be cribiform, having numerous small openings through a solid mucosal plate. On rare occasions, the hymen may be imperforate; thus, no communication between the vagina and the vestibule is present (Fig. 1-10).

The hymen varies somewhat in thickness and elasticity. It may be quite elastic and easily stretched without laceration at the initial intercourse, or it may be so tough and rigid as to prevent intercourse. As a rule, the intact hymen is present only in the virgin; after coitus it is represented by small, membranous elevations referred to as the *carunculae myrtiformes*.

The hymen is lined on both sides by a thin mucous membrane composed of stratified squamous epithelium (Fig. 1-11). This epithelium covers a rather variable thickness of connective tissue containing many small blood vessels.

Bartholin's glands

Bartholin's glands, which are homologous to Cowper's glands in the male, lie deep beneath the fascia, one on each side of the vestibule, posterolateral to the vaginal orifice (Fig. 1-12). They are lobulated, racemose glandular structures about the size of small peas, and contain multiple acini grouped around the termination of each of their many branching ducts. The acini are lined by a cuboidal epithelium in which the cells

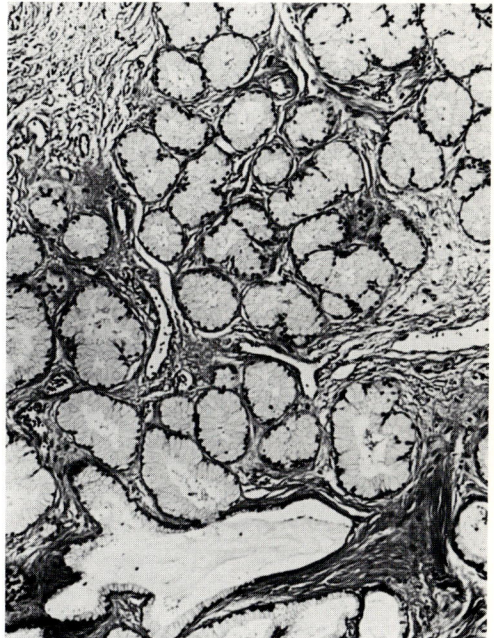

Fig. 1-13. Bartholin's gland. The acini are typical. In lower portion of the picture, a terminal duct enters several acinar structures. (H & E × 117)

have a clear cytoplasm and dark, basally situated nuclei (Fig. 1-13). The cells contain mucin, which is secreted during sexual excitation, and which serves to lubricate the vaginal orifice and canal. The main duct of a Bartholin's gland opens slightly posterior to the midportion of the lateral margin of the vaginal orifice, just outside the hymeneal ring. The duct is lined by stratified transi-

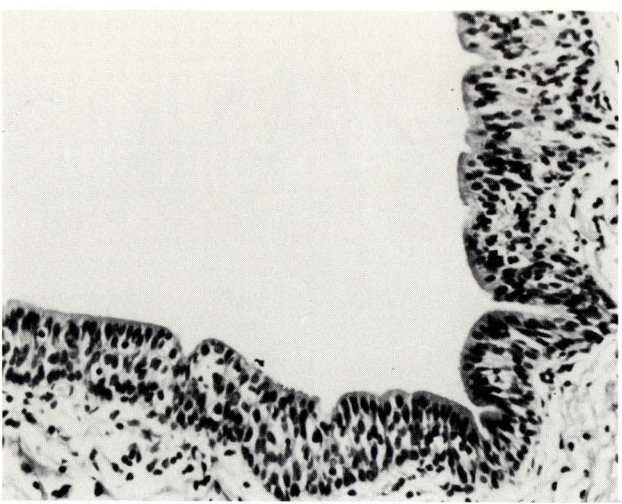

Fig. 1-14. Main Bartholin's duct. The lining is composed of transitional epithelium. (H & E × 286)

tional epithelium (Fig. 1-14) with the exception of the portion near the orifice; this portion is lined by stratified squamous epithelium. As the branching ducts approach the gland, they gradually become smaller and the epithelium becomes flatter, and in their finest, most terminal branches, they are lined by a single layer of cuboidal epithelium. As a rule, so-called Bartholin's gland cysts are actually cysts formed within the main duct of the gland following obstruction to the flow of secretion from this gland. Correctly, these cysts should be referred to as Bartholin's duct cysts.

The bulb of the vestibule

Two oval masses of erectile tissue, called the *bulbi vestibuli* (Fig. 1-12), are incorporated within the bulbocavernosus muscles beneath the floor of the vestibule on each side of the vaginal opening. The bulbi vestibuli are homologous to the bulbus penis of the male. A Bartholin's gland lies in the base of the bulb on each side. Unless affected by trauma, these structures are seldom related to vulvar disease.

The urethra

The urethra opens into the vestibule just anterior to the vaginal introitus. Immediately within the meatus, the urethra is slit-like, with its long axis lying ventrodorsally. The edge of the external orifice is everted and may have two or three overhanging lips; because of these lips, the orifice is occasionally difficult to find. The most distal paraurethral ducts, *Skene's ducts*, open into the urethral canal just within or external to the meatus. According to Huffman, the majority of paraurethral ducts empty into the distal third of the urethral canal, then turn cephalad and divide into many smaller branches (Fig. 1-15). These smaller branches terminate as small bud-like outpocketings and tubular glands, chiefly in the lateral and inferior urethral walls. It is Huffman's opinion that the presence of two lateral ducts, as described by Skene, are the exception rather than the rule.

The *paraurethral glands* are branched tubular glands that empty into the paraurethral ducts. They are lined by epithelium that varies from the low columnar to the cuboidal type. Most of the smaller and many of the larger branches of the paraurethral ducts are lined by pseudostratified or true stratified columnar epithelium. Near the orifices the lining is identical to that of the urethra at that level. If infection develops within the ducts and glands, obstructing the outlet of the duct, abscesses of the anterior vaginal wall may form and rupture into the urethra, ultimately enlarging into diverticula.

The urethra, which measures from 3 to 5.5 cm. in length, extends from the neck of the

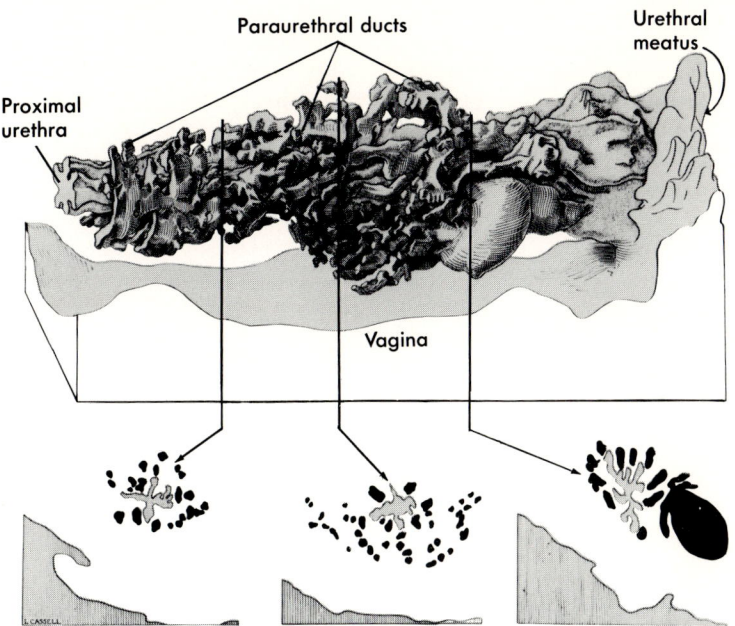

Fig. 1-15. Drawing of a wax model of an adult human female urethra with periurethral ducts and glands, as viewed from the right side. Tissues from which this model was reconstructed were obtained at necropsy of a 20-year-old virgin. The model represents the distal 2.4 cm. of a urethra having a total length of 2.8 cm. No periurethral ducts open at or immediately within the urethral meatus. Thirty-one ducts empty into the urethra, the majority into the distal third; others empty into the middle and proximal thirds. After leaving the urethra, the ducts turn cephalad and extend parallel to the urethral canal. One large duct on the right develops into a cyst of considerable size. At the midpoint in the urethra, many ducts and glands extend laterally far from the canal. At a more proximal level, the urethra is surrounded by many small tubules, and on the right, it is encompassed by a thin, compact, semicircular sheet of ducts and glands. (Huffman, J. W.: Amer. J. Obstet. Gynec. 55:86, 1948.)

bladder to the external urethral orifice. Its proximal two-thirds is usually lined by a stratified transitional epithelium and the outer third by a stratified squamous epithelium. The upper half of the urethra is separated from the anterior vaginal wall by connective tissue, whereas its lower half is firmly adherent to the musculature of the vaginal wall.

Blood, lymph, and nerve supply

The arterial blood supply to the vulva is abundant, coming from branches of the internal pudendal artery, which derives from the internal iliac artery (hypogastric), as well as from branches of the external pudendal artery, which derives from the femoral artery. The veins within the vulva form a large plexus, ultimately emptying into the internal pudendal and external pudendal veins.

The anterior superior portion of the vulva is supplied by the cutaneous branches of the ilioinguinal nerve. The posterior inferior portion receives its nerve supply from the pudendal branches of the posterior femoral cutaneous nerve. Between these two groups of nerves, branches from the posterior labial and perineal branches of the pudendal nerve also extend into the vulva.

The primary lymph channels of the vulva empty into the superficial inguinal lymph nodes. Lymph vessels also pass from the posterior portion of the vulva to the perianal lymph nodes.

THE VAGINA

The vagina extends from the vestibule to the uterus and connects the two. It is directed obliquely upward and backward at an angle approximately 45 degrees to the horizontal; its long axis is parallel to the plane of the pelvic brim and at a right angle to the uterus.

The anterior and posterior walls of the vagina are slack and remain in contact, whereas the lateral walls remain fairly rigid and separated. On cross section, this gives an H-shaped appearance to the vaginal canal. The anterior vaginal wall averages 6 to 7 cm. in length, whereas the posterior wall is approximately 7.5 to 8.5 cm. The upper third of the anterior vaginal wall is in contact with the base of the bladder, and the entire lower two-thirds is in contact with the urethra. The cervix enters the anterior vaginal wall, dividing the upper vagina into the anterior, posterior, and two lateral fornices. The upper third of the posterior wall is covered by cul-de-sac peritoneum, the midportion is separated from the lower end of the rectum by fibrofatty tissue and the rectovaginal septum, and the lower third is separated from the anal canal and anal sphincter by the rectovaginal septum and the muscles of the perineal body.

The vagina consists of three principal layers: an outer fibrous layer, which derives from the pelvic fascia; a middle muscular layer; and an inner mucosal layer. The mucous membrane consists of wavy stratified squamous epithelium that is superimposed upon a tunica propria of fibrous tissue (Fig. 1-16). Small epithelial folds dip down into the tunica propria. In the prepubertal child, the vaginal mucosa is thin, perhaps consisting of only four to eight layers of basal and parabasal cells. Under the influence of estrogenic stimulation at the time of puberty, the mucosa thickens as the squamous cells mature; thereafter, it responds cyclically to the ovarian production of estrogen and progesterone. These cyclic changes are not evident grossly, although they are reflected fairly accurately in the vaginal smear. Under the influence of estrogen alone, the mucosal cells undergo a process of maturation, becoming progressively thinner and flatter, and their nuclei become smaller and more pyknotic. Progesterone inhibits this maturation to some degree, causing the epithelium to mature up to the superficial intermediate cell layer. Testosterone also tends to inhibit this maturation process to some extent. These cellular changes are reflected in the cyclic variation in the shedding of squamous cells from the vagina; this fact is useful in the evaluation of the hormonal status of the woman and is reflected in the vaginal cytogram. Immediately prior to ovulation, when the output of estrogen is at its peak, superficial cells are predominant in the vaginal smear. Following ovulation and throughout pregnancy, the intermediate cells predominate. As the menopause is approached and the output of hormones from the ovaries decreases, the vaginal epithelial cells undergo less maturation, as indicated by a shedding of cells largely from the deeper layers of the epithelium.

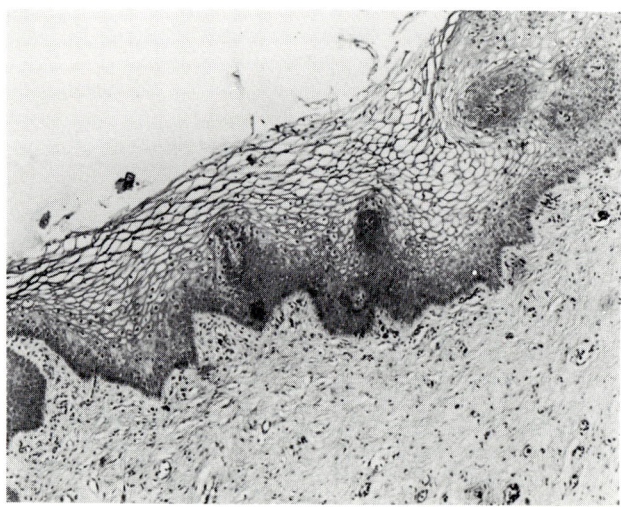

Fig. 1-16. Normal vagina. The mucosal lining consists of a wavy, stratified squamous epithelium overlying a tunica propria of fibrous tissue. (H & E × 88)

Although the vagina itself contains no glands, remnants of the mesonephric (wolffian) and paramesonephric (müllerian) ducts may often be found at almost any location within its walls. The mesonephric remnants are usually located along the anterior lateral aspect of the vagina, whereas the remnants of the müllerian ducts may persist in any area. Cervical glands are only rarely present in the vaginal fornices.

Blood and lymph supply

The uterine and pudendal arteries, both of which are branches of the internal iliac arteries, are the chief sources of blood supply of the vagina. They form a plexus around the vagina, and from this plexus a median artery arises on the anterior and posterior walls. These arteries are sometimes referred to as the *azygos vaginal arteries*. A rich venous plexus also surrounds the vagina and communicates with the vesicle, pudendal, and hemorrhoidal venous plexuses, which empty into the internal iliac veins.

The lymph vessels empty primarily into the internal and external iliac lymph nodes. Those from the upper part of the vagina join the uterine lymph vessels and enter the external and internal iliac glands. Those from the middle third parallel the vaginal vessels to the internal iliac glands. Some of the lymph vessels from the lower third enter the sacral and common iliac lymph nodes, while others end in the superficial inguinal glands.

REFERENCES

Anson, B. J.: Morris' anatomy, ed. 12, New York, 1966, The McGraw-Hill Book Co.

Huffman, J. W.: The detailed anatomy of the paraurethral ducts in the adult human female, Amer. J. Obstet. Gynec. 55:86, 1948.

Kistner, R. W.: Gynecology, principles and practice, Chicago, 1964, Year Book Medical Publishers, Inc.

Lever, W. F.: Histopathology of the skin, ed. 3, Philadelphia, 1961, J. B. Lippincott Co.

Montes, L. F., Baker, B. L., and Curtis, A. C.: The cytology of the large axillary sweat glands in man, J. Invest. Derm. 35:273, 1960.

Novak, E. R., and Woodruff, J. D.: Gynecologic and obstetric pathology, Philadelphia, 1962, The W. B. Saunders Co.

Odland, G. F.: The fine structure of the interrelationship of cells in the human epidermis, J. Biophys. Biochem. Cytol. 4:529, 1958.

Selby, C. C.: An electron microscopic study of thin sections of human skin, J. Invest. Derm. 29:131, 1957.

Smout, C. F. V., and Jacoby, F.: Gynecological and obstetrical anatomy, London, 1948, Edward Arnold & Co.

Zellickson, A. S.: Electron microscopy of skin and mucous membranes, Springfield, Ill., 1963, Charles C Thomas, Publisher.

Chapter 2

Embryology

Arnold A. Zimmermann, Ph.D.

EMBRYONIC AND EARLY FETAL STAGES OF THE INTERNAL GENITAL TRACTS

The embryonic period proper of man covers the first 8 weeks of postovulatory development, that is 10 weeks of postmenstrual age. During that stage there are no differentiating signs of either uterus, cervix, or vagina. In both sexes, a bilateral and dual set of ducts arises that characterizes the neutral or indifferent phase in the development of the human internal genital tracts. Concurrently, the genesis of external sex organs also passes through an undifferentiated, neutral stage.

The establishment of the external body form *(morphogenesis)* with recognizable human features and the formation of all or most organ primordia *(organogenesis)* take place in the truly embryonic period.

The minute size of such basic organ anlagen ("that which is being laid down") is reflected, in a measure, by the overall size of 25 mm. (1 in.) attained by the human embryo at the end of the eighth week. External body sex is recognizable only in the early fetal stage (third month), when the size of the developing organism has reached 50 to 60 mm. (2 in.).

The fetal period lasts from the beginning of the third month to term. Its main characteristics are those of growth, earliest endocrine activities, and histodifferentiation of the organ primordia. The uterus, cervix, and vagina become established rather late in this developmental period.

The embryonic dual duct systems of both sexes comprise the mesonephric (wolffian) and the paramesonephric (müllerian) ducts. The mesonephric ducts represent caudal extensions of the nephric ducts, temporarily consisting of solid epithelial cords, formed by tubules of the pronephros and mesonephros. These are transitory, nonfunctional "kidneys" of mammalian and human embryos. Near their caudal end the mesonephric ducts form an outgrowth, the *ureteric bud,* which is destined to develop into the entire collecting system of the permanent kidneys (metanephros): ureters, renal pelvis, and collecting tubules up to and including the medullary rays. In the developing male fetus, the main portion of the mesonephric duct becomes the ductus deferens and epididymal and ejaculatory ducts, the definitive genital conducting tract that opens into the urethral portion of the urogenital sinus.

In the female fetus, the mesonephric ducts degenerate. Epithelial remnants may be retained along the lateral walls of the uterus, cervix, and vagina, the latter generally being known as *Gartner's ducts.* Their epithelium may proliferate and become stratified, or it may form cysts, especially in the vaginal wall and sometimes at the level of the hymen. Hymenal cysts probably arise from degenerated distal ends of the wolffian ducts which, in their normal course of development, terminate in the dorsal wall of the urogenital sinus at the site of the developing hymen. Meyer and Vilas described vaginal, hymenal, and cervical cysts at various fetal stages, as well as in the newborn. It has been estimated that remnants of mesonephric ducts may be present in 25 percent of adult females. Neurohistochemical staining methods appear to indicate that most cysts without connective tissue walls of their own are derived from müllerian epithelium. Others may be merely the result of faulty canalization of the vaginal epithelial plate.

In the fifth week of the embryonic period, the paramesonephric (müllerian) ducts arise as shallow invaginations of the coelomic epithelium of the mesonephros. The lips of the groove meet and form a solid epithelial cord; this grows caudad, crossing the wolffian ducts and following their lead to the dorsal wall of the urogenital sinus. The sinus itself represents the ventral portion of the original cloaca and thus is lined by endodermal epithelium, as are its derivatives, the bladder, urethra, and prostatic and vestibular (Bartholin's) glands.

By the eighth week of postovulatory age, the caudal portions of the müllerian ducts lie close together, flanked by the wolffian ducts, and begin to fuse. However, they fail to open into the urogenital sinus; instead, they form a protrusion, the *müllerian tubercle* (Fig. 2-1). This marks the junction of three types of epithelia: the blind ends of the fused müllerian ducts, the open distal ends of the wolffian ducts, and the sinus epithelium on the underside of the protrusion. Through 100 years of research, the developmental events at this minute and crucial area of the müllerian tubercle have been variously interpreted. The many attempts to clarify the origin of the vaginal epithelium and of the portio vaginalis of the cervix have led to antagonistic views; even now investiga-

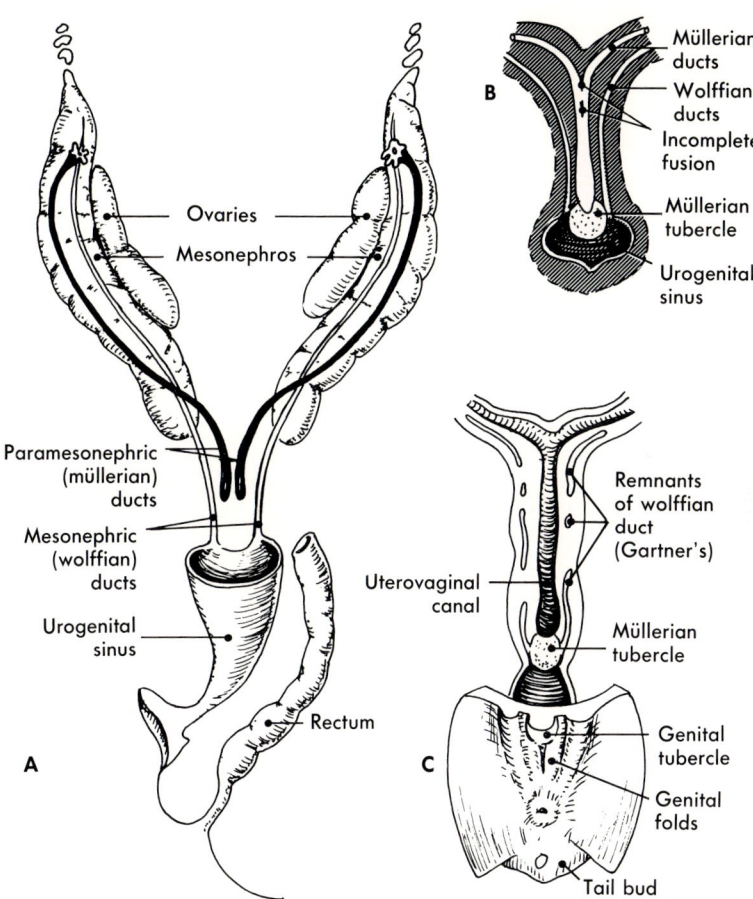

Fig. 2-1. **A**, Diagram showing the relationship of the müllerian and wolffian ducts to the mesonephros, urogenital sinus, and each other near the end of the embryonic period. Embryo of about 25 mm. (Adapted from Hunter, R. H.: Contrib. Embryol. 22:91, 1930.) **B**, The uterovaginal canal, formed by fusion of the müllerian ducts. Fetus of the third month, 33 mm. C.R.L. (Adapted from Koff, A. K.: Contrib. Embryol. 24:59, 1933.) **C**, Fetus of 50 to 60 mm. C.R.L., late third month. (Adapted from Hunter and Koff.)

tors do not agree upon this point. Special attention will be directed toward this complex area later in this review.

It is clearly established, nevertheless, that in the normal female human fetus of the third month, fusion of the distal, tubular portions of the paramesonephric ducts is complete. This is the primordium of the *uterovaginal canal,* consisting of müllerian epithelium and investing visceral mesoderm. The latter supplies the tunica propria of the endometrium and of the vaginal mucosa, as well as the fibrous and muscular tunics.

In the male fetus, the müllerian ducts undergo a pronounced regression under the influence of androgenic hormones produced by the fetal testes.

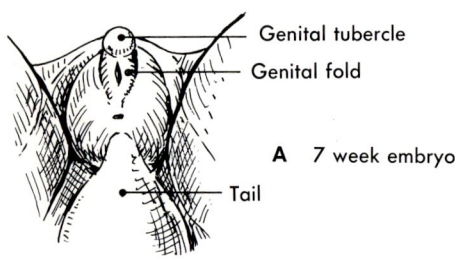

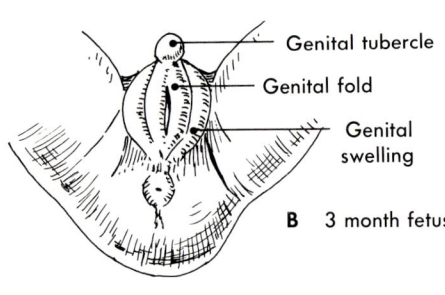

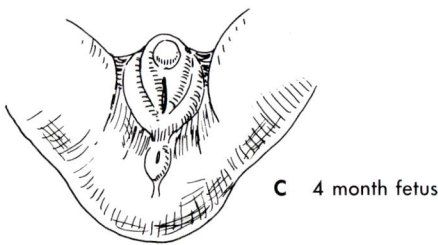

Fig. 2-2. Development of the female external genitalia. **A,** Embryo of the seventh week; **B,** fetus of the third month; **C,** fetus of the fourth month. (Adapted from Spaulding, M. H.: Contrib. Embryol. **13:**67, 1921.)

DEVELOPMENT OF THE FEMALE EXTERNAL GENITALIA

During the sixth and seventh embryonic weeks (embryos of 16 to 18 mm. in length), the cloaca becomes divided by the urorectal septum into ventral and dorsal portions. These represent, respectively, the *urogenital sinus* and the *primitive rectum.* By the eighth week, the original cloacal membrane is perforated by urogenital and anal openings.

The first signs of the neutral stage of external genitalia appear concurrently in the minute perineal region between the broad attachment of the umbilical cord and the tail. They are somatic derivations, consisting of an unpaired protrusion, the genital tubercle in front of the urogenital orifice, and of paired genital folds flanking the most distal portion of the urogenital sinus and narrowing it to form the vestibule of the emerging vulva. The tubercle represents the phallic portion, becoming the clitoris; the genital (urethral) folds are the primordia of the labia minora. Further mesenchymal proliferations produce additional skin folds, the genital swellings or labioscrotal folds, which are destined to form the labia majora (Fig. 2-2).

By the twelfth week, the female and male external genitals are definitely recognizable. Internally, there is as yet no hymen in the female. Histodifferentiation of the definitive vaginal epithelium and the formation of the fornices and of the portio are further delayed until the midfetal period. The major vestibular glands, however, arise in the third month from the entodermal epithelium lining the vestibule.

Temporarily, the glans and body of the clitoris are relatively large. This represents the phallic phase. Normally, the degree of separation or of relative fusion of the lesser and greater lips is variable. This will be reflected in the size and arrangement of the clitoral prepuce, of the frenulum or fourchette of the labia minora, as well as of the posterior commissure of the labia majora and of the pudendal cleft itself. None of these minor variations should be considered as true anomalies nor ascribed to special hormonal influences.

Wilson found that the differentiation of the external genitalia often proceeded more slowly than the general development of the embryo and early fetus. It was slower in male than in female specimens, with wide variations in individual specimens. Wilson could not confirm Spaulding's contention that there is practically no indifferent stage in the development of the external sex organs. Sex determination by examination of the external genitalia in embryonic and early fetal stages remains unreliable. In the light of experimental evidence obtained from rabbit embryos, it would seem probable that variability and delay in the development of the male pudendum may be due to variations in the output of androgenic hormones by the fetal testes.

GENETIC AND HORMONAL FACTORS: MAJOR FEMALE SEX ANOMALIES

Both genetic and endocrine factors are involved in determining and regulating embryonic development and fetal differentiation of organ systems such as the female reproductive tracts and sex characteristics. Aberrations in either factor or imbalance between the two will result in major congenital anomalies.

During the early indifferent stage, there is no evidence of a purely male or female constitution. With histodifferentiation of the testes in the seventh week, events take a definite turn toward the development of maleness. In female embryos, the undifferentiated condition of the gonad and sex ducts is retained a little longer. The female sex is generally considered to be the basic or primary one.

Genetic or chromosomal sex is determined at the moment of fertilization, when twenty-two pairs of autosomes and two sex chromosomes reassemble into the diploid number and supply the full hereditary endowment, including the genetic sex *(genotype)*. The complement of forty-six chromosomes designated as karyotype 46/XX determines the female, and karyotype 46/XY determines the male direction of sexual development. Sex chromosomes X and Y carry the *genes* or messenger codes for sex characteristics. They determine primarily the type of gonad —ovary or testis—to be developed. The exact nature and mode of activity of this control is still unknown. So far, neither specific enzymes nor hormones have been detected in this phase of gonadal sex differentiation.

The Y chromosome definitely is "testis producing." Although it is dominant in its coding effects over a single X chromosome, normal testes will not develop if the Y chromosome is accompanied by extra X chromosomes. Such abnormalities in the number or constitution of sex chromosomes result in various *intersex syndromes*, also called *chromosomal intersex*. An example is complete *primary agonadism* or *Turner's syndrome*. Generally, these intersex fetuses are of karyotype 45/XO. They are genetic females in whom ovaries fail to arise. The paramesonephric (müllerian) ducts nevertheless develop into an immature uterus and vagina of the castrate type. Such "agonadal women" usually have webbing of the neck and often have congenital aortic stenosis. Their external genitals are normal but immature. There are no secondary sexual characteristics either in the breasts or in the distribution of the pubic hair. Usually there is mental deficiency and, of course, sterility.

Some persons exhibiting Turner's syndrome have been found to be of karyotype 46/XX, with one of the X chromosomes being definitely abnormal and the ovaries hypoplastic. Other clinically similar intersex conditions apparently have a mosaic type of chromosomal constitution. *Mosaicism* represents a genetic aberration incident to errors in chromosomal dysjunction, either during maturation division (meiosis) or in ordinary cell division (mitosis). The genetic constitution of some body cells then differs from that of others—the chromosomes are distributed as a mosaic in the same individual. Some somatic cells of a patient with a Turner-like syndrome may be of karyotype 45/XO and others of the type 46/XX. Most individuals with this type of Turner's syndrome are also sterile.

A further example of chromosomal intersex is the congenital form of the *adrenogenital syndrome*. It is caused not by aberrant chromosomal numbers but by a gene defect and consequent metabolic error. In such genetic females (46/XX), adrenal hyperplasia and masculinization take place early; for this reason, the condition is also classified as *hereditary female pseudohermaphroditism*. Bruner-Lorand suggested that the anomaly may derive from recessive genetic factors carried by autosomes, rather than from aberrations in sex chromosomes. He stated that if the suprarenal malfunction—abnormal synthesis of cortisol—begins during fetal life, masculinization is pronounced. The uterovaginal canal remains underdeveloped, the wolffian ducts may be retained, and prostatic glandular tubules may be formed. The genital tubercle develops into a phallic clitoris and the labia minora may fuse to form a partial phallic urethra. The true sex may be mistaken at birth, hence upbringing and psychologic sex may take a course contrary to the genetic sex.

If the suprarenal malfunction begins late —at or after puberty—the symptoms are less severe. Armstrong classified such cases of the adrenogenital syndrome as purely *hormonal intersex*. He based the anomaly upon excessive formation of endogenous adrenal androgens, which is induced by overproduction of ACTH. Nevertheless, among the various types and degrees of virilization of females, Armstrong recognized an "inborn" metabolic error in the congenital form, as well as definite genetic factors in the so-called "constitutional virilism syndrome" (Ferriman, Page, and Newnham). Such persons have a masculine body build (broad shoulders and narrow hips), with male distribution of pubic hair and hirsutism on the face and chest. Ovulation may be irregular, although conception is possible.

In some persons with abnormal sex development, it is difficult to ascertain the genetic sex (genotype) on the basis of their aberrant chromosomal patterns. The identification of the so-called *sex chromatin* then becomes a helpful adjunct. In most somatic cells of the female, a small mass of chromatin is present adjacent to the nuclear membrane. Such cells, and the person in whom they are found, are designated as *chromatin-positive*. Generally, cells of a male constitution are *chromatin-negative*. The sex chromatin or "intranuclear satellite"—also called *Barr body* after its Canadian discoverer—is considered to be an inactivated X chromosome, with only one of the pair being functional in female cells (karyotype 46/XX) and none in male cells (XY). Thus, there will be one less Barr body or sex chromatin than the number of X chromosomes in any combination of X or Y. Some persons with Turner's syndrome are chromatin-negative, others are positive.

Jacobs and others identified two Barr bodies in somatic cells (oral mucosa) of a female patient with an aberrant chromosomal pattern 46/XXX. The symptoms were amenorrhea, underdeveloped breasts, and infantile genitalia. They are hardly impressive as so-called super-females.

In the rare person with *true hermaphroditism*, both testicular and ovarian tissues are present in one or parts of both gonads (ovotestis). The external genitalia may be of either sex or of an intersex type. The apparent chromosomal pattern may be normal. Some persons have been identified as genetic females 46/XX, although mosaicism is suspected. Undetected chromosomal defects, perhaps hormonal factors, may be present and interfere with normal gonadal histodifferentiation. The true etiology of this anomaly, as well as that of some other intersex condition, remains uncertain.

Hormonal factors and intersex

During the past twenty years it has become experimentally established that gonadectomized mammalian embryos of either sex develop in the direction of the female body (somatic) sex. This concerns the differentiation of the internal genital tracts and of the external genitalia. The presence or absence of ovaries is of little importance in the development of the uterovaginal primordium from the paramesonephric (müllerian) ducts. The presence of testes definitely imposes masculinity on the emerging internal and external genitalia. The differentiation of the müllerian ducts is repressed by fetal testicular androgens and that of the wolffian ducts is enhanced.

Ingenious and crucial surgical castration experiments on rabbit fetuses done by Jost supplied incontestable evidence of specific hormonal effects on fetal target organs. Raynaud and Raynaud and Frilley destroyed the fetal male gonad with x-rays and observed the emergence of the female pattern of genital tracts. Both Wells and Jost proved experimentally that the fetal testes are able to affect sexual differentiation for only a short period of time. A critical stage of receptivity in the target organ thus becomes established, and thereafter sexual development is not influenced by castration. In rabbit embryos, for example, the wolffian ducts regress only if orchiectomy is performed before day 24. Bruner and Witschi obtained various effects on the sex development of female hamsters, depending upon the time and dosage of testosterone propionate injected into the pregnant animals. A small dose (1 mg. q.d.) administered on the ninth day of gestation produced faster development of the entire female genital tract. A larger dose (5 mg.) given between the tenth and twelfth days of gestation inhibited the lengthening and downgrowth of the vagina. The masculinization effects included enlargement of the prostatic and urethral glands. Other investigators obtained similar responses to androgen injections in female embryos of the guinea pig, mouse, rat, and opossum.

Signs of the *testicular feminization syndrome* may be present at birth, incident to early failure of the fetal testes to produce androgenic hormones. Jacobs and others reported several cases of such sex reversion in males. The external genitalia of these patients were of the female type; they had scant pubic and axillary hair, and after puberty they exhibited typical female sex behavior, though they had primary amenorrhea. During hernial repair, testicular tissue was found either in the inguinal canal or within the abdomen. No evidence of a corpus or cervix was discovered, although a small blindly-ending pouch measuring several centimeters in length was identified as an incompletely developed vagina. These apparent females were all chromatin-negative. The condition appears to be associated with either a sex-linked recessive gene or an autosomal dominant gene.

If the fetal testes fail to produce adequate hormones at a later stage, female type of micturition caused by hypospadias may be associated with male somatic and psychologic sex characteristics. The karyotype of such persons is 46/XY; they are chromatin-negative and have no uterovaginal canal.

Virilization of females in utero may also take place through exogenous androgens from the mother—the administration of 19-norsteroids for progestational effects—or it may be incident to maternal endocrinopathy. A general consideration of sex inversions in the male is beyond the scope of this review.

It is clear that the exquisitely timed sequence of developmental events (chronology) and hormonal effects in utero are interdependent. In this interplay of regulating factors, the stage of receptivity of various components of the female reproductive organs appears to be more important than the specific nature of the hormone. The time of the latter's influence is of the essence in the course of normal differentiation, as well as in causing anomalies by interference. Much further research is needed to elucidate the specific process involved.

General teratogenic effects produced by various noxious agents are also known to depend on the *time* when they interfere with the establishment of organ primordia that have a high metabolic rate, a need for abundant oxygen, and a rapid synthesis of nucleoproteins (DNA). The disturbances lead to inhibition or arrest of development during crucial stages of organogenesis. Thus far, such congenital anomalies have not been proved to be attributable to either genetic or hormonal factors.

During the development of the female reproductive tracts, incomplete fusion of the distal portions of the müllerian ducts may be followed by various forms of partial or total duplication of the uterus: uterus bicornis, uterus septus duplex, uterus subseptus unicollis. A uterus unicornis may arise if the paramesonephric duct of one side fails to develop. These anomalies, all examples of arrested development, originate between the eighth and twelfth week of the fetal period. The possible mode of formation of a septate vagina will be considered later in this chapter (p. 21).

Differentiation of the uterine and vaginal portions from the primary genital canal

The uterus and vagina slowly arise as recognizable entities during the fourth and fifth fetal months. Their primordium is the previously described uterovaginal canal. The cranial segments of the paramesonephric ducts remain divergent and develop into the uterine tubes. The epithelial (müllerian) lining of the canal itself becomes invested by mesenchymal tissue of the urogenital fold from which arise the muscular and fibrous components of the internal genital tract, as well as the broad, round, and cardinal ligaments.

Gross morphogenetic processes

In a 2 in. fetus—the size at the end of the third month—the primitive genital canal meets the urethral portion of the urogenital sinus directly below the bladder and behind the developing pubic symphysis. By the seventeenth week (5 in. fetus, sitting height or crown-rump length [C.R.L]), lengthening and downgrowth of the vaginal portion has become pronounced, and the fetal urethra is relatively shortened. A gentle forward curve between the emerging uterine and vaginal portions becomes recognizable. The peritoneum extends over the posterior portion of the uterus, almost to the level of the future fornix. The caudal end of the vaginal portion, represented by the müllerian tubercle, now lies well below the pubic symphysis and protrudes into the developing vestibule of the urogenital sinus.

During the fifth month (6 in. fetus, C.R.L.), the vagina expands to a remarkable degree through rapid proliferation of an invading epithelium. It originates on the müllerian tubercle and, by its upgrowth through the primary genital canal, is destined to replace parts or all of its müllerian epithelium. The free lips of the portio vaginalis of the cervix become recognizable by developing fornices. Most strikingly, the cervix itself enters a temporary phase of rapid growth, surpassing that of the corpus uteri until birth.

Hunter's study of the female genital tract in a dozen embryos and 120 fetuses of the Carnegie Collection (Baltimore) established the differences in growth of the cervix and the corpus uteri. The major portion of cervical growth takes place in two phases, one extending from about the twenty-first to the twenty-eighth week, and the other, which is more pronounced, lasting from the thirty-second to the fortieth week (ninth and tenth lunar months). Through the eighth month the cervix grows more slowly. At term, the cervix measures more than twice the length of the corpus (38 mm./17 mm.). It grows in thickness and weight as well as length incident to a generalized enlargement of all cervical layers, rather than by mere hypertrophy of the mucosa and excessive production of mucus. Fluhmann believed that cervical growth is attributable chiefly to epithelial proliferation; Hunter, after comparing fetal cervical growth with that of the cervix of pregnancy, concluded that the former was induced by placental hormones.

During the neonatal period, the length and bulk of the cervix rapidly decrease, the length becoming less than half its maximum at birth (from 38 mm. to 15 mm.). This regression is believed to be brought about by withdrawal of placental hormones at birth. The resulting infantile type of uterus thus differs from the fetal type; though small, its proportions more closely resemble those of the adult uterus.

The postnatal reduction of the length and weight of the uterus had been recognized by several authors at the beginning of this century, yet little was known of its prenatal growth. Scammon was the first to show that the neonatal growth rate of the uterus is practically identical to that of the fetal uterus before the cervical enlargement begins. A straight line drawn through the growth curve before the twenty-first week extends directly into that representing the neonatal growth gradient. A basic component of growth seems to have remained uniform, as though the cervix had never enlarged. The development of the uerus thus reaches a temporary climax at birth. The large cervix of late fetal months obviously is less a sign of functional needs than the likely product of exogenous hormonal stimulation. In some of the earliest studies on endocrine effects on female reproductive organs, Frank and Rosenbloom induced growth in the cervix of the rabbit uterus by injecting placental hormones. Hunter's conclusions were based, in part, on their results. After the rapid regression of the human cervix in the neonatal period, the uterus does not become as large again until puberty; at that time it attains functional competence through regulation of the individual's own hormones.

Histogenetic processes

The formative process of the vagina has been more difficult to determine than that of any other part of the female reproductive system. Despite a vast amount of research in an attempt to clarify the origin of the ultimate epithelial lining of both the vagina and the portio, no definite answer has been found. The opinions of investigators differ as to the specific source of the epithelium, in whole or in part—whether it is derived from the original müllerian lining of the primary uterovaginal canal, from adjacent epithelia of the wolffian ducts, or from the urogenital sinus. All three merge temporarily in the minute area of the müllerian tubercle. They may differentiate into almost identical types of lining cells, their boundaries becoming indistinct; in addition, one or the other possible components involved may be displaced and undergo degeneration.

Some of these changes take place during a limited period near the end of the third month, in fetuses of about 50 to 60 mm. C.R.L. Ordinary histologic staining methods appear inadequate, and thus far even histochemical studies have not proved wholly successful in solving this complex problem. A closely graded series of well-preserved specimens of the particular developmental phase is a prime requisite for such studies. Experimental methods, of course, are impossible on human embryos, and conclusions drawn from studies of various mammalian species have, at times, added to the confusion of divergent interpretations. Rather than present detailed accounts of such investigations, I shall attempt to group the more important interpretations according to their emphasis and concurrence on one or another prime source of the definite vaginal and cervical epithelium.

It is of historical interest that Müller, after whom the paramesonephric ducts were named, believed that they formed only the uterine tubes and the corpus, whereas the cervix and vagina were direct derivatives of the urogenital sinus. This interpretation was accepted through the first half of the nineteenth century. The emphasis then shifted to the müllerian ducts as the sole source of the uterine and vaginal epithelia; this was the classical view through the end of the nineteenth century and the first quarter of this century. Bloomfield and Frazer gave it strong support in England as late as 1927. However, Pozzi had suggested in 1884 that the lower part of the vagina must be derived from the urogenital sinus. This view was strongly confirmed by Retterer in 1891 and especially by Koff's careful study in 1933. Meanwhile, contrary interpretations were again forthcoming. Hart, in 1901, maintained that the wolffian "bulbs" supplied the vaginal epithelium by a secondary invasion of the "müllerian vagina," extending even into the cervical canal. Mijsberg's extensive work (1924-26) confirmed such a contribution by wolffian epithelium to the caudal part of the vagina. The latest study of this subject, reported by Forsberg in 1963, again favored this theory, for Forsberg postulated that "the vaginal plate is a wolffian derivative."

Between 1930 and 1960, the prevalent concept of the origin of the permanent vaginal epithelium was based upon extensive investigations by Vilas (1932-1933), Meyer (1934-1938), Bulmer (1957), and others (Figs. 2-3 and 2-4). It was their opinion that an upgrowth of sinus epithelium replaced the müllerian epithelium throughout the length of the

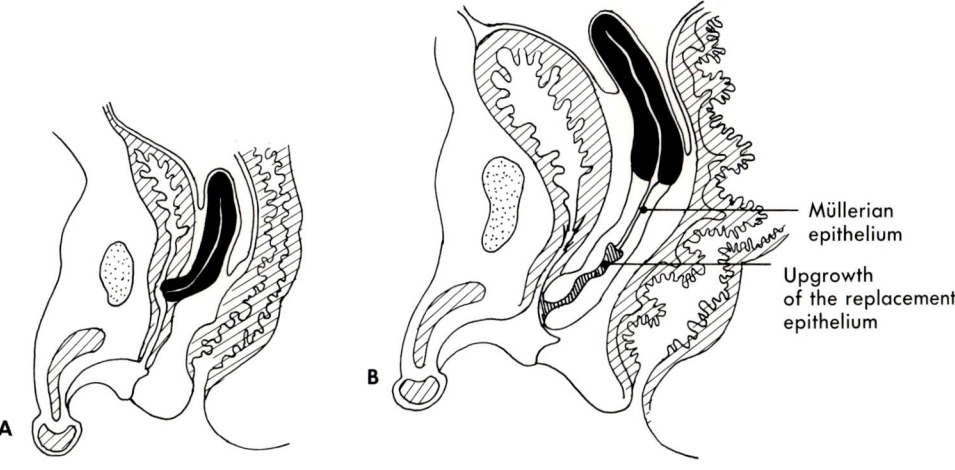

Fig. 2-3. Development of the uterovaginal canal, **A**, in the third month and **B**, in the fourth fetal month, midsagittal aspects. No vaginal portion is recognizable in **A**; replacement in the müllerian epithelium has begun in **B**. (Adapted from Meyer, R.: Arch. Gynaek. 165:504, 1938.)

20 Benign diseases of the vulva and vagina

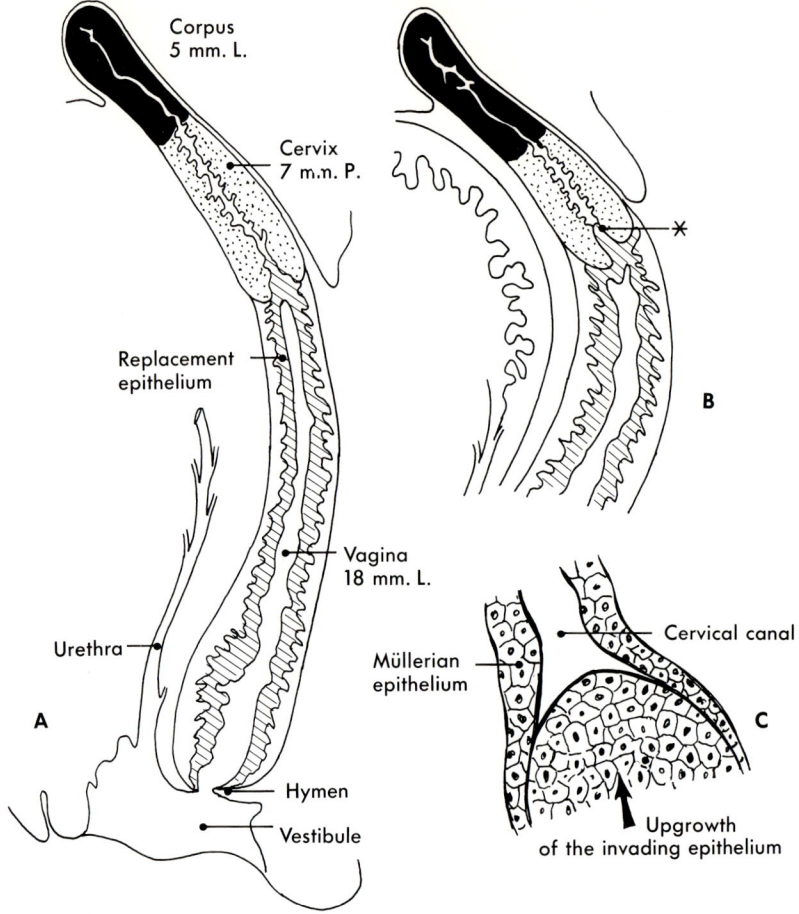

Fig. 2-4. Development of the uterovaginal canal, **A**, in the fifth fetal month (adapted from Koff, A. K.: Contrib. Embryol. 24:59, 1933), and **B** and **C**, in sixth fetal month (adapted from Meyer, R.: Arch. Gynaek. 165:504, 1938). In **A** and **B** the original müllerian epithelium has been replaced throughout the vagina and has reached the cervical canal. **C** is an enlargement of the area marked * in **B**.

vagina and entered the cervical canal to a variable degree. These opinions revived, in a sense, the century-old concept of Müller, which had been abandoned when the fusion of the müllerian ducts became known. Such is the maze of contradictory evidence reflecting the unsatisfactory status of the problem under discussion. The broad principles have been delineated. Special points of interest are highlighted below.

It is generally agreed that the caudal end of the fused müllerian ducts recedes from the tubercle and that a solid vaginal plate comes to occupy the increasing distance between the lumen of the uterovaginal primordium and urogenital sinus. The true origin of that plate, its persistence or disappearance, are points of divergence in the interpretations of different authors. No convincing proof has been offered that it is formed solely by a proliferation from the caudal tip of the uterovaginal canal, or that this median cell strand is retained and contributes to the formation of any part of the vagina.

Various investigators have observed paired dorsal evaginations at the müllerian tubercle. They flank the primary vaginal plate on each side, fuse, and thus contribute to the permanent vaginal canal. Koff called these evaginations "sino-vaginal bulbs" and agreed with Retterer, Vilas, Meyer, and Bulmer that they originate in sinus epithelium. Spuler first recognized them as a single structure—a little late, since they are already fused in a fetus of 85 mm.—and called it "conus vaginalis." On the contrary, Hart, Mijsberg, and Forsberg believed the upgrowth was derived from the caudal ends of the wolffian ducts and designated them as wolffian bulbs, wolffian tubercles, or "dorsolateral projections." Wood-Jones had maintained, instead, that paired bulbar downgrowths arose from the fused müllerian ducts. One is tempted to resolve the confusion by suspecting that these authors observed and interpreted the same important beginnings from an identical structural source, variable and transitional in their differentiation, and most difficult to identify by ordinary histologic methods. Granted, assumptions are hardly part of respectable scientific reasoning.

Pozzi's view that a sinus contributes to the formation of the vagina was based solely upon an abnormal case in which the larger upper part of the vagina was absent, although a hymen and, above it, a small pouch were present. McKelvey and Baxter described an opposite anomaly, in which a double uterus and cervix opened into a closed sac. Both the lower portion of the vagina and the hymen were lacking. The condition appeared to favor the view of a dual source in the establishment of a normal vagina. Defects in other pelvic organs (bladder) were associated, from which the authors concluded that the development of the urogenital sinus may have been arrested, leading to the incomplete vagina. Incomplete fusion of the müllerian ducts may result not only in a dual or septate uterus, referred to previously, but also in septation of the upper portion of the vagina. The lower segment of the vagina might become septate, perhaps through incomplete fusion of the paired sinovaginal bulbs (of Koff) or of their equivalents by another derivation.

The progressive invasion by sinus epithelium and the replacement of the müllerian epithelium of the uterovaginal primordium has been studied, especially by Vilas, Meyer, and Bulmer. According to Bulmer's observations on excellent material, the upgrowth begins in the twelfth week, extends through the lower half of the vagina in the fourteenth week, and reaches the portio by the fifteenth week. A marked proliferation of the invading sinus epithelium begins around the sixteenth week, with the vaginal segment becoming widely expanded, especially in its caudal portion. The invading sinus epithelium arises from a dorsal recess of the urogenital sinus and attains special differentiation on the müllerian tubercle. Its remarkable potentiality for proliferation into a squamous stratified epithelium may be induced by maternal estrogens. The enormous enlargement of the vaginal bulk at the end of the fourth fetal month may well represent a hormonal response by the "differentiated" type of sinus epithelium. Bulmer suggested that it may be sensitive to such hormonal factors, whereas the müllerian epithelium of the uterus and the undifferentiated sinus epithelium of the vestibule remain inactive. Knowledge of hormonal reactions in female human fetuses still is rudimentary and answers to such complex problems of development remain tentative.

The "differentiated" type of the invading sinus epithelium consists of darkly staining basal cells and of lightly staining superficial cells. Periodic acid-Schiff (PAS) staining reveals much glycogen in the basal cells during the fetal months, though none in postnatal specimens. According to Fluhmann, from the twenty-sixth week to term the epithelia of the cervical canal and of the vagina react strongly to the PAS stain, whereas the lining cells of the müllerian endometrium do not stain. Zuckerman postulated that any epithelia derived from the urogenital sinus respond to estrogens by a squamous reaction (proliferation, keritinization, desquamation). A secretory response would indicate an origin from müllerian epithelium. Bulmer later pointed to a fallacy in this "evidence," emphasizing that in many mammals the upper vaginal segment is a müllerian derivative yet gives a squamous response to estrogenic stimulation.

The vaginal expansion, by accumulating squamous stratified epithelium during the fourth and fifth months, produces a bulging contact area with the urogenital sinus. The intervening tissues become compressed, rolled out as it were, into a sickle shaped fold first appearing in the dorsolateral wall of that junction. The hymen is thus being established as a thin mesenchymal plate. It is lined above by "differentiated" sinus epithelium of the vagina and below by the undifferentiated sinus epithelium of the vulvar vestibule. A ventral hymenal fold arises later and contributes to the formation of the disk shaped or *annular hymen*.

During the fifth fetal month (180 mm. C.R.L.), the expansion and canalization by degeneration of central cells takes place throughout the length of the vagina. The posterior and anterior portions of the fornix also acquire lumina by delamination within the previously solid epithelial out-growths from the cranial end of the vaginal tract.

According to Meyer, there is much individual variation in the spread of sinus epithelium into the fornix and upon the portio vaginalis uteri. The upper portion of the cervical canal remains lined by müllerian epithelium, becomes secretory (mucus), and may secondarily displace the squamous stratified epithelium from the cervical canal and extend to the underside of the portio. In a group of postnatal cervical canals studied by Meyer, squamous stratified epithelium lined the lower segment of half the number, yet no trace of it was found in the upper half (it was said to have "disappeared"). By the ninth and tenth fetal months, the histologic features of the cervical canal are definitely established. Meanwhile, the placental output of estrogens and progesterone increases until term. Hunter described the epithelial realationships of this area in a full term fetus and in a 3½-year-old child (Fig. 2-5).

Fluhmann doubted that the epithelium of the cervical mucosa might be of müllerian origin; rather, he believed it to be of the same entodermal origin as the vaginal epithelium, that is, a derivative of the urogenital sinus. He further suggested that the so-called "epidermization" of the cervix epithelium—which may reveal squamous metaplasia at all ages—be called "squamous prosoplasia" and be considered an inherent property of that epithelium.

The latest important contribution in this field by Forsberg again clouded this issue. He compared enzyme patterns in the vaginal plate with those of the wolffian and sinus epithelium. In particular, the distribution of acid phosphatase, esterase, arylsulfatase, and leucine aminopeptidase were studied. He showed a higher degree of correspondence in their activity between wolffian epithelium and that of the vaginal plate than between the latter and sinus epithelium. For this reason, Forsberg favored the view that the vaginal plate is derived from the caudal end of the wolffian ducts, although he recognized the possibility that the very marked proliferation of the vaginal plate may affect its enzyme pattern, and that the wolffian epithelium may induce the upgrowth of sinus epithelium.

These latest conclusions will need confirmation before it can be definitely stated whether the vaginal lining is of entodermal (sinus) or of mesodermal origin (from the wolffian ducts). Nevertheless, secondary re-

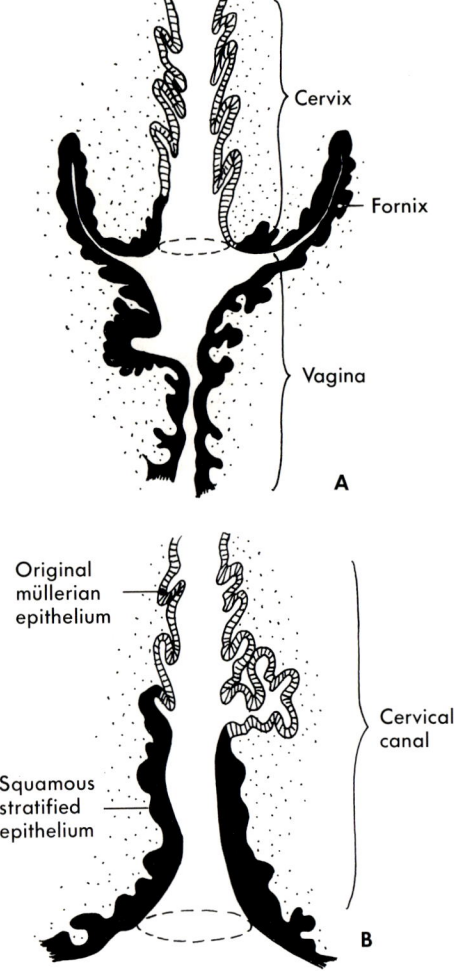

Fig. 2-5. Junction areas of the vaginal replacement epithelium and müllerian epithelium of the external os and within the cervical canal. **A,** Full-term fetus. **B,** Child of 3½ years. (Adapted from Hunter, R. H.: Contrib. Embryol. **22:**91, 1930.)

placement of the original müllerian epithelium in the vagina remains accepted as an established fact.

REFERENCES

Armstrong, C. N.: Intersexuality in man. In Armstrong, C. N., and Marshall, A. J., editors: Intersexuality in vertebrates including man, London, 1964, Academic Press.

Bloomfield, A., and Frazer, J. E.: The development of the lower end of the vagina, J. Anat. **62:**9, 1927.

Bruner, J. A., and Witschi, E.: Testosterone-induced modifications of sex development in female hamsters, Amer. J. Anat. **79:**293, 1946.

Bruner-Lorand, J.: Intersexuality in mammals. In Armstrong, C. N., and Marshall, A. J., editors: Intersexuality in vertebrates including man, London, 1964, Academic Press.

Bulmer, D.: The development of the human vagina, J. Anat. **91:**490, 1957.

Ferriman, D., Page, B. H., and Newnham, R.: Studies bearing on the nature of androgyny, J. Endocr. **25:**351, 1962.

Fluhmann, C. F.: The developmental anatomy of the cervix uteri, Obstet. Gynec. **15:**62, 1960.

Forsberg, J.-G.: Derivation and differentiation of the vaginal epithelium: Dissertation, University of Lund, Sweden, 1963.

Frank, R. T., and Rosenbloom, J.: Physiologically active substances contained in the placenta and in the corpus luteum, Surg. Gynec. Obstet. **21:**646, 1915.

Hart, D. B.: A contribution to the morphology of the human urogenital tract, J. Anat. Physiol. **35:**330, 1901.

Hunter, R. H.: Observations on the development of the human female genital tract, Contrib. Embryol. **22:**91, 1930.

Jacobs, P. A., Baikie, A. G., Court Brown, W. M., Forrest, H. R., Jr., Stewart, J. S., and Lennox, B.: Chromosomal sex in the syndrome of testicular feminization, Lancet **2:**591, 1959.

Jacobs, P. A., Baikie, A. G., Court Brown, W. M., MacGregor, T. N., Maclean, N., and Hernden, D. G.: Evidence for the existence of the human "super female," Lancet **2:**423, 1959.

Jost, A.: The role of fetal hormones in prenatal development, Harvey Lect. **55:**201, 1960.

Koff, A. K.: Development of the vagina in the human fetus, Contrib. Embryol. **24:**59, 1933.

McKelvey, J. L., and Baxter, J. S.: Abnormal development of the vagina and genitourinary tract, Amer. J. Obstet. Gynec. **29:**267, 1935.

Meyer, R.: Zur Frage der Entwicklung der menschlichen Vagina, Arch. Gynaek. **165:**504, 1938.

Mijsberg, W. A.: Ueber der Entwicklung der Vagina, des Hymen und des Sinus urogenitalis beim Menschen, Z. Anat. Entwicklungsgesch. **74:**684, 1924.

Mijsberg, W. A.: Ueber die formale Genese einiger Entwicklungsfehler der weiblichen Genitalien beim Menschen, Z. Anat. Entwicklungsgesch. **77:**630, 1925.

Müller, J.: Bildungsgeschichte der Genitalien aus anatomischen Untersuchungen an Embryonen des Menschen und der Thiere, Dusseldorf, 1930, Arnz.

Pozzi, S.: De la bride masculine du vestibule chez la femme, et de l'origine de l'hymen, à propos d'un cas d'absence du vagin, de l'uterus et des ovaires chez une jeune fille, Ann. Gynec. **21:**268, 1884.

Raynaud, A.: Intersexualité provoquée chez la souris femelle par injection d'hormone mâle à la mère en gestation, Compt. Rend. Soc. Biol. **126:**866, 1937.

Raynaud, A.: Repartition topographique histologique du glycogène dans le tractus urogénital de la souris nouveau-née, Compt. Rend. Soc. Biol. **134:**574, 1940.

Raynaud, A., and Frilley, M.: Effets sur le développement du tractus génital des embryons de souris, de la destruction des ébauches de leurs glandes génitales, par une irradiation au moyen des rayons, à l'âge de 13 jours, Compt. Rend. Soc. Biol. **141:**1134, 1947.

Retterer, E.: Sur l'origine du vagin de la femme, Compt. Rend. Soc. Biol. **43:**291, 1891.

Scammon, R. E.: The prenatal growth and natal involution of the human uterus, Proc. Soc. Exp. Biol. Med. **23:**687, 1926.

Spaulding, M. H.: The development of the external genitalia in the human embryo, Contrib. Embryol. **13:**67, 1921.

Spuler, A.: Ueber die normale Entwicklung des weiblichen Genitalapparates. In Veit, L., editor: Handbuch fur Gynakologie, Munich, 1908, Bergmann.

Vilas, E.: Ueber die Entwicklung der menschlichen Scheide, Z. Anat. Entwicklungsgesch. **98:**263, 1932.

Vilas, E.: Zur formalen Genese der Fehlbildungen der Scheide und der Gebarmutter, Arch. Gynaek. **152:**655, 1933.

Wells, L. J.: Effects of androgen upon reproductive organs of normal and castrated fetuses with note on adrenalectomy, Proc. Soc. Exp. Biol. Med. **63:**417, 1946.

Wilson, K. M.: Correlation of external genitalia and sex-glands in the human embryo, Contrib. Embryol. **18:**23, 1926.

Wood-Jones, F.: The nature of the malformations of the rectum and urogenital passages, Brit. Med. J. **2:**1630, 1904.

Zuckerman, S.: The histogenesis of tissues sensitive to estrogens, Biol. Rev. **15:**231, 1940.

# Chapter 3

Developmental anomalies of the vulva and vagina

Robert R. Franklin, M.D.
L. Russell Malinak, M.D.

Anomalies of the female genital tract, although rare, are of major significance for both the patient and her family. Parents invariably experience great anxiety upon discovery of abnormalities of sexual differentiation in their child; hence, the earlier the diagnosis is made and proper treatment is instituted, the better the immediate and long-term outcome for all concerned. The parents' understanding of the child's condition at an early stage can allay their fears and permit them to provide a healthy environment for the child's development. In addition, an early diagnosis allows the physician to plan the proper reconstructive surgery at the least traumatic time for the child. Occasionally, unrecognized and thus neglected minor anomalies, such as an imperforate hymen, may lead to infertility. Also, ambiguous external genitalia may be the only visible manifestation of severe congenital adrenal hyperplasia with consequent loss of salt; in this event, prompt diagnosis may be life-saving.

On the basis of experimental studies of congenital anomalies in laboratory animals and their counterpart in human beings, it is now accepted that the development of the genitalia in the embryo or fetus may be arrested or altered at any time. The resulting anomalies may be obvious at birth, or they may not become apparent until later in life, particularly at the time of puberty.

Since the embryology and early development of the female genital tract have been covered in Chapter 2, the clinical aspects of congenital anomalies alone will be reviewed herein. Further, it is beyond the scope of this book to consider in detail developmental abnormalities of the upper genital tract. It must be stressed, however, that problems of this nature are frequently associated with anomalies of the lower tract and may be of even more clinical significance.

The anomalies discussed are classified as follows:

A. Developmental abnormalities of external genitalia
  1. Clitoris
    a. Hypertrophy
    b. Hypoplasia
  2. Vulva
    a. Hypoplasia
    b. Labial fusion
    c. Hypertrophy of the labia minora
  3. Vagina
    a. Imperforate hymen
    b. Agenesis
    c. Hypoplasia
    d. Duplication
    e. Transverse vaginal septum
    f. Prolapse of the urethral mucosa
    g. Persistence of the wolffian duct (Gartner's duct cyst)
  4. Female pseudohermaphroditism
B. Genetic-chromosomal abnormalities
  1. True hermaphroditism
  2. Testicular feminization
  3. Mixed gonadal dysgenesis
  4. Male pseudohermaphroditism
C. Abnormalities of vulva and vagina associated with anomalies of urinary tract and intestinal tract

1. Ectopic ureteral orifices
2. Exstrophy of bladder with vulvovaginal defects
3. Epispadias with vulvovaginal defects
4. Ectopic anus
5. High rectovaginal fistula

DEVELOPMENTAL ABNORMALITIES OF EXTERNAL GENITALIA
Clitoris

Hypoplasia of the clitoris is so unusual as to have been mentioned only occasionally in medical literature. It has been observed as an isolated finding in a few patients who complain of difficulty in obtaining sexual arousal from clitoral manipulation. The local application of testosterone is of value in increasing the vascularity, size, and sensitivity of the structure. The systemic administration of testosterone is beneficial, although its side effects preclude long-term therapy.

Hypertrophy of the clitoris, when extensive, is the most striking abnormality of the female genital organs and is found in approximately half of all patients with anomalous external genitalia. It may be present alone but is usually associated with varying degrees of labioscrotal fusion. The term "intersex" has been applied to this abnormality. The most common cause is congenital adrenal hyperplasia. This and other causes of female pseudohermaphroditism will be discussed later in this chapter.

Vulva

Hypoplasia, or infantilism, of the vulva alone is uncommon, since the development of vulvar structures generally is proportionate to the size of the individual's body. This abnormality appears in conjunction with hypoplasia of all genital structures, as in hypopituitary dwarfism and in Turner's syndrome. Hypoplasia of the vulva responds to adequate replacement of estrogen.

Fusion of the labia majora, or more appropriately of the labioscrotal folds, is found in varying degrees in patients with female pseudohermaphroditism. The etiologic factors will be discussed under that topic. The condition results from androgen influence prior to complete development of the external genitalia. Exposure of the female fetus to androgen after the twelfth week of gestation will give rise to clitoral hypertrophy, though not to fusion of the labioscrotal folds. As in all teratogenic effects, there is

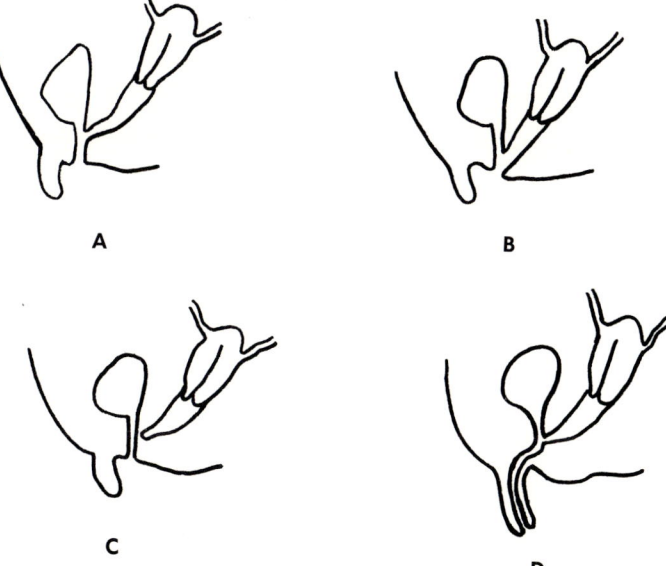

Fig. 3-1. Intersex: some variations in the type of urogenital sinus. **A,** Most common abnormality—perineal opening resembling hypospadial urethral orifice. **B,** Less common abnormality—larger opening resembling a small vaginal introitus. **C,** Occasional abnormality—small urethral opening with no vaginal communication. **D,** Rare abnormality—penile urethra with or without vaginal communication.

a critical time-dose relationship; hence, the earlier the exposure, the more complete will be labioscrotal fusion and, thus, retention of the urogenital sinus. If exposure takes place at a critical moment, a penile urethra will develop (Fig. 3-1). In addition to fusion, the vulvar skin may have a scrotal appearance and the mons pubis may be hypertrophied.

Labial adhesions, which resemble labioscrotal fusion, have often been mistaken for congenital anomalies in infants and young children (Fig. 3-2). These adhesions most often follow vulvovaginitis, or they may develop in the absence of a known inciting factor. The usual complaint is that of partial urinary obstruction. More significant is the anxiety on the part of the mother that this may represent abnormally developed external genitalia.

Local applications of estrogen cream several times daily will bring about resolution of the adhesions over a period of several days to a few weeks. Manual separation of the fused labia has been recommended; this is painful, however, and may be followed by a recurrence of the adhesions. Only rarely does local treatment with estrogens prove ineffective, necessitating surgical intervention.

Hypertrophy of the labia minora is not an uncommon developmental anomaly (Figs. 3-3 and 3-4). Usually it has no clinical significance, although an occasional patient will complain of the cosmetic aspects, as well as of mechanical problems during intercourse. This anomaly can be easily corrected by simple excision. However, it may be a sign of a deep psychologic disorder, since some patients with hypertrophy of the labia mi-

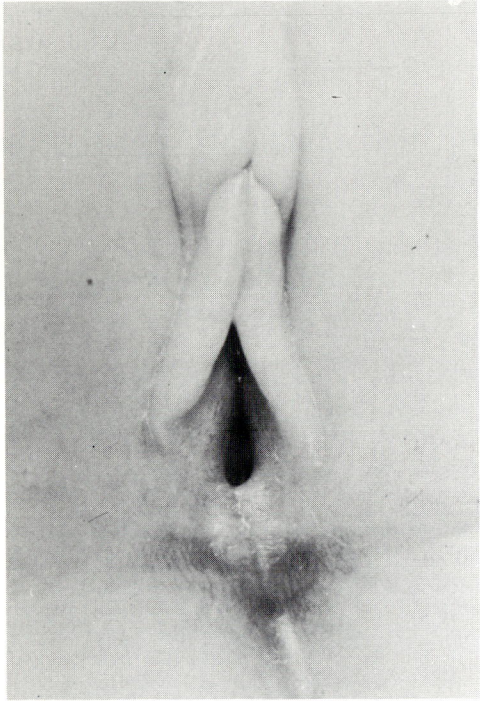

Fig. 3-2. Acquired labial agglutination in a 2-year-old girl. This might easily be mistaken for a congenital anomaly. Repeated applications of estrogen cream brought about resolution of the adhesions. (Courtesy Dr. Herman L. Gardner, Houston.)

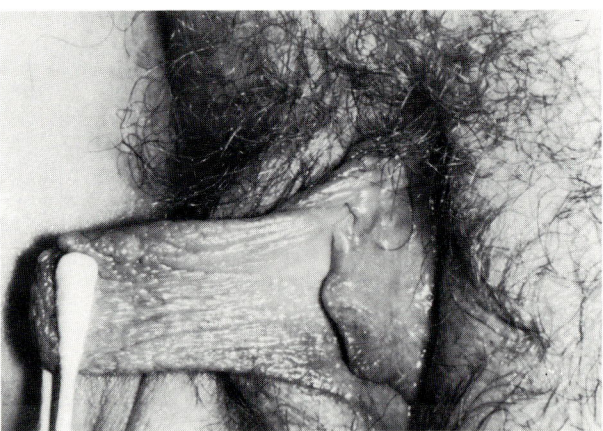

Fig. 3-3. Hypertrophy and elongation of right labium minus. (Courtesy Dr. Herman L. Gardner, Houston.)

Developmental anomalies of the vulva and vagina

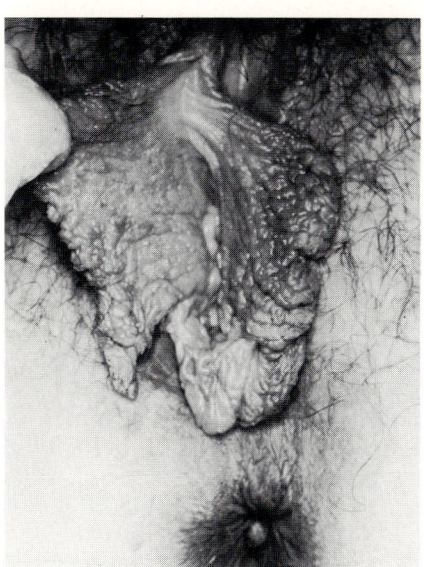

Fig. 3-4. Bilateral hypertrophy of labia minora. (Courtesy Dr. Herman L. Gardner, Houston.)

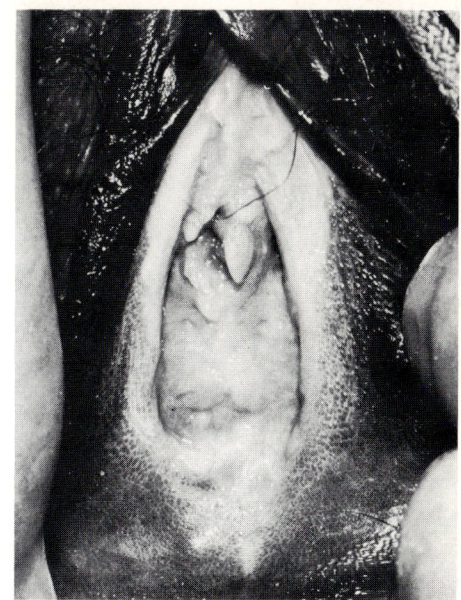

Fig. 3-5. Imperforate hymen in a 13-year-old girl. The thickened membrane bulges. Incision of this structure resulted in drainage of approximately 100 ml. of dark blood and relieved the patient of cyclic cramping, which she had experienced for 3 months. (Courtesy Dr. Herman L. Gardner, Houston.)

nora relate a history of excessive masturbation. In these cases, hypertrophy is apparently a response to chronic irritation. The Hottentot women are extreme examples of changes in the labia that can develop from chronic manipulation.

Vagina

An *imperforate hymen* is discovered in one of approximately two thousand gynecologic patients. This malformation is not likely to be suspected in young children unless a mucoid vaginal secretion distends the vagina and causes protrusion of the hymen. Most often, it is not recognized until after puberty, when retention of menstrual detritus becomes troublesome. As progressively larger amounts of blood accumulate with each menstrual period, the vagina is distended to form a large sausage shaped hematocolpos (Fig. 3-5). The discharge is generally confined to the vagina for a long period of time because of the resistance of the cervix and body of the uterus to distention. Eventually, the cervix becomes dilated, with the accumulation of retained secretions often giving rise to hematometra and hematosalpinx. The patient usually complains of progressively more severe cyclic lower abdominal pain. Occasionally, the presence of a large abdominal mass is the chief complaint. Bladder pressure, dysuria, frequency, and urinary retention may also be reported. The diagnosis can be readily determined if an imperforate hymen is considered. The presence of amenorrhea, urinary retention, lower abdominal discomfort, and a palpable pelvic mass necessitates investigation of the external genitalia and a rectal examination. Failure to recognize this condition may lead to an unnecessary laparotomy for an abdominal mass. If it is neglected, infertility may follow. Also, the possibility of fimbrial adhesions should be kept in mind when infertility follows correction of an imperforate hymen.

The external and internal genitalia of these patients are strongly susceptible to infection because of the presence of old blood. For this reason, a strictly aseptic technique should be maintained during both the corrective procedure and convalescence of the patient.

Congenital absence of the vagina (agenesis), in our experience, is found in approximately one out of five thousand female hospital patients, with the exact incidence being unknown. This condition, which arises from incomplete development and fusion of the müllerian ducts, is usually associated with absence or maldevelopment of the uterus and with anomalies of the urinary tract. Occasionally, the external genitalia appear normal. In most cases, a shallow pouch, representing the lower end of the vagina, is present. Since the ovaries do not develop from the müllerian system, they are normal and their function promotes the normal development of secondary sexual characteristics.

As a rule, the only symptom of complete vaginal agenesis in the absence of a functioning uterus is amenorrhea. Occasionally, futile attempts at coitus may be the patient's chief complaint. If a uterus with functioning endometrium is present, the patient may have recurrent lower abdominal pain incident to trapped uterine blood.

Since 25 percent of patients with vaginal agenesis have a uterus, some procedure to establish drainage and to prevent the trapping of blood is necessary at the time of puberty. Definitive surgery, consisting of construction of an artificial vagina, should be carried out at this time; partial operations lead to scarring and constrictions, which make a subsequent definitive operation difficult and less likely to succeed. Although patients whose complaint is primary amenorrhea usually have no functioning uterus, a rudimentary uterus may be palpated rectally. Previously, construction of an artificial vagina in these patients immediately prior to anticipated marriage was considered the most suitable procedure. Currently, however, repair in the early teens is recommended because of the possible profound psychologic effect upon the patient. If the patient is not having frequent coitus, she must wear an obturator, and this inconvenience must be considered before repair is undertaken. Proper selection of a patient for repair at this time is extremely important, as only the most mature teen-agers will persevere in the long-term use of an obturator.

Many techniques of vaginal construction have been recommended; these have included use of segments of the rectum, sigmoid, and ilium, and in some cases indentation of the vulva with an obturator to invaginate this introital tissue over a long period of time. At present the most popular technique consists of the insertion of a split-thickness skin graft (McIndoe procedure) over a polyacrylic mold into a surgically created defect between the bladder and the rectum. The graft may be obtained from the medial portion of the thigh or abdomen. During the late postoperative period, an obturator, preferably of soft material, is inserted into the artificial vagina.

Complete duplication of the vagina (double vagina), with a septum extending from the upper portion to the introitus (Fig. 3-6), is usually accompanied by complete duplication of the uterus and cervix. Partial longitudinal septa, even more often observed, may or may not be associated with uterine anomalies. Symptoms associated with the longitudinal septa are minimal, although primary dysmenorrhea may be severe, incident to uterine dysfunction. Obviously, the malformations may be overlooked during a cursory pelvic examination and may not be discovered until a patient is married and has dyspareunia or becomes pregnant, or even until the postpartum period. Patients with a longitudinal vaginal septum have often progressed through labor and vaginal de-

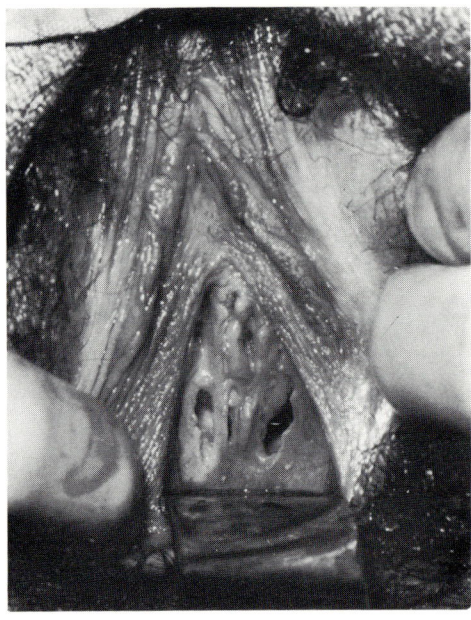

Fig. 3-6. Introitus of a patient with duplication of the vagina, cervix, and uterus. Two vaginal orifices with separate hymenal rings are apparent. (Courtesy Dr. Raymond H. Kaufman, Houston.)

livery without difficulty; others, however, experience soft tissue dystocia or sustain lacerations of the vagina.

Excision of a septum is rarely indicated. Simple division is sometimes necessary when dystocia becomes apparent during labor, or if the inadequate vaginal caliber leads to dyspareunia. In making the incision, care must be taken to avoid injury to the bladder and rectum.

Transverse vaginal septa appear chiefly at the junction of the upper and middle third of the vagina, although they may be present at any level. The septum may be complete or partial, and the symptoms depend upon its extent. A complete septum gives rise to symptoms similar to those of an imperforate hymen. Minor constrictions produced by a partial transverse septum may not be suspected until dystocia or a laceration at the time of childbirth leads to its discovery.

This condition calls for surgical treatment according to the size and location of the septum. In the presence of a constricting partial septum, its division is usually adequate. More extensive transverse malformations may require excision, together with correction of any associated anomaly of the upper genital tract.

Prolapse of the urethral mucosa, which is believed to arise from a congenital weakness of the perivaginal and periurethral supporting structures, is discussed in Chapter 4. Another congenital anomaly, Gartner's duct cyst, is discussed in Chapter 5.

Female pseudohermaphroditism

"Female pseudohermaphroditism" is a term used to describe ambiguity of the external genitalia only in genetic females. As mentioned earlier, it applies to clitoral hypertrophy and labioscrotal fusion accompanied by a scrotal appearance of the labia majora (Figs. 3-7 to 3-11). Since the external genitalia of a fetus develop along female lines in the absence of testes, a female is masculinized only in the presence of androgens.

In the majority of affected infants, pseudohermaphroditism arises from congenital adrenal hyperplasia. Further, this abnormality of the adrenal gland is responsible for approximately half of all developmental anomalies of the external genitalia. Because of its importance, a more detailed discussion of the problem is appropriate.

The biochemical defect in congenital adrenal hyperplasia is impaired cortisol production and subsequent hyperplasia of the adrenal cortex resulting from hypersecretion

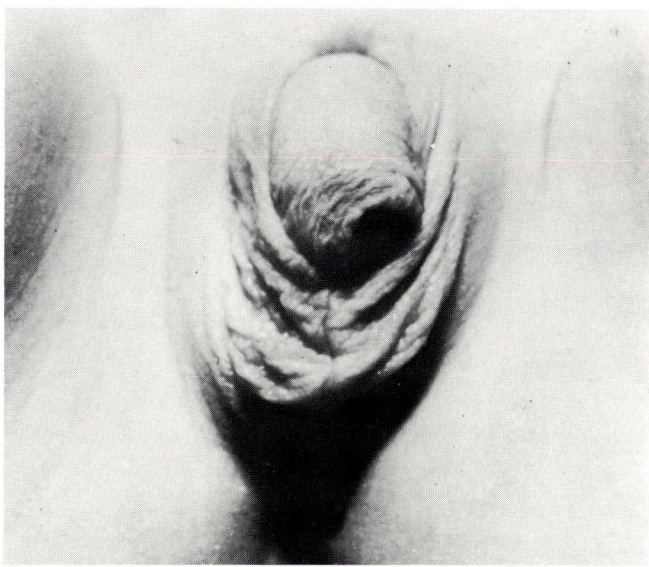

Fig. 3-7. Moderately severe congenital adrenal hyperplasia in a 4-year-old girl. The scrotal-appearing fused labia majora contained no gonads. A urogenital sinus was present at the base of the enlarged phallus. (Courtesy Dr. George W. Clayton, Houston.)

30 Benign diseases of the vulva and vagina

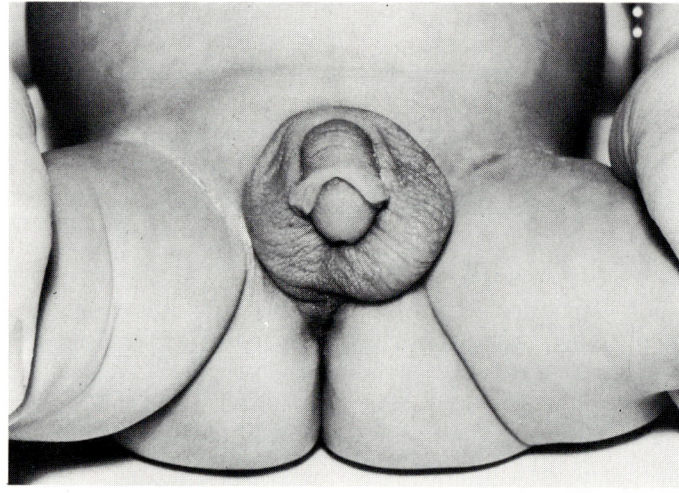

Fig. 3-8. Severe congenital adrenal hyperplasia with salt-losing syndrome in a 1-year-old girl. The patient was mistaken for a boy and was circumcised shortly after birth. No gonads were palpable in the labia majora. (Courtesy Dr. George W. Clayton, Houston.)

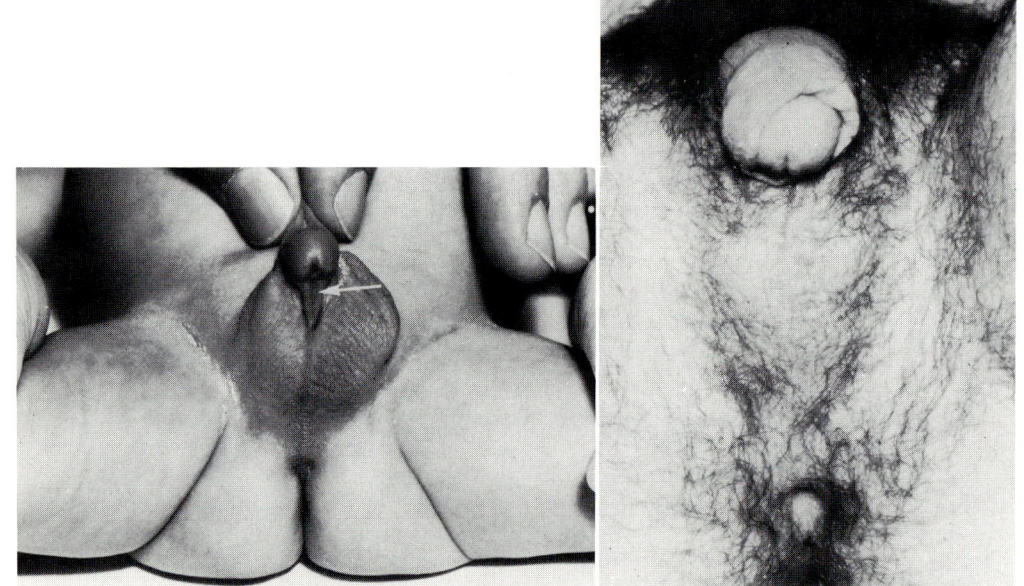

Fig. 3-9. A, Ventral surface of phallus of patient in Fig. 3-8. The hypospadic appearance was actually the opening of a urogenital sinus (arrow). This closely resembles a penile urethra. Labioscrotal fusion was almost complete. (Courtesy Dr. George W. Clayton, Houston.) **B,** Severe congenital adrenal hyperplasia with salt-losing syndrome. Marked virilization of ambiguous external genitalia in a 9-year-old girl. A perineal opening to a urogenital sinus was present at the base of the clitoris. (Courtesy Dr. George W. Clayton, Houston.)

Developmental anomalies of the vulva and vagina 31

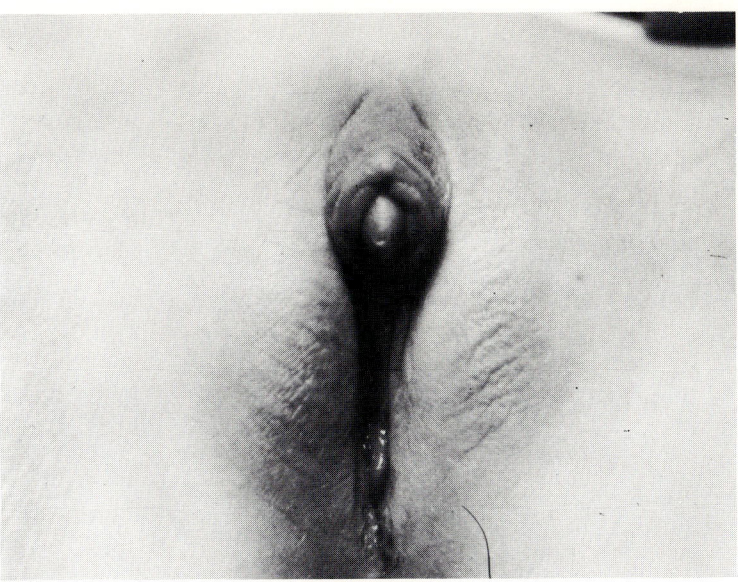

Fig. 3-10. Mild congenital adrenal hyperplasia in a 9-year-old girl. Moderate enlargement of the clitoris and minimal scrotal appearance of the labia majora are apparent.

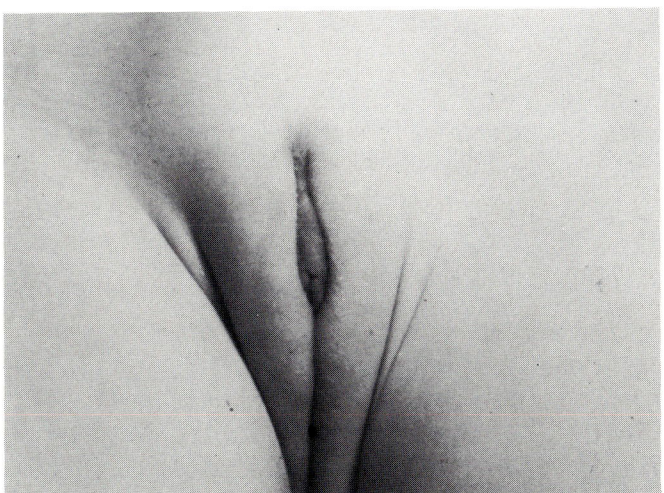

Fig. 3-11. Vulva of patient in Fig. 3-10, 8 weeks after a clitoral recession operation.

of ACTH from the pituitary gland through the negative feedback system. Because of the hyperstimulation of the adrenal gland, androgens are produced that exert their adverse influence upon the infant.

The adrenal cortex may exhibit three primary enzyme defects of clinical significance to the gynecologist. Although others have been described, their rarity precludes discussion herein. The most common defect is that of 21-hydroxylation. Partial inability of the adrenal gland to hydroxylate the carbon-21 compounds leads only to virilism. More severe or complete block of carbon-21-hydroxylation is followed by impaired aldosterone secretion and the consequent salt-losing syndrome in addition to virilization. The second most common enzyme defect is that of 11-hydroxylation, which not only results in hyperproduction of adrenal androgens but also leads to the hypersecretion of 11-desoxycorticosterone and 11-desoxycortisol. Patients with this defect have hypertension in addition to virilization. Finally, the 3-beta-ol-dehydrogenase enzyme deficiency is a less common biochemical error in congenital adrenal hyperplasia. It gives rise to less masculinization than the previously mentioned enzyme defects, yet is accompanied by loss of salt, with its high risk to life. Since this enzyme is active in an earlier stage of steroid synthesis, adrenal physiology is more seriously disturbed.

The medical treatment for congenital adrenal hyperplasia consists of adequate substitution therapy with cortisone to suppress function of the adrenal gland and thus prevent further virilization. In severe forms of this disease process, particularly in the presence of the salt-losing syndrome, the medical treatment is considerably more complicated. If the diagnosis is made early and proper treatment is instituted and continued throughout the patient's life, the prog-

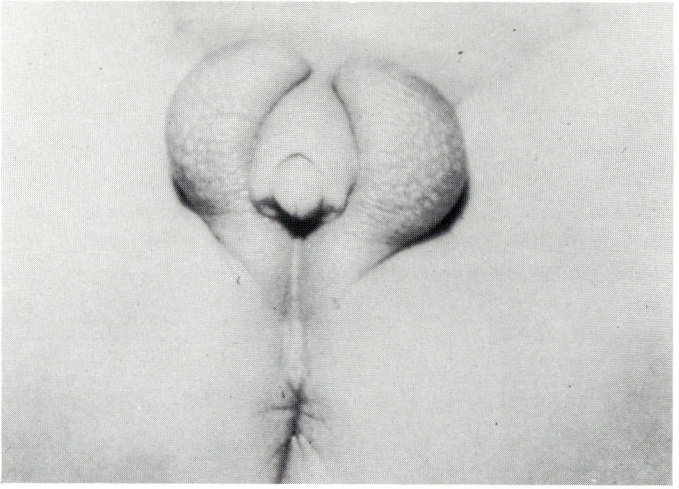

Fig. 3-12. Ambiguous external genitalia in a 1-year-old girl whose mother received norethindrone during the first trimester of pregnancy.

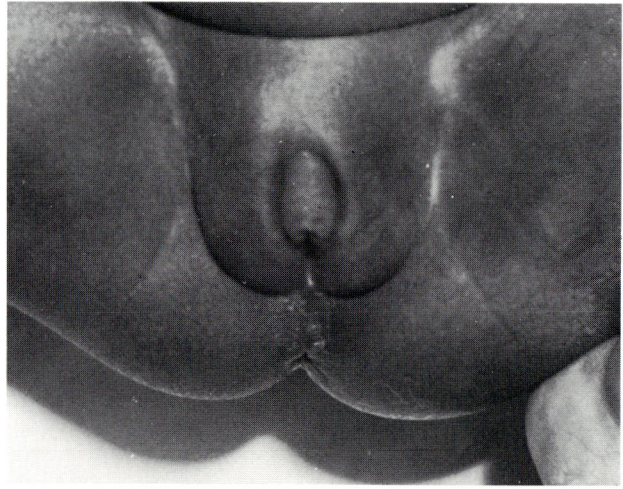

Fig. 3-13. Clitoral hypertrophy in a newborn girl whose mother had bilateral, multicentric ovarian luteomas of pregnancy. The maternal 17-ketosteroids on the day of delivery were 125 mg. every 24 hours. (Malinak, L. R., and Miller, G. V.: Amer. J. Obstet. Gynec. 94:266, 1965.)

nosis is favorable. During times of crisis or illness, additional cortisone is necessary to meet physiologic demands. In more severe cases, hospitalization on multiple occasions can be expected. Therefore, each hospitalization should be made as pleasant and as atraumatic as possible for the patient. The surgical treatment for the abnormal external genitalia will be discussed later.

Female pseudohermaphroditism may also be associated with exposure to exogenous maternal androgen during the first trimester of pregnancy (Fig. 3-12). The usual offending agents are testosterone and synthetic progestational agents, specifically those metabolized to androgens. The latter may be administered orally or parenterally to patients with threatened or habitual abortion. Norethindrone and ethisterone have been the drugs most often responsible for this anomaly.

In rare cases, the external genitalia of the female fetus may be masculinized incident to the presence of an androgen-secreting ovarian tumor, particularly an arrhenoblastoma. Other tumors, however, such as maternal luteomas (Figs. 3-13 and 3-14), have been reported to be the causative factor.

Female pseudohermaphroditism caused by androgen exposure from an external source is the most easily corrected form of abnormal sexual development in the female. No hormonal therapy is necessary. Surgical treatment affords most patients normal female sexual function and reproductive potential.

Genetic-chromosomal abnormalities

In considering known genetic or chromosomal factors responsible for developmental abnormalities of the vulva and vagina, two

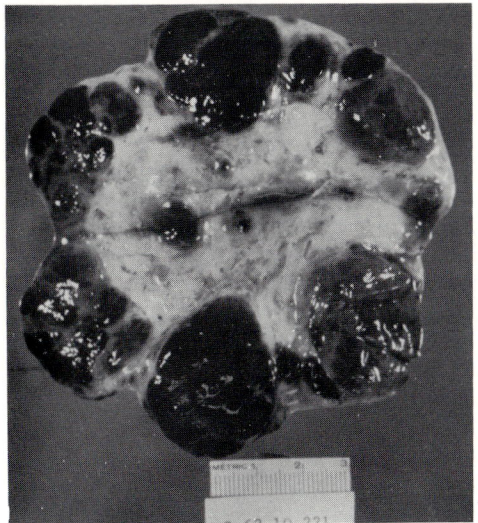

Fig. 3-14. Luteomas of pregnancy in right ovary of the mother whose infant is shown in Fig. 3-13.

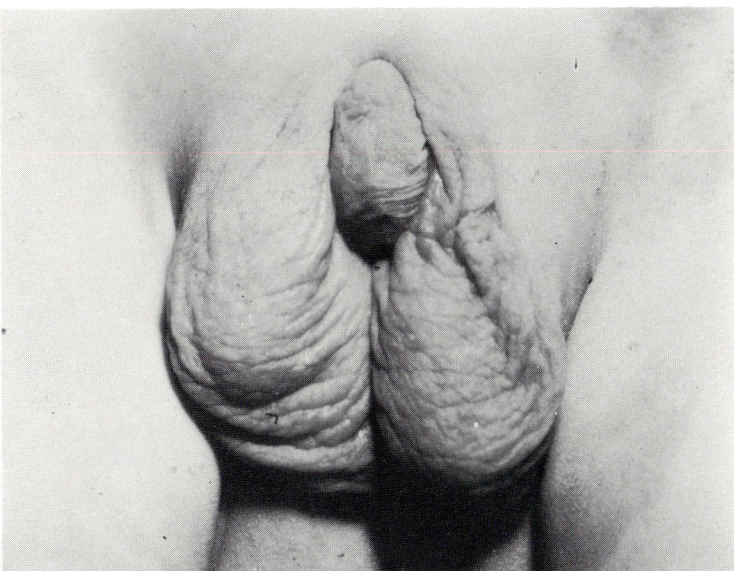

Fig. 3-15. True hermaphrodite. Complete labioscrotal fusion and hypospadias. (Courtesy Dr. George W. Clayton, Houston.)

well-defined conditions are of importance: true hermaphroditism and the syndrome of testicular feminization. Also discussed in this section are mixed gonadal dysgenesis and male pseudohermaphroditism. Although the latter may not necessarily be associated with a chromosome defect per se, it is included here for convenience.

True hermaphroditism

The structure of the genital tract in the true hermaphrodite is highly variable. The external genitalia may appear to be distinctly male or female; most often, however, they are ambiguous. Approximately 75 percent of patients with true hermaphroditism are reared as males because of the size of the phallus. At puberty, the male secondary sex characteristics usually predominate, although the female secondary sex characteristics may be partially developed. Gynecomastia is commonly associated. Periodic hematuria or perineal bleeding depend upon the anatomic relationships of the genital and urinary tracts and the degree of development of the uterus. Hypospadias is often present. Fusion of the labioscrotal folds may be complete with a penile urethra (Fig. 3-15) or partial with a persistent urogenital sinus (Fig. 3-16). The testes lie in the abdomen or in the inguinal canal; as a result, the external genitalia are unlikely to be distorted by an underlying gonad.

It must be stressed that the appearance of the external genitalia cannot be used as a criterion for precise diagnosis in true hermaphroditism. Detailed histologic examination of the gonads is necessary to establish the diagnosis. Determination of the karyotype by study of leukocytes in the peripheral blood usually reveals a 46/XX pattern. If other bodily tissues are examined, however, XY cellular lines are generally discovered.

The treatment of patients with true hermaphroditism is covered on p. 38.

Testicular feminization

Another genetic disorder exhibited by abnormalities of the external genitalia is that of the testicular feminization syndrome. This anomaly, which is attributable to a familial insensitivity of the target tissue to stimulation by androgens, arises in genetic males who are phenotypic females with normal secondary sex characteristics. The vulva appears to be essentially normal, although hypoplasia is frequently present. The entire body hair is diminished and genital hair is usually sparse. More than half the patients have inguinal hernias, and the gonads are often situated in the inguinal canal. If the

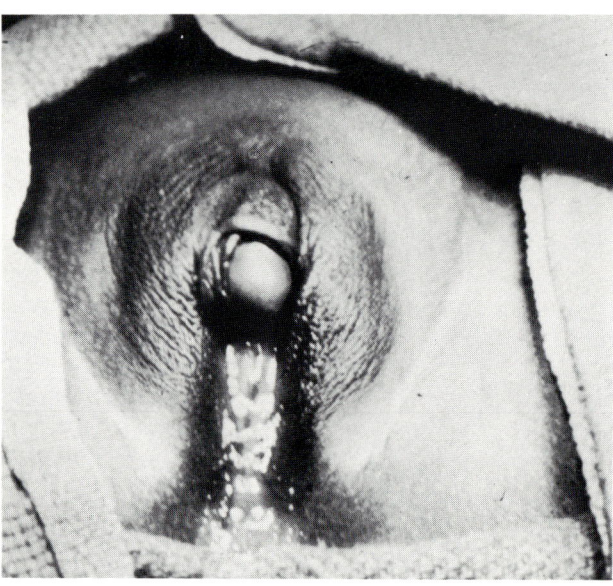

Fig. 3-16. True hermaphrodite. Minimal labioscrotal fusion and clitoral enlargement. A urogenital sinus was present. (Coutresy Dr. George W. Clayton, Houston.)

testes lie in the vulva, the labia majora are prominent. The vagina is shallow and ends in a blind pouch. Laparotomy with gonadal biopsy is usually necessary to establish the diagnosis.

Because of the malignant potential of the abnormal gonads in this condition, castration and subsequent hormone replacement are indicated. The possibility that natural feminization might take place at puberty has led several authors to advocate postponement of castration until after that time. In our opinion, the gonads should be removed when the diagnosis is made, even though the patient has not reached puberty. The reasons are: first, an additional laparotomy is not necessary; second, tissues having a high malignant potential are extirpated; and third, female patients may acquire irreversible masculine characteristics, rather than the anticipated feminization, at puberty. It is difficult, if not impossible, to predict the exact hormone potential of abnormal gonads. Following castration, estrogens may be given at the appropriate time to stimulate the development of normal secondary sex characteristics.

A variation of the testicular feminization syndrome is known as "incomplete testicular feminization syndrome." Patients with this condition are indistinguishable from those classified as male pseudohermaphrodites in that they undergo masculinization at puberty. There is no evidence that they are affected with testicular feminization as opposed to male pseudohermaphroditism other than the fact that they have been reported as siblings of patients with the complete syndrome.

Patients with mixed gonadal dysgenesis (intra-abdominal testes together with "streak ovary") and male pseudohermaphroditism exhibit a spectrum of changes in the external genitalia similar to that found in female pseudohermaphroditism. The changes, however, are associated with sterility. Treatment for these patients consists of castration and reconstruction of the external genitalia. This is generally performed so that the child can be reared as a female, since phallic repair will seldom provide an adult organ of adequate size for sexual intercourse. Castration is indicated because of adverse hormonal secretion at puberty and because of the malignant potential of the abnormal gonad. After puberty, construction of an artificial vagina may be necessary.

ABNORMALITIES OF THE VULVA AND VAGINA ASSOCIATED WITH ANOMALIES OF THE URINARY TRACT AND INTESTINAL TRACT

Anomalies of the urinary tract

As has been previously mentioned, anomalies of the urinary tract frequently appear in patients with malformation of the genital tract. For this reason, every patient with a congenital anomaly of the vulva or vagina should have a thorough evaluation of the urinary tract.

Ectopic ureteral orifices, although highly exceptional, may be present at any level of the perineum, vulva, or vagina. They are usually manifested by incontinence of urine or by a thin, uriniferous vaginal discharge. The diagnosis of this condition may be established by intravenous injection of a dye, which is transmitted to the vagina or the ectopic ureteral opening by way of the urinary tract.

Exstrophy of the bladder and epispadias are the more obvious anomalies of the urinary tract associated with vulvar and vaginal abnormalities. In complete exstrophy, failure of development of the abdominal wall between the umbilicus and the genitalia is obvious and is accompanied by failure of development of the musculature of the lower abdomen, the anterior wall of the bladder, the roof of the urethra, the symphysis pubis, the mons pubis, and the clitoris. Lesser forms of bladder exstrophy may be associated with a bifid clitoris, or the labia minora may be folded over the surface of half the clitoris. The urethral orifice is usually absent, the lowest point of the trigone is exposed, and the posterior urethral wall can usually be visualized. The vagina is displaced forward and may be located at the level of the clitoris. In addition, the anus may occupy a more anterior position than is normal. When the defect involves only the roof of the urethra, the anomaly is known as *epispadias*.

In addition to the foregoing anomalies of the urinary tract associated with congenital defects of the genitalia, such problems as renal agenesis, pelvic kidney, and duplication of the collecting system may be present, though not apparent upon physical examination. This possibility adds to the necessity for a thorough evaluation of the urinary tract.

Ectopic anus

Anomalies of the intestinal tract may also be associated with congenital defects of the genitalia. It has been reported that an ectopic anus is found in one of every five thousand newborn infants. Most often, the anus lies in the lower portion of the vagina (Fig. 3-17) at the introitus ("anus vestibularis") or in the perineum adjacent to the introitus. In many cases, the anus, although somewhat stenotic, is normally developed, having the proper nerve supply and an intact sphincter mechanism. Symptoms of obstruction of the intestinal tract may accompany the more severe forms of the anomaly, whereas lesser constrictions may give rise merely to constipation. The anus and the colon usually function well. Two problems are associated with this condition, the chief one being the esthetic aspects of sexual life. The other is the possibility of disruption of the anal mechanism during the second stage of labor. Cesarean section has been performed to preclude this contingency. Other points of congenital communication between the rectum or the rectosigmoid and the vagina, such as a high rectovaginal fistula, may be present. If so, as in any situation in which the intestinal tract communicates with the genital tract, the symptoms consist of inability to control flatus and the stool or of a chronic vaginal discharge.

The diagnosis might be established simply by administration of an enema of a proper dye solution after insertion of a tampon into the vagina. The actual extent of the anomaly, however, might not be apparent until an exploratory operation is performed.

DIAGNOSTIC APPROACH TO ABNORMALITIES OF FEMALE GENITAL TRACT

All gross anomalies of the external genitalia should be discovered at birth or shortly thereafter by the obstetrician or pediatrician. Abnormal sexual development should be suspected not only when anomalies are obvious but also in the presence of slight enlargement of the clitoris or any abnormality of the urinary or intestinal tract, an inguinal mass, or an inguinal hernia.

Thorough physical examination of the external genitalia should include *gentle* probing of the introitus and anus to determine the patency of the hymen or a possible imperforate anal canal. Careful examination of a newborn will usually rule out an imperforate hymen. Should one be in doubt, a rectal thermometer may be used to test the adequacy of the vaginal opening. If this is performed gently, no trauma or bleeding will be induced.

If abnormal sexual development is suspected, an initial laboratory study of a buccal smear for the number of cells exhibiting nuclear sex chromatin (Barr bodies) is indicated. Although the number varies, in most laboratories buccal smears from the normal female contain not less than 25 percent of these bodies. In timing this test, one should keep in mind that Smith found a lower incidence of cells with nuclear sex chromatin in normal females during the first two days of life. If the Barr body count is inconsistent with the appearance of the infant's external genitalia, karyotype determinations should be performed to ascertain chromosomal sex. With few exceptions, sex

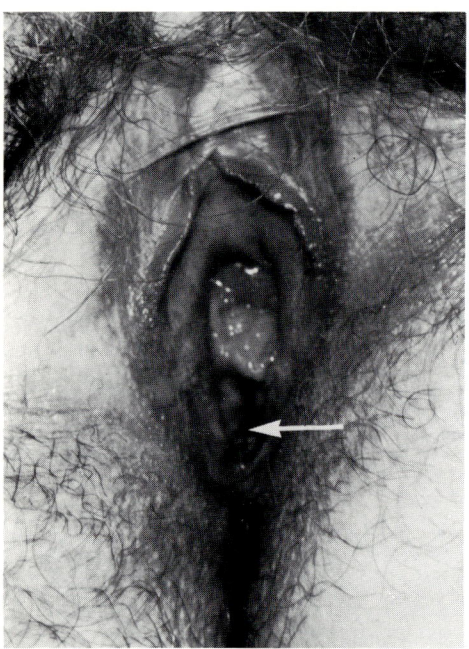

Fig. 3-17. Anus vestibularis. The anus (arrow) and vagina open into the vestibule. (Courtesy Dr. Herman L. Gardner, Houston.)

Developmental anomalies of the vulva and vagina 37

of rearing can be determined prior to studies of the child's karyotype.

In addition, all infants who have chromatin-positive cells should have a 24 hour urine evaluation for 17-ketosteroids and pregnanetriol to distinguish the patient with congenital adrenal hyperplasia from one with other types of hermaphroditism. Jones and Scott outlined methods of collection of 24 hour urine specimens in infants. The 17-ketosteroids are consistently elevated in congenital adrenal hyperplasia. The normal level for children between 3 weeks and 2 years of age is less than 1 mg. per 24 hours; during the first 3 weeks of life the value may be as high as 2.5 mg. per 24 hours. An elevation of pregnanetriol above 0.2 mg. per 24 hours in children up to 6 years of age is considered diagnostic of congenital adrenal hyperplasia. If the infant vomits persistently

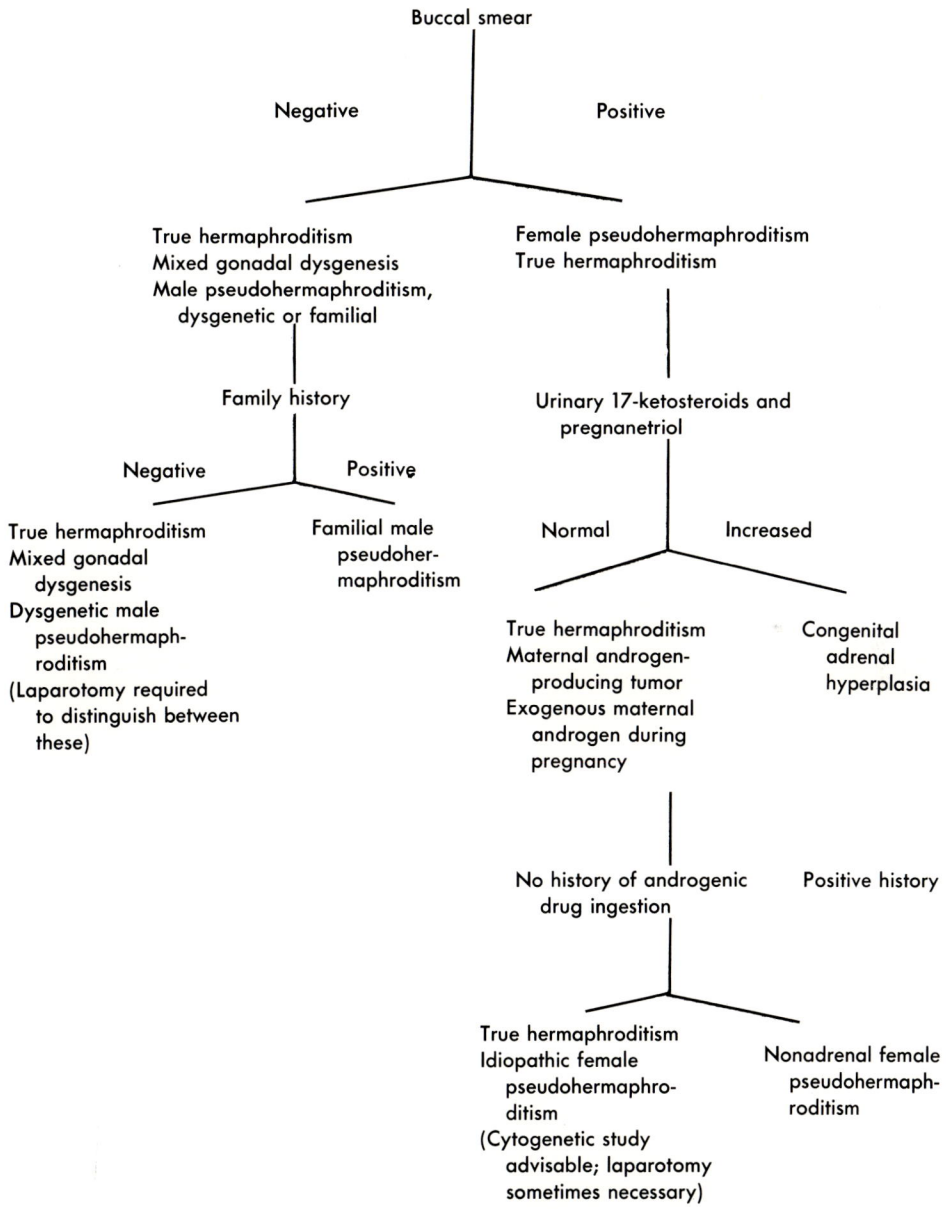

Fig. 3-18. Flow sheet for differential diagnosis of ambiguous external genitalia.

and becomes dehydrated, has electrolyte imbalance, or otherwise fails to thrive, he should be regarded as having the salt-losing type of congenital adrenal hyperplasia until the contrary is proven. Immediate institution of cortisone therapy may be life-saving; this must be maintained for a lifetime.

If congenital adrenal hyperplasia is excluded in chromatin-positive infants with ambiguous external genitalia, the mother must again be questioned as to whether she received progestin or androgen therapy during pregnancy. The possibility of an androgen-secreting tumor in the mother must also be ruled out, particularly if she gives a history of virilization during the pregnancy.

Since approximately 70 percent of patients with true hermaphroditism are chromatin-positive with 46/XX when the blood alone is studied, other body tissues should be examined for karyotypes; 46/XY will usually be discovered. Other diagnostic measures such as radiologic examination, pelvic endoscopy, or laparotomy with gonadal biopsy should serve to establish the correct diagnosis.

Rarely, female pseudohermaphroditism will be present and the etiology will remain obscure; such cases have been designated "idiopathic female pseudohermaphroditism."

Patients with ambiguous external genitalia who are chromatin-negative may be male pseudohermaphrodites, true hermaphrodites, or may fall into the category of those with mixed gonadal dysgenesis. In this group, the diagnosis can be determined only by laparotomy and biopsy of the gonads.

Whatever the type of genital abnormality, a meticulous search should be conducted for anomalies of the urinary and intestinal tracts as well.

The diagram (Fig. 3-18) demonstrating the differential diagnosis of ambiguous external genitalia is a modification of that presented by Federman.

GENERAL PRINCIPLES OF TREATMENT FOR CONGENITAL ANOMALIES

The general principles of treatment of patients with anomalous external genitalia depend primarily on the time at which they are observed by the physician. An organized plan should be kept in mind when the diagnosis is made, whether in the neonatal period or during infancy, in order that the psychologic factors involved in the sex of rearing may receive proper attention. If the condition has been neglected by the parents or previously overlooked, however, sexual orientation may have reached an irreversible stage, thus complicating treatment.

In general, when abnormal genital development has been recognized in infancy and the diagnosis established, surgical correction is not recommended until the child is 18 months to 2 years old. This is generally considered the age of memory; therefore, the child has no recollection of the genitalia prior to this time. In most female children with pseudohermaphroditism, plastic repair can restore normal function and a reasonably normal appearance of the external genitalia. Growth and development, puberty, and sexual and reproductive capability should all be normal (although most of these women are delivered by cesarean section) following proper medical and surgical care. Obviously, the degree of the defect will determine the degree of success of the surgical procedure. Conservation of the clitoris is important; every attempt should be made to keep this organ as a functional unit of the external genitalia. When the phallus is unusually large, only clitorectomy is likely to afford a reasonable cosmetic result. Procedures are advocated wherein the shaft is split longitudinally and resutured in the opposite plane, thus shortening the clitoris. This leaves a large glans, which is difficult to hide, as well as a painful erectile organ. If the phallus is only slightly or moderately enlarged, a clitoral recession procedure is easily accomplished. Exteriorization of the vagina, with plastic repair of the labioscrotal folds to form an introitus, can usually be performed when the child is 18 months to 2 years of age. The genital structures, although small, are for the most part sufficiently large to be handled surgically. In the more severe forms of virilization in the female pseudohermaphrodite, several procedures over a period of time may be required to achieve the desired result. The details of the techniques of plastic repair of ambiguous external genitalia are presented in the reference material for this chapter, being beyond the scope of this book.

The choice of sex of rearing is perhaps

the most important consideration in the treatment. With the proper choice, most individuals with abnormal development of the external genitalia should be able to participate in a satisfactory marriage. In addition, the majority of patients with female pseudohermaphroditism should be able to conceive and bear children. An essential adjunct to surgical correction is the psychologic support of these patients. Continued hormonal therapy may also be necessary.

Aside from those with female pseudohermaphroditism, most patients with ambiguous external genitalia are sterile. The choice of sex of rearing thus depends upon the ease with which a functional sexual unit may be reconstructed from the anomalous organs. If the phallus is large and proper correction of the urethral defect can be anticipated, the child may be reared as a male. In general, however, it is easier to reconstruct the genitalia along female lines; fewer social problems arise, and the long-term result is more acceptable if the patient is reared as a female. Ancillary procedures, such as construction of an artificial vagina and resection of the gonads because of harmful endocrine function or potentially malignant change, may be carried out before or at puberty.

A final but nevertheless significant point in discussing the treatment for abnormal sexual development is the constant awareness by the physician and his nursing personnel of the extreme sensitivity of the patients and their parents. Many tragedies have followed the careless and ill-advised use of incorrect terms such as "morphedite" or "hemaphrodite" in the presence of a patient or the family. Continued psychologic support is always necessary to reassure patients that their birth defect need not be a serious threat to a happy and complete life.

REFERENCES

Armstrong, C. N., and Marshall, A. J., editors: Intersexuality in vertebrates including man, New York, 1964, Academic Press.
Bain, A. D., and Scott, J. S.: Mixed gonadal dysgenesis with XX/XY mosaicism, Lancet 1:1035, 1965.
Bongiovanni, A. M., and Rott, A. W.: The adrenogenital syndrome, New Eng. J. Med. 268:1283, 1342, 1391, 1963.
Bretnall, C.: A case of arrhenoblastoma complicating pregnancy, J. Obstet. Gynaec. Brit. Comm. 52:235, 1945.
Brooks, R. V., Mattingly, D., Mills, I. H., and Prunty, F. T. G.: Postpubertal adrenal virilism with biochemical disturbance of the congenital type of adrenal hyperplasia, Brit. Med. J. 1: 1294, 1960.
Bryan, G., Kliman, B., and Bartter, F.: Impaired aldosterone production in "salt-losing" congenital adrenal hyperplasia, J. Clin. Invest. 44: 957, 1965.
Carpentier, P. J., and Potter, E. L.: Nuclear sex and genital malformation in 48 cases of renal agenesis, with especial reference to nonspecific female pseudohermaphroditism, Amer. J. Obstet. Gynec. 78:235, 1959.
Court Brown, W. M., Harnden, D. G., Jacobs, P. A., Maclean, N., and Mantle, D. J.: Abnormalities of the sex chromosome complement in man, Medical Research Council, Special Report Series 305, London, 1964, Her Majesty's Stationery Office.
Dewhurst, C. J., Warrack, A. J. N., Blank, C. E., Bishop, A. M., and Heslop, W. B.: Chromosome mosaicism in an hermaphrodite, J. Med. Genet. 2:246, 1965.
Dunn, W. J., and Malinak, L. R.: Spontaneous urethral prolapse. Calif. Med. 99:338, 1963.
Engel, E., and Forbes, A. P.: Cytogenetic and clinical findings in 48 patients with congenitally defective or absent ovaries, Medicine 44:135, 1965.
Federman, D. D.: Abnormal sexual development, Philadelphia, 1967, W. B. Saunders Co.
Ferguson-Smith, M. A., Alexander, D. S., Bowen, A. P., Goodman, R. M., Kaufman, B. N., Jones, H. W., Jr., and Heller, R. H.: Clinical and cytogenetical studies in female gonadal dysgenesis and their bearing on the cause of Turner's syndrome, Cytogenetics 3:355, 1964.
Ferrier, P., Gartler, S. M., Waxman, S. H., and Shepard, T. H., II: Abnormal sexual development associated with sex chromosome mosaicism, Pediatrics 29:703, 1962.
French, F. S., Baggett, B., Van Wyk, J. J., Talbert, L. M., Hubbard, W. R., Johnston, F. R., and Weaver, R. P.: Testicular feminization: Clinical, morphological and biochemical studies, J. Clin. Endocr. 25:661, 1965.
Gartler, S. M., Waxman, S. H., and Giblett, E.: An XX/XY human hermaphrodite resulting from double fertilization, Proc. Nat. Acad. Sci. U. S. A. 48:332, 1962.
Greenblatt, R. B.: Clinical aspects of sexual abnormalities in man, Recent Progr. Hormone Res. 14:335, 1958.
Griffin, W. T., and Smith, J.: Congenital vaginal Occlusion, Missouri Med. 65:297, 1968.
Grumbach, M. M.: Some considerations of the pathogenesis and classification of anomalies of

sex in man. In Astwood, E. B., editor: Clinical endocrinology, New York, 1960, Grune & Stratton, Inc.

Grumbach, M. M., and Barr, M. E.: Cytologic tests of chromosomal sex in relation to sexual anomalies in man, Recent Progr. Hormone Res. 14:255, 1958.

Grumbach, M. M., and Ducharme, J. R.: The effects of androgens on fetal sexual development, Fertil. Steril. 11:157, 1960.

Grumbach, M. M., Ducharme, J. R., and Moloshok, R. E.: On the fetal masculinizing action of certain oral progestins, J. Clin. Endocr. 19:1369, 1959.

Hampson, J. L., and Hampson, J. G.: The ontogenesis of sexual behavior in man. In Young, W. C., editor: Sex and internal secretions, Baltimore, 1961, The Williams & Wilkins Co.

Ingersoll, F. M., and Finesinger, J. E.: A case of male pseudohermaphroditism: The importance of psychiatry in the surgery of this condition, Surg. Clin. N. Amer. 27:2, 1947.

Jacobs, P. A., Harnden, D. G., Buckton, K. E., Court Brown, W. M., King, M. J., McBride, J. A., MacGregor, T. N., and Maclean, N.: Cytogenetic studies in primary amenorrhea, Lancet 1:1183, 1961.

Jenkins, M. E., Surana, R. B., and Russell-Cutts, C. M.: Ambiguous genitals in a female infant associated with luteoma of pregnancy, Amer. J. Obstet. Gynec. 101:923, 1968.

Jones, H. W., Jr., and Scott, W. W.: Hermaphroditism, genital anomalies and related endocrine disorders, Baltimore, 1958, The Williams & Wilkins Co.

Jones, H. W., Jr., and Wilkins, L.: Gynecological operations in 94 patients with intersexuality, Amer. J. Obstet. Gynec. 82:1142, 1961.

Josso, N., DeGrouchy, J., Aubert, J., Nezelof, C., Jayle, M. F., Moullec, J., Frezal, J., DeCasaubon, A., and Lamy, M.: True hermaphroditism with XX/XY mosaicism, probably due to double fertilization of the ovum, J. Clin. Endocr. 25:114, 1965.

Jost, A.: Problems of fetal endocrinology: The gonadal and hypophysical hormones, Recent Prog. Hormone Res. 8:379, 1953.

Kase, N., and Morris, J. M.: Steroid synthesis in the cryptorchid testes of three cases of the "testicular feminization syndrome," Amer. J. Obstet. Gynec. 91:102, 1965.

Lattimer, J. K.: Relocation and recession of enlarged clitoris with preservation of glands: An alternative to amputation, J. Urol. 86:113, 1961.

Lewis, F. J. W., Mitchell, J. P., and Foss, G. L.: XY/XO mosaicism, Lancet 1:221, 1963.

Lipsett, M. B., and Riter, B. D.: Urinary steroids in postnatal adrenal hyperplasia with virilism, Acta Endocr. 38:481, 1961.

Lubs, H. A., Jr., Vilar, O., and Bergenstal, D. M.: Familial male pseudohermaphroditism with labial testes and partial feminization: Endocrine studies and genetic aspects, J. Clin. Endocr. 19:1110, 1959.

Maclean, N., Harnden, D. G., and Court Brown, W. M.: Abnormalities of sex chromosome constitution in newborn babies, Lancet 2:406, 1961.

Malinak, L. R., and Miller, G. V.: Bilateral multicentric ovarian luteomas of pregnancy associated with masculinization of a female infant, Amer. J. Obstet. Gynec. 91:251, 1965.

Maxted, W., Baker, R., McCrystal, H., and Fitzgerald, E.: Complete masculinization of the external genitalia in congenital adrenal hyperplasia: Presentation of two cases, J. Urol. 94:266, 1965.

Merrill, J. A., and Ramsey, J. E., True hermaphroditism, Obstet. Gynec. 22:505, 1963.

Mischell, D. R.: Familial intersexuality, Amer. J. Obstet. Gynec. 35:960, 1938.

Money, J., Hampson, J. G., and Hampson, J. L.: An examination of some basic sexual concepts: The evidence of human hermaphroditism, Bull. Johns Hopk. Hosp. 97:301, 1955.

Money, J., Hampson, J. G., and Hampson, J. L.: Hermaphroditism: Recommendations concerning assignment of sex, change of sex and psychology management, Bull Johns Hopk. Hosp. 97:284, 1955.

Moore, J., Franklin, R. R., Wills, S. H., and Clayton, G. W.: Diagnosis and management of individuals with hermaphroditic external genitals, Amer. J. Obstet. Gynec. 83:1175, 1962.

Morris, J. M., and Mahesh, V. B.: Further observations on the syndrome, "testicular feminization," Amer. J. Obstet. Gynec. 87:731, 1963.

Nelson, W. O.: Sex differences in human nuclei with particular reference to the Klinefelter syndrome, gonadal agenesis and other types of hermaphroditism, Acta Endocr. 23:227, 1956.

Overzier, C., editor: Intersexuality, New York, 1963, Academic Press.

Philip, J., and Sele, V.: Testicular feminization (karyotypic-linkage and endocrine studies in three sibs with the complete syndrome), Acta Endrocr. 48:297, 1965.

Philip, J., and Trolle, D.: Familial male hermaphroditism with delayed and partial masculinization, Amer. J. Obstet. Gynec. 93:1076, 1965.

Rabkin, M. T., and Frantz, A. G.: Hypopituitarism: A study of growth hormone and other endocrine functions, Ann. Intern. Med. 64:1197, 1966.

Richardson, G.: Ovarian physiology, New Eng. J. Med. 274:1008, 1064, 1121, 1183, 1966.

Rosenberg, H. S., Clayton, G. W., and Hsu, T. C.: Familial true hermaphroditism, J. Clin. Endocr. 23:203, 1963.

Smith, D., Marden, B., McDonald, M., and Speckhard, M.: Lower incidence of sex chromosomes in buccal smears of newborn females, Pediatrics **30:**707, 1962.

Sohval, A. R.: The syndrome of pure gonadal dysgenesis, Amer. J. Med. **38:**615, 1965.

Sohval, A. R.: Hermaphroditism with "atypical" or "mixed" gonadal dysgenesis, Amer. J. Med. **36:**281, 1964.

Southern, A., Tochimoto, S., Carmody, N. C., and Isurugi, K.: Plasma production rates of testosterone in normal adult men and women and in patients with the syndrome of feminizing testes, J. Clin. Endocr. **25:**1441, 1965.

Talbot, N. B.: Functional endocrinology from birth through adolescence, Cambridge, Mass., 1952, Commonwealth Fund.

Taylor, A.: Sex chromatin in the newborn, Lancet **1:**912, 1963.

Turner, H. H.: A syndrome of infantilism, congenital webbed neck and cubitus valgus, Endocrinology **23:**566, 1938.

Van Wyk, J. J., and Grumbach, M. M.: Disorders of sex differentiation. In William's textbook of endocrinology, Philadelphia, 1968, The W. B. Saunders Co.

Warkany, J., Cj, E. H. Y., and Kauder, E.: Male pseudohermaphroditism and chromosomal mosaicism, Amer. J. Dis. Child. **104:**172, 1962.

Weldon, V., Blizzard, R., and Migeon, C.: Newborn girls misdiagnosed as bilaterally cryptorchid males, New Eng. J. Med. **274:**829, 1966.

Wilkins, L.: The diagnosis of the adrenogenital syndrome and its treatment with cortisone, J. Pediat. **41:**860, 1952.

Wilkins, L.: Diagnosis, selection of sex of rearing, and treatment of various types of abnormal sex differentiation. In Astwood, E., editor: Clinical endocrinology, Vol. 1, New York, 1960, Grune & Stratton, Inc.

Wilkins, L.: The diagnosis and treatment of endocrine disorders in childhood and adolescence, ed. 3, Springfield, Ill., 1965, Charles C Thomas, Publisher.

Wilkins, L.: Masculinization of female fetus due to use of orally given progestins, J.A.M.A. **172:**1028, 1960.

Wilkins, L., and Fleischmann, W.: Ovarian agenesis: Pathology, associated clinical symptoms and bearing on the theories of sex differentiation. J. Endocr. **4:**357, 1944.

Wilkins, L., Jones, H. W., Jr., Holman, G., and Stempfel, R. S., Jr.: Masculinization of the female fetus associated with administration of oral and intramuscular progestins during gestation: Non-adrenal female pseudohermaphroditism, J. Clin. Endocr. **18:**559. 1958.

Wolf, R. B., and Allen, W. M.: Concomitant malformation: The frequent, simultaneous occurrence of congenital malformations of the reproductive and urinary tracts, Obstet. Gynec. **2:**236, 1953.

Young, W. C., editor: Sex and internal secretions, ed. 3, Baltimore, 1961, The Williams & Wilkins Company.

Chapter 4

Solid tumors

A proposed classification of neoplasms can vary according to the tissue of origin, embryologic derivation, morphologic findings, and gross appearance, depending upon the inclination of the investigator. The purpose for which such an outline is proposed should certainly be considered. Upon discovering a tumor of the vulva or vagina in a patient, the clinician seeks the answers to three questions: (1) Is this a cystic or solid tumor? (2) What is its origin? (3) Is it benign or malignant? We prefer a classification of tumors in these locations that can be of some practical use to the clinician in providing the correct answers. The following classification, based upon the tissue of origin, follows this concept. We realize the shortcomings in such a grouping of tumors and the criticism that will be offered by the embryologists, pure morphologists, and dermatologists. Our outline is as follows:

  A. Epidermal origin
   1. Condyloma acuminatum
   2. Papilloma
   3. Acrochordon
   4. Seborrheic keratosis
   5. Nevus
  B. Epidermal appendage origin
   1. Hidradenoma
   2. Sebaceous adenoma
   3. Basal cell epithelioma
  C. Mesodermal origin
   1. Fibroma
   2. Lipoma
   3. Neurofibroma
   4. Leiomyoma
   5. Granular cell myoblastoma
   6. Hemangioma
   7. Pyogenic granuloma
   8. Lymphangioma
  D. Bartholin's gland origin—Adenofibroma
  E. Urethral origin
   1. Caruncle
   2. Prolapse of urethral mucosa

TUMORS OF EPIDERMAL ORIGIN
Condyloma acuminatum

This tumor is discussed in Chapter 16.

Papilloma

Although it is referred to in most textbooks of gynecology, the true squamous papilloma must be extremely rare; we have never seen a true squamous papilloma of the vulva. According to Knox (1965), the term should be discarded in favor of one more specific. A papilloma is described as a single lesion which occasionally may be multiple. These tumors may arise anywhere on the vulva but are found most often on the labia majora. They are tumors of adult life, particularly of the "middle years."

Clinical features

According to the descriptions of other observers, the squamous papilloma is a soft, warty, fleshy growth. It is usually small, although it may attain a diameter of several centimeters. The outer surface has a wrinkled appearance, and small finger-like projections may develop on the surface. Repeated trauma and irritation may lead to ulceration. Reportedly, 2 to 3 percent of papillomata undergo malignant change.

Histopathology

Numerous folds of squamous epithelium cover a finger-like structure having a loose fibrous stroma (Fig. 4-1). The squamous epithelium is thickened and has an arborescent arrangement. A slight hyperkeratosis may be apparent. The cytoplasmic vacuola-

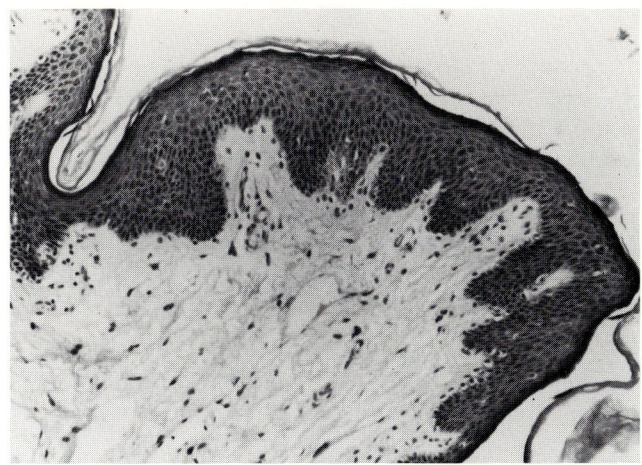

Fig. 4-1. Papilloma. Folds of squamous epithelium covering a loose, fibrous stroma. (H & E × 100)

tion frequently present in condyloma acumininatum is absent in this tumor. Little if any inflammatory reaction is observed beneath the epithelium.

Treatment

Papillomata should be excised together with a small ellipse of surrounding skin. If no evidence of atypia or malignant change is discovered within the tumor, further treatment is unnecessary.

Acrochordon

An acrochordon is a polypoid fibroepithelial lesion often arising on the vulva and adjacent medial aspect of the thigh or perianally. This usually is referred to as a "skin tag." We suspect that many of the so-called squamous papillomata are in reality no more than acrochordons. The cause of acrochordons is unknown; they do not become malignant.

Clinical features

An acrochordon is a soft, flesh-colored, gray-tan, wrinkled polypoid structure devoid of hair. It may be pedicled or sessile. Its size varies from several millimeters to 1 cm. (Fig. 4-2).

Histopathology

The acrochordon is covered by gentle folds of mature, slightly hyperkeratotic epithelium. The stalk and substance of the tumor are composed of loose fibrous tissue containing scattered capillaries. Occasionally, a mild chronic inflammatory reaction is apparent within the stroma.

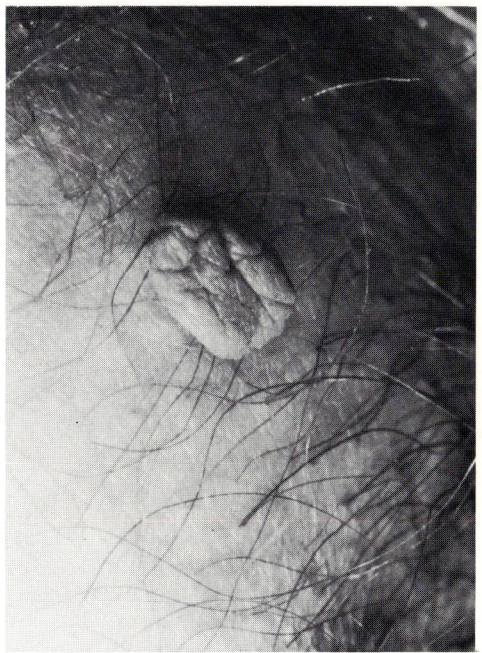

Fig. 4-2. Acrochordon, often referred to as "skin tag," represented by a soft, polypoid structure.

Treatment

The tumor may be left untreated, or it may be removed for cosmetic reasons or because of chronic irritation. Removal usually can be accomplished under local anesthesia by cutting flush with the skin surface with scissors. If bleeding is troublesome, the raw base can be treated with Monsel's solution or a single stitch can be placed to approximate the skin edges.

Seborrheic keratosis

Seborrheic keratosis, a form of papilloma, frequently arises on the trunk, face, neck, and arms. Only occasionally does the lesion appear on the vulva, either as a solitary tumor or in association with similar growths elsewhere.

Clinical features

Seborrheic keratoses are sharply circumscribed, slightly raised, verrucose lesions that are usually papular but which may be macular. They vary in diameter from minute to several centimeters, and they may appear singly or in clusters. They may be flesh colored or black, though the majority are dark brown and have a greasy appearance (Fig.

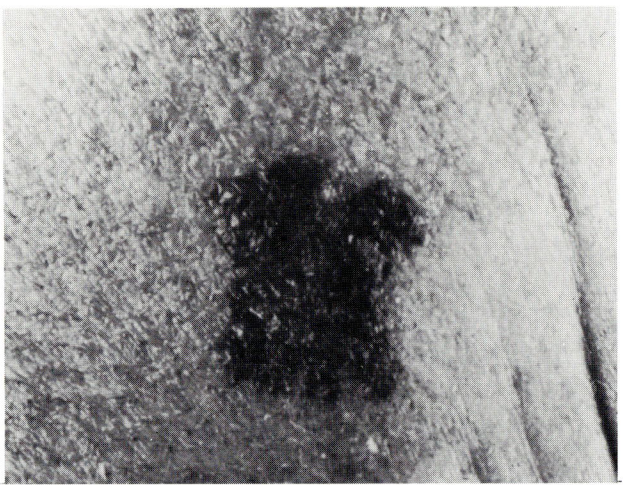

Fig. 4-3. Seborrheic keratosis. A sharply circumscribed, verrucose lesion, usually flesh-colored or black.

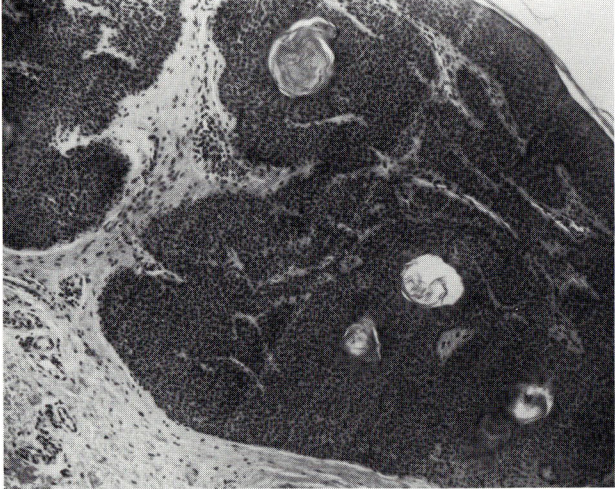

Fig. 4-4. Seborrheic keratosis. Solid sheets of epithelial cells with cystic inclusions of keratinized material. (H & E × 63)

4-3). Often they seem to be pasted to the surface of the skin.

Histopathology

Seborrheic keratoses exhibit considerable hyperkeratosis, acanthosis, and papillomatosis. The epidermal cells grow upward, with the lower borders of the tumor lying above a line between the normal skin on each side of the tumor. The tumor consists of solid sheets or masses of epithelial cells surrounding connective tissue. The horny layer tends to invaginate the lesion, and cystic inclusions of horny material are observed in some areas (Fig. 4-4). Infrequently, thin tracts of double rows of basal cells extend down from the epidermis, branching and interweaving to give the tumor an adenoid appearance.

Treatment

Seborrheic keratoses are limited in their growth potential and do not become malignant. Therefore, no treatment is required unless the tumors become so large as to cause disfiguration or discomfort. When removal is deemed advisable, simple surgical excision will suffice. Small lesions are easily removed with a dermal curette following freezing with ethyl chloride. Bleeding is readily controlled by pressure, although Monsel's solution may be applied or superficial electrodesiccation may be used.

Pigmented nevus

The chief significance of the pigmented nevus lies in its possible development into malignant melanoma. Holland reported that a pigmented nevus (junctional or compound) is the starting point for 40 percent of malignant melanomas. Despite the fact that malignant melanoma of the vulva is an uncommon lesion (constituting, according to Hertig and Gore, 1 to 3 percent of all malignant vulvar neoplasms), its virulence and associated mortality makes its prevention, if possible, important.

Pack and Scharnagel have pointed out that pigmented nevi are highly sensitive to the stimulating effect of the steroid hormones and that they often undergo enlargement and darkening at puberty. They emphasize the importance of prophylactic removal of pigmented nevi in pregnant women. On the contrary, Allen and Spitz doubted the presence of any causal relationship between pregnancy and the development of malignant

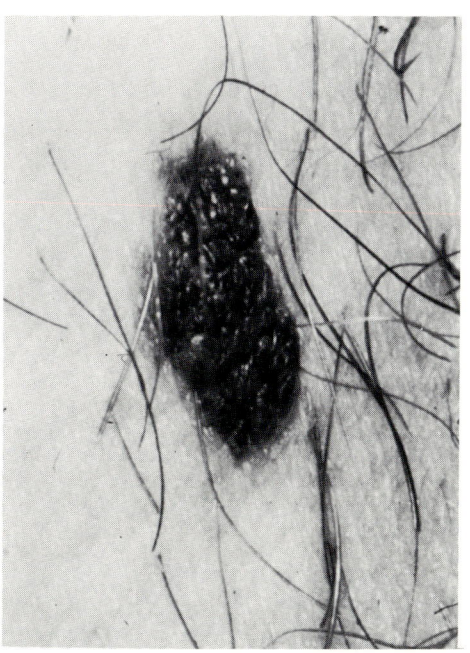

Fig. 4-5. Compound nevus. Usually, a slightly elevated pigmented lesion.

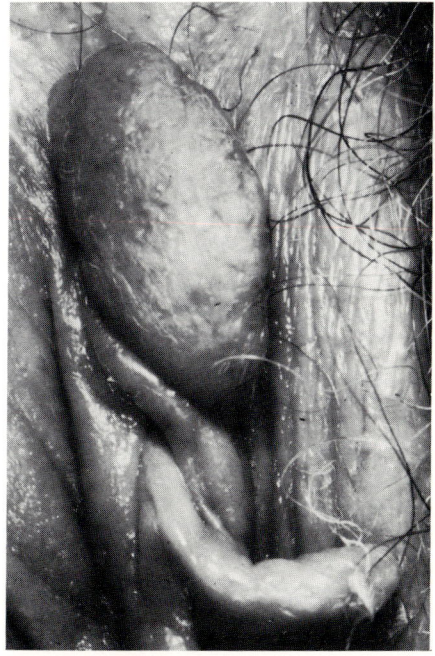

Fig. 4-6. Intradermal pedunculated nevus to right of clitoris.

46 Benign diseases of the vulva and vagina

melanomas. The actual evidence linking malignant melanomas to pregnancy is nebulous.

Clinical features

Lever divides pigmented nevi into five clinical types:

1. Flat nevi—usually junctional type
2. Slightly elevated nevi—usually compound in type (Fig. 4-5)
3. Papillomatous nevi—may be compound, though the majority are of the intradermal type
4. Dome shaped nevi—usually intradermal in type
5. Pedunculated nevi—intradermal in type (Fig. 4-6)

The pigmented nevi vary in color from a light tan to a dark brown to black. They may vary in diameter from 1 mm. to 2 cm.

Histopathology

Nevi are classified into three main groups: junctional, intradermal (Fig. 4-7), and compound (Fig. 4-8). According to Masson, the nevus cell derives from two sources: from the melanocytes in the epidermis and from the Schwann cells of the dermal nerves. Masson has suggested that junctional nevi come from melanocytes and that compound and intradermal nevi arise from both sources. The junctional nevus is characterized by an active formation of cells in the basal layer of the epidermis. These cells form more or less circumscribed nests. The nests may ap-

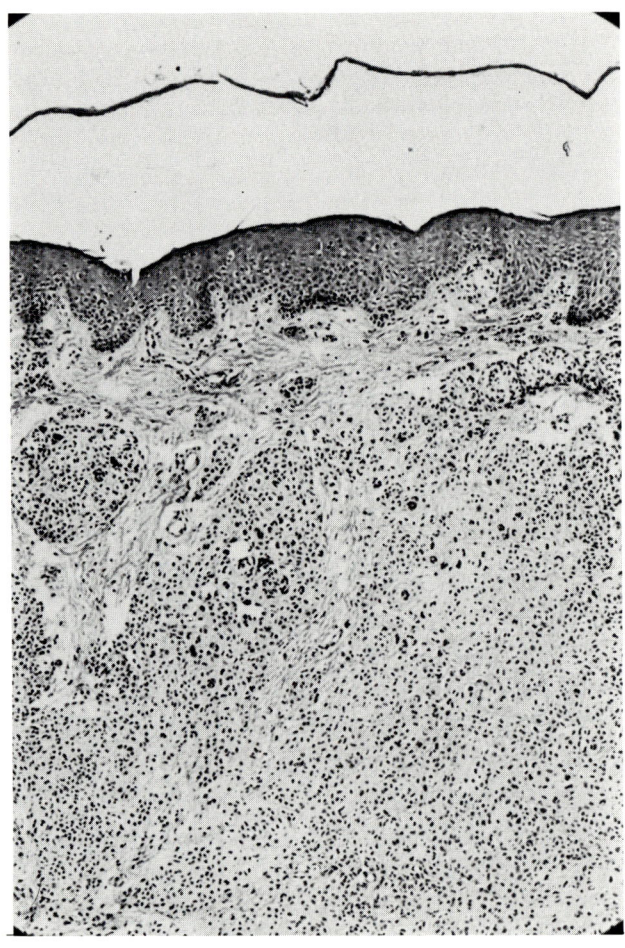

Fig. 4-7. Intradermal nevus. Nests of nevus cells lie within the dermis. No junctional activity is apparent. (H & E × 77)

pear to be "dropping off" the epidermis, yet remain in contact with it. Although this type of nevus is the one most likely to become malignant, the danger of its transformation is slight if the nests of cells are well circumscribed.

The compound nevus exhibits junctional activity, yet nests of nevus cells are present within the dermis. This tumor may also have malignant potential.

The cells in the intradermal nevus are located within the dermis. Careful sectioning of the tissue, however, will generally reveal some foci of junctional activity, even though none have been suspected from routine sections.

The nevus cell is oval or cuboidal. Its membrane is quite distinct, and the cytoplasm has a homogeneous appearance. The cytoplasm of scattered cells may contain dark brown melanin. The nuclei, which may be round or oval, are large, vesicular, and pale. The nevus cells lying deep in the dermis may be spindle shaped and embedded in fibrous tissue. In addition, the dermis may contain multinucleated nevus cells.

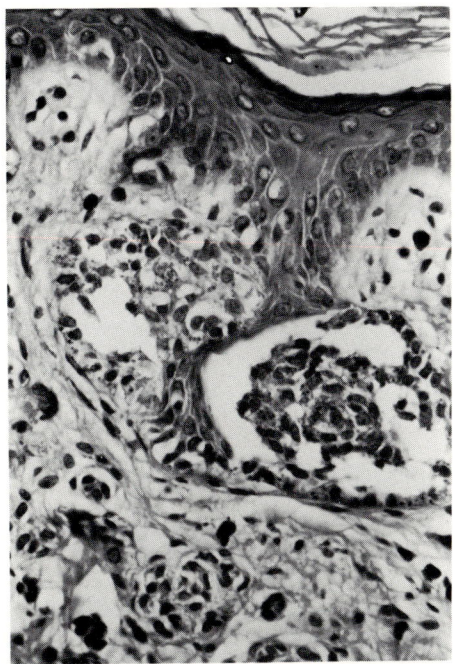

Fig. 4-8. Compound nevus. Nests of nevus cells lie within the dermis and in contact with the basal layer of epithelium. (H & E × 250)

Treatment

Since pigmented nevi of the vulva are frequently irritated, they should usually be surgically removed. This is especially true of the flat junctional nevus, which has the highest malignant potential. At least 0.5 to 1 cm. of the surrounding skin and subcutaneous tissue should be excised with the nevus. Reynolds has advocated the removal of pigmented moles from pregnant women when such lesions are subject to irritation, when they are smooth, blue, black, or dark brown, when pigmentation or rate of growth increases, or when associated with ulceration, bleeding, or pain.

Since obviously raised or hairy moles rarely become malignant, their removal is not particularly urgent. If constantly irritated, painful, or bleeding, however, they should be excised.

An ideal time to remove nevi is at the time of delivery, curettage, or other pelvic surgery. Nevi may also be readily excised in the office under local anesthesia. They should not be removed by desiccation or cauterization. The removed tissue should always be examined microscopically.

TUMORS OF EPIDERMAL APPENDAGE ORIGIN
Hidradenoma

The hidradenoma of the vulva may be either cystic or solid. Being more often cystic than solid, it is discussed in Chapter 5.

Sebaceous adenoma

Usually present beneath the epithelium of the labia minora are raised, yellow-tan nodules, 1 to 3 mm. in diameter, consisting of groups and clusters of mature sebaceous glands. On rare occasions, a true tumor may develop from these sebaceous glands. The distinction of such tumors from the other solid tumors arising in this area can be established only by histologic examination following their excision.

Clinical features

The sebaceous adenoma is a solitary, smooth, firm, elevated, round or oval nodule, usually less than 1 cm. in diameter. At times, it may be pedunculated. It may closely resemble a hidradenoma, epidermal inclusion cyst, sebaceous cyst, or a small cyst of embryonic origin.

Histopathology

Microscopic examination reveals lobules of varying size and shape consisting of two types of cells. One type is identical with the cells found at the periphery of normal sebaceous glands; the other type is a mature sebaceous cell that has developed from the generative cells. The relative number of each type of cell in each lobule varies considerably, with transitional cells from the generative to the mature sebaceous type often being present. The tumor is sharply demarcated from the adjacent tissue and is usually surrounded by a connective tissue capsule.

Treatment

Treatment consists of local excision, primarily to establish the diagnosis. The tumor is readily shelled out of the bed in which it lies. The likelihood of recurrence is negligible.

Basal cell epithelioma

Basal cell epithelioma has a much more onerous significance in gynecologic than in dermatologic literature. Although it is generally recognized as primarily a locally invasive lesion, the gynecologist has advocated a more aggressive therapeutic approach to this tumor and has been more concerned about its capacity to spread and recur. We are inclined to accept the point of view of the dermatologist that basal cell epithelioma does not represent a carcinoma in the usual sense of the term, and we have followed Lever's example of describing this tumor as one of epidermal appendage origin, rather than with the intraepithelial carcinomas.

The incidence of basal cell epithelioma of the vulva has been reported as 2 to 4 percent of the neoplasms in this site. Marcus, combining his cases with those of thirteen other authors, listed forty-one basal cell epitheliomata among 1,499 vulvar carcinomata, or an incidence of 2.7 percent. The tumor arises most often in postmenopausal women. Siegler and Greene reported an average age of 63 years among sixty-five patients in a collected series. The youngest patient was 42 and the oldest was 86 years old.

Histogenesis

Several theories regarding the histogenesis of basal cell epitheliomata have been proposed, but that of Lever is most widely accepted today. Lever believes that basal cell epitheliomata, rather than being carcinomata, are nevoid tumors (hamartomata) derived from immature, incompletely differentiated pluripotential cells. These immature pluripotential cells, which form continuously during life, may differentiate into sebaceous glands, apocrine glands, and hair. Thus basal cell epitheliomas can differentiate toward any or all three of these structures.

Formerly, these tumors were considered to be of embryonal basal origin. Some observers still hold this view, which was based largely upon the frequent observation of nests of basal cell epithelioma in direct continuity with the basal cells of the epidermis. Mallory favored the theory that basal cell epitheliomata developed from hair matrix cells. Wallace and Halpert suggested that they originate in either the hair matrix or hair anlage and proposed the term "trichoma." Willis postulated a multicentric origin from the epidermis per se, from the pilosebaceous apparatus, or from both.

Clinical features

Pruritus, burning, and chronic ulceration are the chief manifestations of basal cell epithelioma. As a rule, bleeding and a dis-

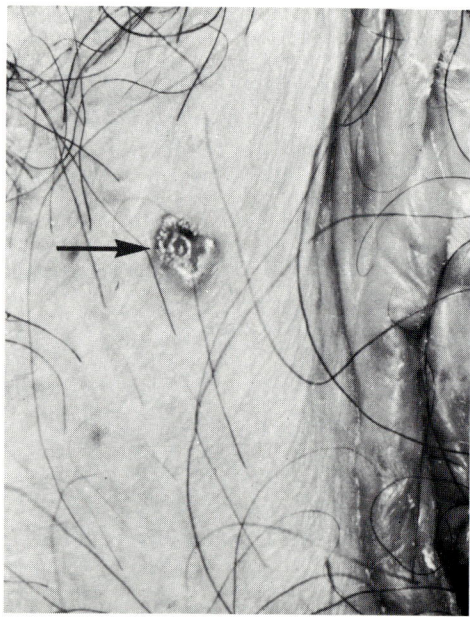

Fig. 4-9. Basal cell epithelioma of vulva. A raised nodule with central ulceration and a pearly, raised border.

charge are associated with large lesions. Occasionally, the presence of a mass is the patient's only complaint. A number of patients have no symptoms, with the tumor being discovered during a routine examination. In Siegler and Green's series, the interval between the appearance of symptoms and treatment averaged 6.6 years.

The labium majus is the most common site of basal cell epitheliomata of the vulva. Of fifteen cases reported by Schueller, in twelve the lesions were in this location, in two on the clitoris, and in one on both the labium majus and mons pubis.

Typically, the vulvar tumors are slightly raised, slowly growing nodules with central ulcerations and pearly, rolled borders (Fig. 4-9). They may or may not be pigmented. The term "rodent ulcer" is frequently applied to this tumor. The base of the ulcers may be covered with a small amount of necrotic debris or small crusts. If untreated, the tumors may erode deeply into the underlying tissues and into the bone of the symphysis pubis. In time, the ulcers may become infected, leading to secondary inguinal adenopathy.

On rare occasions, these tumors have been found to metastasize. This was documented by Binkley and Rauschkolb in a review of forty-two cases of metastasizing basal cell epitheliomas.

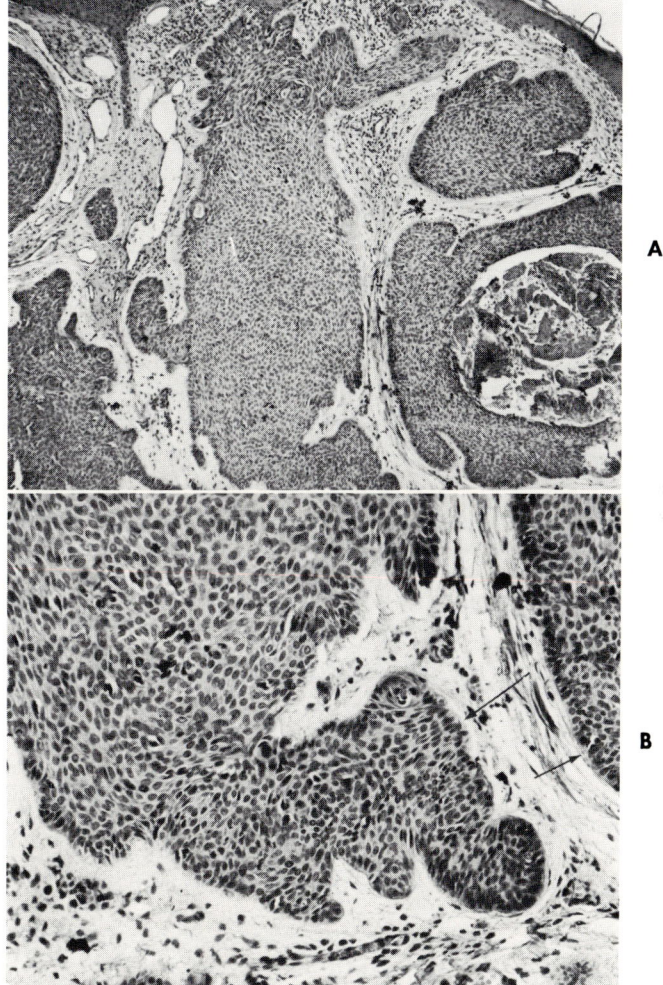

Fig. 4-10. Basal cell epithelioma. **A,** Nests of closely packed, uniform cells within the dermis. (H & E × 60) **B,** The nuclei are uniform and there is peripheral palisading of cells (arrows). No intracellular bridges are present. (H & E × 130)

Histopathology

Basal cell epithelioma is composed of nests of closely packed, uniform cells of oval or fusiform shape (Fig. 4-10, *A*). The clusters of cells appear as single or multiple growths arising from the basal layer of the epidermis or from a hair shaft or glandular apparatus. Many are rimmed by a single layer of cells arranged in a radial pattern, that is, peripheral palisading (Fig. 4-10, *B*). The nuclei of the cells are deeply basophilic and are surrounded by a small rim of cytoplasm. Frequently, the latter is difficult to identify. The cells resemble the basal cells of the epidermis, although they do not have intercellular bridges. Mitotic figures are often present. Lever states that the tumors are both differentiated and undifferentiated. The former exhibit differentiation toward primary epithelial germ structures—sebaceous glands, apocrine glands, or hair—having a cystic, adenoid, or keratotic pattern. Tumors composed of the undifferentiated cells are usually solid and composed of sheets of uniform cells. The two groups cannot be sharply distinguished, and elements of both often are detected in the same tumor.

Mixed basal-squamous cell epitheliomas have been reported. Marcus believes that the cells of the basal cell epithelioma may undergo transformation to squamous cells and, if so, that the lesion carries a poorer prognosis than that of the pure basal cell tumor. Schueller has suggested that the foci of mature squamous cells found in the center of basal cell nests develop from maturation of the basal cells. Lever, however, does not accept the existence of basal-squamous cell epithelioma; rather, he believes that the mixed type of basal-squamous cell epithelioma represents a keratotic basal cell epithelioma. The tumors contain cells differentiating toward cells forming the hair matrix, which have the capacity to develop into keratinized cells. These tumors must be distinguished from mixed basal cell epithelioma and squamous cell carcinoma. When present, a squamous cell carcinoma is contiguous to a basal cell epithelioma and has the same capacity to spread and metastasize as any squamous cell carcinoma.

The distinction of basal cell epithelioma from squamous cell carcinoma is usually easily established, although it may become difficult. The cells of basal cell tumors stain basophilic, whereas those of squamous cell carcinoma are eosinophilic. The cells of undifferentiated squamous cell carcinoma are severely atypical and many atypical mitoses are present. Also, the cell masses of basal cell epitheliomata may appear to retract from the surrounding stroma, a feature not observed in true carcinomata.

Treatment

Because of the tendency of basal cell epitheliomata to recur locally, they should be radically excised, with a wide margin of surrounding normal skin as well as a considerable depth of underlying tissue also being removed. The specimen must be carefully evaluated in the laboratory, with the study including the margins of the specimen to ensure a complete excision. Multiple sections through the tumor should be taken to rule out the presence of an adjacent squamous cell carcinoma. Schueller even reported a case of a melanoma associated with a basal cell epithelioma. If removal of the tumor is not complete, it will eventually recur locally. Since these tumors seldom, if ever, metastasize, a lymph node dissection is not necessary. In our opinion, vulvectomy is not essential, although some authors disagree. Marcus recommended a wide complete vulvectomy because of the possibility of multicentric origin and the propensity for local recurrence. Barclay and Collins also favored this approach. Actually, an informed estimate of the prognosis of this lesion on the vulva is not possible because of the paucity of reported cases, a lack of follow-up in many of these, and differences of opinion regarding the histologic diagnosis and treatment. If one relies upon the extensive experience of the dermatologist with this disease elsewhere in the body, however, it would seem that wide excision of the tumor would afford a favorable outlook for the patient.

VULVAR TUMORS OF MESODERMAL ORIGIN

Tumors of mesodermal origin arise infrequently in the vulva and even less often in the vagina. They may originate in fibrous tissue, fat, smooth muscle, blood vessels, and nerves. Although the inclusion of tumors of neurogenic origin may be open to question it appears justified, since mesodermal nerve

Solid tumors 51

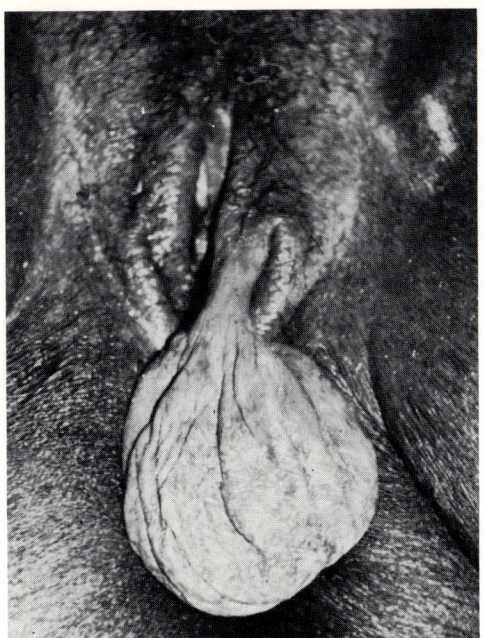

Fig. 4-11. Fibroma arising from labium majus. (Kaufman, R. H., and Gardner, H. L.: Clin. Obstet. Gynec. 8:953, 1965.)

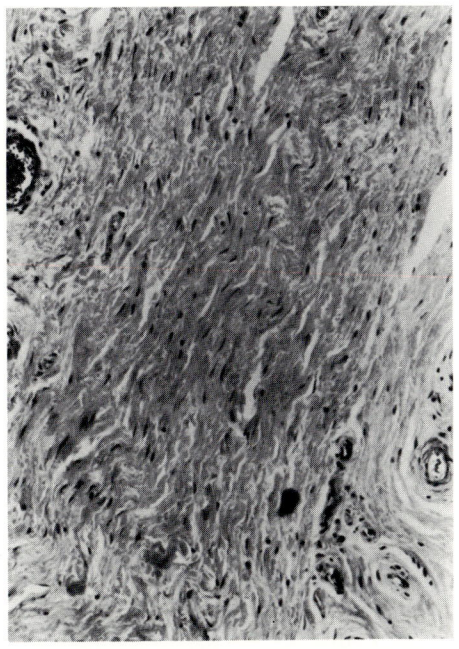

Fig. 4-12. Fibroma. Microscopic section of lesion in Fig. 4-11. The bundles of fibrous tissue are parallel. (Masson trichrome stain × 100) (Kaufman, R. H., and Gardner, H. L.: Clin. Obstet. Gynec. 8:953, 1965.)

sheath cells play an important part in the histogenesis of some of these neoplasms.

Fibroma
Clinical features

Fibromata of the vulva are usually firm, pedunculated masses (Fig. 4-11) and less often small, firm, subcutaneous nodules. The fibromata reported by Lovelady, McDonald, and Waugh varied from 0.6 cm. to 8 cm. in diameter, with the surfaces of the larger tumors being ulcerated. As elsewhere in the body, fibromata arise in the vulva by a proliferation of fibroblasts and often undergo myxomatous degeneration. On cross section, they exhibit a dense, firm, gray-white, fibrous stroma.

The majority of fibromata are asymptomatic; however, the large, pedunculated tumors may produce a sensation of heaviness and pain. If the overlying skin becomes ulcerated, bleeding and a discharge may be associated.

Histopathology

Microscopic examination demonstrates parallel and intertwining bundles of fibrous tissue (Fig. 4-12). No mitotic figures are present. A Masson stain will readily reveal the nature of the tumor.

Treatment

Fibromata should be excised locally. The likelihood of recurrence is quite small.

Lipoma
Clinical features

Lipomata of the vulva are soft, either sessile or pedunculated masses of different sizes (Fig. 4-13). The largest of seven lipomata reported by Lovelady, McDonald, and Waugh was 17 cm. in diameter. Like fibromata, lipomata are asymptomatic unless they become sufficiently large to produce a sensation of heaviness or to cause ulceration of the overlying tissue.

Histopathology

Lipomata are composed of mature fat cells and usually have no well-defined connective tissue capsule. Interspersed between individual and clusters of fat cells are varying amounts of connective tissue. A tumor containing abundant fibrous tissue is more correctly referred to as a *fibrolipoma*.

Treatment

Excision is the correct treatment for large, symptomatic lipomata. Otherwise, if the diagnosis is clinically apparent, they may be left undisturbed.

Neurofibroma

Neurofibromata, which arise from the neural sheath, are observed much more often than most textbooks of gynecology and pathology indicate. This is explained by the fact that they are asymptomatic and remain more or less stationary in size; thus, they are not removed and examined microscopically. The solitary neurofibroma is often referred to as a *neuronevus*.

Clinical features

The tumors appear as small, fleshy, frequently flabby, pink-tan, polypoid masses (Fig. 4-14). Seldom do they reach a large size. Being asymptomatic, the tumors are usually found incidentally upon examination of the patient. If associated with von Recklinghausen's disease, the presence of tumors elsewhere will confirm the diagnosis. Otherwise, the correct diagnosis will usually be suspected by the clinician if he is aware that they arise in this location. A distinction between neurofibromata, fibroepithelial polyps, fibromata, acrochordons, or pedunculated molluscum contagiosum may be necessary. Although neurofibromata may be confined to the vulva, they are more likely to be associated with neurofibromata elsewhere on the body (von Recklinghausen's disease); if so, other stigmata of this condition may be seen, such as café au lait spots. None of the rather numerous vulvar neurofibromata we have encountered have been part of a generalized disease. Schreiber, however, reported finding vulvar lesions in 18 percent of fifty-three female patients with von Recklinghausen's disease. The incidence of the

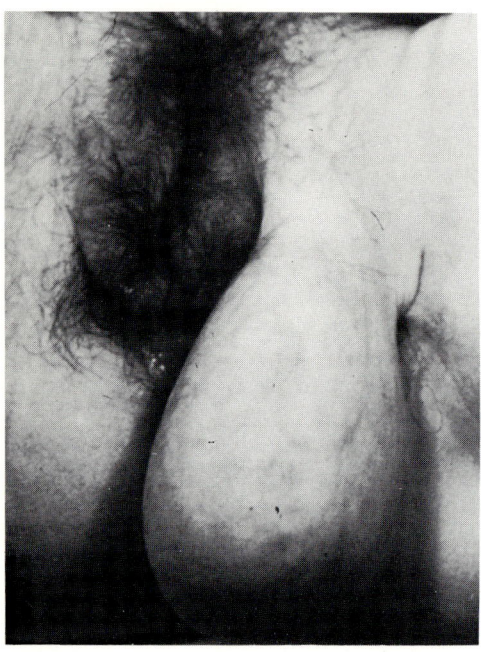

Fig. 4-13. Lipoma arising from genitocrural fold. (Courtesy F. Bayard Carter, Durham, N. C.)

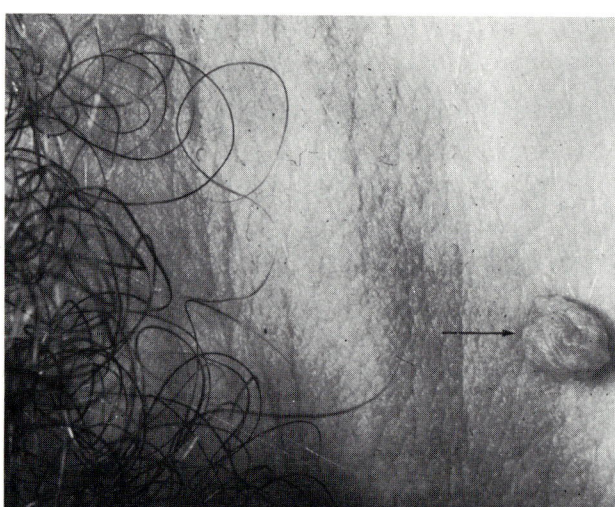

Fig. 4-14. Neurofibroma appearing as a soft, fleshy polypoid mass. (Kaufman, R. H., and Gardner, H. L.: Clin. Obstet. Gynec. 8:953, 1965.)

vulvar lesions is highest in Negro patients; vulvar lesions were found in 28 percent of thirty-three Negro patients observed by Schreiber.

Histopathology

Neurofibromata are well circumscribed, though not encapsulated. They are composed of loose, wavy fibrils of pale blue-staining cells that tend to form whorls (Fig. 4-15). Typically, the nuclei of the cells exhibit a palisaded arrangement.

Treatment

In the absence of symptoms, no treatment is necessary. If the diagnosis is in doubt, however, local excision is easily performed in the physician's office. On rare occasions, vulvectomy may be required because of the presence of multiple symptomatic tumors. Of sixty vulvectomies for benign lesions performed at Tulane University, two (3.3 percent) were for vulvar neurofibromatosis.

Leiomyoma

Leiomyomata of the vulva, in contrast to the uterine counterpart, are rare tumors. In 1964, Palermino reported the thirty-third case in the medical literature to that time. His personal communication with the Armed Forces Institute of Pathology revealed that they had twenty examples of vulvar leiomyomata in their files. Lovelady, McDonald, and Waugh reported two leiomyomata of the vulva; they were 4 to 6 cm. in diameter and grossly and microscopically were similar to the uterine tumor.

As a rule, leiomyomata arise from the smooth muscle of the erectile tissue in the vulva, although they may also arise from the round ligament of the uterus. In the latter case, they are located in the anterior portion of the vulva.

Clinical features

Leiomyomata appear as solitary, firm masses varying in size from less than 1 cm. to over 10 cm. The tumor may progressively enlarge until symptoms of pressure and ulceration appear. Frequently, the only symptom is the recognition of the tumor mass by the patient.

Histopathology

The diagnosis of leiomyoma is seldom made until the tumor has been excised and

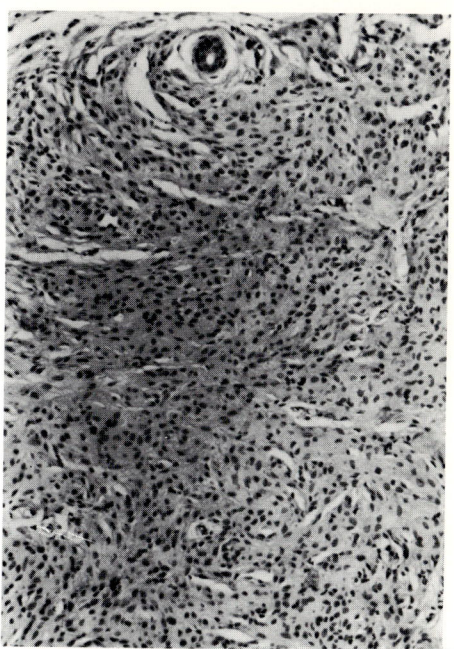

Fig. 4-15. Neurofibroma. Microscopic section of tumor in Fig. 4-14. Whorls and eddies are formed by wavy fibrils of cells. (H & E × 100) (Kaufman, R. H., and Gardner, H. L.: Clin. Obstet. Gynec. 8:953, 1965.)

examined microscopically. The histologic picture is identical with that of the uterine leiomyoma, consisting of bundles of smooth muscle intertwining with fibrous tissue and producing a whorled pattern (Fig. 4-16). The smooth muscle element usually predominates, as demonstrated by a Masson trichrome stain.

We have recently observed two patients with vulvar leiomyomata, one a 13-year-old girl and the other a 35-year-old woman. The tumor in the 13-year-old patient enlarged rapidly, reaching a diameter of 8 to 9 cm. within 6 months (Fig. 4-17). The tumor in the woman was 2.5 cm. in diameter when excised. Of special interest was the pronounced cellularity and nuclear activity in both these tumors (Fig. 4-18). Occasional bizarre and giant cells were present, although careful study of multiple sections failed to reveal more than a rare mitotic figure. Both neoplasms were considered to be cellular leiomyomata rather than leiomyosarcomata. No evidence of recurrence of either tumor was apparent at 15 months and 44 months following wide local excision.

54 Benign diseases of the vulva and vagina

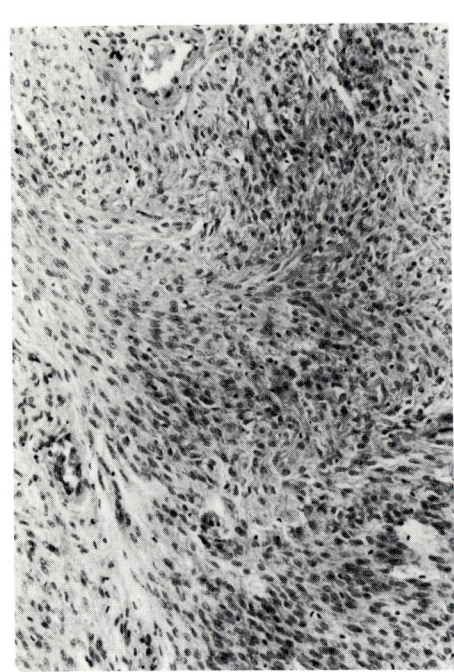

Fig. 4-16. Leiomyoma exhibiting bundles of smooth muscle and scant fibrous tissue arranged in whorls. (H & E × 100)

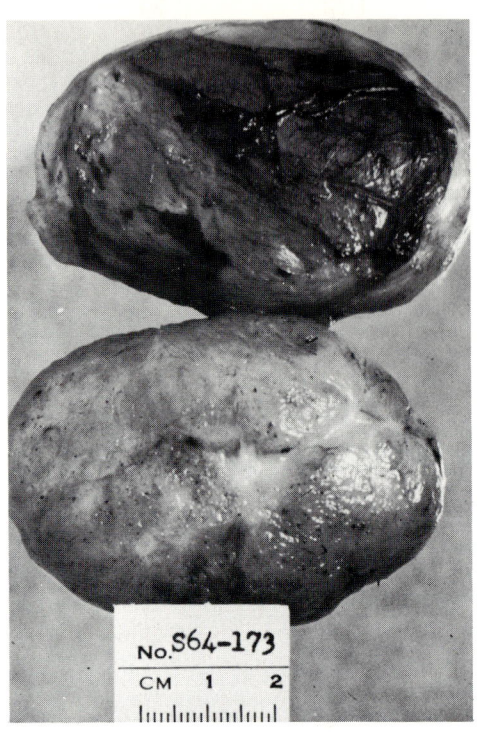

Fig. 4-17. Leiomyoma removed from vulva of 13-year-old child. (Courtesy Robert R. Franklin and H. S. Rosenberg, Houston.)

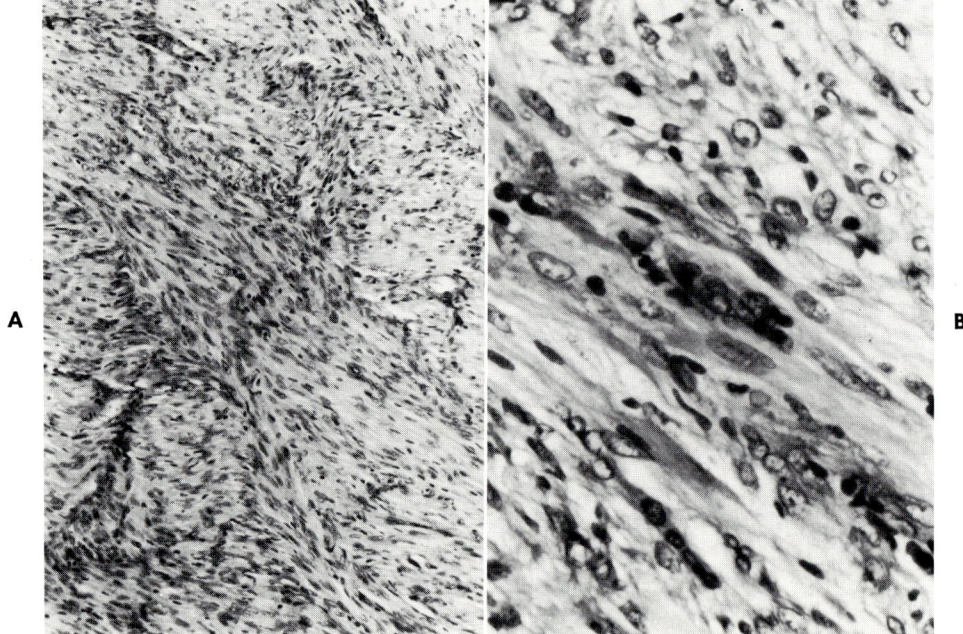

Fig. 4-18. A and **B**, Leiomyoma, showing pronounced cellularity and an occasional pleomorphic cell. (**A**, H & E × 100; **B**, H & E × 400)

Treatment

Treatment consists of wide local excision. This is especially important if the tumor grows rapidly.

Granular cell myoblastoma

The granular cell myoblastoma may be found in almost any location in the body. In a review of the medical literature in 1961, Birch and Sondag found that 35 percent of the lesions involved the tongue, 30 percent the skin or nearby tissues, and 35 percent various other sites. Seven percent of the tumors were found on the vulva. They have no predilection for persons of any age or race. Bishop and Wagner reported the case of a granular cell myoblastoma in a 6-year-old girl.

Histogenesis

Since this tumor was first described by Abrikossoff in 1926 under the name "myoblastenmyoma," a voluminous literature has accumulated, especially regarding its histogenesis. In his first report (1926), Abrikossoff suggested that these tumors might arise by degeneration of adult striated muscle. In 1931, he adopted the view that they originated from embryonic muscle fibers, this theory being based upon a presumed analogy between the granular cells of the tumor and myoblasts and their purported continuity with altered skeletal muscle. In 1939, Leroux and Delarue postulated that granular cell myoblastoma was not actually a true neoplasm but was composed of mesenchymal cells (histiocytes) containing an unknown product. Their view was later supported by Azzopardi. From histochemical observations, Pearse rejected the theory that this tumor was possibly of neural (Schwann) cell, muscular, or histiocytic origin; instead, he believed that the fibroblast was the precursor of the granular cell. Fust and Custer suggested that the tumor might be of neurogenic origin and proposed the name "granular cell neurofibromata." Bangle (1952, 1953) was of the same opinion; he had little doubt that the granular cell tumor arose within a peripheral myelinated nerve. Fisher and Wechsler, in a well-documented report published in 1962, stated that the results of electron microscopic and histochemical studies provided strong evidence of a neural origin of this lesion, and considered the term "granular cell schwannoma" more appropriate. These authors believed that the tumor cells represented altered Schwann cells and that the cytoplasmic granules probably represented altered myelin or axoplasm, or both, or metabolic products of these structures. They could not say definitely whether the tumor was a true neoplasm or a histiocytic response, though they suggested that Schwann cells may assume a histiocytic function.

As the preceding discussion indicates, it has been hypothesized that this tumor originates in mature striated muscle, immature striated muscle, the histiocyte, fibroblast, and nerve sheath cell. According to the preponderance of more recent evidence, the nerve sheath is the source of the neoplasm. In our opinion, however, common usage and knowledge makes retention of the term "granular cell myoblastoma" advisable.

Clinical features

A granular cell myoblastoma is a benign, usually solitary, slowly growing, discrete nodule that tends to infiltrate the adjacent tissues. On occasion, multiple nodules may be present, involving the vulva, or even several sites in the body. Chiodi and others reported the case of a patient with a granular cell myoblastoma of the vulva as well as the lower respiratory tract.

Granular cell myoblastomata rarely attain a large size, varying in diameter from 1 to 4 cm. Those of the vulva may lie deep within the tissue, though they are more often superficial and elevated, and occasionally the overlying skin is depigmented. Rarely, it is a pedunculated tumor and resembles a papilloma. At times, the epidermis may ulcerate, leading to an erroneous clinical diagnosis of carcinoma. Grossly, the tumor is often mistaken for a fibroma or epidermal cyst, or other benign vulvar neoplasm.

The clinical story is that of a slowly growing, firm, nontender, painless nodule on the labia majora. If the overlying skin becomes ulcerated, the patient may complain of pain and a discharge.

The tumor is firm in consistency, is poorly encapsulated, and on section has a glistening surface that is gray-white to pale yellow in color.

Histopathology

Microscopic study reveals irregularly arranged bundles of large, pink-staining, round and polyhedral cells, with indistinct cell

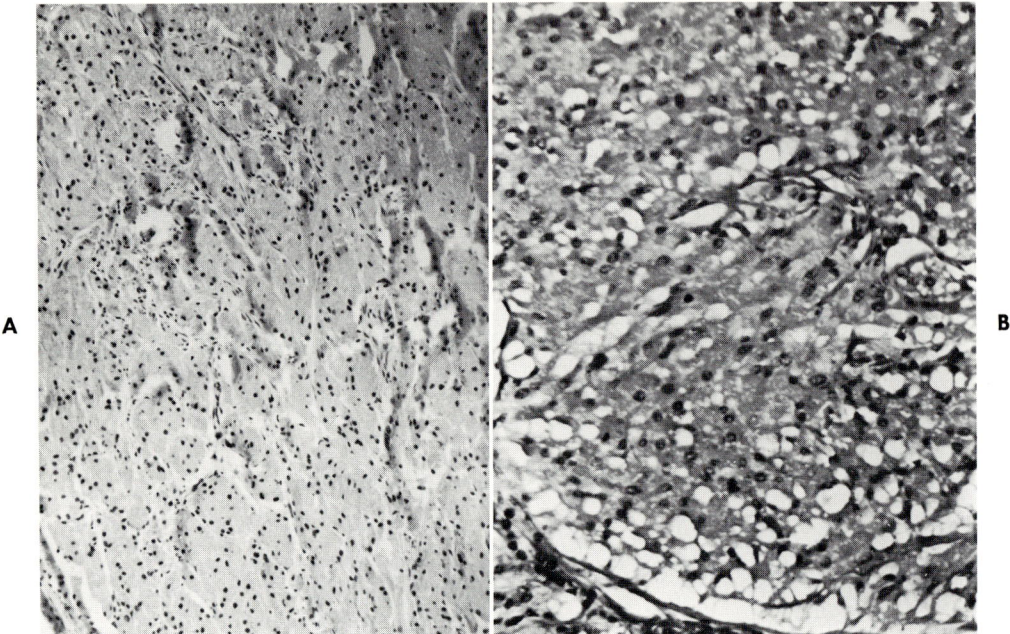

Fig. 4-19. **A,** Granular cell myoblastoma. Bundles of large, round, and polyhedral cells have indistinct cell borders. The nuclei are uniform, small, and darkly staining. (H & E × 100) (Kaufman, R. H., and Gardner, H. L.: Clin. Obstet. Gynec. 8:953, 1965.) **B,** Granular cell myoblastoma. The nuclei are larger and the cytoplasm is more granular. (H & E × 180)

borders, the bundles being separated by bands of collagen fibers (Fig. 4-19). Because of the indistinct cell borders, it often appears that many multinucleated cells are scattered throughout the substance of the tumor. The cytoplasm of the cells contains numerous eosinophilic granules 0.1 to 3.0 μ in diameter; this cytoplasmic picture has been in part the basis for the name of the tumor. The nuclei vary from small to large and are dark-staining, centrally placed structures containing one or two nucleoli. The margins of the tumor are irregular, with bands of tumor cells extending out into the contiguous tissues. On careful search, clusters of granular tumor cells may be found within the sheaths of nerve twigs at some distance from the tumor proper. The squamous epithelium overlying the tumor may be normal or atrophic, or it may exhibit a hyperplastic response that produces a "pseudo-epitheliomatous" hyperplasia. This response may be pronounced, with rete pegs extending down into the tumor mass, thus presenting the appearance of squamous cell carcinoma. The reason for this epithelial response is not clear, although it has been postulated that it is stimulated by some substance elaborated by the tumor cells.

The granular cell myoblastoma is almost invariably benign, although locally infiltrative. Sadler and Dockerty reported one case of a malignant myoblastoma of the vulva with metastasis. They divided the tumors into a uniform and a pleomorphic type; the few metastasizing tumors reported are of the latter variety. Actually, the rare "malignant granular cell myoblastoma" is probably a rhabdomyosarcoma, rather than a variant of the tumor under discussion.

Treatment

Treatment consists of wide local excision. Birch and Sondag, in their review of medical literature, found that in twenty-eight previously reported cases, five tumors persisted following excision, requiring a second excision. Of four granular cell myoblastomas observed by Rubin, three were incompletely removed as confirmed upon removal of additional tissue. In one patient, inadequate excision was followed by local recurrence on two occasions. If one remembers that these tumors are not encapsulated and are locally infiltrative, the rationale for wide excision becomes apparent. If a local recurrence develops, however, it can be re-excised; if the excision is adequate, the likelihood of a second recurrence is small. Since the tumors are benign, extensive surgery with resection of regional lymph nodes is not indicated. The margins of the excised tissue should be carefully examined microscopically, preferably by frozen section, and if evidence of incomplete removal is found, a wider local excision is indicated. Since the tumors are radioresistant, radiotherapy plays no part in their treatment. In view of the multicentric origin of granular cell myoblastoma, the lungs occasionally being involved, radiograms should be made of the chest of all patients with this tumor.

Hemangioma

Hemangiomata are, in reality, "malformations" of blood vessel origin rather than true neoplasms. They are much more common than is suggested by the paucity of cases reported. We have observed numerous hemangiomata of the vulva of different types: the nevus vasculosus (strawberry mark), the cavernous hemangioma, the so-called senile hemangioma, angiokeratomata, and granuloma pyogenicum. Apparently, no classification of these vulvar tumors, either grossly or histologically, has been attempted. Lovelady and others describe them as definite tumors composed of large vascular spaces without intervening smooth muscle. They indicated that the majority were of the cavernous type.

The significance of and treatment for the different varieties of hemagiomata depend upon their gross and histologic characteristics, location, and size.

Strawberry hemangioma

Clinical features. The strawberry mark, so called because of its resemblance to the strawberry, is usually observed shortly after birth. It is an elevated, bright red to dark red soft tumor, varying in diameter from a few millimeters to several centimeters (Fig. 4-20). After an initial period of growth in early infancy, it frequently undergoes spontaneous involution over several years. Andrews and others followed 153 untreated children with strawberry hemangiomata; in 63 percent, involution or improvement of the tumor was apparent within 5 years. In view of the pos-

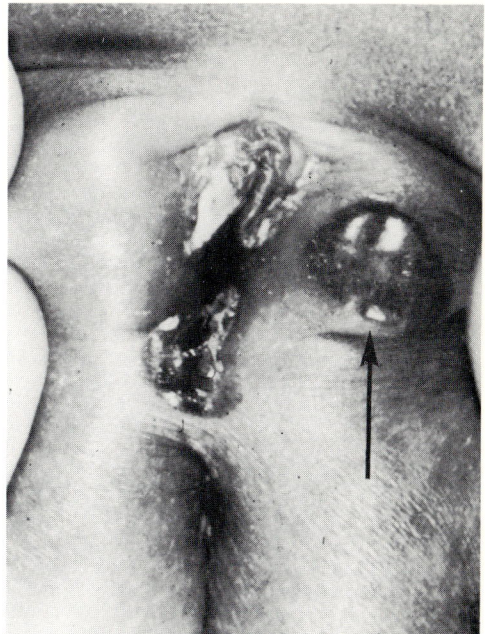

Fig. 4-20. Strawberry hemangioma on vulva of 4-month-old infant. Similar lesions were present on back and over sternum.

sibility of their disappearance, treatment for these hemangiomata in most areas of the body may be unnecessary. Because of their tendency to ulcerate and bleed, however, those on the vulva are an exception to this rule.

Histopathology. Microscopic examination of the tumor reveals dilation of the normal capillaries in the upper dermis as well as the presence of newly formed vessels. In the early stages of growth, considerable capillary proliferation is present, with the endothelial cells being large and prominent. In older lesions, the endothelial cells flatten out and the lumina of the capillaries widen. Later, fibrosis replaces the vessels and leads to gradual shrinkage of the tumor.

Treatment. The simplest and most effective treatment for vulvar lesions is cryotherapy with the use of solid carbon dioxide. A carbon dioxide stick can be shaped to cover the entire surface of the lesion, or different segments of the tumor may be treated separately. The stick is held in contact with the hemangioma for 10 to 30 seconds, with mild to moderate pressure being applied. Excessive blistering should be avoided. The treatment may be repeated after 4 to 6 weeks, and two to four applications may be required. Regression of the strawberry mark illustrated in Fig. 4-20 was induced by this method. This hemangioma is rarely excised. It has responded to the local application of gamma radiation, although generally radiotherapy should be avoided in the region of the genitalia, especially if the patient is a child.

Cavernous hemangioma

Cavernous hemangiomata frequently appear during the first few months of life and increase in size until the child reaches the age of about 18 months; thereafter they may remain static, or they may begin to regress and eventually may almost disappear. Lesions that rapidly enlarge during the first 6 to 8 months of life are prone to spontaneous involution. This process often begins when the child is 12 to 18 months old and is maximal at the age of about 5 years. Hemangiomata present at birth that grow slowly seldom undergo spontaneous regression.

Clinical features. Lesions of the vulva frequently are deep purple in color and multilobular. In size and shape they vary widely, covering only a few square millimeters to several centimeters of the surface of the skin (Fig. 4-21). The tumor masses may extend up into the vagina and bulge from beneath the vaginal mucosa into the vaginal canal. They are round or flat, lobulated or nodular, and extend deep into the subcutaneous tissue. In undergoing spontaneous involution, they may become fibrous.

The symptoms of vulvar lesions in the adult depend upon their exact location and size. Smaller lesions are frequently asymptomatic, and even extensive hemangiomata may cause no difficulty other than pressure and deformity. If overlying skin becomes ulcerated, pain and discomfort as well as hemorrhage are likely to follow. On occasion, hemorrhage may be excessive. Perineal heaviness and discomfort may be associated with the larger hemagiomata. Once a cavernous hemangioma reaches enormous size, it may distort and encroach upon the vaginal passage; the pregnant patient with such a lesion will require cesarean section for de-

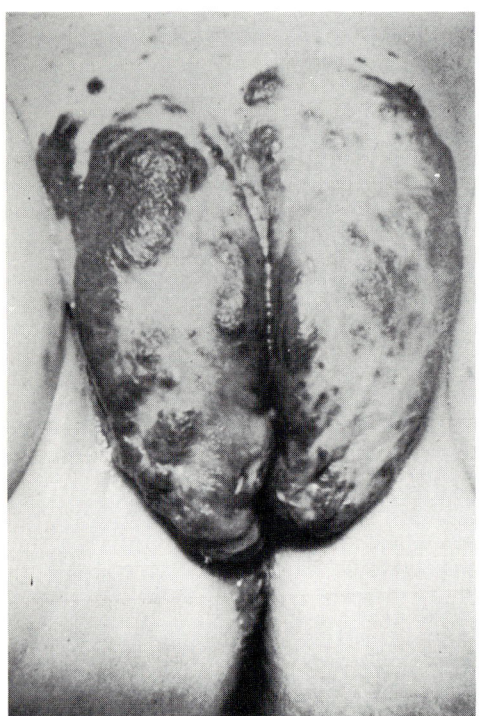

Fig. 4-21. Cavernous hemangioma involving entire vulva. (Novak, E. R., and Woodruff, H. D.: Novak's gynecologic and obstetric pathology, ed. 6, Philadelphia, 1967, W. B. Saunders Co.)

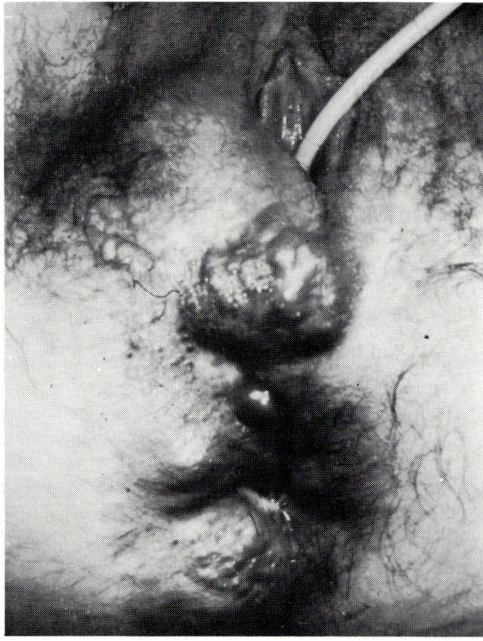

Fig. 4-22. Massive cavernous hemangioma extending perianally and paravaginally in a pregnant patient. A cesarean section was necessary. (Courtesy Charles E. Bancroft, Houston.)

livery without hazardous complications. One of our pregnant patients had a massive hemangioma involving the perineum and extending up around the rectum and high into the vagina (Fig. 4-22). Because of the possibility of laceration of the hemangioma during labor and delivery and consequent uncontrollable hemorrhage, a cesarean section was performed at term.

Histopathology. Microscopically, this tumor exhibits large, irregular blood spaces lined by a single layer of endothelial cells. The walls of the blood vessels are thickened by an overgrowth of adventitial cells. The dilated vessels may progressively ramify in the subcutaneous fat and into the underlying fascia and intermuscular septa.

Treatment.

Treatment of the child. Numerous factors influence the choice of treatment for these tumors in children. Treatment may be expectant and conservative unless ulceration and bleeding occur or unless the tumor grows rapidly, distorting the surrounding tissue. Andrews and others, however, are of the opinion that treatment should be carried out while the lesion is small, rather than waiting until it becomes large and possibly infected; the earlier the treatment, the better the end results. They recommend the use of radium plaques, with gamma radiation, applied directly to the lesion. If the tumor grows rapidly and the overlying skin becomes ulcerated, hemorrhage may be profuse and even threaten life. Local infection and secondary sepsis may also develop. If, on this basis, aggressive treatment is deemed advisable, the more commonly used modalities are radium and x-ray, solid carbon dioxide, and injection of sclerosing solutions into the tumor.

Radium and x-ray are usually preferable for tumors elsewhere on the body; for those of the genitalia, however, they should be used with great caution. If this form of therapy is selected, treatment should be instituted as soon as possible, since the older the lesion, the more radioresistant it becomes. The smallest possible dose sufficient to promote involution should be administered. For small shallow lesions, solid carbon dioxide may be used, as described for the strawberry hemangiomata. Small isolated lesions may also be injected with a sclerosing solution at intervals of 2 to 4 weeks. On rare occasions, the tumor may require surgical extirpation. Isolated small lesions can be excised without difficulty, whereas excision of extensive, deep tumors is usually accompanied by severe blood loss and risk to the child.

Treatment of the adult. In the adult woman, if the cavernous hemangioma is asymptomatic, it may be left untreated, since irradiation is of little value at this stage and complete surgical excision is extremely hazardous and difficult. Sclerosing solutions are also of little value for large tumors. Treatment should be expectant unless bleeding or ulceration, or both, appear. For large tumors that invade the underlying muscle, a subtotal resection may be indicated. If the lesion is small, total excision may be attempted, provided it will not produce mutilation.

Senile hemangioma

The senile hemangioma is observed on the vulva fairly often. The term "senile hemangioma" is not entirely correct, since this lesion is frequently observed in premenopausal women.

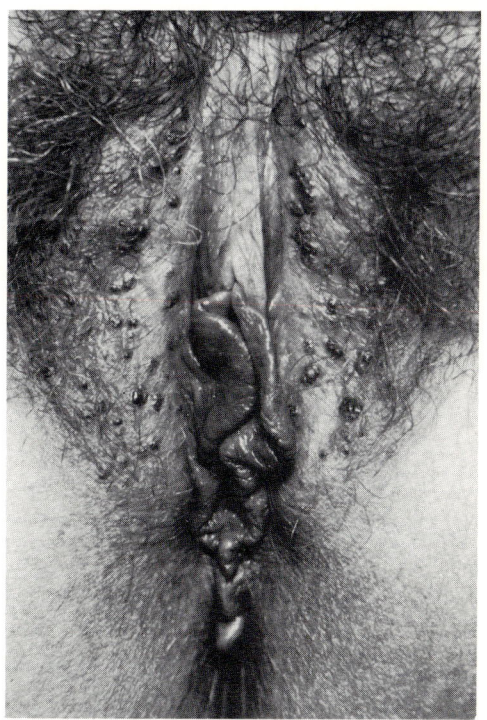

Fig. 4-23. Senile hemangioma. Multiple dark blue, compressible papules. Most patients have fewer lesions.

Clinical features. The tumors are composed of soft, bright red to dark blue, compressible papules, usually no more than 2 to 3 mm. in diameter (Fig. 4-23). The large majority produce no symptoms unless subjected to trauma and consequent bleeding. If a postmenopausal woman complains of bleeding, this possibility should be remembered.

Histopathology. Microscopic study of a senile hemangioma reveals the presence of numerous dilated capillaries lined by flattened endothelial cells. The capillaries are located in the superficial corium, near the epidermis, frequently encroaching upon the lining epithelium (Fig. 4-24). The collagen around the vessels may exhibit some homogenization.

Treatment. Usually, no treatment is necessary for senile hemagiomata. Repeated episodes of bleeding may call for their destruction with a finely pointed CO_2 pencil or by electrodesiccation. They may also be excised.

Angiokeratoma (Fordyce type)

In addition to our two cases of angiokeratoma of the vulva recently reported, we have been able to find only one recent report of vulvar lesions of this type in the medical literature. Despite this, we have observed this to be a fairly common vulvar lesion, having seen several patients with angiokeratoma in private practice. The majority of these lesions develop during the childbearing years and are often associated with and aggravated by pregnancy. They probably arise on the same basis as telangiectasias.

Clinical features. Angiokeratomata may be single or multiple. They are usually dark red in color, although they may be bright red, brown, blue, or black. In shape, they may be slightly lobulated, irregular, or papular and may have a verrucose surface (Fig. 4-25). In diameter, they may vary from 0.2 to 2.0 cm., though the majority are quite small. Unless they become irritated, ulcerate, or bleed incident to trauma, they are seldom symptomatic. These lesions occasionally are confused with melanomata, vulvar warts, or nevi.

Histopathology. The upper dermis contains enormously dilated capillaries, usually within the papillae, and the epidermis exhibits hyperkeratosis, parakeratosis, papillomatosis, and irregular elongation of the rete pegs (Fig. 4-26). In areas, the dilated capillaries high in the papillae may be surrounded by a downward proliferation of the epidermis. Thrombosis, with organization and recanalization of the blood clot, is often a feature.

Treatment. Local excision is recommended only if the true nature of the tumor cannot

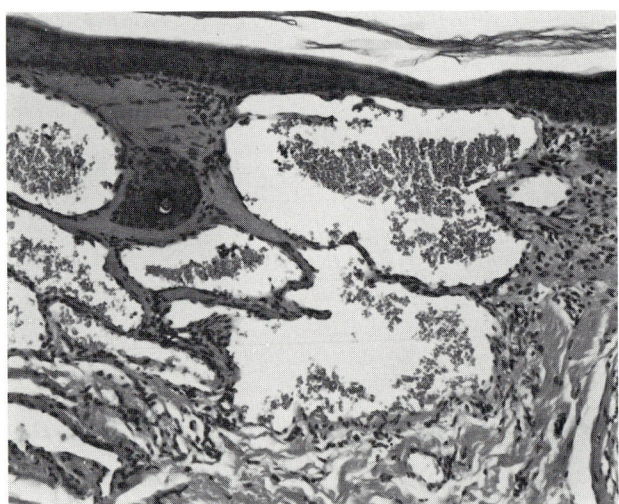

Fig. 4-24. Senile hemangioma. Numerous dilated capillaries lie in superficial corium and encroach upon the surface epithelium. (H & E × 110) (Kaufman, R. H., and Gardner, H. L.: Clin. Obstet. Gynec. **8:** 953, 1965.)

be determined or if trauma causes bleeding or discomfort to the patient. If the clinician is confident of the clinical diagnosis, the tumor may be destroyed by solid carbon dioxide or electrodesiccation.

Pyogenic granuloma

Granuloma pyogenicum is a form of capillary hemangioma that may, on rare occasions, appear on the vulva. Opinion still differs as to whether this lesion represents a form of angioma or is nothing more than a specific reaction to the presence of pyogenic bacteria. We are inclined to agree with Lever that it is a variant of the capillary hemangioma.

Clinical features. The tumor, usually single, may be sessile or pedunculated, and dull red to red-brown in color (Fig. 4-27). It may grow rapidly, attaining a diameter of 0.5 to 2.0 cm., and thereafter remain stationary. The surface may be smooth, although it is frequently covered with a crust. The nodule bleeds easily upon being traumatized. A variant of this tumor is the granuloma gravidarium, which may arise on the gums during pregnancy. It is important that the tumor be differentiated clinically from a malignant melanoma.

Histopathology. Microscopic study reveals a circumscribed, raised lesion covered by a thinned-out epidermis. The stroma contains numerous newly formed capillaries in varying degrees of dilation, surrounded by a loose, edematous stroma (Fig. 4-28). The early lesions may not exhibit any inflammatory reaction, whereas the older lesions often are inflammatory and perhaps ulcerated, resulting from erosion of the thinned epidermis.

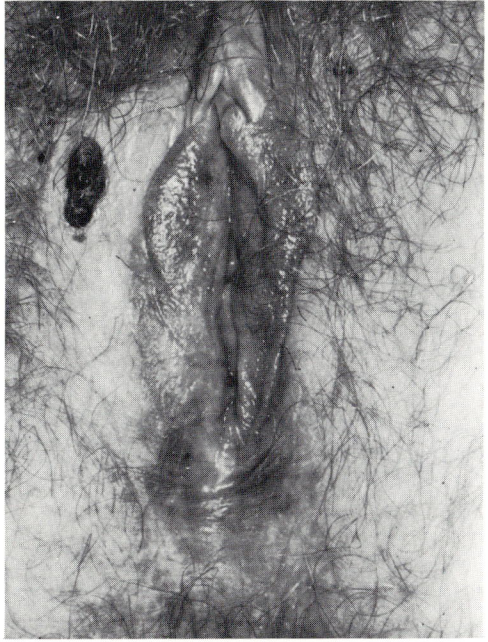

Fig. 4-25. Large angiokeratoma, represented by a dark red, lobulated mass. (Kaufman, R. H., and Gardner, H. L.: Clin. Obstet. Gynec. 8:953, 1965.)

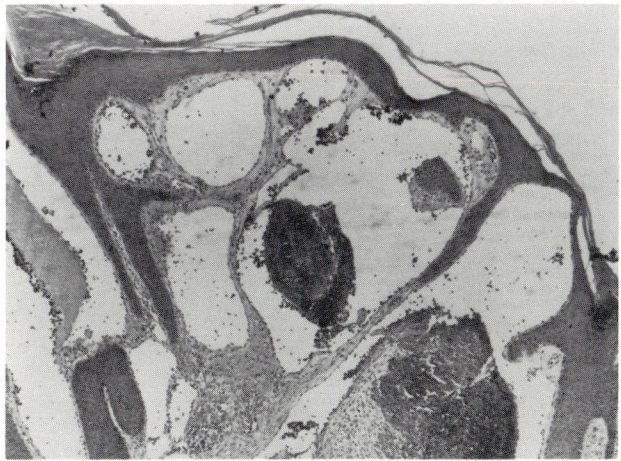

Fig. 4-26. Angiokeratoma. Section from lesion in Fig. 4-25. Numerous dilated capillaries are visible in upper dermis, and in some areas rete pegs are elongated and partially surround vessels. Hyperkeratosis is associated. (H & E × 40) (Kaufman, R. H., and Gardner, H. L.: Clin. Obstet. Gynec. 8:953, 1965.)

62 Benign diseases of the vulva and vagina

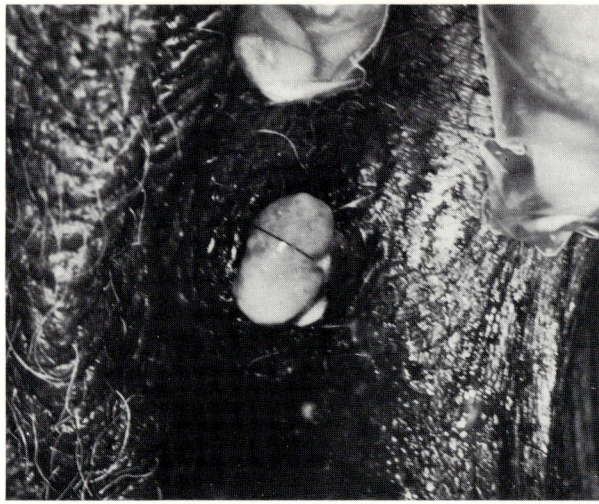

Fig. 4-27. Pyogenic granuloma on labium majus. A typical raised, fleshy, glistening, brownish-red nodule. (Kaufman, R. H., and Gardner, H. L.: Clin. Obstet. Gynec. 8:953, 1965.)

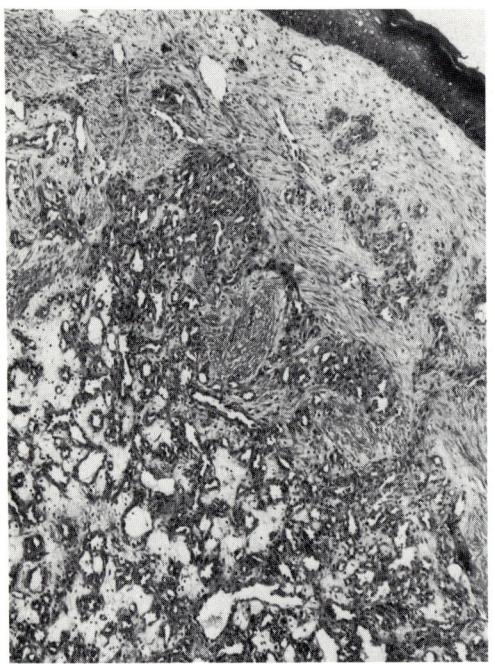

Fig. 4-28. Pyogenic granuloma. Numerous dilated capillaries are surrounded by a loose, edematous stroma. (H & E × 40) (Kaufman, R. H., and Gardner, H. L.: Clin. Obstet. Gynec. 8:953, 1965.)

An inward growth of the epidermis at the neck of the pedunculated lesion may produce an "epidermal collarette."

Treatment. Wide excision of these lesions is the preferred treatment. By this means, the tumor may be examined microscopically and thus distinguished from malignant melanoma.

Lymphangioma

Lymphangiomata, which are tumors of the lymphatic vessels, are analogous to tumors of the blood vessels. In many cases, the two can be distinguished only by the presence or absence of blood or lymph within the vessels.

Allen describes several types of lymphangiomata: (1) lymphangioma simplex; (2) lymphangioma cavernosum, which usually produces diffuse enlargement of the areas affected; and (3) lymphangioma circumscriptum, in which localized groups of small, thin-walled vesicles may be observed.

Lymphangioma simplex

Lymphangioma simplex is the usual type of lymphangiomata involving the vulva. Actually, according to Allen, the skin of the genitalia is a common site of this lesion.

Clinical features. Lymphangiomata simplex are soft, compressible, either solitary or multiple gray-pink nodules. Swelling is usually diffuse. At times, a few straw-colored vesicles are apparent on the surface of the mass. As a rule, the tumors are asymptomatic. Occasionally, a superficial vesicle may rupture, discharging lymph.

Histopathology. The dermis contains lymph vessels of various sizes, in which

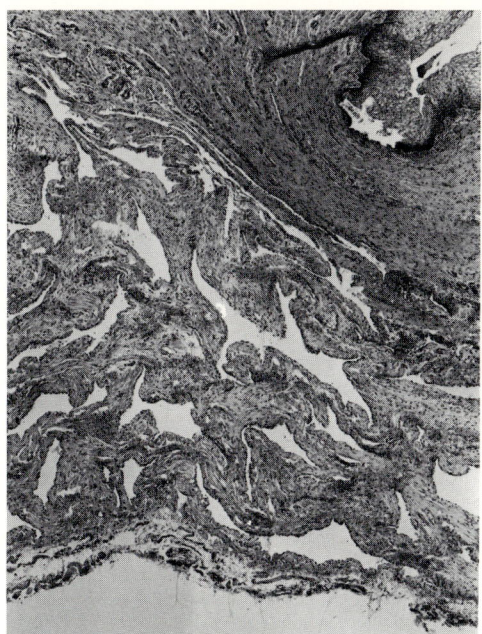

Fig. 4-29. Lymphangioma. Grossly, a soft, compressible mass of the vulva. Empty channels of varying size are lined with endothelium. (H & E × 29) (Kaufman, R. H., and Gardner, H. L.: Clin. Obstet. Gynec. 8:953, 1965.)

lymph may or may not be present. The vessels have thin walls lined by endothelium (Fig. 4-29).

Treatment. Usually treatment is neither necessary nor successful. If the tumor causes pressure or discomfort, or if the overlying skin becomes ulcerated, excision may be necessary.

Lymphangioma cavernosum

Clinical features. This soft, compressible tumor may produce diffuse enlargement of the affected side of the vulva and extend down over the perineum and even up into the vagina. The overlying skin is relatively normal.

Histopathology. Large, cystic spaces filled with lymph and lined by a single layer of endothelial cells are present in the dermis and subcutaneous tissue and may extend into the muscle. The connective tissue surrounding the lymphatic channels is hypertrophied.

Treatment. No treatment is required unless the lymphangioma causes the patient discomfort and pressure. In this event, it may be removed surgically. If the tumor is extensive, the excision required may mutilate the vulva.

Lymphagioma circumscriptum

We have never observed a case of lymphangioma circumscriptum involving the vulva.

Vaginal tumors of mesodermal origin

Theoretically, all mesodermal tumors of the vulva may arise within the vagina; in reality, however, such tumors are seldom discovered in this location. We have observed only three groups of vaginal mesodermal tumors: leiomyomata, fibromata, and cavernous hemangiomata (the last in association with a lesion of the vulva). Hertig and Gore quote Wharton as finding 260 vaginal tumors in 47,500 gynecologic specimens studied. Of these, six were fibromata and four were myomata. Hertig also presented an example of a granular cell myoblastoma of the vagina. Norris and Cooper reported the case of a pregnant patient with a neurofibroma in the vaginal wall.

The histogenesis and gross and microscopic pathology of mesodermal tumors of the vagina, as well as the treatment, are similar to their vulvar counterparts (see preceding discussion). The symptoms, which depend upon their size and location, are dyspareunia and a sense of pressure and heaviness in the pelvis. If the tumors are near the urinary tract or rectum, symptoms referable to these structures may be associated.

Leiomyoma

Although leiomyomata are observed more often than any other vaginal mesodermal tumor, only about 250 cases had been reported in world medical literature until 1961. Strangely, most authorities agree that vaginal myomata are most common in Caucasian patients, whereas the frequency of uterine leiomyomata in the Negro is relatively high.

Clinical features. Leiomyomata may be of any size from extremely small to those that completely occlude the vaginal canal (Fig. 4-30). They may arise anywhere within the vagina, though they are most often located on the anterior wall. In this site, they may be confused with a cystocele, diverticulum of the urethra, developmental cyst, or even a uterine leiomyoma. Those on the posterior

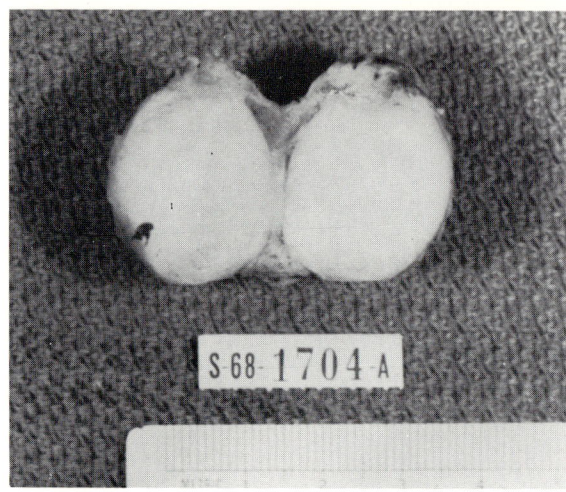

Fig. 4-30. Leiomyoma from upper third of vagina of a 32-year-old patient.

vaginal wall must be distinguished from a rectocele, enterocele, and inclusion cyst. Unlike its uterine counterpart, the vaginal tumor is almost invariably single.

The symptoms of this neoplasm are similar to those of other benign vaginal tumors. An occasional leiomyoma may ulcerate the overlying mucosa and cause bleeding. Dystocia has also been mentioned as a complication of the tumor.

The diagnosis of a leiomyoma may be suspected upon discovery of a semicystic to solid vaginal mass. The consistency of the tumor depends upon the degree and type of degenerative change present.

Histopathology. The typical pattern of whorled bundles of smooth muscle fibers and fibrous tissue is usually observed. The same degenerative changes observed in leiomyomata elsewhere in the body may also be seen —hyaline degeneration, calcification, and so on.

Treatment. Treatment usually consists of simple excision. After the vaginal mucosa has been incised and the tumor substance reached, it can be shelled out of its bed without difficulty. Caution should be exercised to prevent injury to the bladder, rectum, urethra, and ureter.

Solid tumors of Bartholin's gland origin

Theoretically, a solid tumor of fibrous or glandular origin may arise in Bartholin's gland, although the only benign solid tumor that we have encountered in this structure

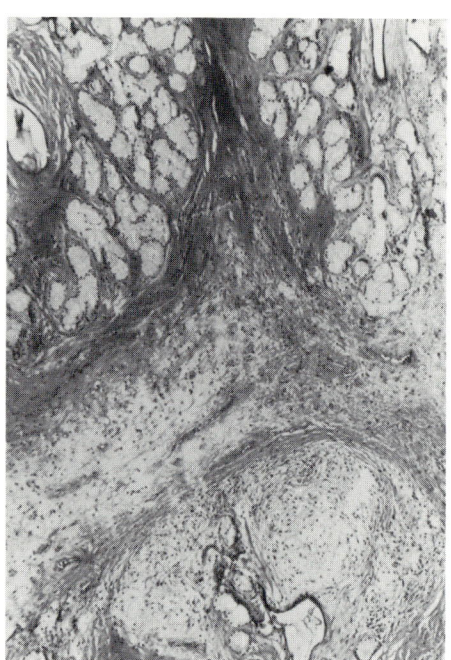

Fig. 4-31. Adenofibroma of Bartholin's gland. Clusters of typical glandular tissue are separated by dense and edematous fibrous tissue. (H & E × 40)

was composed of both glandular and fibrous elements (Fig. 4-31) and was in some respects akin to an adenofibroma of the breast. The tumor measured 4 cm. in diameter, was firm, and on cut section had a gray-white, fibrous appearance. It was composed of clusters of racemose glands lined by tall columnar epithelium whose cells contained clear cytoplasm. The nuclei were dark and were located near the basal portion of the cells. The clusters of glands were separated by bands of dense fibrous stroma, and in areas the fibrous tissue around and between the glands was edematous.

These neoplasms are benign, as are adenofibromata found elsewhere in the body, and are easily removed by local excision. They should be removed, chiefly to establish the diagnosis and particularly to disprove the presence of carcinoma.

Solid tumors of urethral origin
Urethral caruncle

Urethral caruncles arise only in the female urethra, primarily in postmenopausal women. Seldom do they appear during the childbearing years, and even less often during childhood. The term "caruncle" has been applied to widely divergent urethral lesions. The lesion most often mistaken for a caruncle is probably prolapsed urethral mucosa. It is likely that most so-called caruncles in children are prolapses of the urethral mucosa.

The urethral caruncle probably develops from ectropion of the posterior urethral wall, incident to postmenopausal shrinkage of the vaginal mucosa. All of the subsequent changes in the everted mucosa are caused by altered environmental conditions and trauma. Other possible causes for the development of a caruncle are chronic irritation and infection of the urethral meatus.

Clinical features. The urethral caruncle is a benign, red, occasionally friable, fleshy tumor in the distal portion of the urethral mucosa, usually at the posterior meatus (Fig. 4-32). Although generally sessile, it may be pedunculated. Most caruncles are only a few millimeters in diameter; rarely do they exceed 1 cm. in diameter. Also, with few exceptions, they are single. The majority are asymptomatic, being discovered only on routine examination. If exceptionally large, a growth or lump at the urinary meatus may be noticed by the patient. The severity of symptoms is not always related to the size of the tumor, since small caruncles at times give rise to extreme discomfort. Pain, dysuria, bleeding, or hematuria may be distressing. At times, because of exquisite tenderness, the patient may find it almost impossible to wear undergarments or to engage in coitus. The tumors seldom interfere with urination, although they may lead to severe dysuria.

Although the physician rarely biopsies this tumor prior to treatment, only microscopic examination of the tissue can confirm the diagnosis. Most urethral neoplasms arise from the outer third of the urethra and are visible at the external urethral meatus. Hemangiomata, varices, condylomata, polyps, periurethral cysts, prolapsed mucosa, and even carcinomata are easily confused

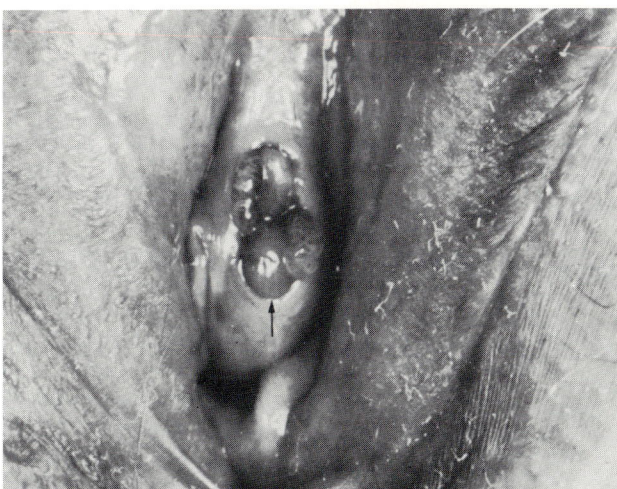

Fig. 4-32. Urethral caruncle, a red, fleshy lesion at urethral meatus.

with caruncles. Tenderness, induration, swelling, and other masses along the entire length of the urethra, as well as the finding of enlarged inguinal lymph nodes, should lead the clinician to suspect the presence of a carcinoma.

Marshall, Uson, and Melicow classified 394 urethral lesions according to their histology. Of these, 356 were caruncles. Of thirty-eight varieties of tumor, twenty were mistakenly regarded clinically as caruncles. Six of fourteen urethral carcinomas were erroneously interpreted as urethral caruncles. Of 376 lesions clinically interpreted as caruncles, nine (2.4 percent) were found to be malignant on biopsy. These observations probably explain why so many clinicians are of the opinion that urethral caruncles may lead to the development of a carcinoma. The tumors were probably carcinoma from the beginning, the diagnosis of urethral caruncles being in error. Marshall, Uson, and Melicow are of the opinion that neither urethral irritation nor urethral caruncle appears to have any causative relation to urethral carcinoma.

Histopathology. Caruncles consist of a core of loose connective tissue, dilated blood vessels, and inflammatory cells covered by an epithelial layer. They are usually divided into three histologic types: granulomatous, angiomatous, and papillomatous, depending upon the degree of inflammatory reaction, hyperemia, and proliferation and infolding of columns of transitional or squamous epithelium. In our experience, most caruncles exhibit features of all three varieties (Fig. 4-33). The core of loose fibrous tissue contains, in addition to a usually heavy infiltration of lymphocytes, some plasma cells and an occasional neutrophil. Columns of transitional or squamous epithelium may extend down into the lesion, at times making a differentiation from carcinoma difficult. The lesion may be covered by a lining of squamous or transitional epithelium, or its surface may be ulcerated and have no surface lining. The degree of vascular dilation varies; when pronounced, it may produce a picture suggestive of a hemangioma.

Treatment. For small, asymptomatic caruncles, no treatment is necessary. If the nature of the lesion is questionable, a small specimen should be removed for microscopic study to establish the diagnosis. For this purpose, a concentrated cocaine solution may

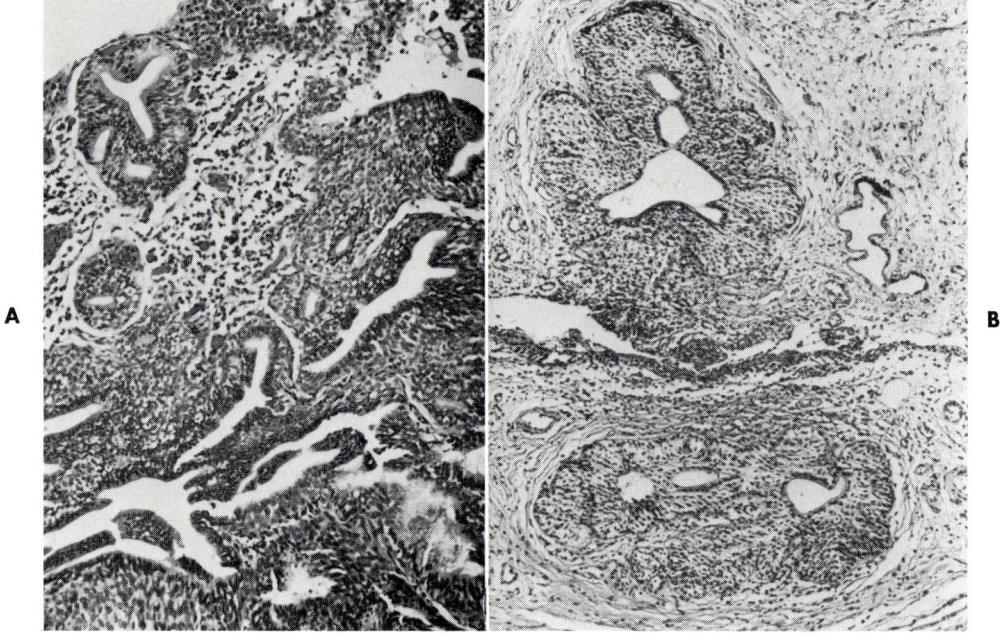

Fig. 4-33. Urethral caruncle. **A,** Hyperemia, inflammation, and some infolding of transitional epithelium. (H & E × 40) **B,** More pronounced infolding of transitional epithelium. (H & E × 30)

be applied to the meatus for a few minutes prior to biopsy. Bleeding may be brisk, though it can usually be controlled with pressure or, if this fails, by cauterization, fulguration, or several fine catgut sutures.

The primary objective of treatment is to afford the patient symptomatic relief, and this should be accomplished by the simplest method available. As a rule, subjective complaints and bleeding can be controlled by topical application of estrogen cream to the vagina and urethra or by giving subbleeding doses orally. This treatment is worthy of trial before surgical correction is attempted. By far the simplest means of destroying small lesions consists of the application of local caustics, such as 75% silver nitrate, usually with a silver nitrate stick. Pedunculated or large lesions are best fulgurated under local anesthesia. For large lesions, surgical removal, including the urethral meatus and a cuff of the adjacent mucosa, is preferable. The mucosal edges of the urethra and vestibule are then united by interrupted sutures with 4-0 chromic catgut. Regardless of the treatment employed, the caruncle may recur.

Prolapse of urethral mucosa

Prolapse of urethral mucosa, which is closely related to the caruncle, has been described as a sliding outward of the mucosa through the external meatus. Practically all patients with urethral prolapse are in the premenarchal and postmenopausal ages, a fact suggesting its relationship to estrogen deficiency. Many other theories, however, have been proposed as the cause of the prolapse. It may suddenly appear after coughing or sudden severe straining. Palmer, Emmett, and McDonald are of the opinion that both mucosal prolapse and urethral caruncle should be classified in the same group, with the term "caruncle" being reserved for localized lesions, in contrast to circumscribed masses of prolapse.

Clinical features. The lesion, which is situated anterior to the introitus, resembles an edematous red ring of tissue at the urinary meatus (Fig. 4-34). Ulceration and necrosis may be present, giving rise to a serosanguineous discharge.

Little pain or discomfort is associated with prolapse of the mucosa. The patients may have difficulty in voiding, especially if con-

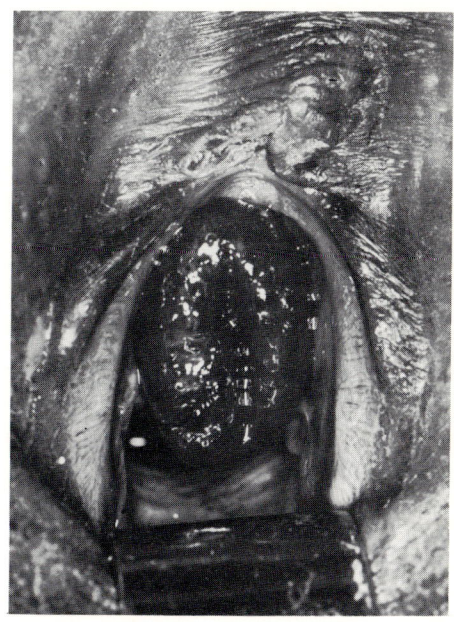

Fig. 4-34. Prolapse of urethral mucosa in a 7-year-old child. Edematous, red collar of tissue surrounds urethral meatus.

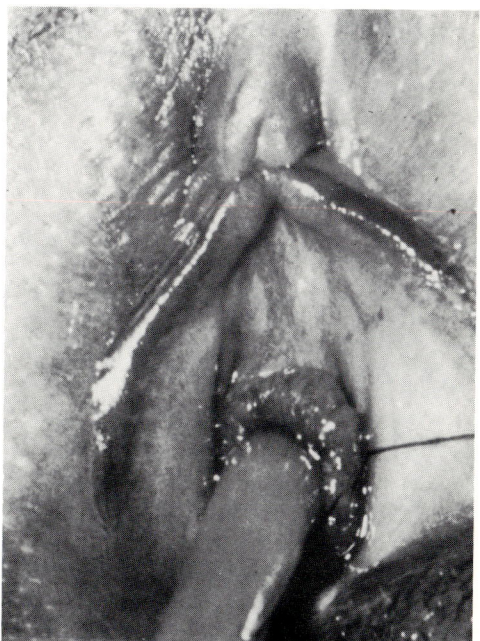

Fig. 4-35. Prolapsed urethral mucosa has been ligated over a Foley catheter.

siderable edema of the prolapsed tissue is present. The correct diagnosis is established by location of the urethra in relation to the mass.

Treatment. Hot sitz baths to reduce congestion and to control infection are followed by either manual reduction of the prolapse under anesthesia or excision of the redundant mucosa. If the latter is performed, the edges of the urethral mucosa should then be attached to the mucosa of the vestibule with interrupted sutures of 4-0 chromic catgut. Complete fulguration with a high frequency cautery has been advocated; since the depth of tissue destruction cannot be controlled, however, this would seem to be a hazardous procedure. Also, convalescence following fulguration is prolonged. Simple ligation of the prolapsed mucosa over a Foley catheter has proved effective and is a logical method if anatomic features permit (Fig. 4-35). Following this measure, the patient's progress should be carefully checked as a safeguard against the development of a urethral stricture.

REFERENCES

Abrikossoff, A.: Über Myome, ausgerhend von der guergistreiften willkurlichen Muskulatur, Virchows Arch. Path. Anat. 260:215, 1926.

Abrikossoff, A.: Über Myome, ausgerhend von der guergistreiften willkurlichen Muskulatur, Virchows Arch. Path. Anat. 280:723, 1931.

Allen, A. C.: The skin, St. Louis, 1967, The C. V. Mosby Co.

Allen, A. C., and Spitz, S.: Malignant melanoma, Cancer 6:1-45, 1953.

Andrews, G. G., Domankos, A. N., Torres-Rodriguez, V. M., and Bembenesta, J. K.: Hemangioma—treated and untreated, J. Amer. Med. Ass. 163:1114, 1957.

Azzopardi, J. G.: Histogenesis of the granular cell "myoblastoma," J. Path. Bact. 71:85, 1956.

Bangle, R., Jr.: Early granular cell myoblastoma confined within a small peripheral myelinated nerve, Cancer 6:790, 1953.

Bangle, R., Jr.: Morphological and histochemical study of the granular cell myoblastoma, Cancer 5:950, 1952.

Barclay, D. L., and Collins, C. G.: Intra-epithelial cancer of the vulva, Amer. J. Obstet. Gynec. 86:94, 1963.

Bennett, H. G., and Ehrlich, H. M.: Myoma of the vagina, Amer. J. Obstet. Gynec. 42:314, 1941.

Binkley, G. W., and Rauschkolb, R. R.: Basal cell epithelioma metastasizing to lymph nodes, Arch. Derm. 86:332, 1962.

Birch, H. W., and Sondag, D. R.: Granular cell myoblastoma of the vulva, Obstet. Gynec. 18:443, 1961.

Bishop, H. C., and Wagner, B. M.: Granular cell myoblastoma in childhood, Pediatrics 19:858, 1957.

Chiodi, N. E., Siegel, I. A., Guerin, P. F., and McCaughan, D. M.: Granular cell myoblastoma of the vulva and lower respiratory tract, Obstet. Gynec. 9:472, 1957.

Collins, J.: Personal communication to M. M., Schreiber, Arch. Derm. 88:320, 1963.

Corscaden, J. A.: Gynecologic cancer, New York, 1951, Thomas Nelson & Sons.

Dodson, A. I., Jr.: Urethral caruncle, gonorrheal infection, and stricture, Postgrad. Med. 33:423, 1963.

Fisher, E. R., and Wechsler, S.: Granular cell myoblastoma, a misnomer, Cancer 5:936, 1962.

Fust, J. A., and Custer, R. P.: Granular cell "myoblastoma" and granular cell neurofibromas, Amer. P. Path. 24:674, 1948.

Fust, J. A., and Custer, R. P.: On the neurogenesis of so-called granular cell myoblastomas, Amer. J. Clin. Path. 19:522, 1949.

Gerbie, A. B., Hirsch, M. R., and Greene, R. R.: Vascular tumors of the female genital tract, Obstet. Gynec. 6:499, 1955.

Hertig, A. T., and Gore, H.: Tumors of the female sex organs, Atlas of tumor pathology, Part 2, Sec. IX, Fascicle 33, 1960.

Holland, E.: A case of transplacental metastasis of malignant melanoma from mother to fetus, J. Obstet. Gynaec. Brit. Comm. 56:529, 1949.

Hyde, W. R.: Sarcoma of the vulva, a case report, J. Nat. Med. Ass. 53:496, 1961.

Imperial, R., and Helwig, E. B.: Angiokeratoma of the vulva, Obstet. Gynec. 29:307, 1967.

Janovski, N. A., Marshall, D., and Tiki, I.: Malignant melanoma of the vulva, Amer. J. Obstet. Gynec. 84:523, 1962.

Kanter, A. E., and Strean, G. J.: Melanoma of the vulva, Obstet. Gynec. 12:516, 1958.

Kaufman, R. H., and Gardner, H. L.: Benign mesodermal tumors, Clin. Obstet. Gynec. 8:953, 1965.

Knox, J. M., and Freeman, R. G.: Symposium on tumors of the vulva and vagina: Epidermal tumors, Clin. Obstet. Gynec. 8:925, 1965.

Knox, W. G., Stanley-Brown, E. G., and Daregon, H. W.: Surgical management of extensive hemangioma associated with severe hemorrhage in the infant, Surgery 49:406, 1961.

Krompecher, E.: Beitr. Path. Anat. 28:1, 1900.

Krompecher, E.: Der Basalzellenkrebs, Jena, 1903, Gustav Fischer.

Leuroux, J., and Delarue, J.: Sur trois cas de

tumeurs à cellules gravidensis de la cavité bucalle, Bull. Cancer 28:427, 1939.

Lever, W. F.: Histopathology of the skin, Philadelphia, 1967, J. B. Lippincott & Co.

Lovelady, S. B., McDonald, J. R., and Waugh, J. M.: Benign tumors of the vulva, Amer. J. Obstet. Gynec. 42:309, 1941.

Lund, H. Z., and Stobbe, G. D.: The natural history of the pigmented nevus, Amer. J. Path. 25:1117, 1949.

Mallory, F. B.: Recent progress in the microscopic anatomy and differentiation of cancer, J.A.M.A. 55:1513, 1910.

Malpas, P.: The recurrence rate of urethral caruncles, J. Obstet. Gynaec. Brit. Comm. 52:367, 1945.

Marcus, S. L.: Basal cell and basal-squamous cell carcinomas of the vulva, Amer. J. Obstet. Gynec. 79:461, 1960.

Marshall, F. C., Uson, A. C., and Melicow, M. D.: Neoplasm and caruncles of the female urethra, Surg. Gynec. Obstet. 110:723, 1960.

Masson, P.: My conception of cellular nevi, Cancer 4:9, 1951.

Mochissi, K.: Myoma of the vagina, Obstet. Gynec. 15:235, 1960.

Neuwirth, R. S.: Urethral prolapse in young girls, Obstet. Gynec. 22:290, 1963.

Norris, J. W., and Cooper, J. R.: Primary neurofibroma of the vagina, a case report, J. Kansas Med. Soc. 51:128, 1950.

Novak, E. R., and Woodruff, H. D.: Gynecologic and obstetric pathology, Philadelphia, 1962, W. B. Saunders Co.

Ormsby, O. S., and Montgomery, H.: Diseases of the skin, Philadelphia, 1954, Lea & Febiger.

Pack, G. T. and Scharnagel, I. M.: The prognosis for malignant melanoma in pregnant women, Cancer 4:324, 1951.

Palermino, D. A.: Leiomyoma of the vulva, Obstet. Gynec. 24:301, 1964.

Palmer, J. K., Emmett, J. L., and McDonald, J. R.: Urethral caruncle, Surg. Gynec. Obstet. 87:611, 1948.

Pearman, R. O.: Snare for removal of urethral caruncle, J. Urol. 84:779, 1960.

Pearse, A. G. E.: Histogenesis of granular cell myoblastoma, J. Path. Bact. 62:351, 1950.

Peters, W. A.: Prolapse of the urethral mucosa, Amer. J. Obstet. Gynec. 84:862, 1962.

Powell, E. B.: Granular cell myoblastoma, Arch. Path. 42:517, 1946.

Quan, A., and Birnbaum, S. J.: Vaginal leiomyoma: Report of a case and review of the literature, Obstet. Gynec. 18:360, 1961.

Reynolds, A. G.: Placental metastasis from malignant melanoma, Obstet. Gynec. 6:205, 1955.

Robinson, S. S., and Tasker, S.: Angiomas of the scrotum (angiokeratoma Fordyce), Arch. Derm. 54:667, 1956.

Rubin, A.: Granular cell myoblastoma of the vulva, Amer. J. Obstet. Gynec. 77:292, 1959.

Sadler, W. P., and Dockerty, M. B.: Malignant myoblastoma vulvae, Amer. J. Obstet. Gynec. 61:1047, 1951.

Schreiber, M. M.: Vulvar von Recklinghausen's disease, Arch. Derm. 88:320, 1963.

Schrum, M.: Leiomyosarcoma of the vagina, Obstet. Gynec. 12:195, 1958.

Schueller, E. F.: Basal cell carcinoma of the vulva, Amer. J. Obstet. Gynec. 93:199, 1965.

Shanahan, R. R.: Large tumor of the vagina, Amer. J. Surg. 56:513, 1942.

Siegler, A. M., and Greene, H. J.: Basal cell carcinoma of the vulva; a report of 5 cases and a review of the literature, Amer. J. Obstet. Gynec. 62:1219, 1951.

Sulzberger, M. B., Wolf, J., Whitten, V. H., and Kopf, A. W.: Dermatology, diagnosis and treatment, Chicago, 1961, Year Book Medical Publishers, Inc.

Symonds, R. E., Pratt, J. A., and Dockerty, M. B.: Melanoma of the vulva, Obstet. Gynec. 15:543, 1960.

Thambiah, A. S., and Rajam, R. V.: A report of two benign vascular tumors in dermatology, Ind. J. Derm. 20:94, 1954.

Tobias, N.: Essentials of dermatology, Philadelphia, 1963, J. B. Lippincott & Co.

Wallace, S. A., and Halpert, B.: Trichoma: Tumor of hair anlage, Arch. Path. 50:199, 1950.

Webster, J. P., Stevenson, T. N., and Stout, A. P.: Surgical treatment of malignant melanoma of the skin, Surg. Clin. N. Amer. 24:319, 1944.

Willis, R. A.: Pathology of tumors, London, 1953, Butterworth & Co., Ltd.

Chapter 5
Cystic tumors

The introductory remarks in Chapter 4 concerning classification of vulvovaginal tumors apply to both cystic and solid tumors. The cysts are classified as follows:

- A. Epidermal origin
    1. Traumatic inclusion cyst
    2. Epidermal cyst
    3. Pilonidal cyst
- B. Epidermal appendage origin
    1. Sebaceous cyst
    2. Hidradenoma
    3. Fox-Fordyce disease
    4. Syringoma
- C. Embryonic origin
    1. Mesonephric (Gartner's) cyst
    2. Paramesonephric (müllerian) cyst
    3. Cyst of canal of Nuck (hydrocele)
    4. Cyst of supernumerary mammary glands
    5. Adenosis (Chapter 7)
    6. Dermoid cyst
- D. Bartholin's duct cyst and Bartholin's abscess
- E. Urethral and para-urethral origin
    1. Skene's duct cyst
    2. Urethral diverticulum
- F. Miscellaneous origins
    1. Endometriosis (Chapter 6)
    2. Cystic lymphangioma (Chapter 4)
    3. Liquefied hematoma (Chapter 23)
    4. Vaginitis emphysematosa (Chapter 17)

CYSTS OF EPIDERMAL ORIGIN
Traumatic inclusion and epidermal cysts

Due to the similarity of the histologic and clinical features, discussions of inclusion cysts and epidermal cysts will be combined. Viable stratified squamous epithelium, if buried beneath either skin or mucosa, may proliferate, secrete, and desquamate, forming an "inclusion cyst." Traumatic inclusion cysts are easily the most common type of vaginal cyst; most follow implantation of fragments of mucosa incident to repair of an episotomy. These cysts have also been attributed to growth of mucosa along suture material before it has been absorbed.

The incidence of traumatic inclusion cysts of the vulva from buried fragments of skin following episiotomy and surgical procedures such as perineorrhaphy is remarkably low. As a matter of fact, the vast majority of epithelial type cysts of the vulva are unrelated to traumatic implantations of fragments of skin. The term "epidermal cyst" has been applied to those epithelial cysts lined by squamous epithelium that are known not to be caused by buried fragments of skin. This is the most common variety of cyst found in the vulva and probably the most common tumefaction of the vulva. These cysts have been and continue to be erroneously called "sebaceous cysts." According to one theory, epidermal cysts arise from embryonic tissues destined to become epithelium that remain in the dermis and subsequently proliferate. Most dermatologists, including Knox, believe that the majority of these cysts arise from pilosebaceous ducts that have become occluded. These ducts are lined with stratified squamous epithelium. As a result of their obstruction, lesions similar to those caused by traumatically buried fragments of the skin develop.

Clinical features

In diameter, inclusion cysts of the vagina vary from microscopic to several centimeters. The largest cyst observed by us was 4 cm. in diameter; it protruded through the introitus as a yellow-orange mass having small blood vessels on its surface. The majority of these cysts are visible through the vaginal mucosa and are round and white, yellow, or orange in color (Fig. 5-1). The contents of the cysts closely resemble a thick, purulent exudate. This may cause some concern to a novice obstetrician who happens to cut into one while making an episiotomy incision. Inclusion cysts are asymptomatic unless they are unusually large.

Inclusion cysts of the vulva are usually situated on the perineum, in the site of a previous operation. They, too, are usually asymptomatic and rarely need treatment. Epidermal cysts of the vulva arise chiefly in the labia majora, particularly the anterior half. As a rule, they are multiple, grow slowly, and are round, nontender, and deep seated (Fig. 5-2). Most are less than 5 mm. in diameter; the largest lesions seldom exceed 2 cm. The skin over the smaller lesions is thickened, whereas over the larger cysts it is frequently loose and thin. The contents are usually inspissated and of a caseous or gritty consistency. These cysts are essentially asymptomatic unless they become infected.

Histopathology

Microscopically, vaginal inclusion cysts are lined with stratified squamous epithelium, similar to vaginal mucosa, though thinner. The cysts contain masses of desquamated epithelial cells.

The lining of epidermal cysts of the vulva consists of all layers of skin but is usually somewhat thin (Fig. 5-3). In older cysts, the walls are sometimes atrophic over wide

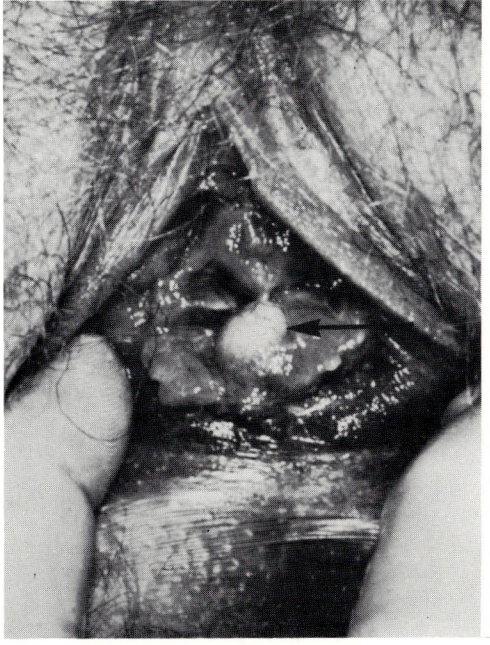

Fig. 5-1. Traumatic inclusion cyst of vagina in episiotomy scar.

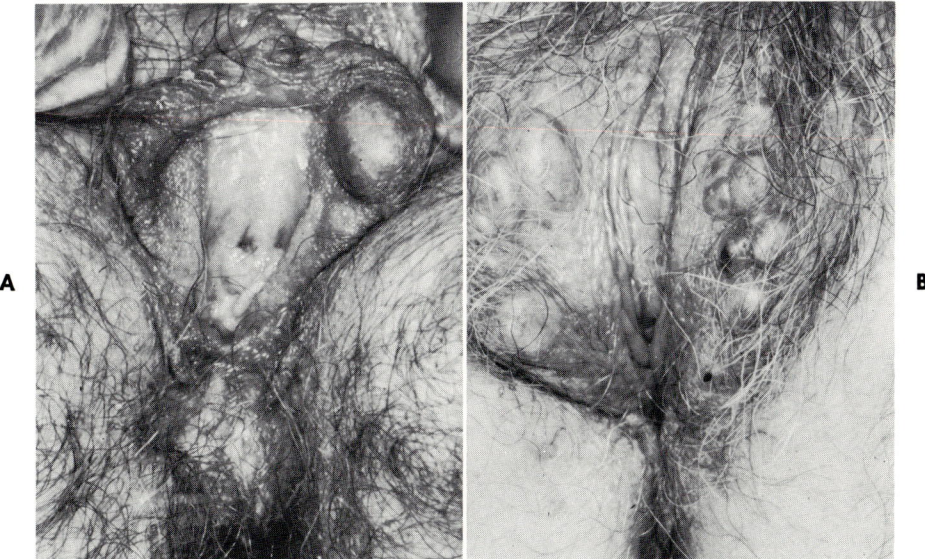

Fig. 5-2. A, Large epidermal cyst of labium minus. **B,** Multiple epidermal cysts in labia majora. These are commonly, though erroneously, referred to as "sebaceous cysts."

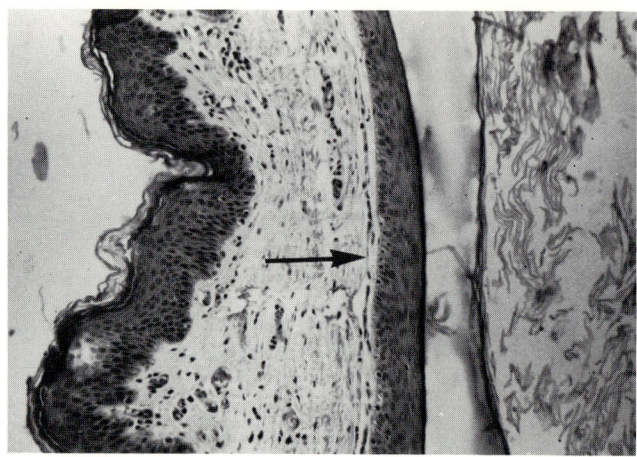

Fig. 5-3. Stratified squamous epithelial lining of an epidermal cyst, indicated by arrow. Desquamated squamous cells in cavity of cyst on right. Normal squamous epithelium of labial skin on left. (H & E × 100)

areas and may consist of only three or four rows of flattened cells. Intercellular bridges as well as rete malpighii are apparent. The surface cells of the lining epithelium are keratinized, and the cysts usually contain laminated keratinized debris.

Treatment

Since vaginal inclusion cysts seldom produce symptoms and their presence is thus unknown to the patient, the majority do not require treatment. Most obstetricians, however, compulsively evulse such cysts when they are discovered at the time of a delivery since they can easily be shelled out intact. Inclusion and epidermal cysts of the vulva are also usually asymptomatic, although their excision occasionally is desirable if they are an annoyance to the patient or if there is a cosmetic reason. They can usually be removed without difficulty under local anesthesia. If infection develops, incision and drainage is sometimes required. Incision of uninfected small and multiple cysts, with expression of the contents, is good therapy, particularly as an office procedure. Anesthesia is frequently unnecessary when a No. 11 Bark-Parker blade is used.

Pilonidal cysts

Unlike their prevalence in the sacrococcygeal area, pilonidal cysts of the vulvar area are unusual. Many recurrent abscesses of the clitoris and periclitoral tissues, although in themselves rare lesions, would perhaps meet the criteria of pilonidal cysts were such tissues excised and appropriately studied. Palmer and Betson, Chiffelle, and George have reported cases of infected cysts of the clitoris that were clinically and histologically identical to pilonidal cysts found in the usual sites. Others have described similar lesions of the mons pubis. We have observed three patients with recurrent periclitoral abscesses, the purulent material in one containing a number of hairs. Smith reported four cases of pilonidal cysts of the perineum.

Although the origin of pilonidal cysts remains debatable, they have generally been considered to be a congenital defect involving either the ectoderm or the neurogenital fold. Patey and Scarff have questioned the congenital origin and, instead have suggested that these cysts represent a foreign body reaction to hair that had become buried beneath the skin surface, causing infection, granuloma, and sinus tracts.

Clinical features

The signs and symptoms of these vulvar lesions consist of pain and swelling in the region of the clitoris or perineum, as well as erythema, induration, and tenderness at the involved site, resembling in most cases an abscess arising from other causes. Spontaneous drainage is usual, and chronic draining sinuses are often associated.

Histopathology

The superficial portion of the sinus tract is lined with squamous epithelium with or without hair follicles, hair shafts, and sebaceous glands. At a deeper level, the tract may be lined with granulation tissue. The tract eventually opens into an abscess filled with purulent exudate and hairs. The granulation tissues exhibit an acute inflammatory reaction throughout, as evidenced by the presence of large numbers of polymorphonuclear leukocytes, lymphocytes, and plasma cells. The contents usually include hair shafts, pus cells, epithelial cells, and necrotic debris. A surrounding cellulitis may be present.

Treatment

In the stage of acute abscess and surrounding cellulitis, incision and drainage are adequate as a temporary expedient. During a period of quiescence, excision of the involved tissues by block dissection appears to be the treatment of choice.

CYSTS OF EPIDERMAL APPENDAGE ORIGIN
Sebaceous cyst

Sebaceous cysts, also referred to as *atheromata* or *steatomata*, are clinically indistinguishable from epidermal cysts. The lesion is actually rare; the majority of cysts clinically considered to be of the sebaceous type prove, upon histologic examination, to be of the epidermal type. Warvi and Gates, in a study of cysts from all areas of the body surface, found only three histologically proved examples of sebaceous cysts, as compared to 556 epidermal cysts. Many authors, including McGavran and Binnington and Kligman, have largely eliminated the myth of the sebaceous cyst.

The exact origin of such cysts, when they do develop, remains debatable. Although embryonal cell rests may explain an occasional lesion, it is probable that the majority result from accumulation of sebaceous secretions incident to obstruction of the ducts of the sebaceous glands.

Clinical features

Grossly, sebaceous cysts are usually spherical, nontender, and firm. The contents are of a cheesy or sebaceous nature. The cysts are often multiple, and are more likely to appear on the inner and anterior aspects of the labia majora, particularly about the clitoris. Since their growth is extremely slow, most of the lesions are less than 5 mm. in diameter. An orifice is sometimes present on the surface. The contents of cysts of the skin, judging from the disagreements among dermatologists, have no diagnostic characteristics, nor does the odor of the contents appear to be distinctive.

The majority of sebaceous cysts are asymptomatic, yet patients are sometimes disagreeably aware of their presence. Pain is experienced only if infection is associated.

Histopathology

These cysts are lined with stratified epithelial cells without intercellular bridges and without keratinization. Because of their lipid content, many of the lining cells appear to be vacuolated. The epithelium exhibits no rete malpighii, as may epidermal cysts. The cysts are filled with an amorphous sebaceous material.

Treatment

For infected cysts, incision and drainage are indicated. Removal may be desirable for esthetic reasons if the cyst is large or if infection recurs.

Hidradenoma

Although a hidradenoma may be solid, the majority are cystic. Frequently called *hidradenoma papilliferum* or, occasionally, *hidradenoma tubulare* or *aprocrine adenoma,* hidradenoma is a rare and essentially asymptomatic small tumor arising from the apocrine sweat glands. The tumor was initially described by Werth in 1878, yet it was Pick, in 1904, who wrote the first significant paper on the lesion and called it "hidradenoma." Theoretically, the tumors can arise from any area containing apocrine glands; however, sixty-five tumors in sixty-three patients reported by Meeker, Neubecker, and Helwig, from the Armed Forces Institute of Pathology, arose from the vulva in fifty-one instances and from the perianal skin in fourteen. All of these lesions were observed in Caucasian women.

Histogenesis

Although it is generally agreed that hidradenomata originate from apocrine sweat glands, it is not known with certainty whether all arise from apocrine glands or whether some may arise from rudimentary glandular structures. It is unlikely, yet possible, that some may originate in the eccrine sweat glands. Additional evidence of an apocrine origin lies in the fact that such glands do not function until after puberty and hidradenomata do not develop until that time. Why hidradenomata appear to be found only in Caucasian women, while apocrine glands are considered to be more numerous in Negroes, is still unexplained. Also unexplained is the rarity of these lesions in other apocrine gland bearing areas such as the axillae, mons veneris, and nipples.

Clinical features

The hidradenoma appears chiefly on the labia majora as a sharply circumscribed, elevated nodule, only occasionally larger than 1 cm. The tumor shown in Fig. 5-4 measured 1.5 cm. in diameter, was firmly adherent to a thin overlying skin, and was partially translucent and dark in color. Such cysts are freely movable, and their consistency varies from hard to soft. Occasionally, pressure necrosis of the overlying skin causes umbilication. Red, granular, papillomatous tissue may protrude through the opening. A protrusion suggests the diagnosis, although it might also point to a pyogenic granuloma or carcinoma. Tumors with intact overlying skin are essential asymptomatic and are usually described by the patient as a lump. If they are umbilicated and infected, bleeding and pain are sometimes associated.

Histopathology

Microscopically, hidradenomata frequently appear to be cystic nodules partially or completely filled with papillomatous growths. Being adenomatous, they consist largely of irregular acini and tubules, usually separated by fine connective tissue septa (Fig. 5-5). Generally, the papillary projections are covered by a single layer of epithelial cells, as are many of the acini. These cells are usually tall columnar or cuboidal; they have a pale eosinophilic cytoplasm and a vesicular nucleus located near the base of the cell. A second layer of myoepithelial cells may lie deep to the secretory cells (Fig. 5-6); these cells may be spindle or cuboidal in shape and have scant cytoplasm. Because of the pronounced glandular proliferation, the tumor may be mistaken for an adenocarcinoma (Fig. 5-7); formerly, this was a common error. Conversely, we recently examined tissues from a metastatic carcinoma of the vulva that had been regarded histologically as hidradenoma. The distinction from carcinoma is based upon a lack of cellular pleomorphism and marked multi-layering of cells in the hidradenoma. Also, unlike carcinoma, invasion of the adjacent tissues is lacking.

Treatment

Local excision is the only treatment required, since these lesions are seldom, if ever, malignant. Because of the occasional firm attachment of the tumor to the overlying skin, a double elliptical skin incision facilitates removal of the tumor intact.

Fox-Fordyce disease

Fox-Fordyce disease is characterized by a chronic, pruritic eruption of multiple microcysts (Fig. 5-8) formed by retention of sweat in the apocrine gland ducts, following their obstruction by excessive keratinization of follicular epithelium. The condition was first

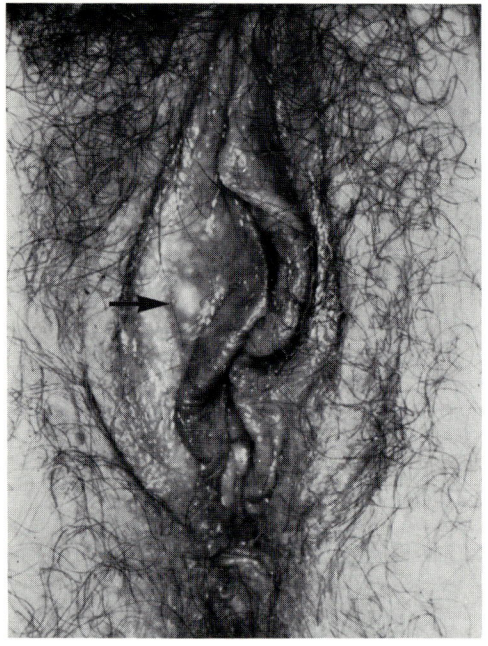

Fig. 5-4. Hidradenoma in sulcus between labium minus and labium majus.

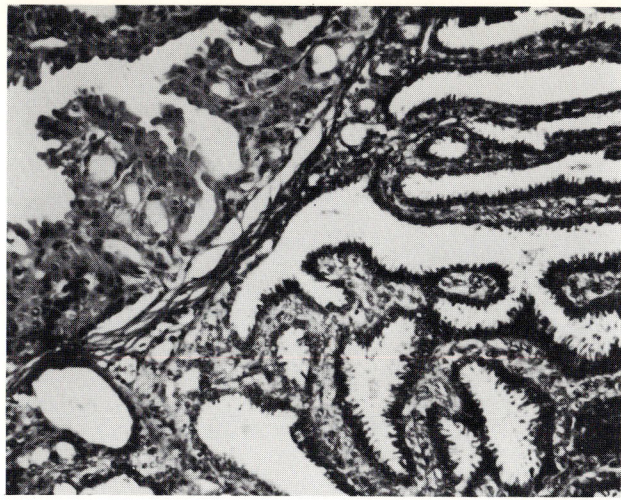

Fig. 5-5. Hidradenoma containing numerous acini. Distinct apocrine gland type of epithelium is present on left. (H & E × 180)

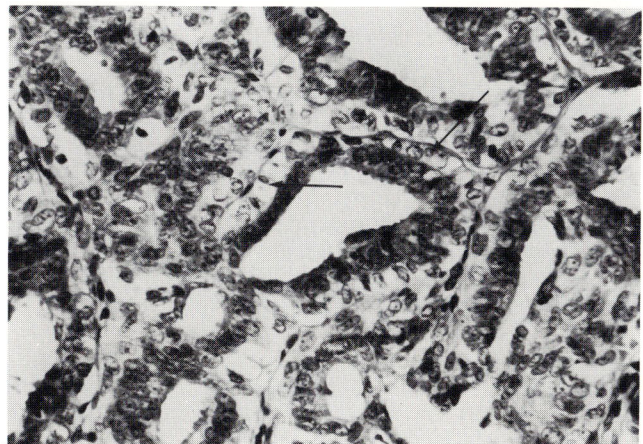

Fig. 5-6. Hidradenoma. Arrows point to second layer of cells around acini. These probably represent myoepithelial cells. (H & E × 250)

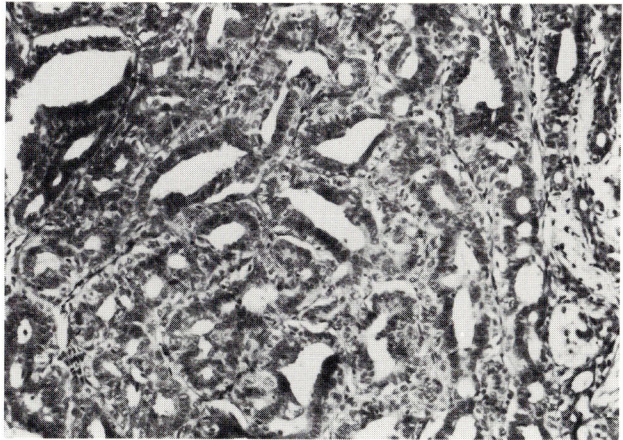

Fig. 5-7. Hidradenoma. The marked proliferation of glandular structures could lead to an erroneous diagnosis of adenocarcinoma. (H & E × 100)

described by Fox and Fordyce in 1902, in a report of two cases in which the axillae were involved. The vulva is second only to the axillae as a site of predilection. Over 90 percent of the reported cases have been in women. Since apocrine function does not begin until sexual maturity, the disease does not appear before puberty. Rarely has it been observed in women beyond the menopausal age.

Etiology

The primary cause of this condition is unknown. Because of its exacerbations with the menstrual cycle and its chronic course between puberty and menopause, hormonal influences seem obvious. Although the follicular hyperkeratinization causing obstruction of apocrine sweat ducts and retention of apocrine secretions explains the formation of the microcysts, the cause of the hyperkeratinization is not apparent.

Clinical features

All apocrine gland bearing areas are often involved simultaneously in the disease process. The closely grouped discrete lesions are 1 to 3 mm. in diameter (Fig. 5-8). Normal skin separates and overlies the individual papules.

Itching is often intense, becoming worse before and during the menses and after emotional crises. The pruritus probably results from leakage of apocrine secretions into tissues through ruptured apocrine ducts, that is, secretions enter the skin rather than reach its surface. The disease usually persists many years. Although pruritus is intensified in association with menstruation, it is relieved

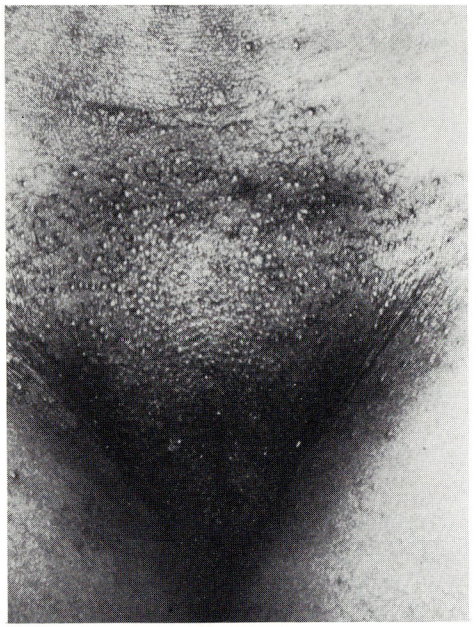

Fig. 5-8. Fox-Fordyce disease. In this patient, typical discrete, minute papules were present over lower abdomen, mons pubis, labia majora, and inner thighs. (Courtesy John M. Knox, Houston.)

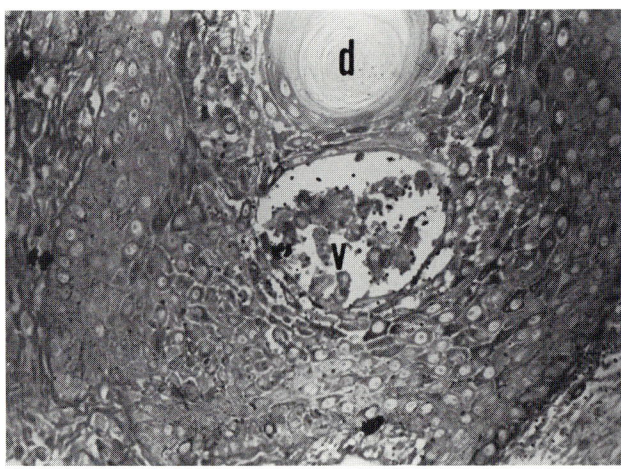

Fig. 5-9. Fox-Fordyce disease. Paraductal intraepidermal apocrine sweat retention vesicle *(V)*. The excretory duct *(d)* is occluded by keratin and is enlarged. (PAS and methylene blue × 798) (Montez, L. S., and others: Arch Derm. **84:**452, 1961.)

somewhat during pregnancy and usually disappears after the menopause.

Histopathology

The small cysts are lined by a flattened epithelium. Rupture of the dilated apocrine ducts into the dermis accounts for the occasional finding of apocrine sweat retention vesicles (Fig. 5-9). Shelley and Levy believe that intradermal sweat retention vescles are the most important microscopic features. These vesicles are sometimes discovered only upon examination of multiple tissue sections. Irritation from the process causes acanthosis and spongiosis of the follicular epithelium and an inflammatory reaction of the dermis.

Treatment

The pruritus of some patients is materially improved by the administration of estrogens. Kronthal has reported benefit from oral contraceptives. It has been suggested that this alleviation of symptoms is attributable to a lower FSH level induced by the estrogens. Regardless of the explanation, the beneficial response to hormones is a bit confusing, since the disease primarily affects women with normal hormonal activity. Local application of corticoids affords relief to some patients. Radiotherapy given in an attempt to reduce apocrine activity is ineffective. Rarely, partial vulvectomy may be indicated for relief of intractable pruritus.

Syringoma

Syringoma is a rather unusual lesion of the vulva frequently mistaken for Fox-

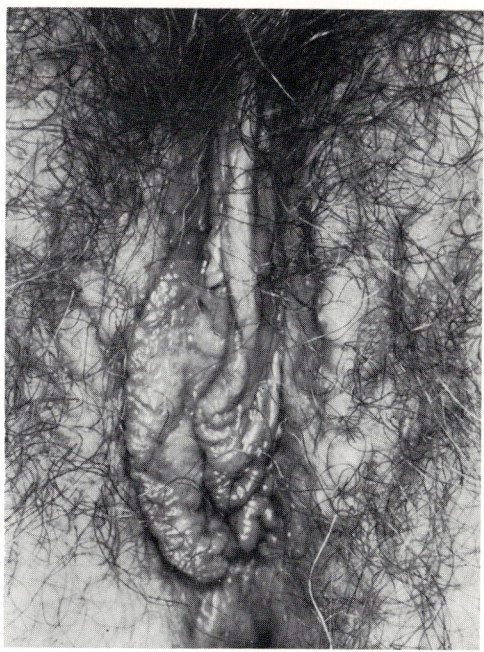

Fig. 5-10. Syringoma. Multiple small cystic structures, indicated by papules on labia majora.

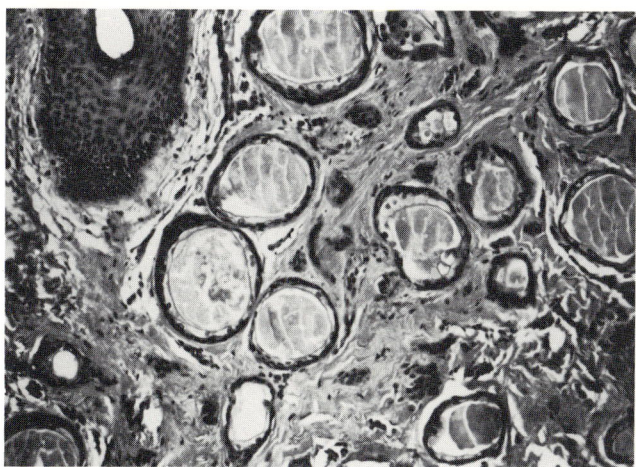

Fig. 5-11. Syringoma. Multiple cystic ducts lined by two layers of cells. Easily confused with Fox-Fordyce disease. (H & E × 100)

Fordyce disease. According to Lever, syringoma represents an adenoma of the eccrine sweat gland structures, although many observers formerly believed it arose in the apocrine glands. The lesion develops at puberty or later in life, most often around the eyelids and less often on the chest, abdomen, and vulva.

Clinical features

Syringoma is exhibited by multiple (or occasionally single) small, firm papules or cystic structures beneath the skin of the labia majora (Fig. 5-10). Although often asymptomatic, it may be associated with pruritus. Since patients are likely to be unaware of asymptomatic lesions, they are usually found incidentally by the physician.

Histopathology

Within the dermis, numerous small, cystic ducts, usually lined by two layers of epithelial cells, are found (Fig. 5-11). The cells tend to be flat, and the inner layer of cells frequently has a clear, vacuolated appearance. Solid strands of epithelial cells may also be seen within the dermis. A secretion is often apparent within the glands; this is one of the reasons why these structures were once believed to be of apocrine origin.

Treatment

If the diagnosis is questionable, one of the small papules may be removed for microscopic examination. Usually, once the diagnosis is confirmed, no treatment is required.

CYSTS OF EMBRYONIC ORIGIN
Mesonephric and paramesonephric cysts

Clinically, mesonephric and paramesonephric cysts are similar; hence, they will be discussed jointly. So-called Gartner's duct cysts of the vagina are simple cysts, usually asymptomatic, and most often are an incidental finding in the vaginal wall. Until recently, practically all vaginal and a few vulvar cysts with a glandular lining were called *cysts of Gartner's ducts,* since it was believed that they had all arisen from the caudal end of the vestigial mesonephric ducts. It has now been found that many, if not the majority, of such lesions have in reality arisen from the remains of the paramesonephric (müllerian) duct system. Distinction between the two types, while perhaps of considerable academic interest, is of little clinical importance.

Histogenesis

True Gartner's duct cysts arise from vestigial remnants of the vaginal portion of the mesonephric (wolffian) ducts in the female, referred to as Gartner's ducts. Normally, during embryonic development these ducts become atretic and lose their glandular lining. If parts of the ducts persist and remain functional, secretory activity gives rise to cystic tumors. The vast majority arise within the vagina, although a few examples of primary lesions of the vulva have been reported. Embryologically, these cysts are related to parovarian cysts.

A second variety of embryonic ductal cyst, clinically indistinguishable from Gartner's duct cysts, arises from vestiges of the paramesonephric ducts and is called a *paramesonephric cyst.* In early embryonic life, the vagina is lined with glandular (müllerian) epithelium. Subsequently, the latter is replaced by stratified squamous epithelium that grows upward from the urogenital sinus. During this process of upward displacement, islands of müllerian epithelium may persist in the vaginal wall or, occasionally, may migrate to the vulva. Because of the potential functional activity in such glandular structures, the formation of paramesonephric cysts in either structure is always possible. Numerous investigators, upon examination of multiple sections of tissues from otherwise normal vaginas, have found persistent islands of glandular tissue that possess the morphologic and staining characteristics of müllerian epithelium. Sandberg observed occult glands, histologically and histochemically identical to those of the endocervix, in nine of twenty-two vaginas of postpubertal patients. Evans and Hughes and other investigators have proved by histologic methods that over 50 percent of simple vaginal cysts in their series were paramesonephric in origin. Janovski found that paramesonephric cysts of the vulva are the most common of the dysontogenetic types. The latter finding is readily understandable if one considers that the mesonephric ducts almost always terminate inside the hymeneal ring, whereas the epithelia of the müllerian ducts and the urogenital sinus merge at the hymen and undoubtedly

Cystic tumors

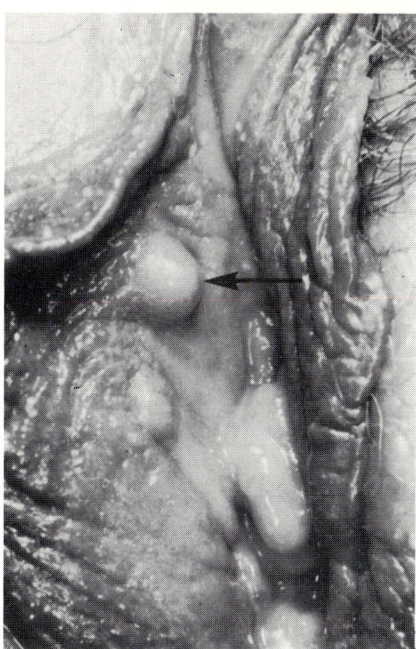

Fig. 5-12. A small vestibular paramesonephric cyst, indicated by arrow.

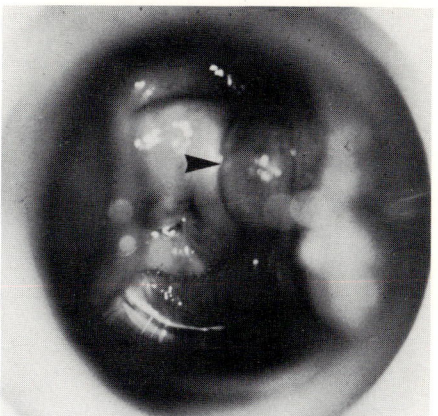

Fig. 5-13. Small Gartner's mesonephric duct cyst in left anterior lateral wall of vagina, just distal to cervix.

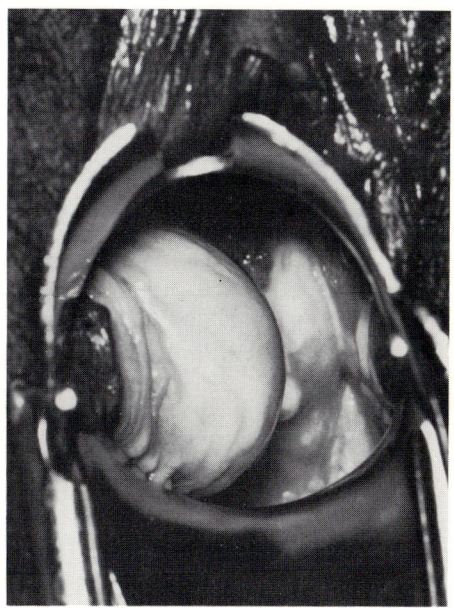

Fig. 5-14. Paramesonephric duct cyst bulging into vagina from right lateral vaginal wall. Found on routine examination; patient was asymptomatic.

mingle to some degree. Sandberg, Danielson, and Prince consider all vaginal cysts having the histologic and staining characteristics of endocervical cells as examples of vaginal adenosis. While not disputing the academic validity of such reasoning, we are inclined to think of a grossly visible cyst, at least clinically, as a separate entity.

Incidence

The incidence of mesonephric and paramesonephric cysts must be higher than reports indicate. Cysts from embryonic vestiges are many times more prevalent in the vagina than in the vulva. Studdiford found only twelve examples, including both types, in 20,000 admissions to Bellevue Hospital. The incidence of these cysts in our own experience has been approximately 1 percent, the majority of these having been small and clinically insignificant. Paramesonephric cysts of the vulva, although extremely uncommon, arise more often than the medical literature suggests, since investigators seem to publish case reports of only the larger cysts. Many small, thin-walled cysts of the vestibule, designated as *mucocele* or *vestibular cyst* (Fig. 5-12), exhibit the histologic and staining characteristics of paramesonephric cysts.

Clinical features

Since the gross appearance and symptomatology of paramesonephric and mesonephric cysts are not sufficiently characteristic to permit their distinction, their exact origin is not of major clinical importance. Usually, mesonephric cysts are located along the route followed by Gartner's ducts,

80 Benign diseases of the vulva and vagina

whereas paramesonephric cysts may arise anywhere in the vaginal wall.

The majority of embryonic vaginal cysts appear in the anterolateral wall of the vagina (Fig. 5-13). They are usually less than 2 cm. in diameter and asymptomatic. Since their presence is unknown to the patient, these cysts are usually found incidentally by the physician. As a rule, they are single and unilateral (Fig. 5-14), although they may be multiple (Fig. 5-15, C) and arise bilaterally. Multiple Gartner's cysts may extend from the cervix to the introitus, having the appearance of link sausage (Fig. 5-15, C). The smaller cysts tend to be ovoid or spherical in shape, whereas the larger ones often assume bizarre shapes and may have finger-like projections.

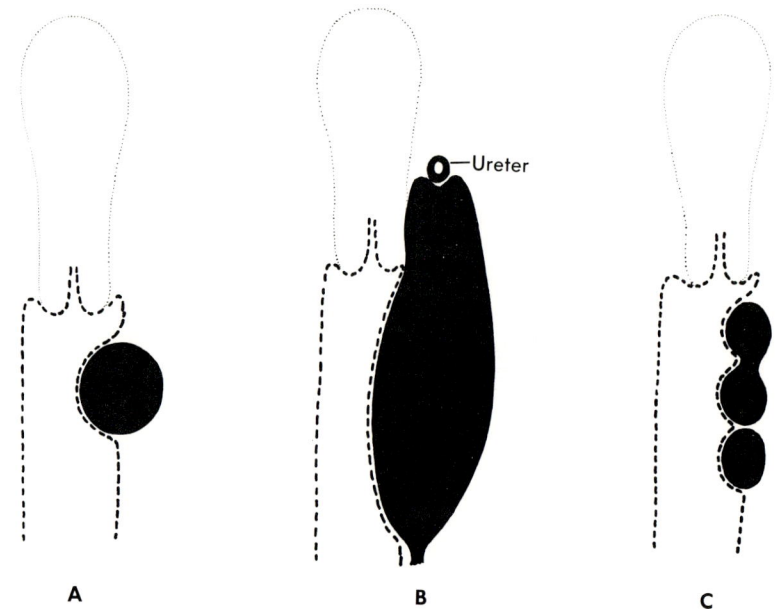

Fig. 5-15. Diagram of several varieties of developmental cysts of the vagina observed by the authors.

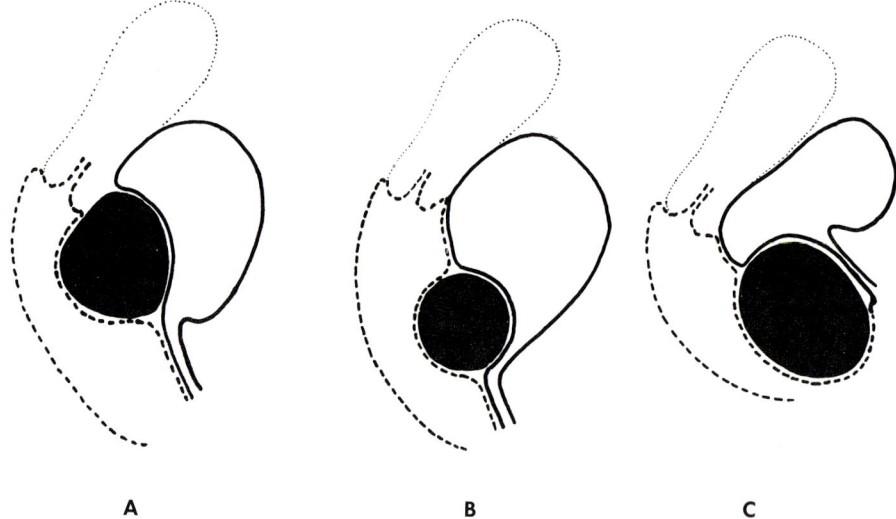

Fig. 5-16. Diagram of developmental cysts impinging upon the bladder and urethra.

A few cysts reach sufficient size to protrude through the vaginal introitus (Figs. 5-16, C and 5-17). During a recent 1 year period, one of us (H.L.G.) found such cysts in three patients. The cysts measured from 4 to 8 cm. in their greatest diameters, all were discovered during pregnancy, and all subsequently required surgical removal. One of the cysts had an anterior projection into the retropubic space. None obstructed labor or interfered with intercourse. One of the patients had been referred for repair of a "large cystocele" (Fig. 5-17). The largest cyst observed in our experience measured 6 cm. by 10 cm. including a finger-like extension that lay in contact with the left ureter (Fig. 5-15, B) in the broad ligament.

Cysts arising at the level of the cervix may extend medially and occupy a position between the bladder anteriorly and the upper vagina and cervix posteriorly (Fig. 5-16, A). If lower in the vagina, they may insinuate themselves between the vagina posteriorly and the bladder and urethra anteriorly (Fig. 5-16, B). Cysts in these positions are likely to provoke urinary symptoms. One patient, who had recently married, experienced such extreme urinary urgency with intercourse that it was necessary to remove the cyst; thereafter, she was completely relieved of this unusual symptom. Two of our patients experienced partial urinary retention incident to cysts impinging on the urethra (Fig. 5-16, C).

The majority of embryonic cysts of the vulva are located in the hymen (Fig. 5-18), vestibule (Fig. 5-12), labia minora, and periclitoral tissues and are usually solitary, superficial, and thin-walled. As a rule, they are less than 2 cm. in diameter, although a few reach 10 cm. When they reach this large size, they tend to be pedunculated. The

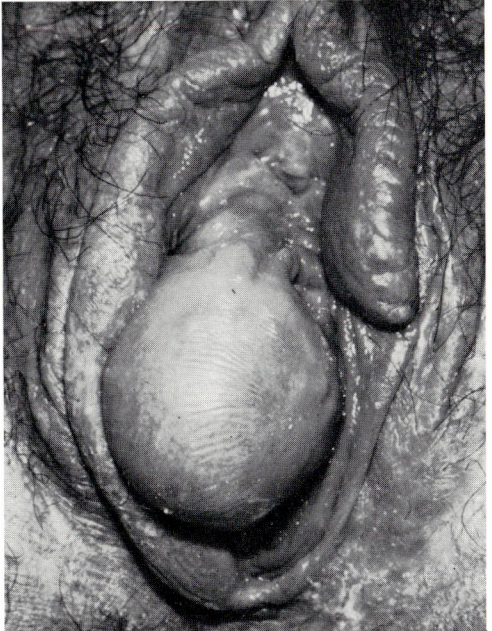

Fig. 5-17. Large mesonephric cyst, which bulged through the introitus when patient strained. Regarded as cystocele by referring physician.

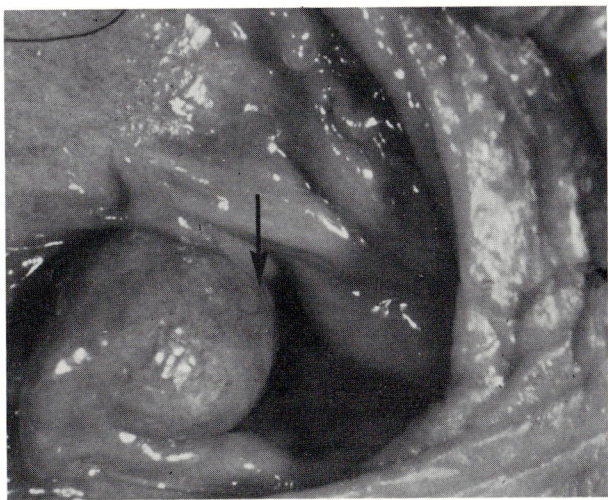

Fig. 5-18. Paramesonephric cyst in hymen, indicated by arrow.

smaller ones frequently resemble clear nabothian cysts, while others are yellow and soft. The contents are mucinous.

The development of carcinoma or infection in either of these two types of embryonic cysts is exceedingly rare. There is little evidence that they ever lead to the formation of urethral diverticula, although this possibility has been suggested.

Histopathology

The majority of mesonephric (Gartner's) duct cysts is lined by nonciliated cuboidal or low columnar epithelium (Fig. 5-19), which generally has a demonstrable basement membrane. Occasionally, a partial lining of squamous epithelium is observed. Mesonephric duct cysts are distinguished from the paramesonephric type by the smooth muscle tissue that surrounds the lining epithelium and by the negative periodic acid, Schiff (PAS) reaction of the glandular epithelium.

Paramesonephric (müllerian) cysts are mainly of two types, endocervical and fallopian. Mucus secreting tall columnar cells with basal nuclei and a clear cytoplasm, sometimes referred to as "picket" cells, are characteristic of the endocervical type that composes the vast majority (Fig. 5-20). The fallopian tube type is ordinarily lined by irregular, columnar epithelium with both ciliated and secretory types of cells and a poorly

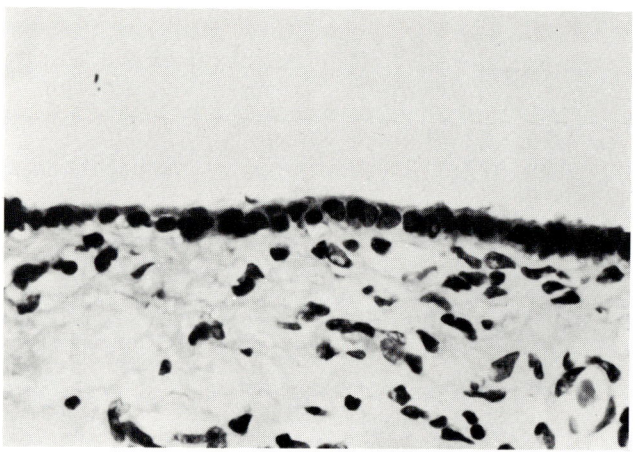

Fig. 5-19. Gartner's duct cyst lined by cuboidal and low columnar epithelium. PAS and mucin stains were negative. (H & E × 400)

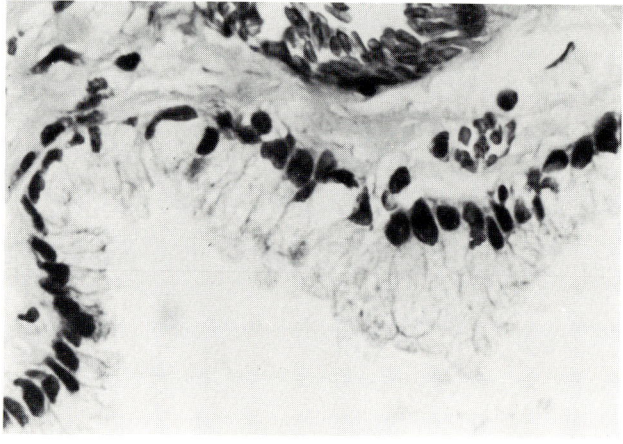

Fig. 5-20. Paramesonephric duct cyst lined with glandular epithelium of the endocervical type. The lining cells are tall columnar, with clear cytoplasm and basally located dark nuclei. Mucin and PAS stains were positive. (H & E × 680)

defined or absent basement membrane (Fig. 5-21). In this type, the nuclei are larger, more vesicular, and more centrally placed. Intercalated cells are sometimes found in the lining of the cyst.

A distinction between mesonephric and paramesonephric cysts by their microscopic morphology alone is not always possible, although the findings are usually highly suggestive. Tall columnar cells or ciliated cells are indicative of a paramesonephric origin. Cuboidal or low columnar cells suggest a mesonephric origin. Smooth muscle fibers adjacent to the lining of the cyst wall are also evidence of the mesonephric type. The most accurate method of identifying the two varieties is by their staining characteristics. Paramesonephric epithelium contains both acid and neutral mucopolysaccharides (mucin) when stained with PAS and alcian blue stain, whereas mesonephric cysts do not contain mucin and are PAS-negative.

Treatment

Since most of these cysts are small, asymptomatic, and benign, the patients usually require no treatment. If, however, the cyst becomes large and protrudes, produces mechanical problems, or causes the patient concern for any reason, its removal may be indicated. Because of the extreme thinness and firm adherence of the vaginal mucosa overlying some areas of mesonephric cysts, it is frequently desirable to make a double epilliptical incision over the cyst, avoiding the thinnest part of the overlying mucosa. The vaginal wall between the incisions provides a convenient area for attaching Allis clamps for traction. It is sometimes difficult to remove these lesions intact, although rupture does not materially hinder complete removal of the lining. Most cysts, particularly the paramesonephric variety, are easily excised. Others are firmly attached to surrounding tissues, necessitating their separation with scissors. A large cyst, or one that arises high in the vagina, may extend into the parametrium and even encroach upon a ureter (Fig. 5-15, *B*). If this relationship is suspected, insertion of a large ureteral catheter might be advisable before the operation is begun. When a cyst encroaches upon the bladder, urethra, or rectum, special precautions are required. Aspiration of the contents of a cyst may be desirable on occasion as a temporary expedient.

Cyst of the canal of Nuck (hydrocele)

The processus vaginalis peritonei, sometimes called the canal of Nuck, is a rudimentary peritoneal sac that accompanies the round ligament through the inguinal canal and, at times, to its terminal attachment in the labium majus. Normally, this peritoneal process becomes obliterated by the third or fourth month of embryonic life. Persistence of the peritoneal canal and an opening at the internal inguinal ring subjects the patient to the danger of an inguinal hernia. Occlusion of a persistent peritoneal sac at any point along its length may lead to the formation of a cyst called a *hydrocele* or cyst of the canal of Nuck. This lesion is homologous to the hydrocele found in males. Histologically, the cysts have a simple serous lining of flattened, cuboidal cells.

Clinical features

Hydroceles are usually limited to the inguinal canal or to subcutaneous tissues in the mons pubis (Fig. 5-22). If, however, a cyst

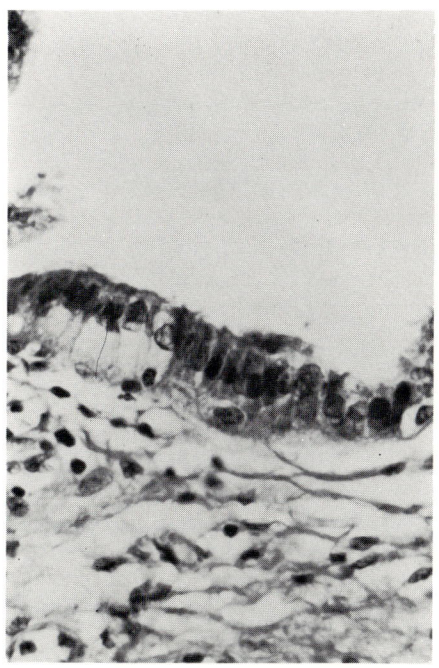

Fig. 5-21. Paramesonephric cyst of fallopian tube type. The tall columnar epithelium resembles that which lines the oviduct. Goblet cells on left. (H & E × 400)

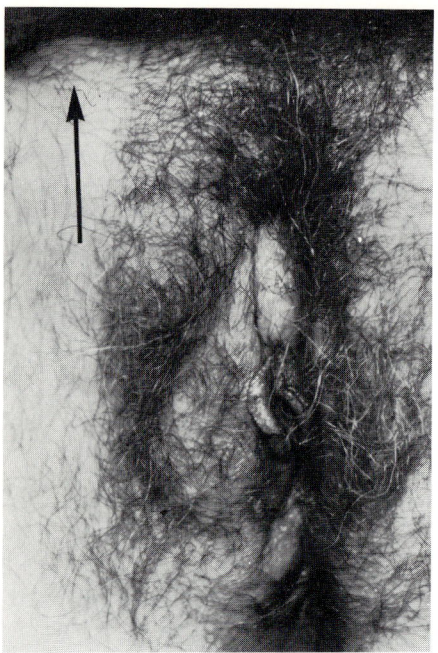

Fig. 5-22. Cyst of canal of Nuck (hydrocele) in right inguinal region.

extends into the labium majus from the latter location, as is possible, it may be referred to as a *hydrocele of the labium majus*. Should the canal of Nuck become obliterated at several levels, multiple cysts may form. One such patient observed by us had five independent cysts extending from the mons pubis to the peritoneal cavity at the internal ring. The diameter of the individual cysts vary from 1 to several centimeters.

Hydroceles in women seldom produce any symptoms other than a mild discomfort in the inguinal area. Although their growth is extremely slow, if they reach a large size they may be subject to tenderness from external pressures. One of our patients reported that she was unable to wear a girdle, and another complained that she was unable to wear a "well-fitted" evening dress because the mass then became apparent.

Lesions that must sometimes be differentiated include inguinal hernia, swollen inguinal lymph nodes, and lipomata. The cardinal signs of hernia are always lacking.

Treatment

Small, asymptomatic hydroceles require no treatment. For cosmetic reasons or because of discomfort, others must be surgically removed. The approach is identical to that for inguinal herniorrhaphy. Usually, and particularly if multiple cysts are present, an incision from the subcutaneous ring to the internal ring is necessary. Since separation from the round ligament is difficult, the ligament and the cysts may be lifted from the inguinal groove and removed en masse. The tissues should be reapproximated according to the technique employed in inguinal herniorrhaphy.

Cysts of supernumerary mammary glands

Breast anlagen along the mammary ridges, extending from the axillae to the inner thighs, form the rudiments of mammary glands. Because of the phylogenetic position of man, these concentrations of anlagen, with two exceptions (one on each anterior chest wall), are normally suppressed. Small supernumerary mammary glands are common along the embryologic "milk lines" in the axillae, lower chest, and upper abdomen, whereas the presence of breast tissue in the human vulva is exceedingly rare. The formation of neoplastic growths and cysts in accessory breast tissue of the vulva is even more rare. Breasts in whales and porpoises are located on the vulva, a fact that suggests an evolutionary inheritance from remote ancestry. The microscopic appearance of accessory breast tissue and lesions developing within such tissues is essentially identical to those of normally placed breasts (Fig. 5-23).

Clinical features

Supernumerary breast tissues are subject to the same hormonal influences and to the same functional and neoplastic diseases as are normal breasts, including fibroadenoma, cysts, and carcinoma. In view of the rarity of supernumerary breasts of the vulva and the lack of a characteristic gross appearance, their preoperative recognition is difficult. An interesting example of a vulvar mammary gland is shown in Fig. 5-24. Enlargement and "mastalgia" in the premenstruum and during pregnancy and postpartum engorgement afford clues to the true nature of the lesion.

Treatment

Local excision should be performed, as for any tumor of the vulva of unknown etiology.

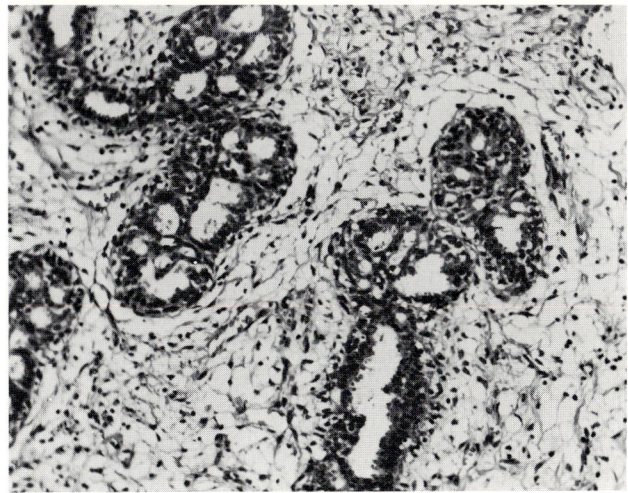

Fig. 5-23. Accessory breast tissue removed from vulva. The globules are composed of acinar and ductal elements in intralobular connective tissue. (H & E × 213)

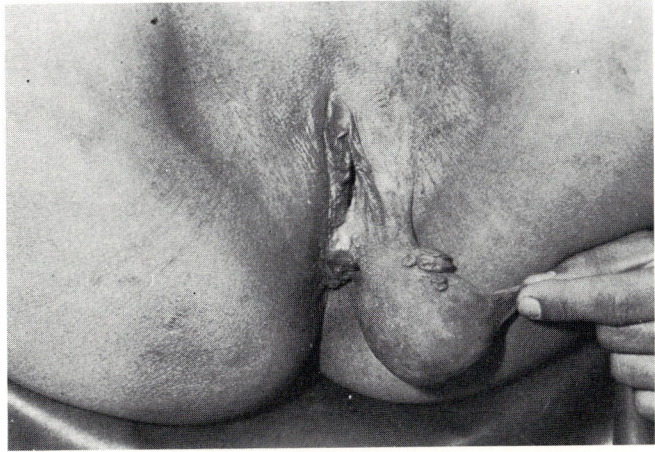

Fig. 5-24. Mass of mammary gland tissue arising from labium majus. (Tow, S. H., and Shanmugaratnam, K.: Brit. Med. J. 2:1234, 1962.)

Dermoid cyst

Dermoid cysts of the vulva and vagina are occasionally mentioned in medical literature, yet authentic tumors of this nature must be medical curiosities. We have never encountered a proved dermoid cyst or teratoma of these structures in practice nor have we had the privilege of examining one microscopically. The presence of skin, sebaceous glands, sweat glands, and hair follicles in a cyst wall, and even of hair and sebaceous material within its cavity, is not complete evidence of a true dermoid cyst, which is comparable to an ovarian dermoid with elements from other embryonic layers. Some cysts of the vulva that are sometimes classified as dermoids represent, perhaps, embryonal or posttraumatic epidermal inclusion cysts or uninfected pilonidal cysts, particularly since osseous and cartilaginous tissues are usually lacking. True dermoid cysts of the skin reportedly develop along embryonic lines of closure which, in the case of the vulva, would be situated chiefly near the perineogenital raphe. Jackman, Clark, and Smith reported twelve retrorectal tumors meeting the criteria of teratoma or dermoid. These tumors cannot be classified as vulvovaginal cysts.

Reportedly, dermoid cysts of the vulva are lined with epidermis and have appendages that include sebaceous glands, sweat glands, and hair follicles. The contents are mainly a mixture of sebaceous material and keratin. Hairs are present in these cysts and occasionally cartilagenous and bony tissue is found. The accuracy of the diagnosis of dermoid cyst might be questioned if elements from embryonic layers other than the ectoderm cannot be demonstrated.

BARTHOLIN'S DUCT CYST AND BARTHOLIN'S ABSCESS
Bartholin's duct cyst

Clinically important cysts of the vulva most often observed are those of Bartholin's duct, appearing in approximately 2 percent of new gynecologic patients. These cysts arise in the duct system of Bartholin's glands. Requisite to formation of these cysts is occlusion of some part of the duct system and continued secretory activity of Bartholin's glands. The occlusion is usually near the opening of the main duct into the vestibule. Since the ducts distend from retention of mucus secreted by the gland, the size and rapidity of growth of the lesions are influenced to some degree by the sexual habits and responsiveness of the individual patient. Most cysts involve only the main duct and thus are unilocular, although occasionally one or more locules lie deep to the main cyst. Such multilocular cysts result from occlusion of deeply placed minor ducts or acini of the ductal system, in addition to occlusion of the main duct.

In an infected cyst, the contents become purulent, thus constituting a *Bartholin's abscess*. Since the wall of the abscess is composed of epithelium rather than stromal tissue, the lesion may be regarded as a type of pseudoabscess. Infection may be suspected if pain and tenderness develop and the overlying skin becomes inflamed. Development of a tumor mass at the site of Bartholin's gland any time after the menopause should arouse suspicions of a solid neoplasm, either benign or malignant.

Etiology and pathogenesis

Ductal obstruction is an essential etiologic factor in Bartholin's cyst, although the cause of obstruction is usually obscure. Before the introduction of antibiotics, most cysts and abscesses were considered to be results of gonorrheal infection, particularly if bilateral. Currently, except in the sexually promiscuous, gonorrhea can seldom be incriminated as a cause of infection, ductal obstruction, and cyst formation. If primary gonorrheal bartholinitis is present, however, it becomes a potent factor in the production of occlusion. Primary bartholinitis from other microbial agents is probably extremely rare and thus unimportant in the etiology of ductal occlusion and cyst formation. While a cause and effect relationship between Bartholin's cysts and abscesses is well-established, it is unknown whether obstruction and cyst formation more often precede than follow bartholinitis. The incidence of these cysts in virgins who give no history of trauma or inflammation suggests that congenital stenosis or atresia of the ducts may play a role. Another factor seldom considered as a cause of obstruction is thickened or inspissated mucus near the ductal opening. Spontaneous disappearance of a cyst after a sudden outflow of uninfected mucus is presumptive evidence of temporary obstruction from this cause. Theoretically, a combination of congenitally narrowed duct and altered consistency of mucus might well account for many cysts. Mechanical trauma from any cause may also give rise to ductal occlusion by disrupting continuity of the duct, by provoking adhesions between opposed surfaces, or from contraction of resulting scar tissue. Poorly placed episiotomies and sutures are responsible for a few cysts; their role is not significant, however, since lateral episiotomies are now seldom performed.

The size of a cyst depends upon accumulation of secretions from Bartholin's gland and thus is influenced by sexual stimulation. This is exemplified by their rapid enlargement during courtship and stationary size or even shrinkage in a woman with diminished libido or sexual inactivity. Although ductal obstruction and glandular secretions are essential to cyst formation, the fact remains that the primary cause of the majority remains unknown.

Clinical features

Symptoms. Most patients with a small Bartholin's cyst have no symptoms, although minor discomfort on sexual intercourse may

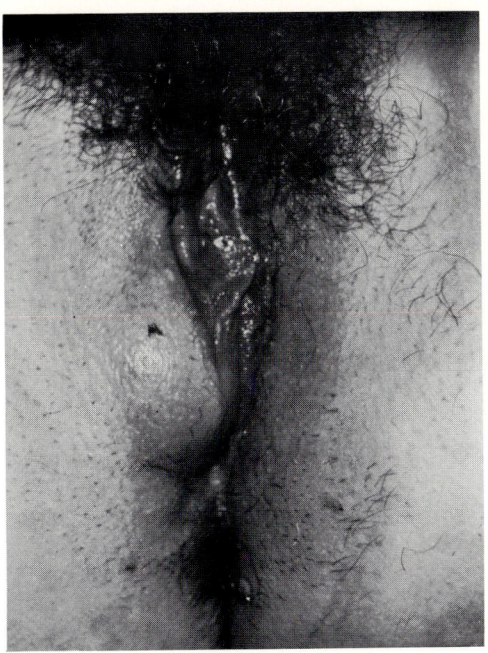

Fig. 5-25. Typical Bartholin's duct cyst.

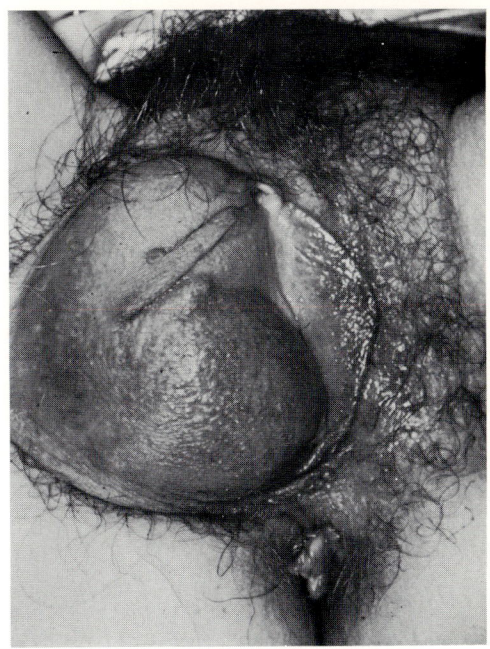

Fig. 5-26. Enormous Bartholin's duct cyst occluding introitus.

be experienced. If the cyst becomes enlarged or infected, other complaints will arise; extremely large lesions can mechanically interfere with walking or with coitus. Distinct discomfort may be associated with rapid enlargement, such as that which might be induced by repeated and prolonged sexual stimulation. Abscess formation gives rise to severe vulvar pain.

Objective signs. All except the smallest cysts cause the entrance to the vestibule to be crescent shaped. The majority are visible, unilateral, nontender, tense, palpable masses situated in the posterior part of the labia majora, opposite the posterior fourchette (Fig. 5-25). The smallest cysts are palpable only between the fingertips. As a rule, they are from 1 to 4 cm. in diameter, although a few become as large as 8 to 10 cm. (Fig. 5-26). Aborjaily and McSweeney reported a cyst 12.5 by 8 by 3 cm. and weighing 183 gm. The larger cysts arise from the main duct and lie immediately beneath the vulvar skin. The skin is loosely attached unless previous infection has caused extensive scar tissue formation. Most cysts are round or ovoid, although a few have a bizarre configuration with finger-like projections. A recently observed virginal patient had an unusual cyst with projections 2 cm. wide that reached the mons pubis anteriorly and the perianal tissues posteriorly. At its widest point this cyst measured only 2.5 cm., yet it was 9 cm. in length.

Histopathology

A cyst that has arisen from the main duct of a Bartholin's gland is lined by transitional (Fig. 5-27) or squamous epithelium, whereas if it originated in an acinus, the lining consists of cuboidal epithelium. Within the cyst wall, the typical acini of the Bartholin's gland are frequently present (Fig. 5-27). These acini are lined by tall columnar epithelium containing clear cytoplasm and dark basally located nuclei. A chronic inflammatory infiltrate is frequently present.

Treatment

The attitude once prevailed that once a Bartholin's cyst was discovered, it should be removed surgically. After it became widely known that most small, deep-seated cysts required no treatment at all, the practice of routine excision was largely abandoned. It is suggested, therefore, that small quiescent, asymptomatic cysts be left strictly alone. Cysts that are subject to recurrent abscess formation and those that cause pressure symptoms or introital obstruction require sur-

88 Benign diseases of the vulva and vagina

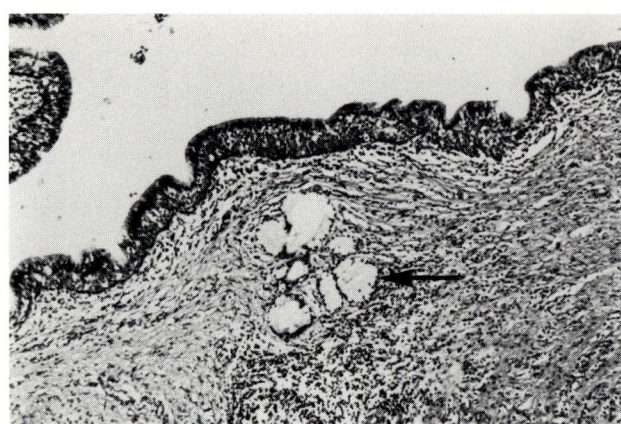

Fig. 5-27. Bartholin's duct cyst lined with transitional epithelium. Arrow points to typical Bartholin's gland acini, commonly observed within wall of cyst. (H & E × 100)

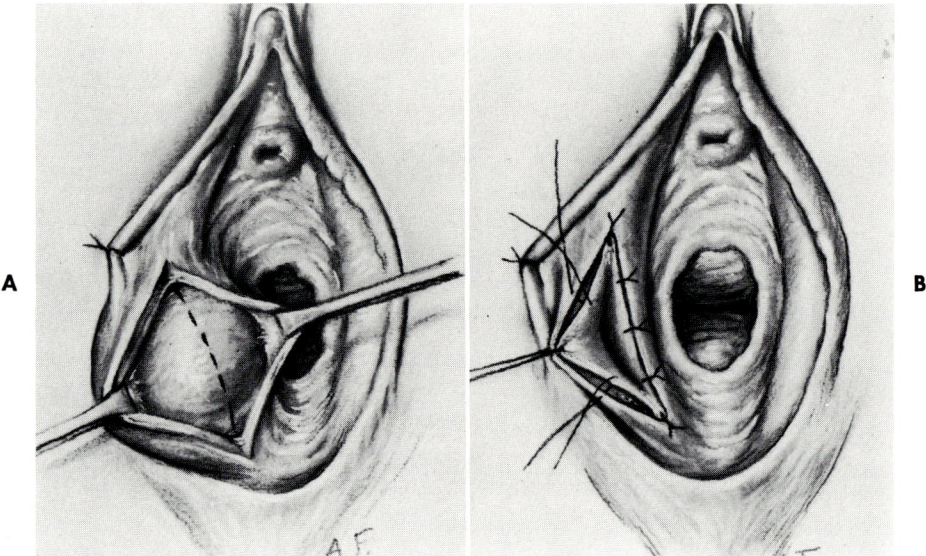

Fig. 5-28. A, Incision for marsupialization of Bartholin's duct cyst. (Tancer, M. L., Rosenberg, M., and Fernandez, D.: Obstet. Gynec. 7:608, 1956.) B, Marsupialization being completed. (Tancer, M. L., Rosenberg, M., and Fernandez, D.: Obstet. Gynec. 7:608, 1956.)

gical attention. Also, perhaps, when the nature of a tumefaction in this area is uncertain, excision should be performed.

The complications and morbidity associated with surgical removal of Bartholin's cyst are well known to experienced gynecologists. They are more frequent than is generally recognized. Mortalities from the operation have been recorded. The complications include cellulitis in the surgical field, recurrence of the cyst following failure to remove the entire gland, postoperative hemorrhage, hematoma, and, at times, the formation of disfiguring and painful scar tissue. Also, removal of the gland deprives the patient of nature's lubricant for sexual intercourse.

Any procedure that preserves function and prevents the formation of a cyst and abscess is far preferable to the excision operation. Marsupialization of Bartholin's cysts, first described by Davies in 1948, was one of the gynecologic milestones. Modifications and improvements were reported by Jacob-

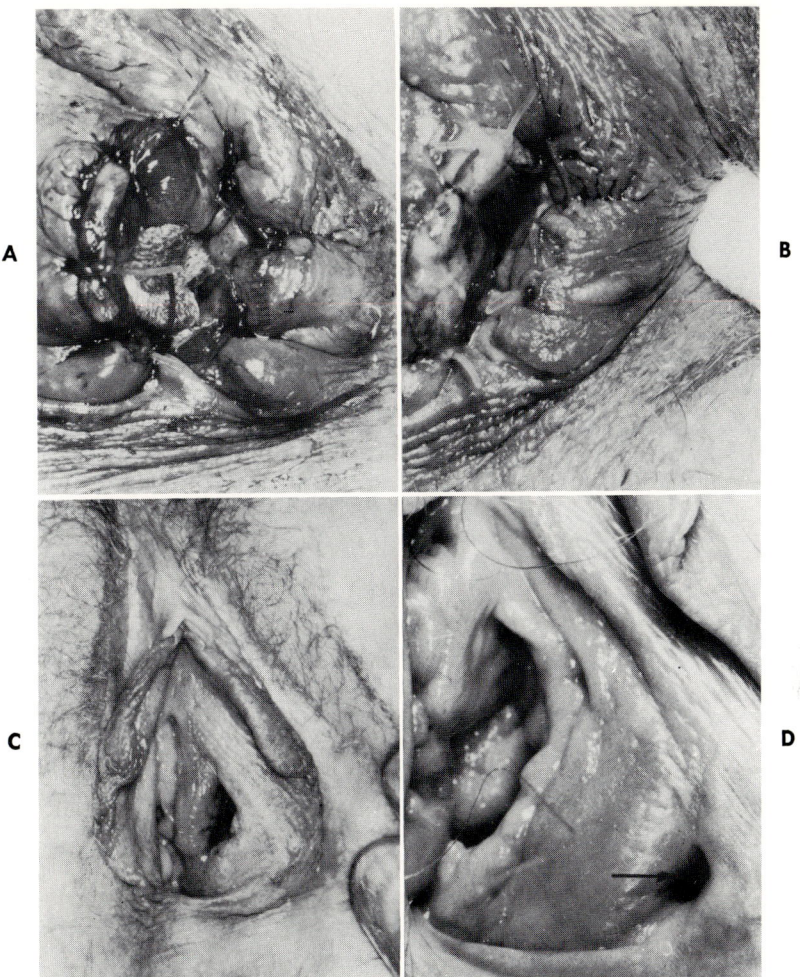

Fig. 5-29. **A**, Marsupialization of cyst completed. Gauze indicates cavity of cyst. Packing of the cavity is unnecessary. **B**, Three days following marsupialization. **C**, One month following marsupialization. **D**, Six months following marsupialization. A small functional opening is indicated by arrow.

son in 1950. Since that time, numerous reports of success with this treatment have been published, although no further major improvement has been described, unless it is that of Word, who described reestablishment of permanent ostia by the use of an inflatable bulb-tipped catheter maintained in the cyst or abscess for 4 or 5 weeks. With only slight planning, marsupialization can be performed effectively and safely in a physician's treatment room or in an outpatient facility of a hospital. Where it is performed is a matter of individual preference, based on experience, local attitude, and available facilities. If the cyst is deeply placed, perhaps a hospital environment would be best.

When marsupialization is performed in the office or outpatient facility, the vulva is shaved, scrubbed, and draped. The surgical tray includes knife, scissors, Addison's tissue forceps, two mosquito hemostats, needle holder, two small Allis clamps, sponges, 3-0 chromic catgut on an atraumatic needle, sterile gloves, and syringe with a 26 gauge needle. One to 3 ml. of an anesthetic solution is injected between the skin and the wall of the cyst at the site chosen for the incision. A longitudinal incision approximately 1.5 cm. in length is made parallel to and outside the hymeneal ring, preferably where the cyst is near the skin surface (Fig. 5-28, *A*). Because of mechanical problems, it is necessary at times to place the incision some distance below the hymeneal ring. The initial incision is carried only down to the cyst wall, and hemostasis is accomplished at this time. The avascular cyst wall is then incised with the knife and extended with scissors to the length of the skin incision. In the presence of an abscess, the ostium tends to close; thus, the initial opening should be slightly longer. With the use of interrupted sutures, the edges of the cyst wall are affixed to the edges of the skin, with the intervening tissues being avoided (Fig. 5-28, *B*). Within 2 or 3 weeks the opening shrinks to a fraction of a centimeter and remains as a permanent outlet for secretions of the gland (Fig. 5-29). This simple operation, successful in practically every case, obviates the disadvantages of excision of the gland. Jacobson (1960) reported only four recurrences of 152 cysts, and none of his patients had complications or unpleasant results. With the exception of one patient with a multilocular cyst, we have found this operation effective as a treatment for all uninfected cysts. Because of friability of tissues and difficulty in identifying the lining of the cyst, the failure rate of the operation for Bartholin's abscesses is higher.

Word's use of an inflatable bulb-tipped catheter in the treatment for Bartholin's cysts and abscesses has been highly successful in his hands (Fig. 5-30). The catheter is the size of a No. 10 Foley catheter and has a stem 1 inch long and a single barrel. A sealed stopper is attached to one end and a 5 ml. capacity latex inflatable balloon is attached to the other. Insertion of the catheter under local anesthesia is an office procedure. Word makes a small stab wound into the cyst or abscess through the mucosal lining of the vestibule below the hymeneal ring (Fig. 5-30, *A*). The catheter is inserted (Fig. 5-30, *B*) and the bulb is then inflated with 2 to 4 ml. of water, depending upon the amount necessary to prevent its dropping out (Fig. 5-30, *C*). The catheter maintains patency of the incision into the

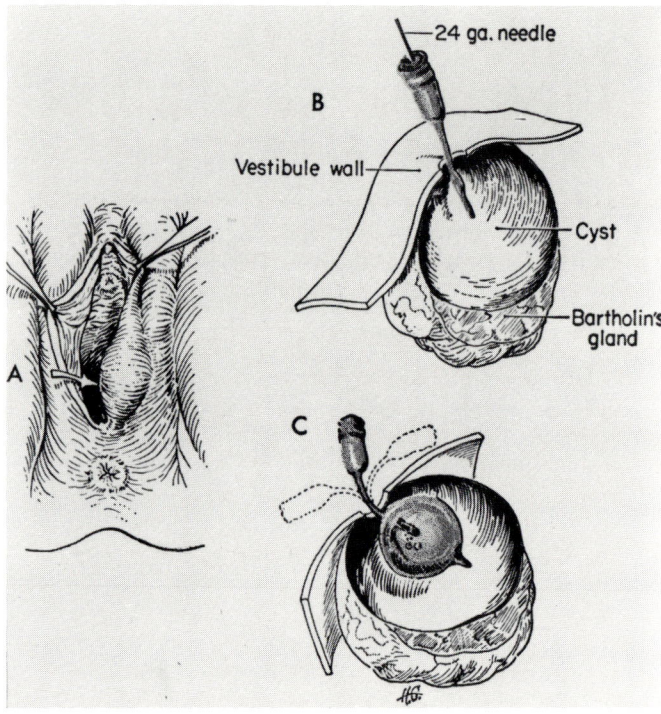

Fig. 5-30. Inflatable, bulb-tipped catheter used in treatment of Bartholin's duct cysts and abscesses. (Word, B.: J.A.M.A. **190**:777, 1964.) **A,** Arrow indicates location for stab wound in cyst or abscess. **B,** Insertion of catheter in stab wound. **C,** Inserted catheter inflated with water.

cavity until epithelialization ensures a permanent ostium. Word (1967) has referred to his method as "fistulization."

Bartholinectomy is seldom preferable to marsupialization as a treatment for Bartholin's cysts. The occasional patient with a massive cyst, with deep seated lesions associated with pronounced periglandular fibrosis, or with a multilocular cyst may be more suitably treated by removal of the cyst and gland.

Needle aspiration is sometimes useful as a temporary expedient. Occasionally, it may also be employed for distinguishing between a cyst and a solid tumor.

Bartholin's abscess

The majority of Bartholin's abscesses, especially if recurrent, develop as a consequence of a nongonorrheal infection of the fluid content of Bartholin's duct cysts. The pathogenesis of Bartholin's cysts has already been discussed. Today, abscesses proved to be incident to gonorrheal infection are rarely observed. Although the route of entry of infectious organisms into a cyst has not been determined, they probably gain admission through a stenotic opening into Bartholin's duct which is, perhaps, too small to allow emission of thick mucus, yet adequate for entry of the bacteria. In addition to the gonococcus, the various types of staphylococci and streptococci, *Escherichia coli, Aerobacter aerogenes,* and perhaps other organisms are often isolated from these abscesses.

Clinical features

Symptoms. The chief symptoms of Bartholin's abscess are varying degrees of pain and tenderness over the affected gland. The rapidity of development and the extent of involvement depends upon the size of the affected cyst and the virulence of the infectious agent. Some abscesses develop slowly, over a week or longer, and may give rise only to mild symptoms. Occasionally, such a smoldering type of infection will ultimately regress, although eventually it is more likely either to drain spontaneously or to require incision and drainage. Usually Bartholin's abscesses develop rapidly, over a period of 2 to 3 days, and are associated with exquisite pain and tenderness. This type tends to rupture spontaneously within 72

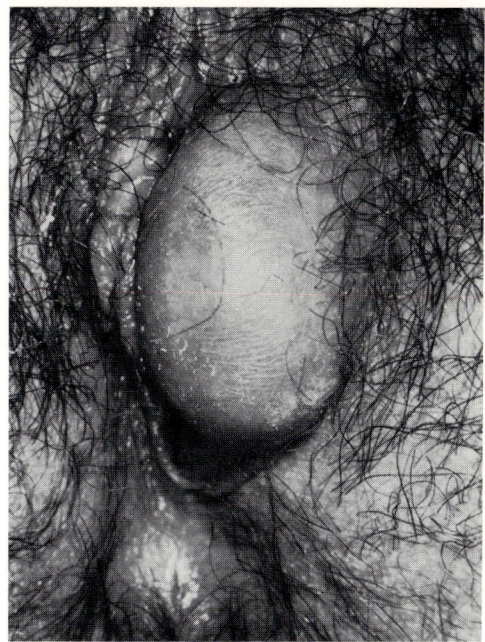

Fig. 5-31. Bartholin's abscess, indicated by fluctuant tender mass.

hours. Meanwhile, the patient often experiences difficulty in sitting and walking.

Objective signs. The objective signs include unilateral swelling over the site of the affected gland, redness of the overlying skin, and, frequently, edema of the labia. The abscess is usually palpable as an exquisitely tender, fluctuant mass (Fig. 5-31). The size of the lesion rarely exceeds 5 cm. in diameter. Impending spontaneous rupture is indicated by an area of softening or pointing on the vestibular aspect of the abscess. Bilateral abscesses, although exceptional, are suggestive of a primary gonorrheal infection.

Treatment

Local applications of heat, preferably by hot, wet dressings or sitz baths, promote spontaneous drainage of the abscess or its development to a stage suitable for incision and drainage. Occasionally, early treatment of an obvious bartholinitis with broad spectrum antibiotics may prevent the formation of an abscess; this, however, could easily delay ripening of the abscess. Many abscesses drain spontaneously within 72 hours. Incision and drainage, if necessary, are easily performed in the physician's office. The skin overlying the site of pointing should first be infiltrated with 1 to 2 ml. of 1% lidocaine. Negative pressure on the syringe is inadvisable, since purulent material may thus be drawn into the anesthetic solution; if reinjected, it might cause severe localized cellulitis. Also, the intravenous injection of such a mixture could lead to uncontrollable septicemia; episodes of this type have been reported. After drainage of the abscess, a wick of iodoform gauze should be inserted into the cavity and left in place for several days to ensure continued adequate drainage. Further applications of heat accelerate resolution and healing. Surgical removal of an abscessed Bartholin's duct and gland is contraindicated.

Marsupialization of Bartholin's abscesses has been advocated, although we prefer to defer the procedure until a new Bartholin's cyst forms; all the circumstances, including the temperament of the patient, are then more favorable. This procedure, especially if performed in the office, is not only difficult but, in our experience, too often fails to establish a permanent ostium. Word has employed his bulb-tipped catheter (Fig. 5-30) in the treatment for abscesses as well as for cysts with equal success.

Recurrent Bartholin's abscess is a distinct indication for active treatment. In general, however, definitive surgical methods are best deferred until a period of quiescence of the lesion.

CYSTS OF URETHRAL AND PARA-URETHRAL ORIGIN
Skene's duct cyst

Skene's ducts, which are 0.5 to 1.5 cm. long, are located in the floor of the terminal end of the urethra and open just within or external to the meatus. The formation of retention cysts within these ducts is secondary to ductal occlusion. Although the majority of patients in whom these cysts develop give no history of infection, skenitis is considered to be the primary cause. Posttraumatic occlusion may also play a role. Regardless of the primary etiology, clinically significant cysts of Skene's ducts are relatively rare.

Clinical features

Cysts larger than 2 cm. in diameter are seldom observed, since symptoms of urethral

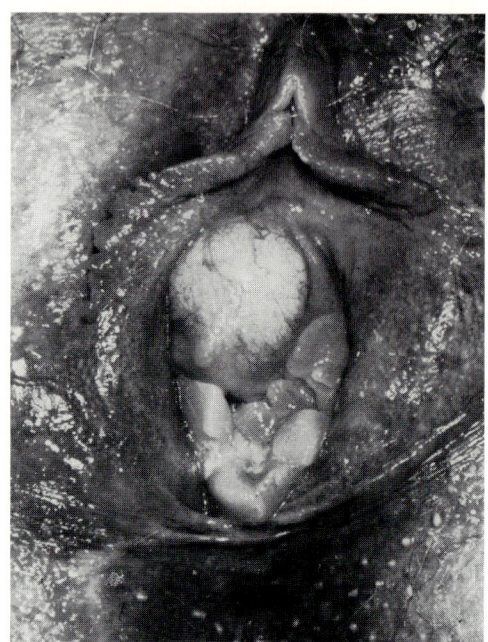

Fig. 5-32. Cyst of Skene's duct. Despite the relatively large size of the cyst, the patient had no symptoms referable to the urinary tract.

obstruction usually prompt patients to seek medical attention before the lesions reach this size (Fig. 5-32). In our experience, some patients with cysts less than 1 cm. in diameter have some degree of urinary retention, whereas other patients with cysts 2 cm. in diameter have no evidence of obstruction. Occasionally, dyspareunia is a prominent symptom. An abscess may be associated with acute pain and urinary retention.

Treatment

Excision is recommended for all except the smallest asymptomatic cysts. This excision should never be undertaken during an inflammatory episode, however. Incision and drainage are preferable for infected cysts, with removal being deferred until the infection subsides and an uninfected cyst reforms. Excision is a relatively simple procedure, yet care must be taken to prevent injury to the urethral wall. The use of an indwelling catheter is of value in this respect. Marsupialization is not advocated since removal of the cyst is simple; the duct, having no useful function, need not be preserved.

URETHRAL DIVERTICULUM

A urethral or suburethral diverticulum is a sac-like protrusion that communicates with the urethra by a small opening. It may appear in persons of any age and is often an unrecognized source of persistent urinary symptoms and recurrent infection. The diagnosis of this lesion seems to depend largely upon awareness of such a possibility and an eagerness to verify its presence. Both Nourse and Brown found urethral diverticula in approximately 0.35 percent of their urologic patients.

Etiology and pathogenesis

Huffman has demonstrated numerous glands and ducts in the paraurethral tissues (Fig. 1-15). The ducts empty chiefly into the distal two-thirds of the floor of the urethra. The glands, for the most part, are lined with columnar cells that possess some secretory function. It seems likely that these structures are the site of origin of most diverticula. Theoretically, obstruction of any of the ducts could lead to the formation of a retention cyst or abscess. Persistent uncomplicated cysts of this origin must be extremely rare, or, if they do exist, they are unrecognized by gynecologists and urologists. Every gynecologist, however, may observe several diverticula during his career. Although the exact pathogenesis of the lesions remains debatable, according to the most prevalent opinion, the following is the sequence of events in their development: ductal obstruction, retention, infection, abscess formation, and rupture into the urethra. Repeated distention with urine and purulent material can ultimately produce a fairly large cavity having a permanently epithelialized communication with the urethra. That a diverticulum may be congenital is also plausible. It is possible, yet questionable, that a true abscess sometimes forms in the urethral supporting tissues from infections such as gonorrhea and from ruptures into the urethral canal; this latter is followed by epithelization of the abscess wall. Some diverticula have been attributed to infected cysts of the mesonephric and paramesonephric ducts that rupture into the urethra and develop a permanent communication.

Clinical features

Symptoms. Symptoms are related chiefly to the lower urinary tract. Small diverticula may be asymptomatic for varying periods, whereas large lesions invariably produce symptoms. Dyspareunia is often reported, and in the absence of other explanations for this complaint, a diverticulum should be suspected. Many patients give a history of urinary "leakage" or of a sudden discharge independent of urination. If the sac is firmly distended, urinary retention of some degree may be associated. Patients with a urethral diverticulum are extremely susceptible to recurrent cystitis and usually have had repeated dysuria with frequency, burning, and tenesmus. Intractable pyuria or cystitis is always suggestive of the lesion. Pyelitis with chills and fever is not uncommon. One exceedingly rare complication is a urethrovaginal fistula incident to temporary occlusion of the orifice, abscess formation, and rupture into the vagina.

Objective signs. Whereas diverticula are usually located between the urethra and vagina, extensions of the sac occasionally surround the urethra entirely or extend to the bladder trigone. The majority of diverticula open into the floor of the distal two-thirds of the urethra (Figs. 5-33 to 5-35). The opening is usually single, although at times multiple openings are present. The diameter of the sac varies from a few millimeters to 6 to 8 cm., with the ultimate size being determined by pressures with-

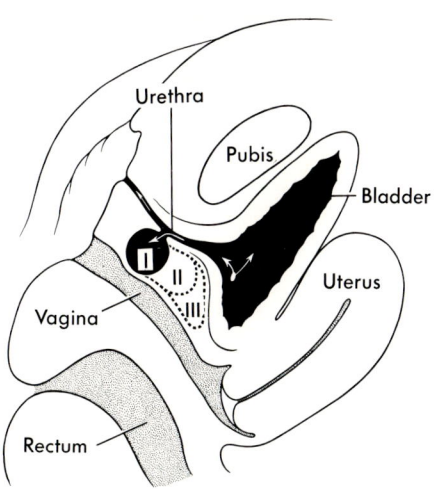

Fig. 5-33. Urethral diverticulum *(I)* and extensions beneath the trigone *(II)* and bladder floor *(III).* (Tancer, M. L.: Clin. Obstet. Gynec. 8: 992, 1965.)

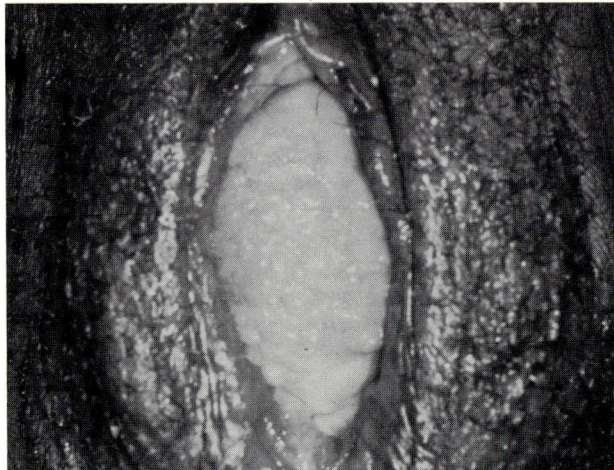

Fig. 5-34. Large urethral diverticulum, resembling a cystocele. The majority are smaller.

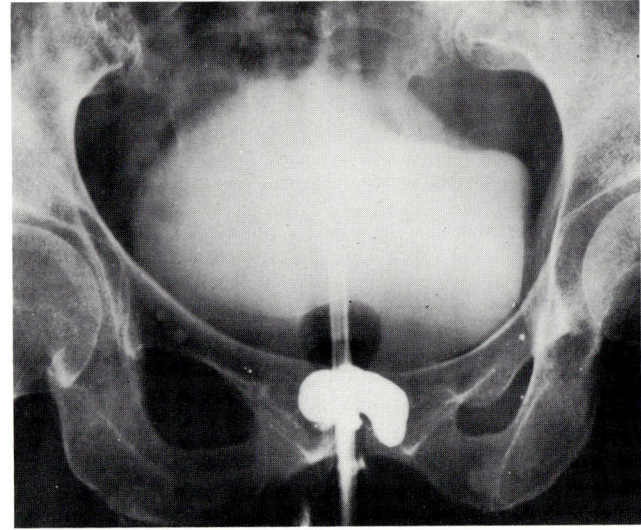

Fig. 5-35. Large urethral diverticulum distended with opaque medium.

in the lesion and the distensibility of the wall. Other factors that perhaps influence the size of a diverticulum are the diameter of the communication, infection, the amount of scar tissue, the duration of the lesion, the secretory activity of the lining cells, and the filling and emptying mechanisms of the particular lesion.

Upon palpation, a thickness or a fluctuant mass of varying degrees of tenderness can generally be detected in the lower part of the anterior vaginal wall. Palpation is facilitated by the insertion of a metal sound into the urethra. Pressure upon the diverticulum will usually force the fluid contents into the urethra and out through the meatus. The contents vary from clear, sterile urine to thick, malodorous purulent material. When present, stones are easily palpable and are diagnostic.

Histopathology

The microscopic picture of this lesion is nonspecific. The lining may consist of columnar, cuboidal, transitional, or stratified squamous epithelium; because of destruction

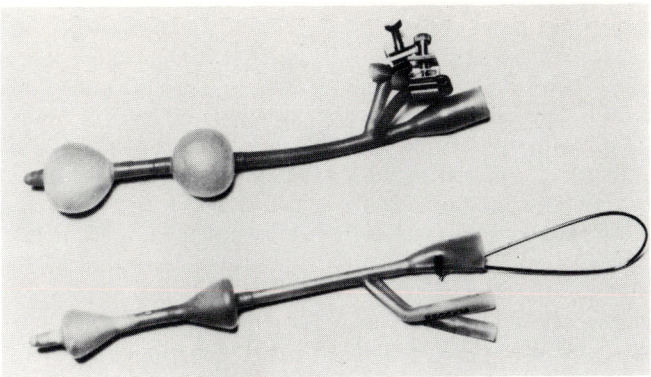

Fig. 5-36. Hyman catheter for positive-pressure urethrography. (Tancer, M. L., and Hyman, R.: Amer. J. Obstet. Gynec. 84:1853, 1962.)

by inflammation, however, many lesions have no demonstrable epithelial lining. The appearance of the supporting tissues is modified by associated inflammation.

Diagnosis

The diagnosis may be suspected from the history alone, and vaginal examination will often provide confirmatory evidence. Diverticula have been confused with urethroceles, cystoceles (Fig. 5-34), and cysts of Skene's ducts or of Gartner's ducts.

Endoscopy will establish the diagnosis if the communication is visualized, although failure to discover the opening does not exclude the presence of a diverticulum. The diameter of the endoscope should be as large as is practical. If visualization is difficult, suburethral pressure will usually force the contents into the field of vision. Special attention should be directed to the lower two-thirds of the floor of the urethra.

Radiography is the most reliable confirmatory diagnostic procedure (Fig. 5-35). Numerous urethrographic techniques have been described. According to one method, a urethral or ureteral catheter is threaded into the diverticulum through the endoscope and the diverticulum is filled with a radiopaque medium. If the diverticulum can be well-delineated by palpation, the contents can sometimes be aspirated through the vagina with a needle and syringe, permitting the introduction of the radiopaque medium. With the use of the same technique, one may also confirm the presence of a diverticulum by injecting sodium indigotindisulfonate (Indigo Carmine) and expressing it through the urethra.

The most successful urethrographic procedure is carried out with a Hyman (Fig. 5-36) or a Davis catheter. Both have balloons at the bladder and meatal ends for retaining the radiopaque medium within the urethra. The Davis catheter has a sliding balloon at the meatal end that can be adjusted according to the length of the urethra. A stylet is useful for placement of the catheter into the bladder. The balloons on each end are filled with air, and a liquid radiopaque medium (10 ml. is usually adequate) is introduced under moderate pressure. Both anteroposterior and lateral views are necessary for accurate delineation of the diverticulum. The air-filled balloons are easily identified (Fig. 5-35).

Treatment

The most successful treatment is surgical excision, though this should be deferred until after an attempt has been made to overcome infection. Since a predominant bacterium is seldom demonstrable, cultures of the diverticular contents are of little value. *Escherichia coli* is most often isolated. The use of broad spectrum antibiotics and repeated expression of the contents of the diverticulum are sometimes beneficial.

Regardless of the surgical technique employed, ideal treatment includes complete removal of the sac and accurate closure of the opening into the urethra. The lining may be so intimately bound to surrounding fibrotic tissues that complete resection becomes exceedingly tedious, if not impossible. Before beginning the operation, it is well to place a large caliber Foley catheter into the bladder to permit easier identification of the urethra and neck of the bladder. The vagina and the diverticulum are incised longitudinally and the sac is entered first to avoid injury to the urethra and bladder and to more easily identify the communication. Under direct visualization, the lining is resected from surrounding fibromuscular tissues. Failure to remove the entire sac may lead to a recurrence of the diverticulum, but this is not inevitable. After the sac has been separated to the edge of the communication, it is completely excised. (To facilitate resection, Hirschorn advocated the use of a silicone compound that hardens after instillation into the diverticulum.) The urethral opening is closed with continuous 3-0 or 4-0 sutures of chromic catgut on a short, small, atraumatic needle. Special care is taken to invert the edges of the urethral mucosa. The urethrovaginal fascia is approximated with a second layer of sutures. Redundant vaginal mucosa is excised, and the edges are approximated with interrupted sutures. Excision of a sac with an anterior urethral communication may require a retropubic approach.

Edwards and Beebe have described a somewhat different surgical technique. The vagina is incised longitudinally from the external urethral meatus to a point near the cervix. The vaginal mucosa is separated from the diverticulum and urethra in a manner similar to the first step in repair of a cystocele. The floor of the urethra is incised with scissors from the external meatus to the opening of the diverticulum and the resection is then performed. We have had no experience with this method; theoretically, it possesses no advantage over the orthodox method of excision to offset the theoretical disadvantages such as urethral granulations, stricture, and fistulae.

In the presence of an ill-defined sac, extensive involvement of the neck of the bladder, or inseparable tissue planes, Ellik has recommended incision, drainage, and packing with oxidized cellulose gauze. The incision into the diverticulum is kept small and is closed with interrupted sutures after the sac has been packed. Ellik claims excellent results, regardless of the physical nature of the diverticulum. In such cases, we prefer to remove as much of the sac as possible without endangering the integrity of the bladder and to close the urethral communication. The patient is usually cured, even though fragments of lining may remain.

We recommend a retention catheter for only 24 hours after the operation. Most patients experience no difficulty in voiding when allowed bathroom privileges. Subsequent catheterization, if necessary, should be performed meticulously, with a well-lubricated catheter.

Excision of a diverticulum that impinges upon the bladder neck and trigone is occasionally followed by urinary stress incontinence. This requires later correction. If the bladder is inadvertently opened and unrecognized, a vesicovaginal fistula may result. A urethrovaginal fistula occasionally develops. If low in the vagina, such a fistula may not be a problem to the patient.

One patient who was treated by excision had recurrent abscesses at the original site of the diverticulum that repeatedly ruptured spontaneously into the vagina. Apparently, the urethral opening had been permanently closed. Marsupialization of the diverticular sac into the vagina effected a cure.

REFERENCES

Aborjaily, A. N., and McSweeny, D. J.: Bartholin cyst of extraordinary size, Obstet. Gynec. **11:** 350, 1958.

Anderson, N. P.: Hidradenoma of the vulva, Arch. Derm. Syph. **62:**873, 1950.

Betson, J. R., Jr., Chiffelle, T. L., and George, R. P.: Pilonidal cyst involving the clitoris, Amer. J. Obstet. Gynec. **84:**543, 1962.

Boatwright, D. C., and Moore, V.: Suburethral diverticula in the female, J. Urol. **89:**581, 1963.

Brown, E. D.: Diverticulum of the female urethra, Southern Med. J. **49:**982, 1956.

Davies, W. B.: Bartholin cyst (a simple method for its restoration to function), Surg. Gynec. Obstet. **86:**329, 1948.

Edwards, E. A., and Beebe, R. A.: Diverticula of the female urethra, Obstet. Gynec. **5:**729, 1955.

Ellik, M.: Diverticulum of the female urethra: A new method of ablation, J. Urol. **77:**243, 1957.

Evans, D. M. D., and Hughes, H.: Cysts of the vaginal wall, J. Obstet. Gynaec. Brit. Comm. **68:**247, 1961.

Fisher, J. H.: Fibroadenoma of supernumerary mammary gland tissue in vulva, Amer. J. Obstet. Gynec. **53:**335, 1947.

Fox, G. H., and Fordyce, J. A.: Two cases of a

rare papular disease affecting the axillary region, J. Cutan. Dis. **20:**1, 1902.

Gardner, G. H., Greene, R. R., and Peckham, B. M.: Normal and cystic structures of the broad ligament, Amer. J. Obstet. Gynec. **55:**917, 1948.

Hendrix, R. C., and Behrman, S. J.: Adenocarcinoma arising in a supernumerary mammary gland in the vulva, Obstet. Gynec. **8:**238, 1956.

Hirschorn, R. C.: A new surgical technique for removal of urethral diverticula in the female patient, J. Urol. **92:**206, 1964.

Huffman, J. W.: The detailed anatomy of the paraurethral ducts in the adult human female, Amer. J. Obstet. Gynec. **55:**86, 1948.

Jackman, R. J., Clark, P. L., and Smith, W. D.: Retrorectal tumors, J.A.M.A. **145:**956, 1951.

Jacobson, P.: Marsupialization of vulvovaginal (Bartholin's) cysts, Amer. J. Obstet. Gynec. **79:**73, 1960.

Jacobson, P.: Vulvovaginal cyst (treatment by marsupialization), Western J. Surg. **58:**704, 1950.

Janovski, N. A.: Dysontogenetic cysts of the vulva, Obstet. Gynec. **20:**227, 1962.

Kligman, A. M.: The myth of the sebaceous cyst, Arch. Derm. **89:**253, 1964.

Knox, J. N.: Personal communication.

Kronthal, H.: Fox-Fordyce disease, treatment with an oral contraceptive, Arch. Derm. **91:**243, 1965.

Lever, W. F.: Histopathology of the skin, ed. 3, Philadelphia, 1961, J. B. Lippincott Co.

McGavran, M. H., and Binnington, B.: Keratinous cysts of the skin, Arch. Derm. **94:**499, 1966.

Meeker, J. H., Neubecker, R. D., and Helwig, E. B.: Hidradenoma papilliferum, Amer. J. Clin. Path. **37:**182, 1962.

Mengert, W. F.: Supernumerary mammary gland tissue on the labia minora, Amer. J. Obstet. Gynec. **29:**891, 1935.

Montes, L. F., Caplan, R. M., Riley, G. M., and Curtis, A. C.: Fox-Fordyce disease, Arch. Derm. **84:**452, 1961.

Nourse, M. H.: Diverticulum of the female urethra, Western J. Surg. **69:**286, 1961.

Novak, E., Woodruff, J. D., and Novak, E. R.: Probable mesonephric origin of certain female genital tumors, Amer. J. Obstet. Gynec. **68:**1222, 1954.

Palmer, E.: Pilonidal cyst of the clitoris, Amer. J. Surg. **93:**133, 1957.

Patey, D. H., and Scarff, R. W.: Pathology of postanal pilonidal sinus: Its bearing on treatment, Lancet **2:**484, 1946.

Pick, L.: Ueber Hidradenoma and Adenoma hidradenoides, Arch. Path. Anat. **125:**312, 1904.

Sandberg, E. C.: The incidence and distribution of occult vaginal adenosis, Amer. J. Obstet. Gynec. **101:**322, 1968.

Sandberg, E. C., Danielson, R. W., Cauwett, R. W., and Bonar B. E.: Adenosis vaginae, Amer. J. Obstet. Gynec. **93:**209, 1965.

Sandberg, E. C., Danielson, R. W., and Prince, E.: Benign vaginal adenosis, Obstet. Gynec. **30:**93, 1967.

Santa, U. V.: Tumors of mesonephric origin in the female genital tract, Amer. J. Obstet. Gynec. **89:**680, 1964.

Shelly, W. B., and Levy, E. J.: Apocrine retention in man, Arch. Derm. **73:**38, 1956.

Siegler, A. M., and Gordon, R.: Fibroadenoma in a supernumerary breast of the vulva, Amer. J. Obstet. Gynec. **62:**1367, 1951.

Smith, T. E.: Anterior or perineal pilonidal cyst, J.A.M.A. **136:**973, 1948.

Studdiford, W. E.: Vaginal lesions of adenomatous origin, Amer. J. Obstet. Gynec. **73:**641, 1957.

Tancer, M. L., Rosenberg, M., and Fernandez, D.: Cysts of the vulvovaginal (Bartholin's) gland, Obstet. Gynec. **7:**608, 1956.

Tow, S. H., and Shanmugaratnam, K.: Supernumerary mammary gland in the vulva, Brit. Med. J. **2:**1234, 1962.

von Preuschen, F.: Ueber Cystenbildung der Vagina, Arch. Path. **70:**111, 1877.

Warvi, W. N., and Gates, O.: Epithelial cysts and cystic tumors of the skin, Amer. J. Path. **14:**765, 1943.

Werth, R.: Anatomy of cysts of the vulva, Zbl. Gynaek. **22:**513, 1878.

Word, B.: New instrument for office treatment of cysts and abscesses of Bartholin's gland, J.A.M.A. **190:**777, 1964.

Word, B.: Office treatment of cyst and abscess of Bartholin's bland duct, Southern Med. J. **61:**514, 1968.

Word, B.: Personal communication, August, 1967.

Chapter 6

Endometriosis

Endometriosis of the lower genital tract was largely unknown until significant reports began to appear in the 1950's. Professional awareness of these lesions partially accounts for the larger number of cases observed, particularly of the superficial cervical disease. The increased incidence is also a real one, being attributed chiefly to the many traumatizing therapeutic and diagnostic procedures performed on the cervix within recent years. In fact, the majority of lesions of the vulva and vagina are the result of injury to these tissues in the course of modern obstetric and gynecologic care. Primary endometriosis of the ectocervix is several times more prevalent than the combined incidence of the lesions in the vulva and vagina.

Endometriosis of the vulva
Incidence and etiology

According to Binder in 1964, thirty-six cases of endometriosis of the perineum and sixteen of the vulva proper had been reported. The majority of perineal endometriomata appear at the sites of healed episiotomy or perineorrhaphy scars. A few lesions have been reported after bartholinectomy and other surgical procedures on the vulva. It is significant that uterine curettage has usually preceded these surgical procedures. Endometriosis in a hernial sac that extends to the vulva or in a round ligament near its labial attachment is not actually an authentic vulvar lesion. Most, if not all, vulvar and perineal endometriomata are clear-cut implantations of viable endometrial fragments from the uterine cavity. Considering the frequency with which endometrial cells must be transplanted during obstetric delivery, it is surprising that the perineum is not involved more often. (In the past, this observation has been used as an argument against Sampson's theory of implantation.) The number of the vulvar and perineal lesions appears to be related to the potential of implanted endometrial tissue to survive, which, in turn, may possibly be inversely proportional to the degree of stimulation by progesterone to which the endometrium has been subjected before implantation. Thus, implanted proliferative endometrium would be more likely to survive than secretory endometrium, and the latter would be more likely to survive than gestational endometrium. Also, successful implantation is partially dependent upon high estrogen levels, which are lacking during the first few weeks after childbirth.

Clinical features

The period between the time of implantation and the appearance of the gross and symptomatic lesion of the vulva varies from a few months to several years. Pain and tenderness of the involved site, particularly during menstruation, are characteristic. According to several reports, pain is experienced by some patients only after menstruation. If the lesion is near the anal canal, defecation is painful. Dyspareunia is associated with all lesions of significant size. A dark brown or bloody discharge from the site of the nodule is reported by an occasional patient.

Grossly, the size of endometrial growths of the vulva and perineum varies from a few millimeters to several centimeters and may noticeably increase at the time of menstruation. Usually one or more firm nodules are present, sometimes projecting above the sur-

Endometriosis

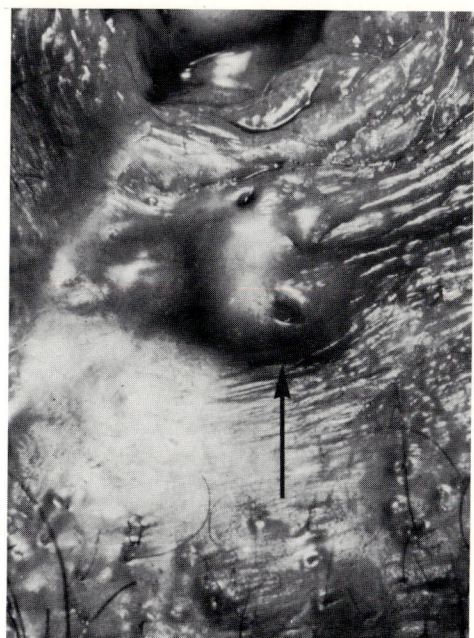

Fig. 6-1. Endometriosis of vulva in a perineorrhaphy scar.

face of the skin (Fig. 6-1). If they are superficial, the overlying skin has a bluish tint and may bleed during the menstrual cycle. Deeply-placed lesions may be difficult to palpate. Sections through excised lesions will ordinarily show cystic structures containing tarry material, similar to the contents of endometriomata of the ovaries.

Histopathology

Endometrial stroma and glands are microscopically demonstrable. The epithelial cells composing the glands are frequently distorted and may be of the cuboidal or low columnar type. Periglandular hemosiderosis is often present; fibrous tissue usually surrounds individual lesions. Not uncommonly, if the lesions are of long duration, the endometrial glands and stroma may be largely or partially replaced by dense fibrous tissue containing many pigment-laden microphages. During pregnancy, a decidual reaction takes place.

Treatment

The lesions should be removed by moderately wide excision. Because of the nature of the disease, recurrences are not uncommon. Long-term administration of a combination of estrogen and progestogen may bring about resolution of smaller lesions; this, however, is hardly worth the effort, since local excision is not a major procedure. For repeated recurrences, this approach to treatment might be considered.

Endometriosis of the cervix
Etiology

Primary cervical endometriosis. Endometriosis that originates on or within the cervix is regarded as primary. The dominant theories of etiology include implantation of fragments from the endometrium, lymphatic and vascular metastases from the endometrium, activation of embryonal cell rests, and metaplasia of cervical epithelium.

The ectocervix is the squamous cell mucosa extending from the external os to the vaginal fornices. Only one explanation of the origin of endometriosis in this site—that the implantation and subsequent growth of shed endometrial cells occurs in recently traumatized sites—seems logical. The trauma can be induced by cauterization, conization, punch biopsy, surgical repair, curettage, or, perhaps, abortion or delivery. *Superficial cervical endometriosis* serves as an example of Sampson's implantation theory of endometriosis, and every investigator who has seen a significant number of cases has attributed their development to this mechanism. Of Williams' 111 patients, seventy-four gave a history of surgical trauma to the cervix, and all except five of the other patients reported having had either a full-term delivery or a prior abortion. Sixty-four of sixty-eight patients with superficial cervical endometriosis observed by one of us (H.L.G.) gave an unmistakable history of trauma to the cervix. Each of the other four women had had either an abortion or a full-term delivery. Of the sixty-eight patients, thirty-four were known to have had no signs or symptoms of endometriosis before the traumatic incident. We have been unable to relate any case of ectocervical endometriosis to extension from the cul-de-sac, although pelvic disease was suspected or proved in thirteen of the sixty-eight patients.

Other personal experience also substantiates the implantation theory. For a number of years one of us (H.L.G.) has indicated more or less routinely on drawings of the cervix the site of biopsy and the site and extent of cauterization. Endometriosis has repeatedly been observed later in these sites of trauma. For example, the patients displaying the lesions in Fig. 6-2 had had multiple punch biopsies and cauterization of the biopsy sites less than 12 months before the endometriosis was discovered. Lesions involving the entire periphery of the external os may develop after conization or whole erosion cauterization (Fig. 6-3). Branscomb, in a 3 to 5 year follow-up of 153 patients whom she had cauterized, found that abnormal premenstrual spotting developed in forty-eight (32 percent). Adequate cervical biopsy specimens were removed from forty of her patients; in eleven of the specimens, endometrial glands and stroma were discovered, whereas two other specimens yielded only endometrial stroma. In Branscomb's opinion, if serial sections could have been made on all of the biopsy specimens, endometriosis might have been found more often. From her experience, it might be concluded that superficial cervical endometriosis develops in at least 10 percent of patients on whom cauterization of the cervix is performed. According to our own "shirt-sleeve" calculation, demonstrable lesions will develop in 5 to 10 percent of patients subjected to moderate cauterization, and in 20 to 25 percent of those who have an electroconization. Without question, if the cervix is traumatized by cauterization or conization, superficial endometriosis will develop in a significant number of patients, in contrast to the few with untraumatized cervices. Repeated packing of the cervix of these patients to control bleeding seems to further predispose the cervix to endometriosis.

For lack of convincing evidence and as a matter of logic, we remain unconvinced that metaplasia explains any case of cervical endometriosis, either superficial or deep. One possibility that cannot be completely ignored is its origin in an embryonic rest. Displaced or persistent nests of embryonal cells of the paramesonephric (müllerian) duct system are of a pluripotent nature (tubal, endometrial, and cervical) and could persist, occasionally giving rise to vaginal adenosis, which is not unlike endometriosis.

Proved examples of *endocervical endometriosis* are few in number. The majority of such lesions probably represent upward extension of the superficial ectocervical disease. We have observed several superficial primary lesions in this location. No proved examples arising from a downward growth of endometrium have come to our attention. The endocervix must be a frequent site of unsuccessful implantation, since at the time of dilatation and curettage it is traumatized, and endometrial fragments are smeared on the injured or partially denuded surfaces, probably being pressed into healthy nidi. In view of the few lesions in this location, the endocervix presumably has a natural hostility to endometrial implants. This is perhaps explained by a competitive, rapid regeneration of the glandular endocervical epithelium. The true incidence of the lesions may be much higher than is apparent, since the endocervical canal is relatively inaccessible to inspection and biopsy, and since implants would be protected from physical trauma likely to produce metrorrhagia (the only significant symptom of the superficial disease).

Deep primary lesions within the fibromuscular matrix of the cervix are seldom diagnosed and then only in the removed uterus. They exhibit no established clinical pattern. Although posttraumatic implantation is the most logical explanation, development from late activation of a deeply displaced remnant of an embryonal müllerian duct would be difficult to disprove. Theoretically, cells from the endometrium could metastasize through lymphatic vessels or veins; however, this would necessarily be statistically rare, and to establish that it is the mode of origin of any single case would be almost impossible.

Secondary cervical endometriosis. Secondary lesions found within the cervix are those that have spread from other sites of endometriosis by direct extension or by vascular or lymphatic metastasis. The usual site or origin is the cul-de-sac.

A large percentage of patients with intrapelvic endometriosis has lesions of the cul-de-sac, particularly at the sites of its uterosacral attachments to the uterus. Much of the posterior fibromuscular matrix of the cervix is separated from the abdominal cavity by a single layer of peritoneum and perhaps by a layer of endopelvic fascia in this area; since these structures are poor barriers, the posterior cervical wall is often involved to some degree. As a rule, these secondary cervical lesions are an insignificant part of the total primary pelvic disease.

Another theoretical source of secondary cervical endometriosis would be the downward extension of adenomyosis into the cervical matrix. If unbroken endometriosis could be followed microscopically from the deep myometrium to a point below the isthmus, presumptive proof of secondary cervical disease from this source might be gained. To our knowledge, no such example has been reported.

The remaining possible origin of secondary disease would be that of lymphatic or hematogenous spread from primary pelvic lesions. Proof of origin by such routes is extremely difficult; nevertheless, one of our patients had a proved endometrioma 1.5 cm. in diameter between the bladder trigone and anterior cervix at a point well below the internal os. This lesion involved both the anterior cervical wall and the bladder musculature. Since no endometriosis intervened between the cul-de-sac and the lesion, a vascular or lymphatic route of spread might be assumed.

Incidence

Cervical endometriosis was first reported by Fels in 1928. Ranney and Chung described sixteen cases in 1952 and could find only twelve previously recorded cases. The apparent rarity of this disorder was convincingly disproved, however, when Williams and Richardson (1955) and Williams (1960) reported 111 cases of the superficial disease accumulated in their private practices. In contrast, Javert, in a retrospective study of pathology reports, found only seven examples in 24,436 hospital dismissals. Other reports, including those of Novak and Hoge, Branscomb, Wolfe, Mackles, Greene, and Gardner, further disproved the opinion that cervical endometriosis is rare.

We include cervical endometriosis in this book because of the embryologic and histologic similarity of the vagina and ectocervix.

Clinical features

Symptoms. Pelvic pain is not a symptom of superficial cervical endometriosis. With respect to the extremely rare primary nodule involving the deep fibromuscular tissues of the cervix, clinical experience is obviously limited. Pelvic pain from secondary cervical lesions arising by extension from the cul-de-sac is only a part of the total clinical picture.

In our experience, superficial cervical endometriosis has been one of the chief causes of persistent or recurrent minimal metrorrhagias, even more so than cervical or endometrial polyps. The type of intermenstrual bleeding most often reported by patients is premenstrual spotting for 3 to 14 days (forty-six of sixty-three patients). Approximately a third of those affected have postmenstrual spotting for 2 to 7 days. Contact bleeding is common, although erratic spotting may be unrelated to either menstruation or coitus. The bleeding pattern of many patients varies from cycle to cycle, and some patients experience all varieties of spotting. Of the sixty-eight patients in one of our series (H.L.G.) with superficial disease, sixty-two gave a clear-cut history of metrorrhagia, whereas Williams (1960) found that only sixty-nine of his 111 patients had abnormal bleeding.

Objective signs. *Superficial cervical endometriosis* constitutes the only clinically characteristic variety of the primary disease. Practically all such lesions are apparent on speculum examination. The lesions have a superficial submucosal position and do not form the large masses typical of pelvic endometriomata. As a rule, the examiner finds round, slightly elevated red to dark blue spots, measuring 2 to 3 mm. in diameter and resembling hemorrhagic nabothian cysts (Fig. 6-2) on the ectocervix. Because of their tendency to cyclic rupture, the rounded, papular lesions seldom reach a diameter of more than 5 mm. Some small lesions resemble hemorrhagic herpetic blebs or "blood blisters," whereas others are macular and only slightly elevated, depending upon cellular and capillary activity from hormonal influences. Macular lesions of a light red color with poorly defined edges are sometimes difficult to visualize, particularly during the early phase of the menstrual cycle, although shortly before menstruation they may become darker, slightly elevated, and enlarged. The macular type is more extensive than the small rounded lesions. They remain flat and superficial and usually do not develop into nodules. Some of the larger macular lesions exhibit bizarre configurations. Occasionally, the external os is surrounded by irregular peripheral extensions

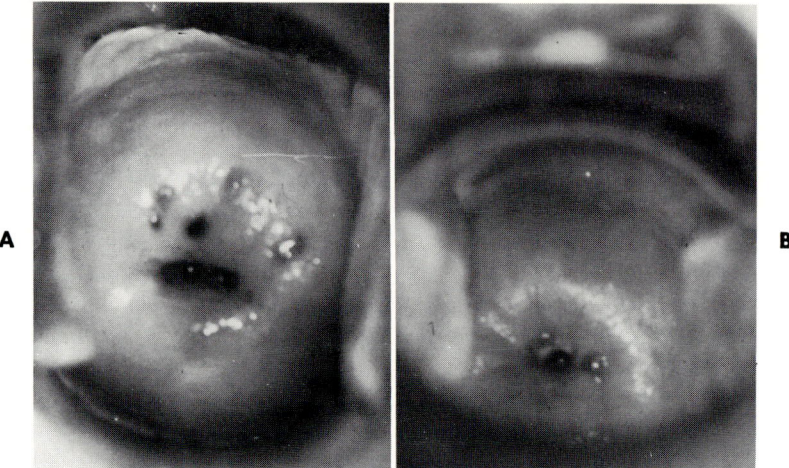

Fig. 6-2. **A** and **B**, Superficial endometriosis of ectocervix, resembling hemorrhagic nabothian cysts. Lesions followed multiple punch biopsies and cauterization. (Gardner, H. L.: Amer. J. Obstet. Gynec. **84:**170, 1962.)

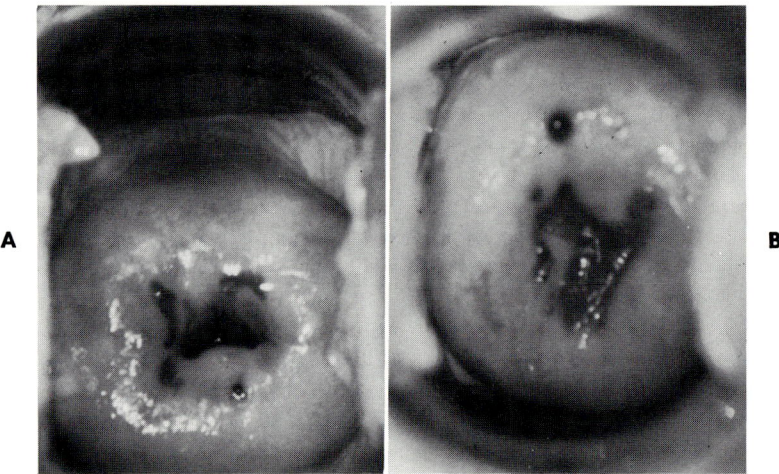

Fig. 6-3. **A**, Superficial cervical endometriosis that developed after cauterization. **B**, Superficial cervical endometriosis that developed after electroconization. (Gardner, H. L.: Amer. J. Obstet. Gynec. **84:**170, 1962.)

for a distance of 1 cm. (Fig. 6-3), particularly in patients who have had a conization or an extensive cauterization. Also, macular lesions of varying shades of redness often develop at a distance from the external os. Grossly, these may resemble areas of localized erythema, whereas lesions about the external os may be mistaken for erosion. Maceration or superficial ulceration of the overlying mucosa can be induced by coitus or other physical trauma, though many lesions rupture spontaneously before or with the menses. Following trauma with the speculum or cotton-tipped applicator, some lesions appear to increase in diameter from submucosal bleeding.

The puckered, scarred appearance characteristic of the intrapelvic disease is rarely, if ever, apparent in cervical lesions. We have never observed such scarring, nor have we observed any similarity of the occasional endometrioma to invasive carcinoma, as has been reported.

A description of the clinical features of primary lesions found deep within the fibromuscular wall of the cervix is unnecessary;

these are extremely rare and usually are not perceptable on physical examination. Secondary deposits in the cervix from intrapelvic disease are usually not independently discernible. Occasionally, speculum examination of a patient without visible ectocervical disease will reveal fresh bleeding from the endocervix. Superficial endocervical disease may be suspected; proof, however, will depend upon adequate biopsy or conization. It is possible that more cases would be found if the endocervix could be adequately visualized and if appropriate specimens of tissue were removed routinely in the presence of prolonged intermenstrual spotting.

Of twelve pregnant patients known to have had cervical endometriosis before pregnancy, Williams (1960) found that ten exhibited clinical evidence of a decidual reaction. We have repeatedly observed gross decidual reactions in patients who had been clinically "cured" of cervical endometriosis before pregnancy. For example, obvious gross decidual reactions developed in ten of fourteen pregnant patients who had previously been found to have cervical endometriosis. Most of these patients had been treated before pregnancy with presumed success. Each of three cervical biopsies taken from patients with clinical deciduomas exhibited a typical decidual reaction, yet none contained endometrial glands. Possibly, in some patients, residual endometrial stromatosis alone is responsible for the gross decidual reaction; however, decidual changes are observable in many biopsy specimens taken during pregnancy from the cervices of patients who had previously exhibited no evidence of endometriosis.

Histopathology

Proof of superficial cervical endometriosis should perhaps depend upon demonstration of both endometrial glands and stroma. From a practical standpoint, however, a grossly characteristic area with an abundance of endometrial stroma might be acceptable as proof of the disease. The proportion of glands to stroma is highly variable, and subserial sections that include the entire specimen are sometimes necessary for the demonstration of both components. Functionally, the superficial lesions usually correspond closely to the phase of the menstrual cycle (Figs. 6-4 and 6-5). The responsiveness to both estrogens and progestogens implies a well-differentiated functional tissue, such as would be expected from implants. The functional activity is best determined premenstrually (Fig. 6-5), when the typical changes of a secretory endometrium are usually apparent. The cyclic response of superficial cervical disease differs somewhat from the less common cyclic changes of encapsulated pelvic lesions.

Intrastromal infiltration with red blood cells and hemorrhage into glandular spaces

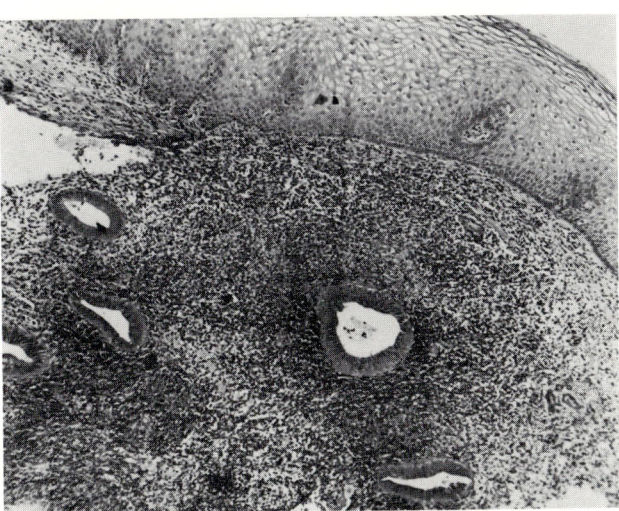

Fig. 6-4. Superficial cervical endometriosis, proliferative phase. (H & E × 45) (Gardner, H. L.: Clin. Obstet. Gynec. 9:358, 1966.)

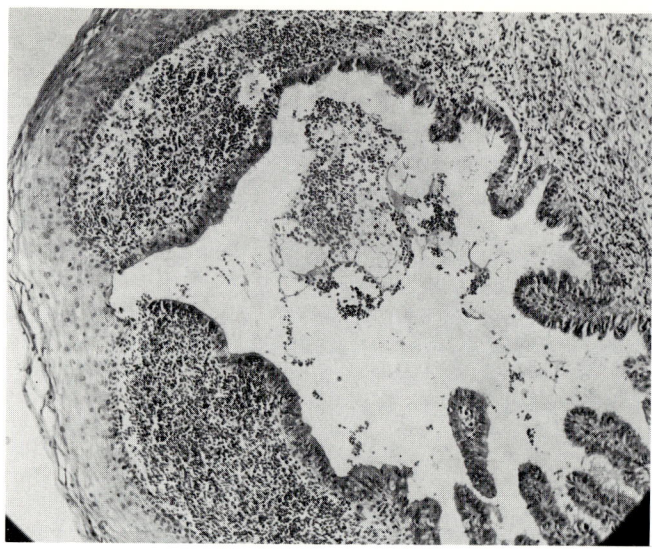

Fig. 6-5. Superficial cervical endometriosis, secretory phase. (H & E × 45) (Gardner, H. L.: Amer. J. Obstet. Gynec. **84:** 170, 1962.)

are frequently observed, particularly around the menstrual phase of the cycle. A minor leukocytic infiltration, slightly peripheral to the lesions or within the endometrial stroma, is often present. The squamous epithelium overlying many individual lesions is thinned or disrupted, or both, from mechanical trauma or spontaneous premenstrual maceration. During pregnancy, patients with cervical endometriosis manifest typical decidual reactions at the sites of endometriosis.

Diagnosis of superficial cervical endometriosis

A large number of patients with hemorrhagic submucosal lesions of the cervix and persistent minimal metrorrhagia will be found to have superficial cervical endometriosis. Such lesions are usually more apparent premenstrually.

Williams (1960) has repeatedly pointed out the necessity of knife excision of the tissues for diagnosis of this condition. He believes that the ordinary technique of biopsy of the cervix can fail, since the small superficial lesions are likely to rupture, allowing escape of the bulk of the glandular mass. With few exceptions, we have established the diagnosis from specimens removed by punch biopsy with the use of the Schubert instrument. Admittedly, however, no microscopic evidence was found in many other patients who were considered clinically to have the disease. Branscomb's experience, as well as our own, might well bear out the validity of Williams' advice.

Treatment

Treatment for the primary superficial disease consists of its excision or destruction. Excision can be performed with a sharp punch biopsy instrument, the scalpel, or the loop electrode. Destruction by cauterization or coagulation is also useful, particularly as an adjunct to excision. Recurrence at the original site takes place surprisingly often. Whether some "recurrences" represent new implants in a susceptible patient or persistence of an inadequately excised lesion may be difficult to determine. Inadequate treatment, however, seems a more logical explanation for most of the failures.

When the lesions recur following treatment, we agree with Williams (1965) that they should be excised immediately after a menstrual period and that subsequent menstrual periods be suppressed with hormones until the operative site has completely healed.

Endometriosis of the vagina
Primary vaginal endometriosis

The varieties, the etiology, the pathology, and the symptoms of primary vaginal endometriosis are essentially identical with those of the cervical disease. Primary vaginal lesions

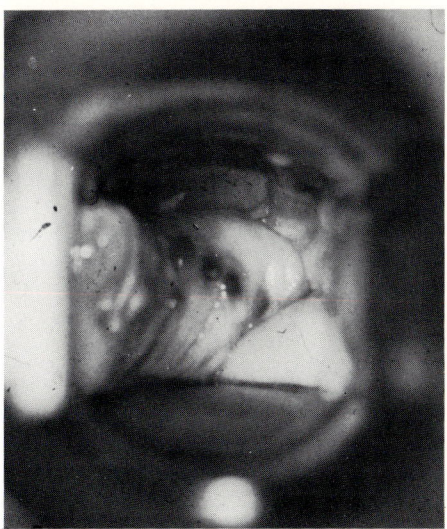 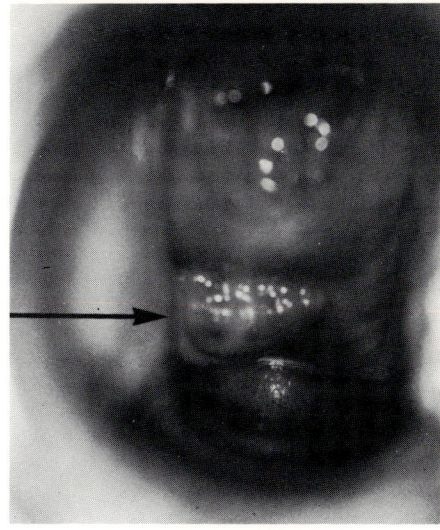

Fig. 6-6. Primary endometriosis of right vaginal wall. (Gardner, H. L.: Clin. Obstet. Gynec. 9: 358, 1966.)

Fig. 6-7. Endometriosis of posterior vaginal fornix, secondary to lesions in cul-de-sac. (Gardner, H. L.: Clin. Obstet. Gynec. 9:358, 1966.)

(Fig. 6-6) arise mainly from implantation of shed endometrial fragments in traumatized areas. In our experience, they have been relatively rare. During the same period of time in which sixty-eight cases of superficial cervical disease were observed by one of us (H. L. G.), only six cases of primary superficial vaginal endometriosis were discovered. Two other patients without pelvic endometriosis were found to have lesions in the vaginal vault after hysterectomy (one complete abdominal hysterectomy and one vaginal hysterectomy requiring morcellation). Because of the rarity of vaginal endometriosis subsequent to hysterectomy, Reich, Nechtow, and Abrams thought it worthwhile to report a single case. Green and Meigs collected twelve cases from a large gynecologic service over a few years' time; in ten of these, intrapelvic disease was associated. Schmid was able to implant endometrial fragments in the vaginal cuff at the time of hysterectomy and obtain an almost 100 percent "take."

Williams (1965) reported a patient with extensive endometriosis of the vagina after a severe chemical burn of the vaginal mucosa. We have observed vaginal endometriosis in the site of deep vaginal ulceration and subsequent exuberant granulation caused by placement of a bichloride of mercury tablet in the vagina.

Endometriosis may develop after vaginal plastic procedures, though its extreme rarity defies explanation. The infrequency of vaginal lesions secondary to obstetric delivery is at least partially explained by the known resistance of gestational endometrium to successful implantation and by the low estrogen levels after delivery. Theoretically, endometrium-destined müllerian cell rests could give rise to primary vaginal endometriosis, yet this would be difficult to prove. Variants of vaginal adenosis might be confused histologically with endometriosis.

Secondary vaginal endometriosis

Secondary vaginal endometriosis is perhaps more common than the primary disease. Many patients with pelvic endometriosis have nodules that are palpable through the posterior vaginal fornix. Visible dark nodulations in the posterior fornix (Fig. 6-7) leave no doubt as to their nature and origin. In microscopic sections through such areas, the fibromuscular layers of the vaginal wall are invaded by endometrial tissue. The number of vaginal lesions that develop after operations for pelvic endometriosis is surprisingly few, considering the number of opportunities for their doing so. Such lesions are classified as secondary, whether they arise from direct extension after operation or from implantation and growth of endometriotic fragments.

Treatment

Treatment for primary superficial vaginal endometriosis is identical with that employed for superficial cervical lesions. Secondary lesions associated with pain or annoying bleeding sometimes require more extensive surgical excision or removal of the ovaries, or both. Often, bleeding and pain can be alleviated by the production of "pseudopregnancy" by treatment of the patient with a combination of estrogen and progestogen.

REFERENCES

Binder, S. S.: Endometriosis of the vulva and perineum, Pacif. Med. Surg. 73:294, 1965.

Branscomb, L.: Habitual premenstrual spotting following electrocauterization of the cervix: A newly observed phenomenon, Amer. J. Obstet. Gynec. 79:16, 1960.

Fels, E.: Endometriose der Portio, Zbl. Gynaek. 52:285, 1928.

Gardner, H. L.: Cervical endometriosis, a lesion of increasing importance, Amer. J. Obstet. Gynec. 84:170, 1962.

Gardner, H. L.: Cervical and vaginal endometriosis, Clin. Obstet. Gynec. 9:90, 1966.

Green, T. H., and Meigs, J. V.: Pseudomenstruation from posthysterectomy vaginal vault endometriosis, Obstet. Gynec. 4:622, 1954.

Javert, C. T.: Observations on the pathology and spread of endometriosis based on the theory of benign metastasis, Amer. J. Obstet. Gynec. 62:477, 1951.

Novak, E. R., and Hoge, A. F.: Endometriosis of the lower genital tract, Obstet. Gynec. 12:687, 1958.

Ranney, B., and Chung, J. T.: Endometriosis of the cervix uteri, Amer. J. Obstet. Gynec. 64:1333, 1952.

Reich, W. J., Nechtow, M. J., and Abrams, R.: Endometriosis of the vagina following vaginal hysterectomy, Amer. J. Obstet. Gynec. 56:1192, 1948.

Schmid, H. H.: Kunstliche Endometriosis, Arch Gynaek. 155:217, 1934.

Williams, G. A.: Endometriosis of the cervix uteri—a common disease, Amer. J. Obstet. Gynec. 80:734, 1960.

Williams, G. A.: Post-surgical and post-traumatic tumors of the vulva and vagina, Clin. Obstet. Gynec. 8:309, 1965.

Williams, G. A., and Richardson, A. C.: Endometriosis of the cervix uteri, Obstet. Gynec. 6:309, 1955.

Wolfe, S. A., Mackles, A., and Greene, H. J.: Endometriosis of the cervix, Amer. J. Obstet. Gynec. 81:111, 1961.

Chapter 7
Adenosis

The definition of vaginal adenosis is controversial. Evans and Paine, as well as others, consider multiple glands or cysts in the subepithelial connective tissues of the vaginal wall to be indicative of the disease. Sandberg and others (1967) have extended the definition to include all varieties of vaginal lesions containing, or being composed of, cells producing mucus and having the morphologic and histochemical characteristics of cells lining the endocervix. This would include vaginal cysts, regardless of their size. We do not completely accept such a broad definition. Rather, we prefer to interpret vaginal adenosis as microscopically or grossly visible lesions formed by replacement of the normal squamous epithelium of the vagina by glandular epithelium.

In 1910, Bonney and Glendining reported a case in which the normal vaginal mucosa had been almost entirely replaced by proliferating mucus-secreting columnar epithelium. They designated this condition "adenomatosis vaginae." Subsequently, Plaut and Dreyfuss suggested the term "adenosis," believing it more appropriate for nonneoplastic lesions of this nature.

Prior to 1967, approximately fifty-five cases of adenosis vaginae had been reported. In 1967, Sandberg, Danielson, and Prince reported ten cases, chiefly cystic lesions, which they designated "adenosis." Although most of these ten cases were clear-cut examples of what we would call small paramesonephric vaginal cysts, the authors offered good reasons for their diagnosis of adenosis. Subsequently, Sandberg reported the discovery of glands in vaginas removed at autopsy from nine of twenty-two postpubertal subjects. He considered such nests of vaginal glands to represent "occult" adenosis. Regardless of the ultimately adopted concept of vaginal adenosis, its incidence is obviously higher than is indicated by the number of cases reported.

Histogenesis

In 1877, von Prueschen reported the discovery of mucus-secreting glandular tissues in the submucosa of four of thirty-six vaginas removed at autopsy. Since that time, numerous reports have been published, including Sandberg's (1968), in which subepithelial nests or islands of glandular tissue in the vaginal wall were described. It has been generally agreed that most of these nests are remnants of the embryonic müllerian (paramesonephric) epithelium. The majority of embryologists believe that the entire vaginal canal was originally lined with müllerian epithelium and subsequently replaced with stratified squamous epithelium growing upward from the urogenital sinus. According to the most widely accepted theory of origin, adenosis arises from these subepithelial islands of persistent müllerian epithelium, either mature or undifferentiated. Sandberg and others (1965) have referred to the islands as the "occult form" of adenosis and regard them as the progenitors of all the clinical forms. As evidence that vaginal adenosis does not arise by extension of glandular epithelium from the endocervix, these authors also point out the lack of gross or histologic continuity of the lesions with the cervix and their frequent localization in the lower vagina. Should a cervical erosion ever spread to the vaginal fornices, however, it would perhaps represent a form of adenosis. Dougherty described such a lesion and called it adenosis.

Metaplasia of either mesodermal or basal

squamous epithelial cells is another, although not widely accepted, theory of the histogenesis of adenosis. Siders, Parrott, and Abell reported that the columnar glandular cells of the lesion were often continuous with and appeared to arise from basal cells of the squamous mucosa; for this reason, they considered adenosis to be a form of prosoplasia.

The conditions that precipitate the appearance of clinical vaginal adenosis are usually not apparent. Thinning and ulceration over the glandular structures, incident to trichomoniasis and candidiasis, seems to be one logical explanation for some cases. This opinion is supported by Evans and Hughes. Excessive physiologic stimulation of the glandular tissues, with consequent secretion, formation of cysts, and rupture into the vagina, has also been suggested as a cause of the fistulization between glandular masses and the vaginal canal. Should sinuses already connect the glandular masses with the vaginal canal, a pronounced alteration of physiology might explain replacement of areas of squamous cell mucosa by glandular epithelium in a manner similar to the formation of cervical erosion.

Types of adenosis

Sandberg and others (1965) proposed dividing adenosis into four different types as follows: the occult, the cystic, the effluent, and the adenomatous.

In the *occult type,* the submucosa contains quiescent noncystic glandular elements that are detectable only by histologic examination. Although such nests of cells may be the progenitors of all other forms, not all pathologists would agree that they constitute vaginal adenosis in the clinical sense.

The *cystic type* of adenosis is described as being exhibited by one or more cystic structures formed by the accumulation of mucinous material within the glandular spaces. This group comprises both large and small grossly apparent cysts. Here again, it is unlikely that all observers would agree that every grossly visible vaginal cyst, regardless of size, lined by a cervical type of glandular epithelium should be considered as an example of vaginal adenosis. We prefer to classify such cystic lesions beneath intact vaginal mucosa as paramesonephric cysts, although this is a purely academic point.

In the *effluent type,* areas of normal vaginal squamous epithelium have been replaced by the subepithelial glands. Sandberg and others (1965) believe that, logically, these lesions develop by outward growth of the glandular epithelium through luminal communications with the vagina, yet they do not propose that this is the only mechanism of their origin. This variety meets the criteria of vaginal adenosis most acceptable to us.

The *adenomatous type,* exemplified by an accumulated overgrowth of glandular epithelium, forms a vaginal mass resembling an endocervical polyp.

Clinical features

The usual rate of development of adenosis has not been determined. Once established, the lesions behave somewhat as a cervical erosion, although they are less likely to regress spontaneously. The observations of Siders, Parrott, and Abell suggest that gradual healing may take place, with the lesions being supplanted by a squamous cell overgrowth that may eventually result in an apparently normal vagina. It is frequently stated in the medical literature that spontaneous regression is unusual.

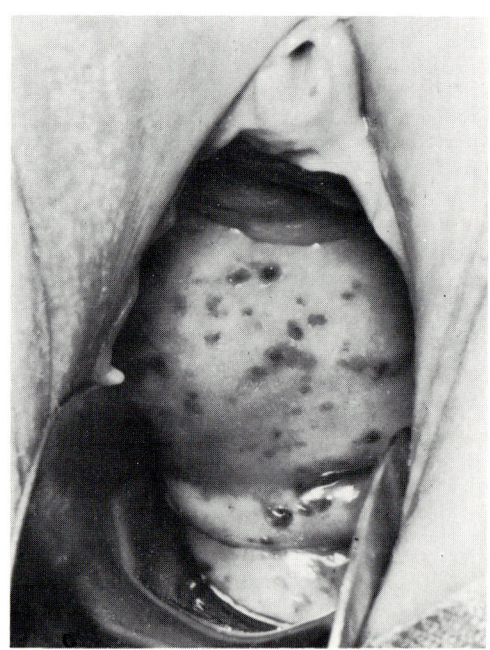

Fig. 7-1. Extensive adenosis of vagina. (Evans, D., and Hughes, H.: J. Obstet. Gynaec. Brit. Comm. 68:247, 1961.)

Symptoms. Vaginal adenosis may or may not be symptomatic. An excessive mucoid vaginal discharge is the most often reported complaint, and next in order is minimal postcoital bleeding. Dyspareunia may be experienced.

Objective signs. According to our preferred criteria of vaginal adenosis, the individual lesions most often consist of red patches resembling an erosion, though they have also been described as granular or ulcer-like. The patches, usually only a few millimeters in diameter, may be scattered over any part of the vaginal surface or, in some cases, even the entire vagina (Fig. 7-1). Again, the lesions may be confluent, producing large red, raw areas. The vestibule is occasionally involved. We have observed vaginal polyps that meet Sandberg and others' (1965) description of adenomatous adenosis, being essentially identical, both grossly and microscopically, to polyps of endocervical origin.

Excessive vaginal mucus is often present, especially if the disease is extensive. Bonney and Glendining reported the case of a patient with lesions that secreted as much as 180 gm. of mucus daily, and Stabler (1967) reported the case of a patient who secreted 381 ml. in 24 hours. The individual lesions bleed rather easily upon traumatization, and spontaneous bleeding is not uncommon. Usually the bleeding is of the nature of minimal metrorrhagia.

Histopathology

Although it is generally agreed that the glandular tissue of these lesions is of the endocervical type, Evans and Paine and others have found that it may occasionally resemble tubal or endometrial epithelium. Should endometrial-destined müllerian epithelial rests proliferate to form gross lesions, the diagnosis of endometriosis would perhaps be more appropriate, especially if endometrial stroma were present. The most characteristic cell of adenosis is the tall columnar type with a basal nucleus, corresponding to the "picket" cells of the cervix (Fig. 7-2). The cellular cytoplasm and the fluid secreted contain mucus, which is recognizable by a positive reaction with mucicarmine and PAS stains. The areas of vaginal mucosa that appear ulcerated or eroded are usually covered by columnar cells. Irregular glandular spaces may be present in the substantia propria. As a rule, the adjacent stroma exhibits no significant inflammatory reaction, nor does it have a characteristic appearance, as does the endometrium or endometriosis.

Since adenosis and other paramesonephric lesions stain with mucicarmine, they are easily distinguished from Gartner's duct cysts, the latter being mucicarmine-negative. Also, Gartner's duct cysts are usually lined with low cuboidal epithelium. Still another feature of Gartner's duct cysts lacking in paramesonephric structures is a layer of smooth muscle adjacent to the glandular lining. Sandberg and others (1965) have distinguished the cervical variety of paramesonephric gland from the tubal and endometrial types by testing for the metachromasia present in cervical cells with toluidine blue O stain.

Treatment

No treatment is required for asymptomatic lesions. Siders, Parrott, and Abell have reported good responses of the multiple lesions to the application of a cautery or silver nitrate. We successfully treated one patient

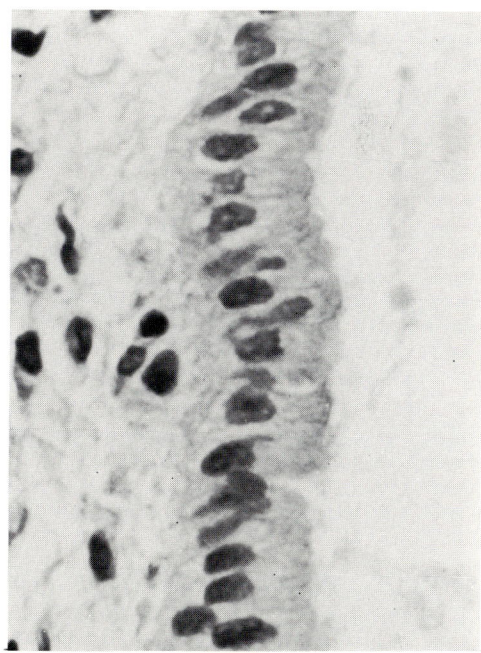

Fig. 7-2. Adenosis of vagina. The lining cells resemble endocervical epithelium. (H & E × 1200)

with a limited number of small lesions by cauterization. Polypoid forms are excised. Sandberg and others (1965) found simple excision of all varieties of lesions effective. They suggested that vaginectomy and hysterectomy may be necessary for the occasional extensive lesions, the vaginal mucosa being replaced by a skin graft if preservation of the vagina is desired. Stabler reported successful treatment of several patients by vaginectomy and a delayed split skin graft of the canal. This procedure allows preservation of the uterus.

Karnaky allegedly eradicates practically all cervical erosions by maintenance of an extremely acid vagina (pH 1.8 to 2.4) with the use of the buffered powder, Tramigill. This treatment for erosion is based upon the theory that cervical glandular epithelium cannot survive in such a highly acid medium, whereas stratified squamous epithelium is stimulated to proliferate and replace glandular epithelium. Since vaginal adenosis is similar to cervical erosion in most respects, it would be interesting to observe the effects of this buffered powder upon the "effluent" type. If the opinion is correct that vaginal infections such as candidiasis and trichomoniasis sometimes stimulate the development of clinical adenosis, a search for these pathogens is indicated and, if found, they should be eradicated.

REFERENCES

Bonney, V., and Glendining, B.: Adenomatosis vaginae, a hitherto undescribed condition, Proc. Roy. Soc. Med. **4**:18, 1910-11.

Dougherty, C. M.: Histopathology of surgically excised lesions of the vagina, Ann. N. Y. Acad. Sci. **83**:328, 1959.

Evans, D. M. D., and Hughes, H.: Cysts of the vaginal wall, J. Obstet. Gynaec. Brit. Comm. **68**:247, 1961.

Evans, D. M. D., and Paine, C. D.: Benign cysts and tumors of developmental origin, Clin. Obstet. Gynec. **8**:997, 1965.

Karnaky, K. J.: A simple, self-administered treatment for the prevention and destruction of cervical ulcers and pre-cancerous lesions, Med. Rec. Ann. **55**:200, 1962.

Plaut, A., and Dreyfuss, M. L.: Adenosis of vagina and its relation to primary adenocarcinoma of vagina, Surg. Gynec. Obstet. **71**: 756, 1940.

Sandberg, E. C.: The incidence and distribution of occult vaginal adenosis, Amer. J. Obstet. Gynec. **101**:322, 1968.

Sandberg, E.: C., Danielson, R. W., Cauwet, R. W., and Bonar, B. E.: Adenosis vaginae, Amer. J. Obstet. Gynec. **93**:209, 1965.

Sandberg, E. C., Danielson, R. W., and Prince, E.: Benign vaginal adenosis, Obstet. Gynec. **30**:93, 1967.

Siders, D. B., Parrott, M. H., and Abell, M. R.: Gland cell prosoplasia (adenosis) of vagina, Amer. J. Obstet. Gynec. **91**:190, 1965.

Stabler, F.: Adenomatosis vaginae, J. Obstet. Gynaec. Brit. Comm. **68**:857, 1961.

Stabler, F.: The treatment of adenosis vaginae, J. Obstet. Gynaec. Brit. Comm. **74**:493, 1967.

von Preuschen, F.: Ueber Cystenbildung in der Vagina, Virchow Arch. Path. Anat. **70**:111, 1877.

Chapter 8

Dermatoses of the vulva

Occasionally, the gynecologist observes a patient with a dermatosis of the vulva that is a part of a more generalized dermatologic disease. Even more rarely is a dermatosis limited to the vulva. For the dermatologist, diagnosis and treatment usually are not difficult; for the clinician who is inadequately trained in the interpretation of diseases of the skin, the affections often present diagnostic problems. Again, the classical appearance of these diseases in the area of the vulva may be modified by friction, occlusion, and maceration. In this event, they may simulate many other dermatoses, leading to further confusion in the diagnosis. More important, several of the so-called dermatoses at times resemble "white lesions" and thus are mistaken for "leukoplakia." As a result, treatment is improper or overdone, with disastrous consequences. In the evaluation of a vulvar lesion, the entire surface of the skin should be examined. The presence of characteristic lesions elsewhere will frequently point to the nature of the vulvar disease.

Of the many affections of the vulvar skin, those most often encountered in our experience have been psoriasis, seborrheic dermatitis, lichen planus, pseudoacanthosis nigricans, neurodermatitis, intertrigo, and contact dermatitis. Only the first four of these dermatoses will be discussed in this chapter; neurodermatitis, intertrigo, and contact dermatitis will be discussed in other chapters.

Psoriasis

The prevalence of psoriasis is higher than most gynecologists realize. In the United States, 2 to 3 percent of the population suffers with this disease. The lesions usually develop in multiple sites, although a form of psoriasis (intertriginous psoriasis) appears wherever apocrine glands are numerous, for example, in the axilla, groin, vulva, and intragluteal folds.

Etiology

The tendency to develop psoriasis is probably inherited. Abel, Dobson, and Graham have indicated that the mode of inheritance is a simple dominance with 60 percent penetrance. No biochemical changes characteristic of psoriasis alone have been reported, although an impressive number of biochemical aberrations have been documented. Van Scott and Ekel were able to demonstrate that increased keratin is related to increased mitotic activity of basal cells and therefore to an increased number of cells to form this substance. The turnover rate of the cells in the lesions is 3 to 4 days, in contrast to 28 days in normal skin. Psoriatic plaques are the result of a temporary local disturbance in genetically susceptible skin.

Clinical features

As a rule, psoriasis develops in the female at an early age. Hellgren reported 16 as the median age of onset in his series, and the average age in Perlman's (1964a) patients was 13 years. Psoriasis appeared at the menarche in 18 percent of the patients in Hellgren's series; in 25 percent it developed during pregnancy, and in 27 percent, at the menopause. Approximately 50 percent of his patients reported an improvement during pregnancy, and 45 percent were adversely affected by menstruation.

One of the puzzling features of this dis-

112 Benign diseases of the vulva and vagina

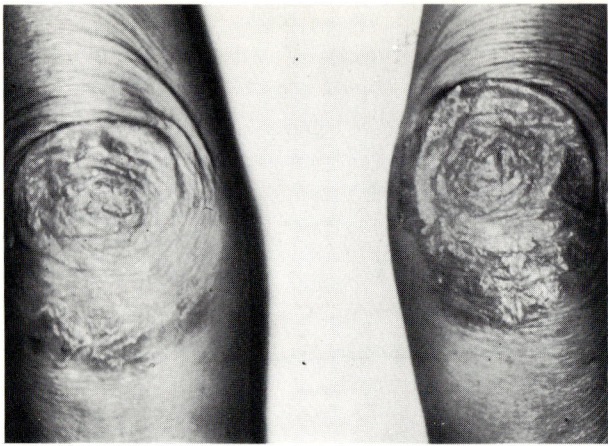

Fig. 8-1. Psoriasis of the elbows, as well as other areas of predilection, gives a clue to the diagnosis of vulvar psoriasis.

ease, and one that makes the evaluation of therapy difficult, is its tendency to spontaneous remission and exacerbation. Lesions may improve during the summer months upon exposure to sunlight or even with change of weight, as well as during pregnancy. Frequently, nervous stress incites an exacerbation of psoriasis.

Psoriasis most often arises on the scalp, behind the ears, over the extensor surfaces of the extremities (especially the elbows and knees; Fig. 8-1), the nails, the trunk, and the sacral and genital areas. The primary lesion is a round, slightly elevated, reddish yellow, squamous papule the size of a pinhead that disappears under pressure. Initially, it may not be scaly, although characteristically it is covered by fine, silvery scales. Gradually, the papule enlarges and becomes a plaque. The lesions are sharply demarcated and, even though covered by scales, the edges are erythematous (Fig. 8-2). When the scales are removed by gentle curettage, fine bleeding points become apparent.

In the genital region, moisture, heat, and friction, characteristic of this location, may give rise to lesions resembling a fungus infection, such as cutaneous candidiasis. Lesions in the vulvar region may exhibit minimal scaling and thus simulate seborrheic dermatitis. Culture of the lesions and examination of scrapings in 20% potassium hydroxide (KOH) solution may aid in differential diagnosis. Of more value is the presence of lesions elsewhere on the body.

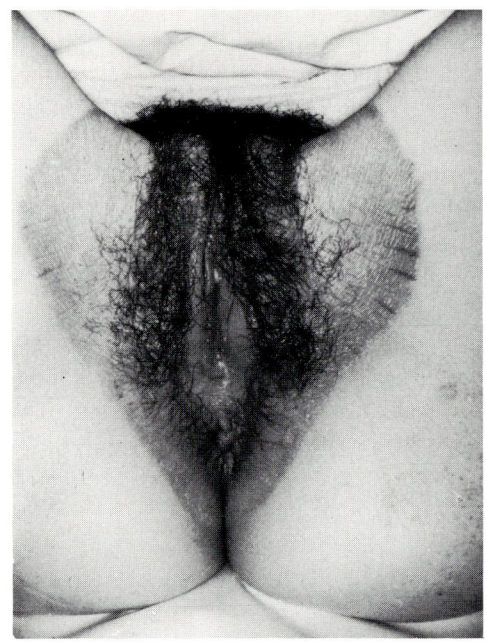

Fig. 8-2. Psoriasis of vulva. Extensive, sharply demarcated lesions. Usually vulvar lesions are less extensive than these.

An interesting phenomenon in psoriasis is the so-called *isomorphic response* (Koebner reaction), which is the appearance of new lesions at the site of an injury to the skin. This usually takes place when new lesions are forming elsewhere on the body or when old lesions are increasing in size.

The subjective symptoms associated with

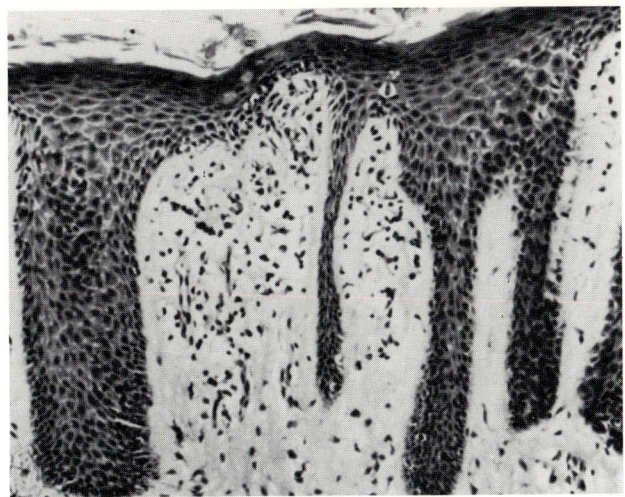

Fig. 8-3. Psoriasis exhibited by a thin suprapapillary plate, edema, clubbing, and hyperemia of the papillae, and elongation of the rete ridges. (H & E × 168) (From case of Dr. Esther Weisfogel, Roslyn, N. Y.)

psoriasis may vary. Pruritus, if associated, may be quite annoying. The unsightly appearance of the lesions is disturbing to many patients.

Histopathology

The epidermal changes of psoriasis consist of parakeratosis, thinning of the suprapapillary plates, edema, clubbing and hyperemia of the papillae, elongation of the rete ridges, and Munro microabscesses (Figs. 8-3 and 8-4). The clinical appearance of the lesions is determined by the predominance of one or another of the various microscopic changes. The horny layer, which is thickened, consists primarily of parakeratotic cells; the consequent scaly surface is the most distinctive feature of the lesion. The silvery appearance of the scales is caused by air pockets in the horny layer. The stratum malpighii over the papillae is thinned, and the rete pegs are elongated, their distal ends being branched and clubbed. These ends may fuse with those of adjacent rete pegs. Between the rete ridges, the papillae are edematous and club shaped. The capillaries are dilated, tortuous, and engorged; this may give a vivid hue to the lesion. The vessels are so near the surface that removal of the scales may tear off the thin suprapapillary area leaving minute bleeding points. The microabscesses of Munro, located in the stratum corneum, consist of small accumu-

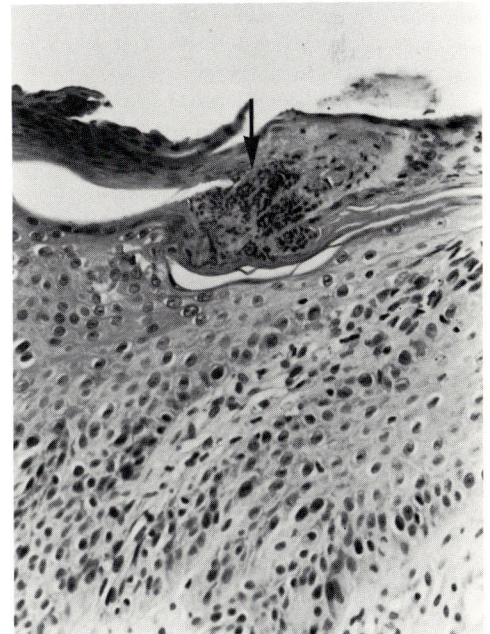

Fig. 8-4. Psoriasis exhibiting microabscess of Munro. (H & E × 160)

lations of neutrophils that have migrated up through the epidermis. Usually, these abscesses are not grossly visible; on occasion, however, they may be predominant, leading to the formation of macroabscesses and the clinical picture of pustular psoriasis.

A mild to moderate inflammatory reaction

is usually present in the upper dermis and papillae. This consists of lymphocytes, histiocytes, and, in the early lesions, polymorphonuclear leukocytes. According to Weddell and others, these so-called inflammatory cells are actually perineural and Schwann cells in all stages of development and degeneration. These authors believe that an excessive proliferation of accessory neural cells in the skin of patients with psoriasis may reflect an increase in the nervous control of growth and differentiation of the skin. As yet, this finding has not been reported by other investigators.

Treatment

The treatment for psoriasis is complicated and difficult and is best left to the dermatologist. Treatment for the vulvar lesions alone is insufficient; it should be directed to the generalized disease. On those rare occasions when the lesions are limited to the vulva, the same measures should be employed.

The general principles of treatment are important. First, it is necessary to gain the confidence of the patient and help her realize that psoriasis is a chronic systemic disease that undergoes spontaneous remissions and relapses. Second, it should be pointed out that, at present, no specific or curative measures are available. All treatment is palliative.

One of the oldest forms of treatment is a modification of the Gaeckerman regime. This consists of local applications of crude coal tar in petrolatum followed by exposure of the lesions to increasing amounts of ultraviolet light. The object of this treatment is to soften and remove scales and to inhibit abnormal keratinization. The development of corticosteroid ointments is one of the major therapeutic advances for psoriasis. These tend to reduce the chronic plaques, especially if applied beneath airtight dressings that are left in place for 8 to 72 hours. Even though the lesions undergo rapid involution, they may reappear in 5 to 7 days after treatment is discontinued; thus, repetition of the applications once or twice weekly may be necessary. Injections of triamcinolone into chronic small lesions may be followed by their complete involution for from 2 to 3 weeks to a year or more. The systemic administration of corticosteroids may bring about a regression of the lesions, although they may recur once treatment is discontinued. In this event, they are extremely difficult to control.

Recently, methotrexate and aminopterin, given orally, have been widely endorsed as therapeutic agents for psoriasis. These drugs, however, should be given only to patients with lesions that are extensive and resistant to other forms of therapy. Aminopterin, in doses of 0.5 gm. daily, or methotrexate, 2.5 mg. daily, has been administered in courses of 7 days, with a rest of 3 days between courses. A total of twenty-one doses is suggested. Callaway, McAfee, and Finlayson have recommended methotrexate in a single weekly dose of 25 to 50 mg. until the lesions are brought under control, and a dose of 10 to 15 mg. per week thereafter. For severe psoriasis, they have combined methotrexate with oral steroids. No recurrence has followed this treatment. The usual careful control of patients receiving any antimetabolite must be observed if these drugs are administered.

Seborrheic dermatitis

Seborrheic dermatitis, although a common disease, seldom involves the vulva. The usual sites are the midportion of the face, the scalp, and the presternal and interscapular regions, the areas most diffusely supplied with sebaceous glands. Eventually, however, the pubic, genital, and perianal regions may become involved. In the majority of cases, the lesions appear first on the scalp. If the vulva is involved, the diagnosis is made by a process of elimination and by the presence of the typical dermatitis in the usual sites.

Etiology

The exact etiology of seborrheic dermatitis has never been determined. Many metabolic causes have been suggested, yet none has been thus far established. The yeast-like fungus *Pityrosporon ovale* and the mite *Demodex folliculorum* have been incriminated, although these organisms are now regarded as probable secondary, rather than causative, invaders. Mental strain and excessive consumption of alcohol or greasy and starchy foods may give rise to exacerbations. Patients with neurologic disorders such as Parkinson's disease often have severe seborrheic dermatitis.

Clinical features

The typical lesions of seborrheic dermatitis are yellow-red and covered with dull, greasy, nonadherent scales and crusts (Figs. 8-5 and 8-6). The lesions are usually poorly defined and superficial, although later they may become infiltrated if an inflammatory reaction takes place in the skin. Initially, one or more erythrematous spots covered with greasy yellow scales may be observed. These tend to increase gradually in size, forming large lesions, often with yellow zones of clearing in the center. On the intertriginous areas, and especially on the vulva, the lesions are likely to become eczematoid because of moisture and friction. Patients frequently complain of mild or moderately severe pruritus.

The disease entities that most often must be differentiated from seborrheic dermatitis are psoriasis, cutaneous moniliasis, tinea cruris, and neurodermatitis. Examination of scrapings of the lesion in 20% potassium hydroxide will usually aid in the differentiation from candiasis and tinea cruris. The similarity to psoriasis is often striking; some dermatologists believe that seborrheic dermatitis and psoriasis are variants of the same disease process. The scales of seborrheic dermatitis are not silvery, however, as are those of psoariasis, and the extragenital sites of the two diseases differ. Moreover, seborrheic dermatitis is usually bilaterally symmetrical and is prone to involve only the hairy surfaces of the vulva. This is not true of psoriasis. Borderline eruptions may appear, making clinical and histologic differentiation difficult. Such lesions are frequently referred to as *sebo-psoriasis*.

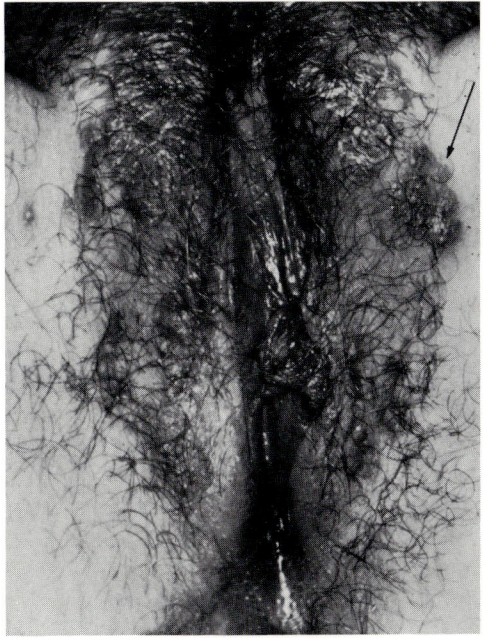

Fig. 8-5. Seborrheic dermatitis. The lesions are greasy and scaly.

Histopathology

Microscopic sections of biopsy specimens of the lesions of seborrheic dermatitis are not

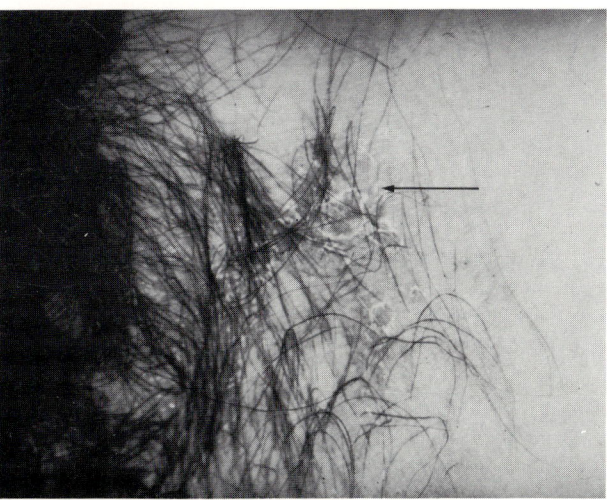

Fig. 8-6. Seborrheic dermatitis. A typical scaly lesion.

116 Benign diseases of the vulva and vagina

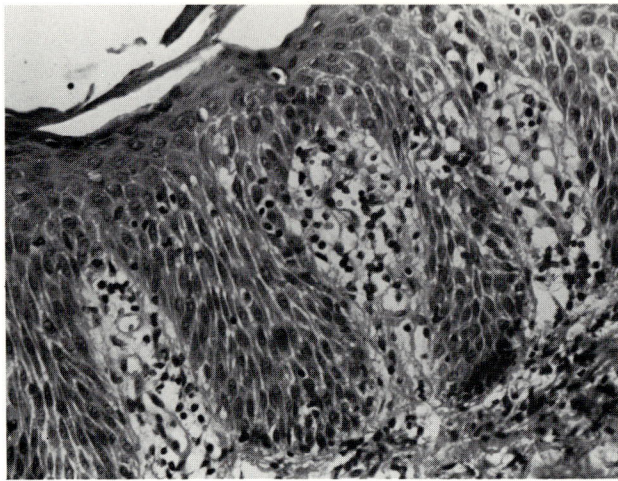

Fig. 8-7. Seborrheic dermatitis. Elongation and clubbing of rete ridges, intracellular edema, and spongiosis. (H & E × 160)

diagnostic; the changes have some of the characteristics of psoriasis and other chronic dermatoses (Fig. 8-7). A poorly developed horny layer with considerable parakeratosis is characteristic, although this is less pronounced than that observed in psoriasis. The epidermis exhibits a slight to moderate acanthosis with elongation and, at times, clubbing of the rete ridges. A slight intracellular edema and spongiosis are also present; these findings, as well as the absence of Munro abscesses, thin suprapapillary plates, and dilated vessels within the papillae, are of value in the distinction of this lesion from psoriasis. The dermis exhibits a mild, chronic inflammatory reaction.

Treatment

Topical corticosteroids, alone or combined with iodochlorhydroxyquin (Vioform) or coal tar, are extremely effective for relief of pruritus and for inducing regression of the lesions, although they are not curative. They should be used daily until the lesions disappear. Regression may last for weeks or months. In severe cases, systemic steroids are indicated. The intake of alcohol and greasy or starchy foods should be restricted.

The scalp usually requires simultaneous antiseborrheic treatment with similar therapeutic agents, and hair should be washed frequently with one of the numerous preparations available for the care of seborrhea. In the presence of an acute, swollen, moist

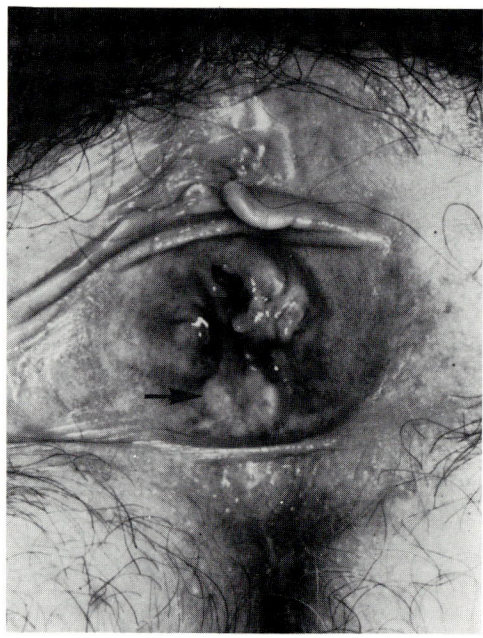

Fig. 8-8. Lichen planus. Arrow indicates discrete, elevated white lesion.

exudative lesion, wet dressings with Burow's Solution (1:20) should first be applied several times daily; thereafter, corticosteroids in the form of a lotion or cream may be used.

Lichen planus

Lichen planus is an inflammatory disease of the skin and mucous membranes characterized by smooth, flat, violaceous papules. On the vulva, it may appear as a "leukoplakic" or white plaque.

Etiology

As is true of many other dermatoses, the etiology of lichen planus is unknown. Microbic, toxic, neurogenic, and constitutional causes have been suggested. Many authorities believe that lichen planus is a functional disease. Emotional factors are also said to be responsible for exacerbations of the lesions.

Clinical features

The lesions of lichen planus arise on the flexor aspects of the wrists, forearms, inner thighs, ankles, waistline, back of the neck, and mucous membranes. In approximately 25 percent of the cases, the mucous membranes are involved, especially those of the oral cavity. The relatively rare lesions of the vulvar mucosa are opaline, elevated papules, either discrete or confluent (Fig. 8-8). They may increase in size, covering extensive areas of the vulva. These white raised lesions may suggest lichen simplex chronicus or the maculopapules of lichen sclerosus et atrophicus. Seldom do they have the shiny, violaceous appearance common to lesions in extragenital sites.

The acute lesions of lichen planus frequently involve many sites on the body and are easily recognized. After 3 to 6 weeks, the acute lesions begin to fade. When the disease becomes chronic, it may be generalized, although on occasion it is limited to areas such as the vulva. In the latter event, the diagnosis may be difficult.

The clinical course of lichen planus is variable. The acute eruptions seem to respond to treatment better than those that develop slowly. Also, the acute lesions frequently run a self-limiting course, although a chronic, recurrent eruption may ensue, and new lesions may continue to appear. Old lesions may heal and leave residual pigmentation. Localized forms involving the vulva have a tendency to chronicity and minimal dissemination. Altman and Perry report that the lesions arose solely in the mucosa in approximately 15 percent of cases; these were the most persistent of all varieties of lichen planus, their average duration being 4½ years. From this, it appears that mucosal lesions are less likely to regress.

Pruritus is the outstanding symptom of lichen planus. It may be severe during the initial stage of the lesions and gradually disappear as the chronic stage is reached. Scratching may cause secondary changes in the vulvar skin resembling those of neurodermatitis.

Histopathology

The microscopic changes of lichen planus are usually characteristic, although in longstanding cases the distinction from lichen simplex chronicus may be difficult. The outstanding features of the former are hyperkeratosis, irregular acanthosis, and irregular lengthening of the rete ridges. Many of the ridges may be pointed, giving the epidermis a saw-toothed appearance. A third and typical finding is a band-like infiltrate of lymphocytes in close approximation to the epidermis above but sharply demarcated at the lower border (Fig. 8-9). This infiltrate may invade the epidermis, causing a haziness of its border with the dermis; the basal layer of epidermis may appear to be destroyed and may be difficult to distinguish. In older lesions, the density of the lympho-

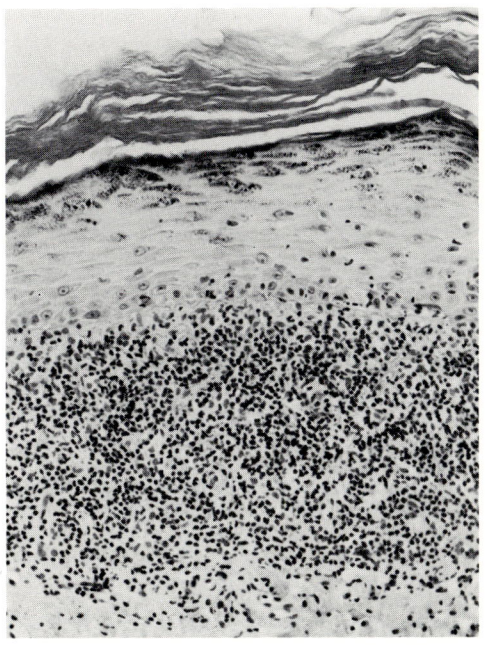

Fig. 8-9. Lichen planus. A band-like infiltrate of lymphocytes is closely approximated to the epidermis. Hyperkeratosis is prominent. (H & E × 243)

cytic infiltrate may decrease, and the number of histiocytes and fibroblasts may increase.

Treatment

In the past, heavy metals were used extensively in the treatment of patients with lichen planus, but they proved to have little effect upon the course of the disease; today their use has been largely discontinued. Pruritus may be relieved by the oral administration of antipruritic agents or by local applications of a corticosteroid cream. Injection of discrete lesions with corticosteroids such as triamcinolone may not only relieve pruritus but also may bring about their regression. For erosive lesions, a short course of systemic steroids may be necessary. If the lesions are more generalized, the patient should be referred to a dermatologist for treatment.

Acanthosis nigricans

A rare dermatosis that may affect the genitocrural area is acanthosis nigricans. In the presence of an unexplained, widespread, pigmented dermatosis of the vulva and surrounding skin, this condition deserves consideration. Several variations of the disease have been described, each of which must be distinguished from the others, since true acanthosis nigricans is associated with a highly lethal internal adenocarcinoma.

Curth and Aschner have described three types of acanthosis nigricans, all of which are somewhat similar in appearance and distribution.

1. *Malignant acanthosis nigricans* is itself a benign condition, although it accompanies an internal carcinoma. It arises during any stage of the malignant lesion, increases in severity with its growth, and may regress temporarily after treatment for the tumor. Unlike the other varieties of acanthosis nigricans, this lesion may occasionally involve the oral cavity.
2. *Benign acanthosis nigricans* is not associated with a malignant tumor. It may be present at birth, yet it more often arises later in childhood or at puberty. After puberty, the lesions become stationary or subside.
3. *Pseudoacanthosis nigricans* develops primarily in darkly pigmented persons. Its distribution may be similar to that of the malignant form, although it is not associated with a malignant tumor. Invariably, the cutaneous changes accompany pronounced obesity

and usually disappear when the weight returns to normal.

Etiology

The exact pathogenesis of malignant acanthosis nigricans is not known. The benign variety, which arises only in pediatric patients, may have a genetic background; recently, however, it has been found that most cases are associated with an endocrine disturbance of some type. Lesions similar to acanthosis nigricans have been reported in patients who receive nicotinic acid in large doses.* Nicotinic acid inhibits the biosynthesis of cholesterol from acetate. Since cholesterol is synthesized in the epidermis, the reported changes may well be based upon alterations of cholesterol metabolism. How this affects the development of acanthosis nigricans remains to be seen. The association of pseudoacanthosis nigricans with obesity is probably related to increased friction in the various folds of the body where this lesion develops.

Clinical features

In all varieties of this disease, the body folds, especially the axilla, neck, thighs, and submammary, cubital, and genitocrural

---
*Reported in an editor's note in the Yearbook of Dermatology, 1964-65.

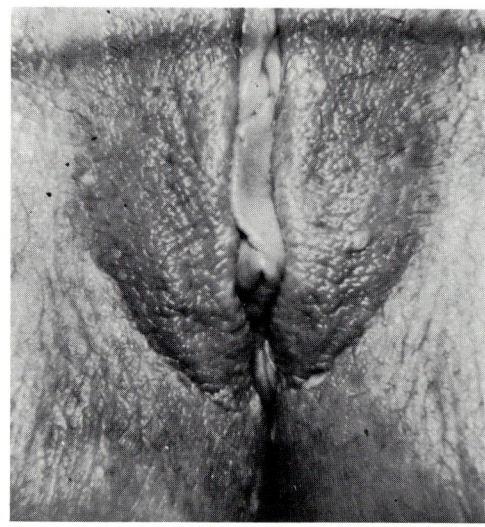

Fig. 8-10. Malignant acanthosis nigricans, represented by a hyperpigmented, verrucoid lesion. (Courtesy Dr. H. O. Curth, New York, N. Y.)

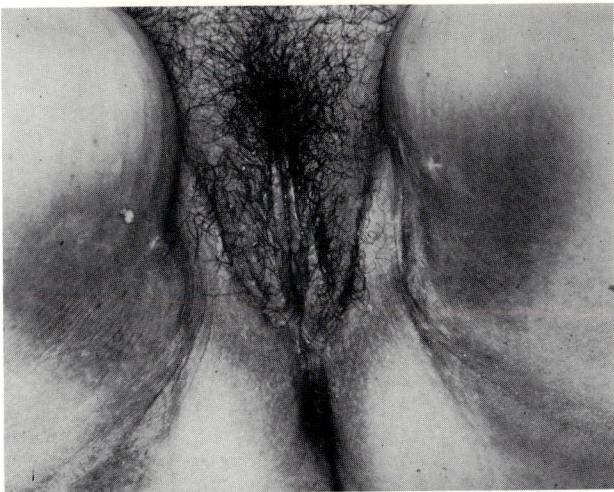

Fig. 8-11. Pseudoacanthosis nigricans. The skin of the inner thighs and vulva is dark and thickened. A small achrochordon is present on inner side of right thigh.

areas, may be involved. In the malignant variety, the lesion appears hyperpigmented and velvety, with elevated ridges, and is associated with a verrucose or papillomatous hypertrophy (Fig. 8-10). The skin of the entire body is only rarely involved. Pigmented nevi and keratoses on the trunk and extremities may also be present. The lesions of the other two varieties of acanthosis nigricans are similar, although the verrucose and papillomatous changes are less prominent (Fig. 8-11). In pseudoacanthosis nigricans, the mucous membrane, plantar, and palmar surfaces are never affected.

Histopathology

The microscopic features of these lesions consist of hyperkeratosis, acanthosis with finger-like projections, and a pronounced increase in pigmentation of the basal layer of cells. The histopathologic changes of pseudoacanthosis nigricans are similar, though less conspicuous.

The tumors associated with malignant acanthosis nigricans are almost invariably adenocarcinomata that ultimately prove fatal. Most of the primary cancers are in the stomach or abdominal cavity. Taffanelli reported one case of acanthosis nigricans associated with lupoid hepatitis. He also noted that the list of diseases associated with this dermatosis appeared to be increasing.

Treatment

No specific treatment for true acanthosis nigricans is available. When the presence of the malignant variety is suspected, a search should be made for an adenocarcinoma within the patient's body. Often, the benign variety in pediatric patients will regress spontaneously after puberty. An endocrine disturbance can sometimes be corrected. In obese patients with pseudoacanthosis nigricans, loss of excess weight will usually be followed by regression of the lesions.

REFERENCES

Abel, D. C., Dobson, R. L., and Graham, J. B.: Heredity and psoriasis, Arch. Derm. 88:38, 1963.

Altman, J., and Perry, H. O.: The variations and course of lichen planus, Arch. Derm. 84:179, 1961.

Baer, R. L., and Kopf, A. W.: Yearbook of dermatology, Chicago, 1965, Year Book Medical Publishers, Inc., p. 340.

Callaway, J. L., McAfee, W. C., and Finlayson, G. R.: Management of psoriasis using methotrexate orally in a single weekly dose, Southern Med. J. 59:424, 1966.

Crotty, R. Q.: Dermatologic lesions of the vulva, Nebraska Med. J. 48:334, 1963.

Curth, H. O.: Problems of acanthosis nigricans, Hautarzt 15:433, 1964. Abstract in Baer, R. L., and Kopf, A. W.: Yearbook of Dermatology, Chicago, 1965, Year Book Medical Publishers, Inc.

Curth, H. O.: Significance of acanthosis nigricans, Arch. Derm. 66:80, 1952.

Curth, H. O., and Aschner, B. M.: Genetic studies on acanthosis nigricans, Arch. Derm. 79:55, 1959.

Curth, H. O., Hillberg, A. W., and Machacek, G. F.: The site and histology of the cancer associated with malignant acanthosis nigricans, Cancer 15:364, 1962.

Curth, H. O., Tovell, M. M., and Janovski, N.: Malignant acanthosis nigricans associated with endometrial adenocarcinoma, Bull. Sloane Hosp. for Women 8:584, 1962.

Eddy, D. C., Ascheim, E., and Ferber, E. M.: Experimental analysis of isomorphic (Koebner) response in psoriasis, Arch. Derm. 89:579, 1964.

Farber, E. M., and Roth, R. J.: Course and care of psoriasis, Mod. Med. 33:100, 1965.

Farber, E. M., Roth, R. J., Ascheim, E., Eddy, D. C., and Eperrette, W. W.: The role of trauma in isomorphic response in psoriasis, Arch. Derm. 91:246, 1965.

Grayson, L. D., and Shair, H. M.: Psoriatic family tree, Arch. Derm. 79:661, 1959.

Hellgren, L.: Psoriasis, Acta Dermatovener. 44:191, 1964.

Kingery, F. A.: Why psoriasis looks that way, J.A.M.A. 195:953, 1966.

Lever, W. F.: Histopathology of the skin, ed. 3, Philadelphia, 1963, J. B. Lippincott Co.

Perlman, H. H.: Psoriasis, Med. Sci. 15:40, 1964.

Perlman, H. H.: Seborrhea, seborrheic dermatitis and the seborrheid reaction, Med. Sci. 15:60, 1964.

Scholtz, J. R.: Topical therapy of psoriasis with fluocinolone acetonide, Arch. Derm. 84:1029, 1961.

Sulzberger, M. B., Wolf, J., Witten, V. H., and Kopf, A.: Dermatology, diagnosis and treatment, ed. 2, Chicago, 1961, Year Book Medical Publishers, Inc.

Taffanelli, D. L.: Acanthosis nigricans with lipoid hepatitis, J.A.M.A. 189:138, 1964.

Tobias, N.: Essentials of dermatology, ed. 6, Philadelphia, 1964, J. B. Lippincott Co.

Van Scott, E. J., and Ekel, T. M.: Kinetics of hyperplasia in psoriasis, Arch. Derm. 88:373, 1963.

Weddell, G., Cowan, M. A., Palmer, E., and Ramaswamy, S.: Psoriatic skin, Arch. Derm. 91:252, 1965.

Wilson, J. F.: Cutaneous diseases of the vulva, Med. Clin. N. Amer. 39:1741, 1955.

Chapter 9

Vulvar dystrophies

Since the introduction of the terms "leukoplakia" and "kraurosis vulvae" during the latter part of the nineteenth century, the number of conflicting opinions expressed on this subject in the medical literature has served to confuse the interested student. Clinically and histopathologically, a variety of conditions has been similarly designated and, conversely, similar changes have been described under different terms. To add to the confusion, the clinician and the pathologist each have often ignored the findings and opinions of the other and have failed to correlate closely the clinical and histopathologic features.

Jeffcoate (1966) suggests that the different terms used by the gynecologist and the dermatologist apply to mere variants in the epithelial response of the vulva to one or more adverse agents. He believes that the special appearance of the reactions of the vulvar skin is explained by its environment of warmth and moisture. The differences in the appearance of dystrophic skin do not necessarily denote separate diseases; rather, they are the environmentally conditioned reactions to adverse agents, whatever they may be. In support of the latter suggestion, Jeffcoate cites evidence to the effect that if the involved vulvar skin is excised and the raw area covered with normal skin from a site not ordinarily subject to the lesions characteristic of the vulvar area, the transplanted epithelium will undergo the changes present in the vulvar skin before its removal. Also, Whimster observed that when vulvar skin with lichen sclerosus et atrophicus and "leukoplakia" were interchanged with healthy skin grafted from the thigh, the vulvar skin in the new site cleared spontaneously, whereas skin from the leg became dystrophic in its new site.

Jeffcoate (1966) states that the same etiologic factors can lead to different epithelial reactions in the vulva or different etiologic factors can be the foundation for similar vulvar changes. He prefers to ascribe the general term of "chronic vulvar dystrophies" to the entire group. These consist of lesions known in the past as leukoplakia, leukoplakic vulvitis, lichen sclerosus et atrophicus, kraurosis vulvae, primary atrophy, sclerotic dermatosis, and atrophic and hyperplastic vulvitis. Although inclined to agree, we have included lichen simplex chronicus (localized neurodermatitis) of the vulva in the group, in view of its close clinical and histopathologic similarity to the hyperplastic lesions that have long been called "leukoplakia."

In any discussion of a thickened or thinned white vulvar lesion, the term "leukoplakia" immediately comes to mind. This term, which merely denotes a visible "white, flat patch" incident to hyperkeratinization of the skin, was first applied to a lesion of the tongue and mouth by Schwimmer in 1887. Later, it was applied to similar lesions of the mucous membrane in other areas of the body. Berkeley and Bonney described four stages of "leukoplakia," beginning with a red, swollen, excoriated vulva and ending with a thin, atrophic, apparently quiescent lesion. Taussig (1923) described three stages, the first being a hypertrophic phase and the third, an atrophic stage. Taussig, as well as Berkeley and Bonney, was of the opinion that "leukoplakia" of the vulva was a premalignant lesion.

Unfortunately, most of the reports of "leukoplakia" are based solely upon a single biopsy or vulvectomy specimen from the untreated patient. To distinguish accurately the progressive stages of a dystrophy, a series of biopsies from the untreated patient over a prolonged period of time would be necessary. Since such observations have rarely, if ever, been made, the authenticity of the description of stages of the disease and the incidence of subsequent carcinoma may well be questioned.

Although the appearance of a vulvar lesion may change in time, and although mixed atrophic and hyperplastic changes may be present simultaneously in the same vulva, we believe the primarily hyperplastic and atrophic lesions probably represent separate disease entities. Also, any malignant potential of such lesions (if it exists) has been found to be more closely related to the degree of cellular atypia, if present, than to any other factor or factors.

The word *dystrophy* has been defined as "abnormal nourishment" or "defective nutrition," which means little to the clinician who is trying to treat patients with vulvar diseases. For this reason, we have attempted to classify the dystrophic lesions in a manner that will be readily understood by both the clinician and the pathologist. Our classification is:

A. Hyperplastic dystrophies
 1. Benign epithelial hyperplasia
    a. Lichen simplex chronicus (neurodermatitis)
    b. Unclassified
 2. Atypical epithelial hyperplasia (dysplasia)
B. Atrophic dystrophy—lichen sclerosus et atrophicus
C. Mixed dystrophy—lichen sclerosus et atrophicus with foci of epithelial hyperplasia
 1. Without atypia
 2. With atypia

The classification of a vulvar disease and its significance with regard to malignant potential demands the cooperative efforts of the pathologist and clinician. The clinician bears the responsibility for clinical recognition of the disease and must provide the tissue for diagnosis and evaluation. The pathologist is responsible not only for the histopathologic diagnosis but, more important, for the recognition of atypia. Determination of malignant potential by the pathologist is highly essential as a guide to the clinical care of the patient, as we shall later demonstrate. Woodruff and Baens have attempted this in their subdivision of hyperplastic vulvitis into three grades (I, II, and III). Grade I lesions exhibit no atypia, and grade III lesions represent carcinoma in situ. Grade II lesions exhibit less cellular atypia than in situ carcinoma. In a further effort to reduce confusion within our group at Baylor College of Medicine, we have classified the dystrophies into three types: those lesions in which the epithelium is thickened or *hyperplastic*, those in which it is thinner than normal or *atrophic*, and those in which both hyperplastic and atrophic epithelial changes are present. Since a distinction between epidermal thickening and thinning is not always possible by gross inspection alone, the classification of a lesion must depend upon its microscopic characteristics. Also, since the histologic appearance may vary in different sites in the vulva, lesions can be accurately classified only if multiple biopsies are taken from several locations.

HYPERPLASTIC DYSTROPHIES
Benign epithelial hyperplasia

We believe that most hyperplastic lesions previously called "leukoplakia" represent examples of *lichen simplex chronicus (neurodermatitis)*. Although all hyperplastic lesions are associated with epithelial thickening and hyperkeratosis, their gross appearance is highly variable. Further, their appearance varies from time to time in the same patient, being influenced by moisture, scratching, scrubbing, and medications. The size of the lesions likewise varies from small to extensive. The areas most frequently involved are the hood of the clitoris, the labia majora, the interlabial sulci, the outer aspect of the labia minora, and the posterior commissure. The lesions may also extend onto the lateral surface of the labia majora and even the adjacent thighs. Many are bilaterally symmetrical.

Gross and microscopic appearance

Frequently, areas of neurodermatitis are localized, elevated, and well-delineated (Fig. 9-1). On other occasions, the vulvar lesions may be extensive and poorly defined. The vulva is most often dusky red in color (Fig. 9-2); however, at times, both red and white patches may be observed in different sites,

Vulvar dystrophies

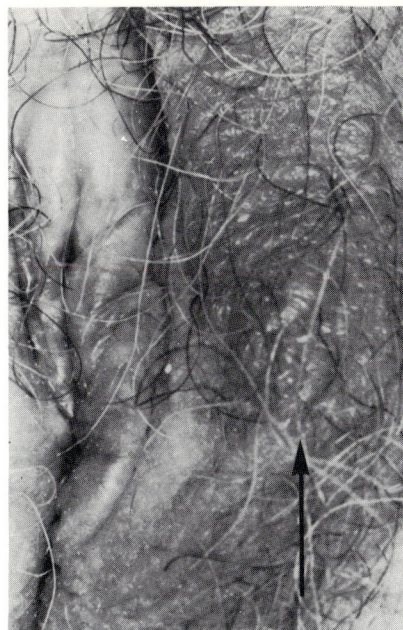

Fig. 9-1. Benign epithelial hyperplasia (neurodermatitis). Demonstrated in this patient by a well-delineated lesion of left labium majus. Lichenification is pronounced. Patient previously had been given a diagnosis of "leukoplakia."

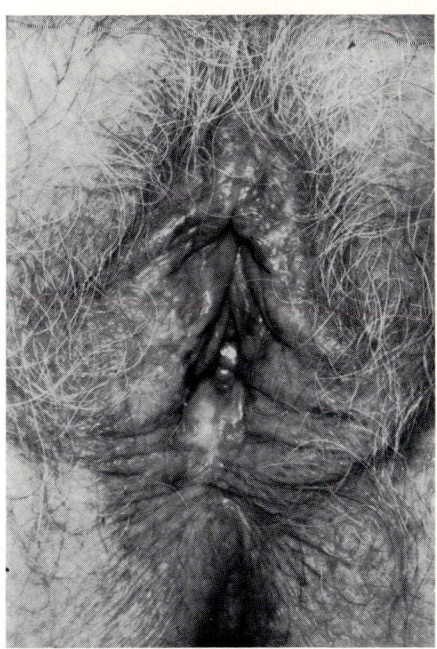

Fig. 9-2. Benign epithelial hyperplasia (neurodermatitis). This patient had an ill-defined, dusky red thickening of the skin which had been interpreted histologically as "leukoplakia."

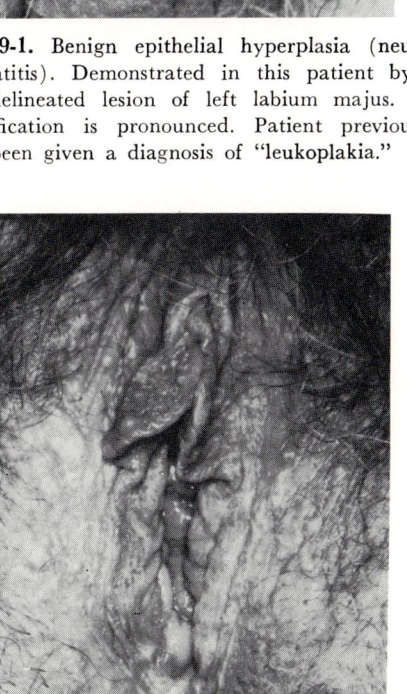

Fig. 9-3. Benign epithelial hyperplasia (neurodermatitis). Numerous raised, white plaques demonstrated. The lesions disappeared after 2 to 3 weeks' treatment with a topical corticosteroid.

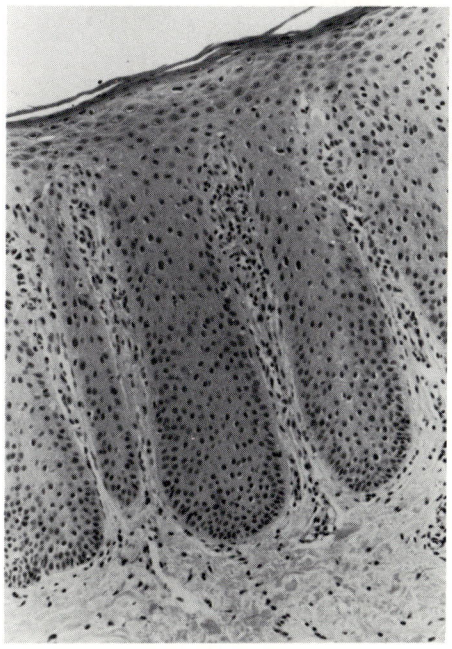

Fig. 9-4. Benign epithelial hyperplasia (neurodermatitis). Elongation and clubbing of the rete pegs and an inflammatory infiltrate of the papillae, as well as slight parakeratosis and hyperkeratosis. This lesion disappeared after the use of topical corticosteroids for 1 month. (H & E × 100)

124 Benign diseases of the vulva and vagina

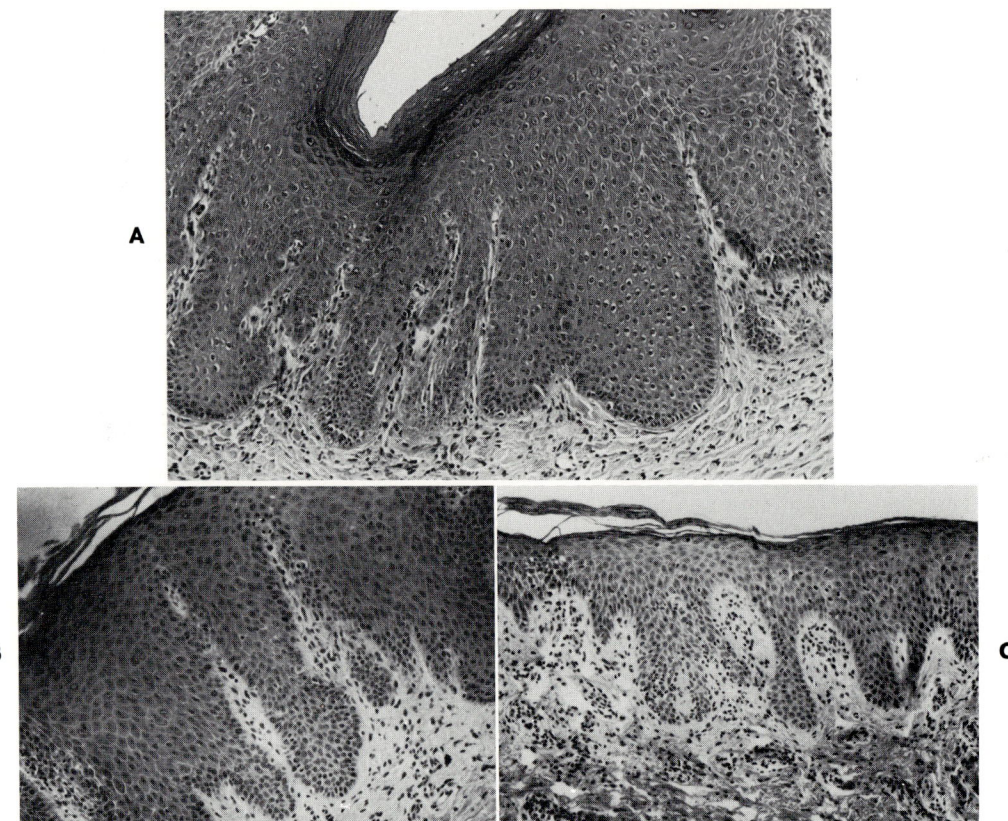

Fig. 9-5. Benign epithelial hyperplasia. Each of the lesions in **A**, **B**, and **C** had been interpreted microscopically as "leukoplakia" elsewhere. They constitute further examples of neurodermatitis. (H & E × 100)

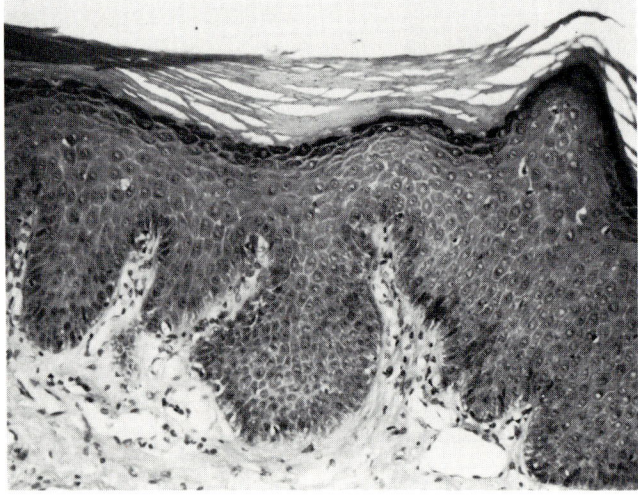

Fig. 9-6. Benign epithelial hyperplasia (neurodermatitis). The granular layer is conspicuous, as are also acanthosis and hyperkeratosis. (H & E × 100)

or the affected areas may appear thickened, white, and lichenified (Fig. 9-3). Edema, especially of the labia minora and hood of the clitoris, may be associated. Fissuring is not uncommon, and excoriations may be present from scratching. Excoriation and fissuring require careful evaluation, since carcinoma may first be exhibited by a minute ulceration.

The essential microscopic finding in lichen simplex chronicus consists of a variable increase in thickness of the horny layer (hyperkeratosis) and an irregular thickening of the malphigian layer (acanthosis), the latter producing a thickening of the epithelium as well as lengthening and distortion of the rete pegs into either a club or pointed shape (Figs. 9-4 and 9-5). Parakeratosis may also be present. The granular layer of the epithelium may be prominent (Fig. 9-6), although we have observed this less often than have other investigators. Because of the elongation of the rete pegs, the papillae became conspicuous and, often, edematous. A variable inflammatory reaction is apparent within the dermis, with the inflammatory infiltrate consisting of lymphocytes and a small number of plasma cells. This is usually quite pronounced in neurodermatitis, as is the clubbing of rete pegs.

Unclassified hyperplasia

There are rare unclassified hyperplastic lesions of the vulva that seem to be localized chiefly on the surfaces of the labia minora, clitoris, and inner aspects of the labia majora. These lesions are usually exhibited by "white patches" with fairly well-demarcated borders. The microscopic picture of such lesions is similar to that already described, although the inflammatory infiltrate within the dermis and the papillary edema is less pronounced than in the majority of cases of lichen simplex chronicus. We find it difficult to classify these lesions as lichen simplex chronicus; for the present we prefer to list them as "unclassified." The absence of cellular atypia places them among the benign hyperplastic dystrophies.

Atypical epithelial hyperplasia (dysplasia)

The vulvar dystrophies that exhibit epithelial atypia (dysplasia) are of far more significance in regard to malignant potential than the benign epithelial hyperplasias. Jeff-

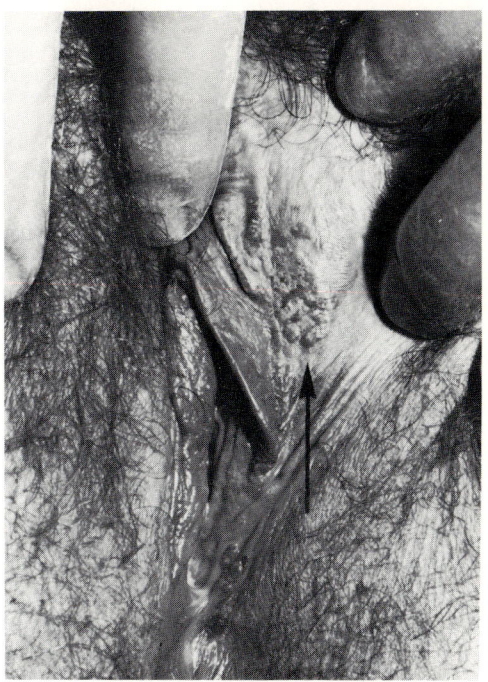

Fig. 9-7. Atypical epithelial hyperplasia, exhibited by a sharply demarcated raised white lesion. The microscopic features of this lesion are shown in Fig. 9-11.

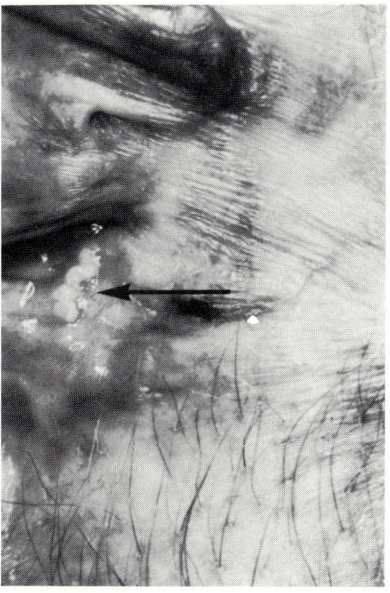

Fig. 9-8. Atypical epithelial hyperplasia. A small, sharply demarcated white plaque on vestibule. The microscopic features of this lesion are shown in Fig. 9-10.

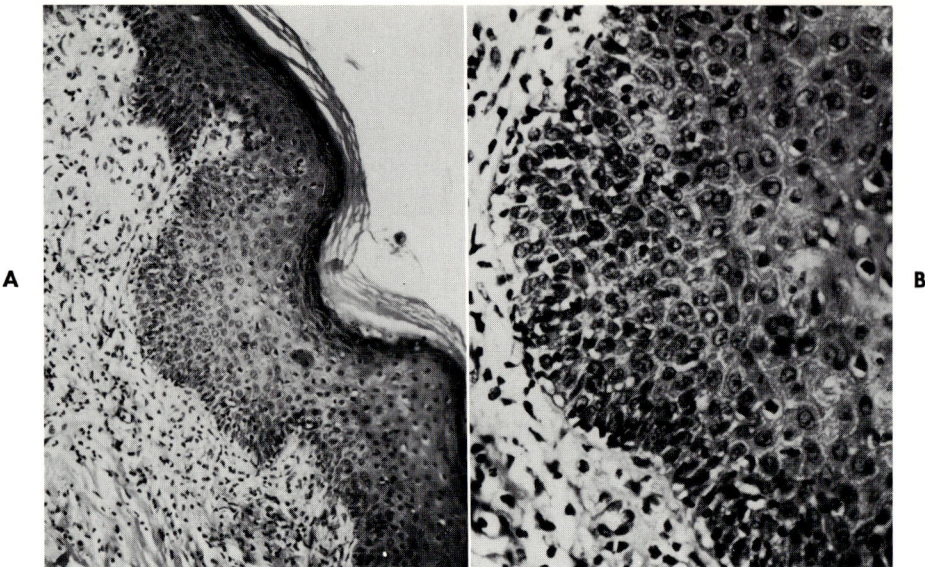

Fig. 9-9. A and B, Mild atypical epithelial hyperplasia. Increased cellularity and mild nuclear atypia in deeper layers of the epithelium. This is best demonstrated in B. (A, H & E × 100; B, H & E × 250)

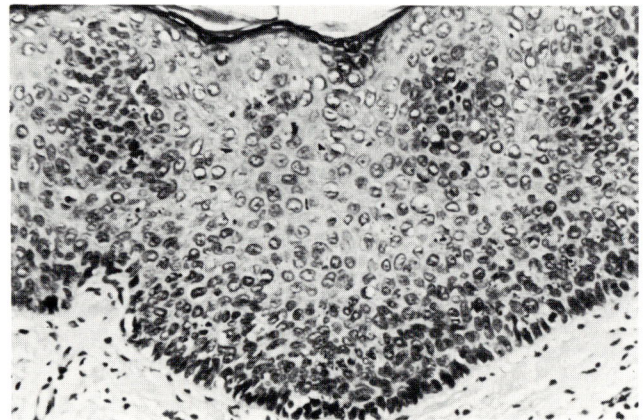

Fig. 9-10. Moderate to severe atypical epithelial hyperplasia. Biopsy from lesion demonstrated in Fig. 9-8. (H & E × 210)

coate (1966) observed such lesions in only a small percentage of the patients he studied, yet they proved to be precursors of carcinoma. Lever and many other authors restrict the use of the term "leukoplakia" to only those lesions demonstrating cellular atypia. This usage of the term would appear to justify its historically onerous reputation. Little purpose is served by clinging to a term subject to misconception, and we believe its use should be abandoned. The malignant potential of the lesions under discussion here is accurately reflected in the term "atypical hyperplasia" or "dysplasia."

Gross and microscopic appearance

The gross appearance of lesions in this category is similar to those without cellular atypia. In our experience, the majority of such lesions are well localized, well delineated, and slightly elevated (Figs. 9-7 and 9-8). They may be white or red, or consist of both red and white patches. The diagnosis is established by histopathologic study. Since

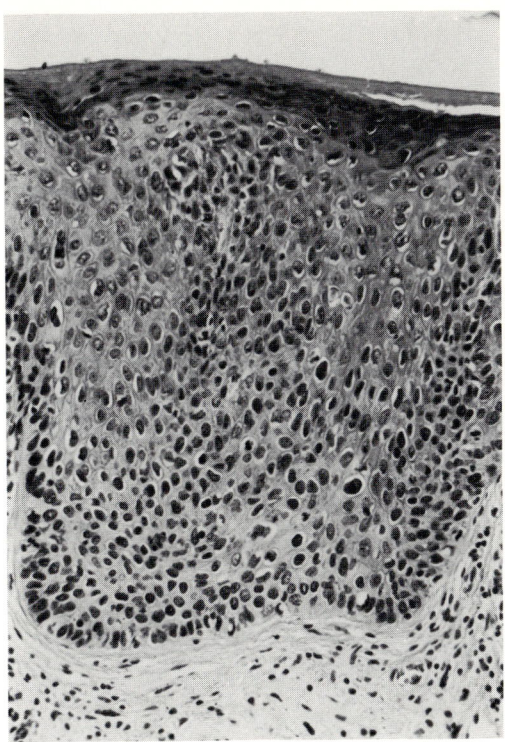

Fig. 9-11. Severe atypical epithelial hyperplasia. Biopsy from lesion demonstrated in Fig. 9-7. Lesion borders on in situ carcinoma. (H & E × 300)

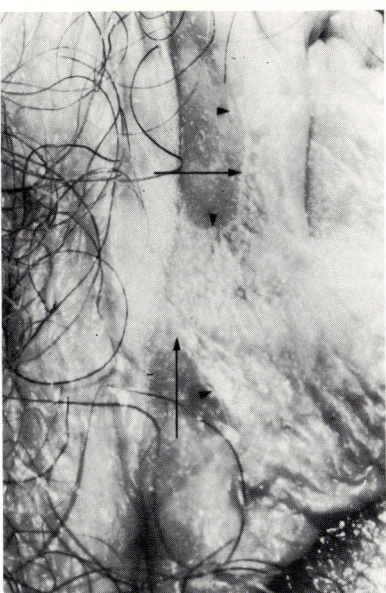

Fig. 9-12. Lichen sclerosis et atrophicus. White, well-circumscribed plaques sometimes present.

lesions of varied histopathologic structure often arise in the same vulva, biopsies should be taken from more than one involved site.

In the presence of only mild atypia, the significant changes are first detected in the deeper layers of the epidermis and rete pegs (Fig. 9-9). The size and shape of the nuclei vary, and many are hyperchromatic. Scattered mitotic figures are also observed. As the cellular atypia progresses, these changes extend toward the surface of the epithelium and are associated with more pronounced degrees of pleomorphism and loss of cellular polarity (Figs. 9-10 and 9-11), until, finally, the picture resembles that of squamous cell carcinoma in situ. In our opinion, these changes are analogous to those found in association with the cervical atypias and are not related to or caused by the benign hyperplasias.

ATROPHIC DYSTROPHY—LICHEN SCLEROSUS ET ATROPHICUS

Almost as much confusion has surrounded this lesion as has been associated with "leukoplakia." The vast majority of lesions interpreted as "kraurosis vulvae," primary atrophy, and the atrophic phase of leukoplakia are probably examples of lichen sclerosus et atrophicus. Oberfield concluded that Taussig's (1923) description of the atrophic phase of leukoplakic vulvitis (which Taussig referred to as "Briesky's kraurosis") was identical to the picture of this condition. Henri Hallopeau, who first described this disease in 1887, called it "lichen planus atrophicus." Jeffcoate (1966) prefers not to consider this disease as a separate entity; rather, he regards it as another dystrophic lesion and only one of several responses of the vulva to the same etiologic factors.

In our opinion, lichen sclerosus et atrophicus represents a specific disease entity, even though it is included in the general group of chronic vulvar dystrophies. Its gross and microscopic appearance and clinical course are characteristic. Further, since identical lesions are located elsewhere on the body, its development is not solely dependent upon the local environment of the vulva. The disease may involve the labia majora, labia minora, the perianal skin, the skin folds adjacent to the thighs, and the clitoris, usually in a bilaterally symmetrical pattern.

128 Benign diseases of the vulva and vagina

Janovski found lichen sclerosus on the labia and fourchette in all twenty-seven of his patients. The perineum was also involved in 89 percent of the patients and the clitoris in 48 percent. In addition, the lesions may arise on the trunk, neck, forearms, under the breasts, and in the axilla. Oberfield observed genital lesions in only twenty-two of fifty-six women with lichen sclerosus et atrophicus. Practically all of the thirty-two examples of this lesion that we have observed have been limited to the vulva. Chernosky, Derbes, and Burks reported that in only 32 percent of their cases in children were the lesions limited to the anogenital region. Clark and Muller found the anogenital area involved in 75 percent of children with lichen sclerosus et atrophicus.

Gross and microscopic appearance

Initially, the lesions may appear as low, irregularly outlined, flat topped, white maculopapules, though they may later coalesce and form well-defined plaques (Fig. 9-12). Comedo-like plugs or depressions, frequently associated, help to distinguish the condition from hyperplastic dystrophies, scleroderma,

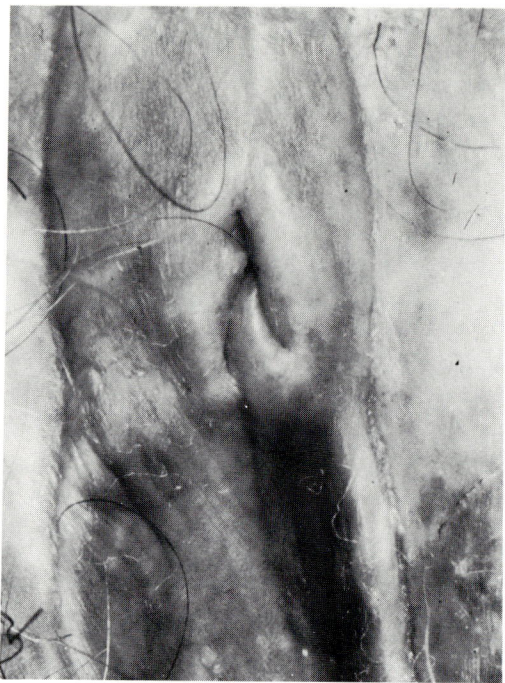

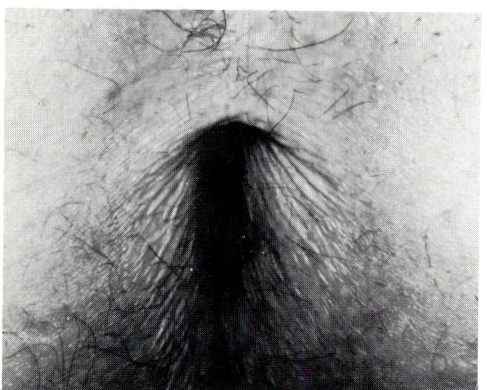

Fig. 9-13. Lichen sclerosus et atrophicus. Typical "cigarette paper" crinkling of skin extends around anal region.

Fig. 9-14. Lichen sclerosus et atrophicus. Edema of foreskin of clitoris, a common early finding.

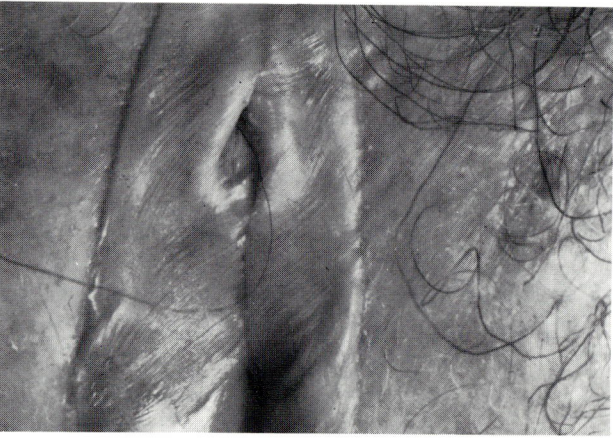

Fig. 9-15. Lichen sclerosus et atrophicus. Phimosis of clitoris, often a late development.

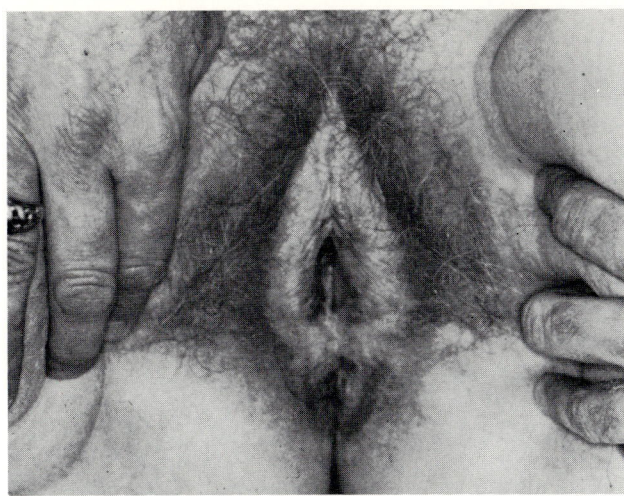

Fig. 9-16. Lichen sclerosus et atrophicus. Pronounced atrophy of labia minora and symmetrical depigmentation. (Kaufman, R. H., Gardner, H. L., and Johnson, P. C.: Amer. J. Obstet. Gynec. 98:312, 1967.)

lichen planus, and vitiligo. In the well-developed and classical lesions, the skin has a crinkled "cigarette paper" or parchment-like appearance; this feature commonly extends around the anal region in a figure eight or keyhole fashion (Fig. 9-13). Often, a rather severe edema of the clitoral foreskin produces a phimosis; we consider this one of the early diagnostic signs of the disease (Fig. 9-14). Subsequently, the foreskin and clitoris may atrophy and adhere, resulting in complete disappearance of the clitoris from sight (Fig. 9-15). At times, the labia minora almost completely disappear as a result of atrophy (Figs. 9-16 and 9-17). Not uncommonly, splitting of the skin in the midline is observed (Fig. 9-18), especially between the clitoris and urethra. Synechiae may develop between the edges of the skin in these locations, causing pain and limiting physical activity. Fissures may also develop in the natural folds of the skin and in the posterior fourchette. The introitus may became so stenotic that the opening barely admits one finger, even in a parous woman (Fig. 9-19). Occasionally, this small opening precludes intercourse. We feel that the contracture stage of this disease accounted for most lesions previously classified as "kraurosis vulvae."

Several authors have divided the lesions of lichen sclerosus et atrophicus into two stages, although the validity of such staging

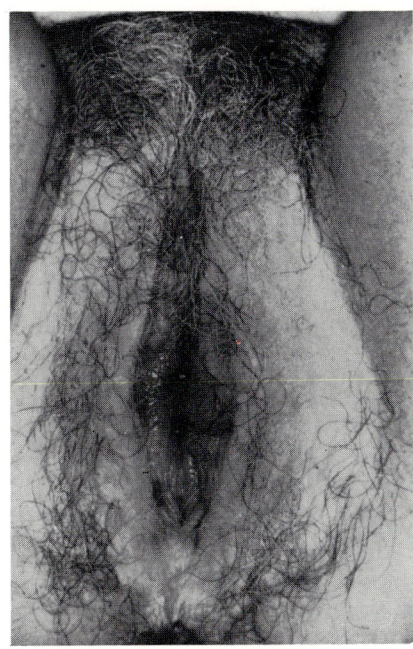

Fig. 9-17. Vitiligo, a condition resulting from absence of pigment in the skin. Can be confused with lichen sclerosus et atrophicus.

is not clear at all. They consider erythematous, edematous lesions with occasional prominent telangiectases and minute hematomas as features of the early stage, and the thin, white, crinkled appearance of the skin as evidence of the late stage. However, we

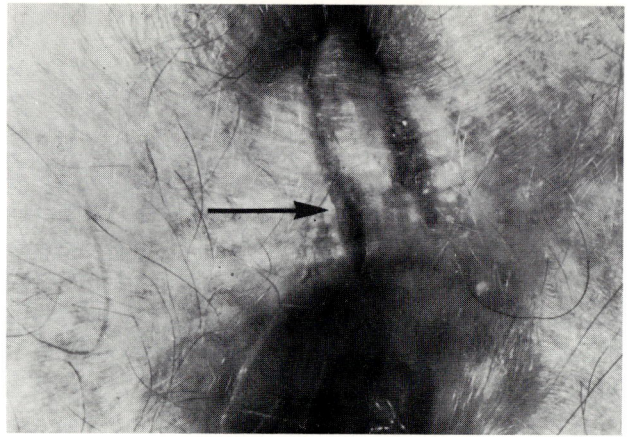

Fig. 9-18. Lichen sclerosus et atrophicus. Splitting of skin of perineum demonstrated.

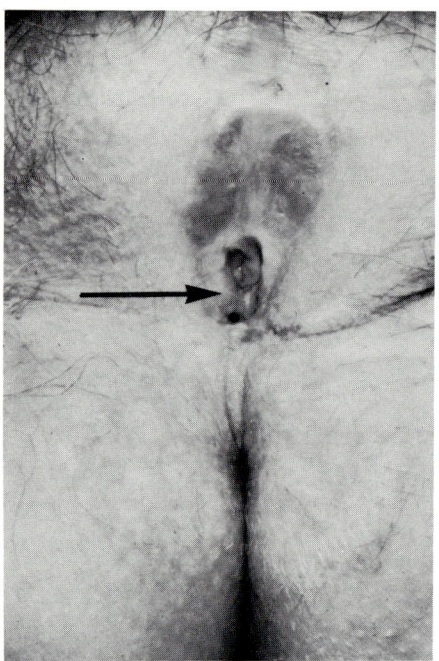

Fig. 9-19. Lichen sclerosus et atrophicus. The introitus (arrow) of this parous patient barely admitted one finger. This condition is sometimes erroneously diagnosed as "kraurosis."

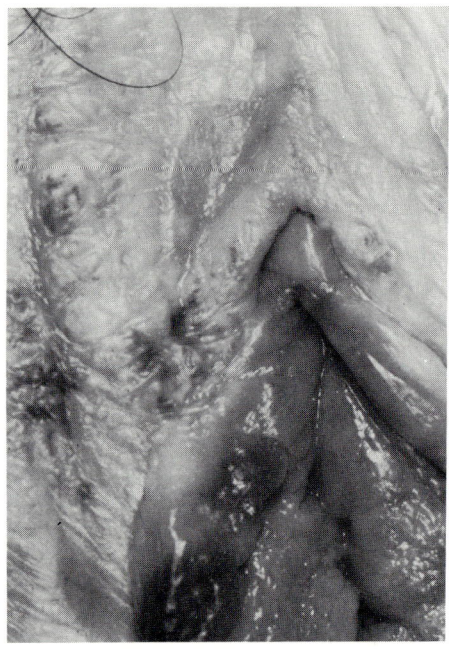

Fig. 9-20. Lichen sclerosus et atrophicus. Telangiectases and small hematomata are sometimes present, especially after trauma.

have found telangiectasia and hematomas in all stages of the disease (Fig. 9-20).

Grossly, the disease in children is essentially the same as that found in the adult (Fig. 9-21). Chernosky, Derbes, and Burks observed a vesiculobullous and edematous lesion early in the course of the disease in children.

The microscopic features of lichen sclerosus et atrophicus are typical. In the early stages, the epidermis may be of normal thickness or even mildly hyperplastic, with very slight elongation of the rete pegs. Hyperkeratosis is also present. A moderate to severe edema of the upper dermis is associated with a clear, pink-staining band of collag-

Vulvar dystrophies 131

enous tissue beneath the epidermis (Fig. 9-22). Below this, a mild, chronic inflammatory reaction may be apparent.

The advanced stages of the disease are exhibited by hyperkeratosis, epithelial atrophy with flattening of the rete pegs, and, frequently, cytoplasmic vacuolation of the basal layer of cells and follicular plugging. Beneath the epidermis lies a zone of homogenized, collagenous tissue having a dull pink, acellular appearance (Fig. 9-23). Special stains reveal an absence of elastic fibers in this zone. Immediately below this, in the middermal area, lies a narrow band of chronic inflammatory cells consisting of lymphocytes and an occasional plasma cell.

MIXED DYSTROPHY—LICHEN SCLEROSUS ET ATROPHICUS WITH EPITHELIAL HYPERPLASIA
Gross and microscopic appearance

Lichen sclerosus et atrophicus is often associated with both foci of hyperplastic epithelium and atrophic changes. Also, during extended periods of observation and medical treatment, the vulva undergoes grossly apparent changes. A grossly hyperplastic vulva may become atrophic in appearance, or the reverse may be true. The

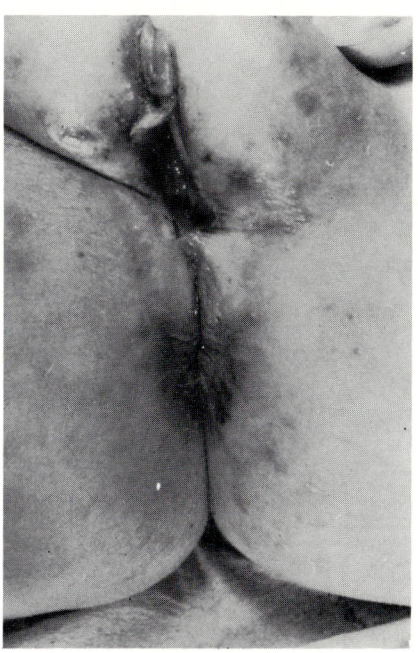

Fig. 9-21. Lichen sclerosus et atrophicus in a 3-year-old child. The microscopic features of this lesion are shown in Fig. 9-23, *A*. (Courtesy Marvin E. Chernosky, Houston.)

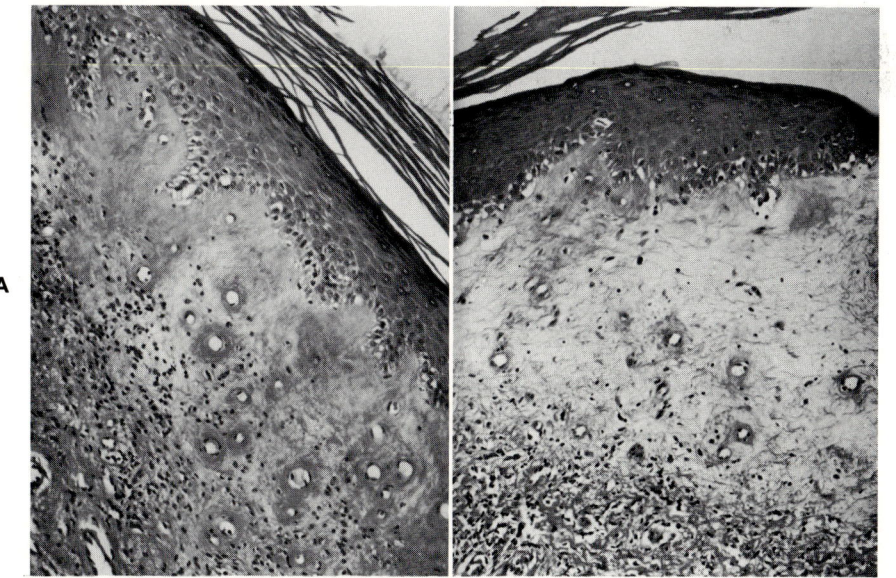

Fig. 9-22. **A** and **B**, Early lichen sclerosus et atrophicus. Edematous, clear zone beneath epithelium, hyperkeratosis, and mild chronic inflammatory infiltrate. The epithelium, especially in **B**, is not yet atrophic. (H & E × 100)

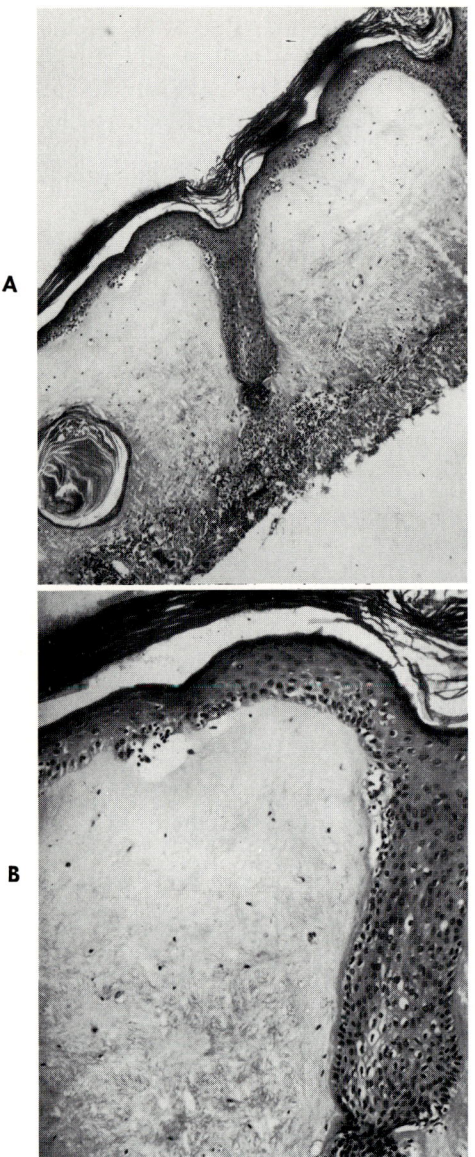

Fig. 9-23. Lichen sclerosus et atrophicus. Typical changes are hyperkeratosis, epithelial atrophy, and an acellular zone. **A,** Follicular plugging and inflammatory infiltrate. **B,** A few basal cells contain vacuoles. (**A,** H & E × 100; **B,** H & E × 40)

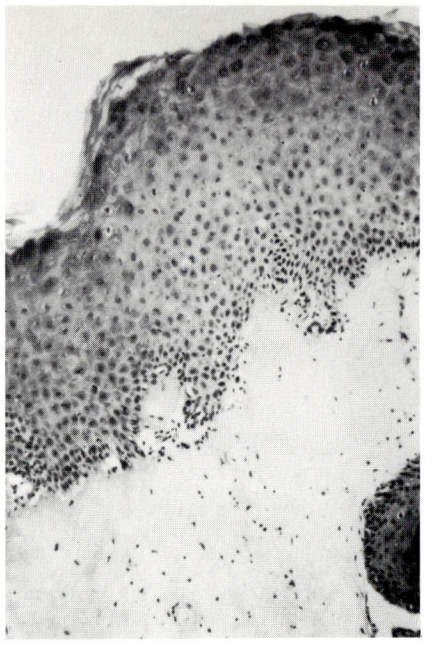

Fig. 9-24. Mixed dystrophy. Areas of epithelial hyperplasia, not uncommonly present in lichen sclerosus et atrophicus. Other areas exhibited epithelial atrophy. (H & E × 115)

plastic islands mixed with the atrophic areas within the lesion per se.

Microscopic study of biopsies of the vulvar lesions will verify the coexistence of both hyperplastic and atrophic changes. Islands of epithelial hyperplasia may be interspersed between areas presenting the classical picture of lichen sclerosus et atrophicus (Fig. 9-24). Within the areas of epithelial hyperplasia, foci of dysplasia may be discovered. If the patient is followed over a long period of time, a variation of the morphology of the lesion may be detected, although we have not observed a gradual progression of an exclusively hyperplastic lesion to a final atrophic phase such as described by Taussig.

ETIOLOGY OF THE DYSTROPHIES

The etiology of the various chronic vulvar dystrophies is obscure. The environment of the vulva undoubtedly influences the pathologic processes involved. The role of chronic trauma, allergy, nutritional deficiency, psychoneurosis, metabolic disturbance, and perhaps other factors is unknown. The relationship of chronic vulvovaginal infections such as candidiasis to neurodermatitis seems ap-

occasional alternating appearance of the vulvar lesion from one examination to the next tends to confound the clinician. Areas of hyperplasia that develop adjacent to an otherwise atrophic lesion may be caused by scratching and may thus represent a form of neurodermatitis, in contrast to the hyper-

parent, particularly in diabetics. The nervous habit of scratching in one location may produce a dermatitis that meets all the criteria of a neurodermatitis. Of Jeffcoate's (1966) 269 patients with chronic vulvar dystrophies, nine had recurrent glycosuria, sixty had histamine-fast achlorhydria, twenty-eight had vaginal moniliasis, and fifteen were found to have deficiency states, such as macrocytic anemia or folic acid deficiency. Thirty-four patients had a fungus infection of the hands or feet.

In 1936, Swift suggested that "leukoplakia" might be the result of a deficiency of vitamin A, usually caused by gastric achlorhydria and lack of absorption of the vitamin or by its deficiency in the diet. Of thirty-five of his patients with "leukoplakia," only four had normal gastric acids following a test meal. Miller and others, however, found a low vitamin A level in the blood of only one of ten patients. Clinical experience with the use of vitamin A and dilute hydrochloric acid as a treatment for vulvar dystrophies has not borne out Swift's theory.

Miller and others, in a well-controlled group of patients, could find no relationship between "leukoplakia" and other systemic diseases, venereal diseases, psychiatric disturbance, blood plasma, ascorbic acid, gastric acidity, or endocrine abnormalities. Jeffcoate (1966) suggested that the lesions might be, in part, an allergic reaction, although this has not been proved. Despite the many theories proposed, no single one, as yet, has stood the test of time and experience.

Relationship to cancer
Hyperplastic lesions

Regardless of the nomenclature used, whether it is leukoplakia, leukoplakic vulvitis, epithelial hyperplasia, white lesion, or vulvar dystrophy, one of the most controversial points in regard to the chronic vulvar dystrophies is that of their malignant potential. The recorded prevalence of "leukoplakia" associated with carcinoma varies from 5 to 80 percent. Taussig (1930) stated that in 50 percent of patients with "leukoplakia" of the vulva, the lesion will become malignant. He believed that if the patients lived long enough, all "leukoplakias" would eventually develop into carcinomas. Taussig (1940) also found that 70 percent of his patients with squamous cell cancer of the vulva had concomitant "leukoplakia." In the opinion of Berkeley and Bonney, "leukoplakia" is a precursor of vulvar carcinoma. With the passage of time and the accumulation of case studies, the onerous significance of lesions called "leukoplakia" in relation to the development of carcinoma has decreased. Unfortunately, early observations of disorders of the vulvar skin do not fulfill our present histopathologic requirements. A reevaluation of the impressions and concepts based upon these studies is therefore necessary. Most of these studies were retrospective; they were based upon the discovery of epi-

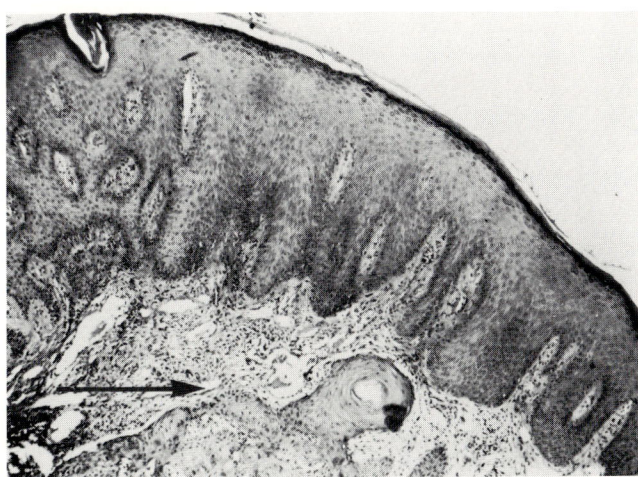

Fig. 9-25. Carcinoma of vulva (arrow). Pronounced benign epithelial hyperplasia overlying focus of squamous cell carcinoma. (H & E × 40)

thelial hyperplasia in association with cancer of the vulva. Quite possibly, the changes reported as "leukoplakia" found adjacent to carcinoma may appear at the same time as the cancer, or their development may even be stimulated by the presence of the carcinoma. In reviewing our cases of vulvar cancer, it was found that the vast majority of patients had no clinical history suggestive of preexistent vulvar dystrophy, although dystrophic changes were discovered adjacent to the carcinoma in most of the patients (Fig. 9-25). Jeffcoate (1966) has also made this observation.

It is noteworthy that in reviewing many of the older studies, some question can be raised as to the type of skin lesions reported in association with carcinoma. From the photomicrographs and the gross descriptions, a variety of lesions, rather than a single entity, was referred to as "leukoplakia."

More recent prospective studies have indicated that the likelihood of the development of carcinoma from "leukoplakia" is small. Woodruff and Baens estimated that approximately 25 percent of hypertrophic lesions of the vulva may become malignant. McAdams and Kistner found that 10 percent of the patients with "leukoplakia" subsequently had carcinoma at the site of the lesion. Langley, Hertig, and Smith reported that "leukoplakia" was followed by carcinoma in only one of 122 patients who were observed for 5 or more years after having a partial or simple vulvectomy, despite the fact that 59 percent of these patients had a recurrence of their symptoms, of the lesion, or of both. In the one patient, the carcinoma developed 12 years after a simple vulvectomy.

Jeffcoate (1966) is of the opinion that the risk of the development of carcinoma in the vulva in the presence of a chronic vulvar dystrophy is less than 5 percent over a period of 3 to 25 years, this estimate being based upon his observation of 138 women over that length of time. He stresses, however, that the risk of carcinoma is serious only if the initial biopsy reveals atypical hyperplasia (dysplasia). McAdams and Kistner have also emphasized this essential point. Jeffcoate states that atypical hyperplasia may be anticipated in 2 to 3 percent of all initial diagnostic biopsies of the vulva. He estimates that carcinoma is already present in 5 percent of women who consult a physician for a chronic vulvar dystrophy.

In Abel's experience, 10 to 20 percent of hypertrophic lesions will become cancerous if not treated. Abel also observed that the dysplasias were more likely to progress to intraepithelial carcinoma.

Lichen sclerosus et atrophicus

Most investigators believe that there is little or no relationship between lichen sclerosus et atrophicus and the development of carcinoma of the vulva. Wallace, however, believes that lichen sclerosus may be complicated by the development of "leukoplakia" and carcinoma. He stated that lichen sclerosus et atrophicus is the most common precursor of vulvar "leukoplakia"; of fifty-two patients with "leukoplakia" complicated by carcinoma, he found that thirty-five had lichen sclerosus et atrophicus as well. We have observed only one patient with carcinoma and lichen sclerosus et atrophicus, both of which were present at her initial visit to the office (Fig. 9-26). None of the thirty-two private patients with lichen sclerosus et atrophicus who have been followed from 5 to 20 years have developed carcinoma. In two recent studies in which tritiated thymidine and acridine-orange fluorescence were used, Woodruff and others and Friedrich, Julian, and Woodruff observed that the metabolic activity of the epithelium in lichen sclerosus et atrophicus appeared to

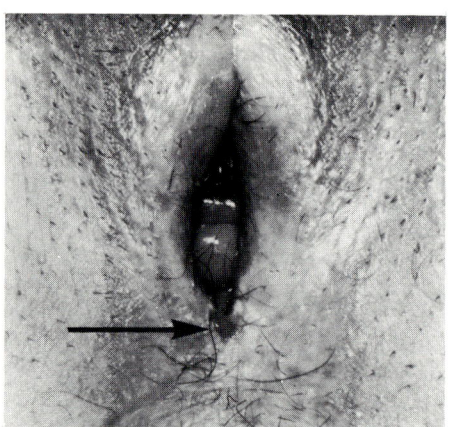

Fig. 9-26. Invasive carcinoma of vulva (arrow) associated with lichen sclerosis et atrophicus. Previously, patient had had a vulvectomy for lichen sclerosis et atrophicus.

be more intense than that of normal tissue. Their findings suggested that the conditions labeled atrophic are, in reality, not inactive or degenerative. On the contrary, Kaufman, Gardner, and Johnson detected no more pronounced uptake of phosphorus-32 in vulvar skin with lichen sclerosus et atrophicus than in normal skin from comparable sites of the vulva. The uptake of phosphorus is related to nuclear activity and is therefore highest where cells are in a growth phase. These latter findings suggest that lichen sclerosus et atrophicus is not necessarily a metabolically excessively active disease.

In summary, the likelihood that a superimposed vulvar carcinoma will develop in a patient with a chronic vulvar dystrophy is small, being in the range of 2 to 5 percent over a prolonged period of time. The patient who is probably destined to develop cancer is the one with microscopically proved atypical hyperplasia at her initial examination by the physician. In the absence of atypia in the dystrophic lesion, the danger of a subsequent carcinoma is almost nil. Any chronic, irritative process of the vulva, however, will add to the risk of carcinoma; thus, patients with any chronic process must be closely followed, with multiple biopsies of the vulva being examined at regular intervals.

Symptoms

The large majority of patients with chronic vulvar dystrophies report that pruritus is the principal symptom. Severe pruritus is probably caused by degeneration and inflammation of terminal nerve fibers. The hyperplastic lesions appear to be associated with the most intense itching; in lichen sclerosus et atrophicus, it is often relatively mild. When pruritus is present, however, a vicious cycle is established; the itching provokes grattage, which in turn increases the itching. The scratching of the vulva frequently produces excoriations and further thickening of the skin and mucosa. On occasion, patients complain of soreness and pain in the vulvar region. Dyspareunia, especially in the presence of lichen sclerosus et atrophicus, is reported fairly often. Shrinkage of the introitus sometimes makes intercourse all but impossible. An occasional patient is free of symptoms; this is especially true of the patient with lichen sclerosus et atrophicus without severe contraction of the vulva.

Treatment

Because of the better understanding of the vulvar dystrophies, treatment for these conditions has been simplified. Since the vast majority of chronic vulvar dystrophies are not premalignant, vulvectomy is recommended only under exceptional circumstances, such as in the presence of significant cellular atypia. In fact, the incidence of recurrence of the dystrophies is so high following a vulvectomy that for most lesions of this type surgical treatment should be condemned. Treatment is based upon several essential principles. First, a thorough evaluation of the disease and a correct diagnosis are required. Second, contributing factors must also be investigated and eliminated. Third, an attempt must be made to relieve the patient's symptoms, and, finally, adequate follow-up of the patient is essential.

Before any treatment is undertaken, multiple punch biopsies should be taken from several areas of the vulva, especially from sites of fissuring, ulceration, induration, and thick plaques. A search should be made for all possible aggravating factors, such as trichomoniasis, candidiasis, allergy, vitamin deficiencies, cervicitis, diabetes, and fungus infections elsewhere in the body; if any are found, the patient should be treated accordingly. The hygienic measures for keeping the vulva clean and dry seem beneficial and should be recommended. Cotton panties should be worn in preference to those made with synthetic materials such as nylon and rayon; this will permit better circulation and evaporation of moisture. Since nervous, emotional women sometimes have vulvar pruritus, which promotes scratching and leads to further secondary changes in the skin, possible emotional factors should be investigated.

After the diagnosis and malignant potential of the lesion have been determined and all possible contributing factors eliminated, local measures for the control of symptoms, primarily pruritus, can be instituted. If an eczematous type of vulvitis, resulting from infected excoriations and ill-chosen medications, is associated, wet dressings with such agents as Burow's Solution, applied frequently, are beneficial. We have observed, however, that lotions and creams containing the combination of an antibacterial agent, such as polymyxin B sulfate (Neosporin), and a corticosteroid afford as rapid a response as wet dressings and are more conveniently applied.

The local application of corticosteroids has been a saving grace in keeping most patients free of symptoms. Application of 0.025% or 0.01% fluocinolone acetomide cream (Synalar), 1% hydrocortisone cream, 0.1% triamcinolone acetomide (Kenalog), or similar products two to three times daily will usually relieve pruritus. Rarely, the intradermal injection of triamcinolone may be tried. A combination of 1% hydrocortisone with 3% iodochlorhydroxyquin (Vioform) is particularly beneficial in the presence of fungi. Complete control of pruritus and burning is no assurance that the lesions will regress. The hyperplastic lesions, however, especially lichen simplex chronicus, may improve to a striking degree or disappear entirely once pruritus is controlled. If so, the histopathologic changes also regress.

Richardson and Williams have reported a pronounced improvement of the tissues, grossly and microscopically, from the use of 500 mg. of testosterone propionate in 10 gm. of white petrolatum jelly massaged into the vulvar tissue two or three times daily. In our experience, testosterone applied topically to the hyperplastic lesions has been of little value for either controlling symptoms or altering the gross and histopathologic changes in the vulvar tissues. As a treatment for lichen sclerosus et atrophicus, however, testosterone has relieved pruritus and brought about improvement of the gross and histopathologic changes. Phimosis and preputial edema are largely controlled. Often, the use of testosterone stimulates libido and causes enlargement of the clitoris. Application of a mixture of 1% hydrocortisone and 2% to 3% testosterone three or four times daily has proved particularly helpful in the relief of the symptoms of lichen sclerosus et atrophicus. This regime may be continued until the patient is asymptomatic; thereafter, the cream may be applied only as necessary to control the symptoms.

Generally, local anesthetic agents such as ethyl aminobenzoate (Benzocaine) should be avoided. Although they may temporarily relieve pruritus, they often provoke severe contact dermatitis. The systemic and local use of estrogens has also been advocated as a treatment for the various vulvar dystrophies; we have found them to be essentially worthless, however, except in the occasional patient with an associated postmenopausal vulvovaginitis. Dystrophies seem largely unrelated to estrogen deficiency. For intractable pruritus, small amounts of alcohol have been injected intradermally into multiple foci throughout the vulva, then rubbed into the tissues. We have had no experience with this method.

Chloroquine has been administered orally for lichen sclerosus et atrophicus. Since the drug may induce changes in the cornea and retina, and since the symptoms are usually readily controlled with topical corticosteroids or testosterone, its use would be seldom, if ever, justified.

The Mehring undercutting operation for relief of pruritus has not been widely accepted. We have not tried this procedure and have seen no patient in whom it seemed indicated.

Since Swift's report, the use of large doses of vitamin A (250,000 to 500,000 U. daily) and dilute hydrochloric acid with meals has been advocated. Although control of symptoms and a regression of the lesions may occasionally follow this treatment, the results are unpredictable.

The administration of x-ray therapy to the vulva is mentioned only to be condemned. It is highly questionable that radiation has a place in treatment of any benign disease of the vulva.

Surgical treatment for the chronic vulvar dystrophies is rarely indicated. If significant cellular atypia is found in a biopsy specimen, however, at least wide excision of a localized lesion, or even vulvectomy, is indicated. Vulvectomy is reserved primarily for the rare patient with uncontrollable disease or for patients with persistent or progressive atypical changes. Should local excision or vulvectomy be neccessary, examination of the margins of the excised tissues is of the utmost importance to ensure removal of all the areas containing atypical cells. Should the skin or mucosal edges exhibit cellular atypia, a more extensive excision should be performed. If vulvectomy is necessary, the high recurrence rate of these lesions calls for regular observation of the patient for a long time thereafter.

The treatment of lichen sclerosus et atrophicus in children is directed primarily to the relief of pruritus. Usually, this can be accomplished with topical corticosteroids. The prognosis of this disease in children differs from that in the adult. Many of the lesions improve or disappear spontaneously during or after adolescence. Resolution usually leaves normal skin. According to Clark and Muller, the clearing of the lesions has no consistent relationship to the menarche, although they have found a general correlation between improvement of the lesions and maturation of the child.

All patients with a chronic vulvar dystrophy should be examined at regular intervals. Biopsies should be taken from areas of ulceration or excoriation or from foci that retain toluidine blue stain (Chapter 10). We strongly urge the use of the toluidine blue test for assisting in the selection of biopsy sites. Following a conservative regime, most patients will remain asymptomatic and need not fear carcinoma. All patients, however, must be impressed with the necessity for regular, adequate follow-up studies, even though they may remain free of symptoms.

REFERENCES

Abel, M. R.: Hyperplastic lesions of the vulva: hypertrophic leukoplakia, dysplasia, intra-epithelial carcinoma, J. Arkansas Med. Soc. 63: 249, 1966.

Berkeley, C., and Bonney, V.: Leukoplakic vulvitis and its relation to kraurosis vulvae and carcinoma vulvae, Brit. Med. J. 2:1739-1744, 1909.

Bonney, V.: Leukoplakic vulvitis and the conditions liable to be confused with it, Proc. Roy. Soc. Med. 31:1057-1060, 1938.

Breisky, A.: Z. Heilk. 6:69, 1885; quoted by Wallace, H. J., and Whimster, I. W., Brit. J. Derm. 63:241-257, 1951.

Chernosky, M. E., Derbes, V. J., and Burks, J. W., Jr.: Lichen sclerosus et atrophicus in children, Arch. Derm. 75:647-652, 1957.

Cinberg, B. L.: Postmenopausal pruritus vulvae, Amer. J. Obstet. Gynec. 49:647-657, 1945.

Clark, J. A., and Muller, S. A.: Lichen sclerosus et atrophicus in children, Arch. Derm. 95: 476-482, 1967.

Clark, W. H., Jr.: A histological study of kraurosis vulvae, lichen sclerosus et atrophicus and leukoplakia of the vulva—a preliminary report, Bull. Tulane U. Med. Fac. 16:123-128, 1957.

Crissey, J. T., Osborne, E. D., and Jordon, J. W.: Lichen sclerosus et atrophicus in children, New York J. Med. 55:2912-2915, 1955.

Ditkowsky, S. P., Falk, A. B., Baker, N., and Schaffner, M.: Lichen sclerosus et atrophicus in childhood, J. Dis. Child. 91:52-54, 1956.

Friedrich, E. G., Julian, C. G., and Woodruff, J. D.: Acridine-orange fluorescence in vulvar dysplasia, Amer. J. Obstet. Gynec. 90:1281-1287, 1964.

Hallopeau, H., quoted by Shelley, W., and Crissey, J. T.: Classics in clinical dermatology, Springfield, Ill., 1953, Charles C Thomas, Publisher, p. 289.

Hunt, E.: Diseases affecting the vulva, London, 1954, Henry Kimpton Co.

Hyman, A. B.: Atrophic and "white" lesions of the vulva, Skin 2:121-125, 1963.

Hyman, A. B., and Falk, H. C.: White lesions of the vulva, Obstet. Gynec. 12:407-413, 1958.

Janovski, N. A., and Ames, S.: Lichen sclerosus et atrophicus of the vulva, Obstet. Gynec. 22: 697-708, 1963.

Jeffcoate, T. N. A.: Chronic vulvar dystrophies, Amer. J. Obstet. Gynec. 95:61-71, 1966.

Jeffcoate, T. N. A.: Dermatology of the vulva, J. Obstet. Gynaec. Brit. Comm. 69:889-890, 1962.

Jeffcoate, T. N. A., and Woodcock, A. S.: Premalignant conditions of the vulva with particular reference to chronic epithelial dystrophies, Brit. Med. J. 15:127, 1961.

Kaufman, R. H., Gardner, H. L., and Johnson, P. C.: P-32 uptake in lichen sclerosus et atrophicus of the vulva, Amer. J. Obstet. Gynec. 98:312-319, 1967.

Kindler, T.: Lichen sclerosus et atrophicus in young subjects, Brit. J. Derm. 65:269-279, 1953.

Langley, I. I., Hertig, A. T., and Smith, G. V. S.: Relation of leukoplakia vulvitis to squamous carcinoma of the vulva, Amer. J. Obstet. Gynec. 62:167-169, 1951.

Lascano, E. F., Montes, L. F., and Mazzini, M. A.: Lichen sclerosus et atrophicus in childhood—report of six cases, Obstet. Gynec. 24: 872-877, 1964.

Lever, W. F.: Histopathology of the skin, Philadelphia, 1967, J. B. Lippincott Co.

McAdams, A. J., and Kistner, R. W.: The relationship of chronic vulvar disease, leukoplakia and carcinoma in situ to carcinoma of the vulva, Cancer 11:740-757, 1958.

Miller, N. F., Parrott, M. H., Stryker, J., Riley, G. M., and Curtis, A. C.: Leukoplakia of the vulva: Preliminary report, Amer. J. Obstet. Gynec. 54:543-560, 1947.

Oberfield, R. A.: Lichen sclerosus et atrophicus and kraurosis vulvae: Are they the same disease?, Arch. Derm. 83:806-815, 1961.

Parrott, M. H., and Miller, N. F.: Diseases of the vulva. In Davis, C. H., and Carter, B., editors: Gynecology and obstetrics, Hagerstown, Md., 1953, W. F. Prior Co.

Richardson, A. C., and Williams, G. A.: Topical androgenic hormones in vulvar kraurosis–leukoplakia syndrome, Amer. J. Obstet. Gynec. **76:** 791-799, 1958.

Schwimmer, E.: Die idiopathischen Schleim haut plaques der Mundhöhle, Vrtljschr. Derm. Syph. **9-10:**510-570, 1877-1878.

Suūrmond, D.: Lichen sclerosus et atrophicus of the vulva, Arch. Derm. **90:**143-152, 1964.

Swift, B. H.: Achlorhydria as an aetiological factor in pruritus vulvae, associated with kraurosis or leukoplakia, J. Obstet. Gynaec. Brit. Comm. **43:**1053-1077, 1936.

Taussig, F. J.: Cancer of the vulva: An analysis of 155 cases, Amer. J. Obstet. Gynec. **40:**764-779, 1940.

Taussig, F. J.: Diseases of the vulva, New York 1923, D. Appleton & Co.

Taussig, F. J.: Leukoplakia and cancer of the vulva, Arch. Derm. Syph. **21:**431-445, 1930.

Taylor, C. W.: Dermatology of the vulva, J. Obstet. Gynaec. Brit. Comm. **69:**881-887, 1962.

Van Geuns, E. J.: Kraurosis vulvae, Nederl. T. Verlosk. **59:**49-61, 1959.

Wallace, H. J.: Vulvar leukoplakia, J. Obstet. Gynaec. Brit. Comm. **69:**865-870, 1962.

Wallace, H. J., and Whimster, I. W.: Vulvar atrophy and leukoplakia, Brit. J. Derm. **63:** 241-257, 1951.

Whimster, I. W.: Personal communication. In Jeffcoate, T. N. A.: The dermatology of the vulva, J. Obstet. Gynaec. Brit. Comm. **69:**888, 1962.

Williams, G. A., Richardson, A. C., and Hathcock, E. W.: Topical testosterone in dystrophic diseases of the vulva, Amer. J. Obstet. Gynec. **96:**21-30, 1966.

Woodruff, J. D., and Baens, J. S.: Interpretation of atrophic and hypertrophic alterations in the vulvar epithelium, Amer. J. Obstet. Gynec. **86:** 713-723, 1963.

Woodruff, J. D., Borkowf, H. I., Holzman, G. B., Arnold, E. A., and Knaack, J.: Metabolic activity in normal and abnormal vulvar epithelia, Amer. J. Obstet. Gynec. **91:**809-819, 1965.

Chapter 10

Intraepithelial carcinoma of the vulva

Intraepithelial carcinoma of the vulva has been defined by a variety of terms, including Bowen's disease, erythroplasia of Queyrat, squamous cell carcinoma in situ, and Paget's disease. Woodruff and Hildebrandt pointed out that there is no characteristic microscopic picture for the various types of intraepithelial carcinoma of the vulva and that it may vary in different areas of a single lesion. We concur with this opinion, although we believe that subtle differences between each of these diseases will become apparent if the gross and microscopic features of each lesion are carefully correlated and evaluated. For practical purposes, separation of intraepithelial carcinoma of the vulva into four types is somewhat academic, since the treatment for all is similar. Some importance, however, must be attached to the fact that Paget's disease is more often associated with an adjacent invasive carcinoma than the other varieties of intraepithelial carcinoma and that the biologic behavior of Bowen's disease differs materially from that of the other lesions in this category.

The general characteristics and gross and microscopic appearance of each of the above types of intraepithelial carcinoma of the vulva are separately discussed. Since the symptoms and the treatment for all four diseases are similar, they are discussed for the group as a whole rather than for each lesion separately.

Bowen's disease

Bowen, in 1912, first described the disease bearing his name. He believed the lesion, which was observed on the arm of one male patient and on the buttock of another, to be a premalignant dermatosis, though it is now believed to be a malignant growth limited to the epidermis. Unfortunately, a variety of gross and microscopic lesions have been erroneously termed Bowen's disease, despite the fact that the gross and microscopic findings in the lesion are quite specific.

Knight found that the age of the average patient with Bowen's disease of the vulva is 48.3 years, the span being between 25 and 73 years. The average duration of symptoms in the twenty-six cases he reviewed was 4.6 years, varying between 3 months and 11 years. In one of the six new cases he reported, Bowen's disease was associated with an invasive carcinoma. In two cases, the patients had a "leukoplakic" lesion involving the vulva.

Clinical features

Bowen's disease is a superficial, noninvasive, intraepithelial carcinoma characterized by chronicity, pruritus, and a typical gross and microscopic appearance. Lever described the disease as a "single lesion characterized by a dull red patch of sharp but irregular outline, showing little or no infiltration. In the patch there are generally areas of crusting beneath which one finds a granular oozing surface. The patch spreads slowly by peripheral extension and shows no tendency to healing in its center." On the skin surfaces of the vulva, the lesion may have a white appearance, although more often it appears red and raw, as described above (Fig. 10-1). It may be grossly confused with eczema, tuberculosis, or other

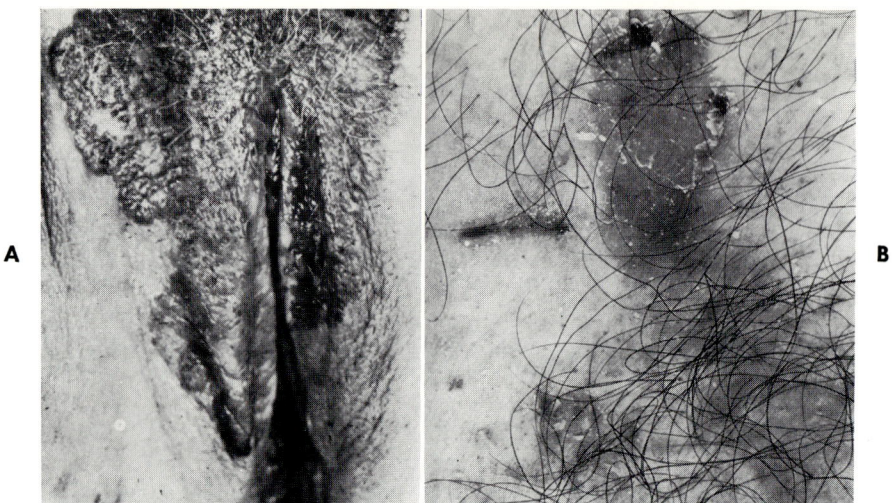

Fig. 10-1. Bowen's disease. **A,** Dull red, crusty lesion with sharp outline. (Courtesy Dr. Lawrence L. Hester, Jr., Charleston, S. C.) **B,** Typical dull red patch covered by scales and crusts. (Kaufman, R. H., and Gardner, H. L.: Clin. Obstet. Gynec. 8:1035, 1965.)

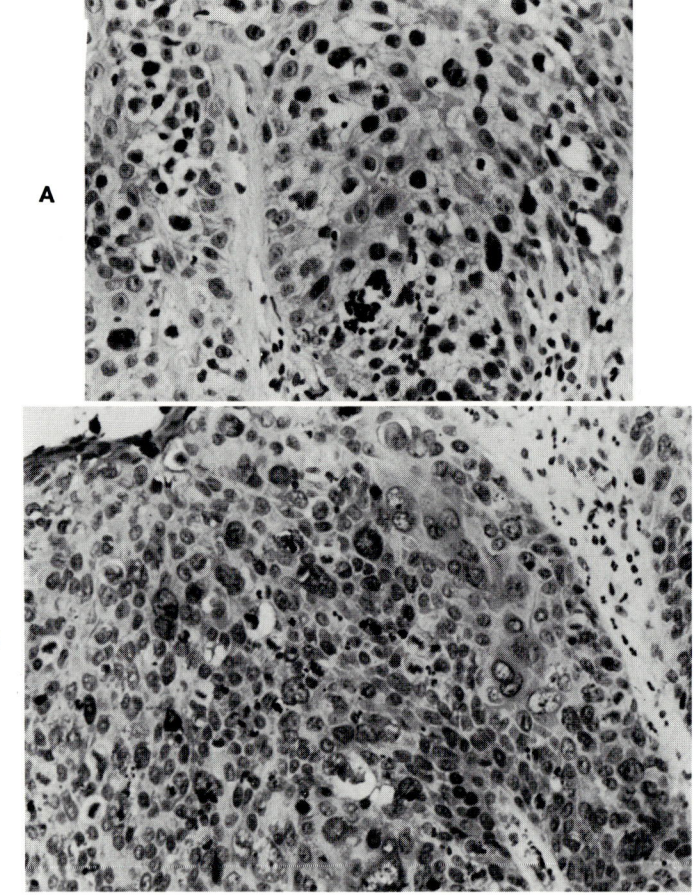

Fig. 10-2. Bowen's disease. **A** and **B,** Large, irregular, hyperchromatic nuclei lie in complete disorder. Cells with vacuolated cytoplasm are also present. (**A,** H & E × 250; **B,** H & E × 300)

benign superficial ulcers and, rarely, with condyloma acuminatum, as reported by Janovski and Barchet.

Histopathology

Hyperkeratosis, parakeratosis, and acanthosis may be observed on microscopic examination of the lesion. Throughout the stratum malpighii, the cells lie in complete disorder and many are atypical, having large and hyperchromatic nuclei (Fig. 10-2). Multinucleated epidermal cells are frequently present. Some cells may contain vacuoles, simulating Paget's cells; in contrast to Paget's cells, however, the intercellular bridges of these cells are preserved. Keratinization of individual cells in the stratum malpighii (dyskeratosis) is commonly found, with each of the cells containing a strongly eosinophilic cytoplasm and a large, irregularly shaped hyperchromatic nucleus. Moderate numbers of lymphocytes and plasma cells are present in the corium and within the papillae. Many small congested vascular channels are apparent.

In true Bowen's disease, the basal layer of the epithelium is intact. Ultimately, the basement membrane may be broken through with the development of a true invasive carcinoma. This usually is a slow process, the lesion being preinvasive for many years prior to infiltration of the dermis. Jeffcoate, Davie, and Harrison have mentioned that progression into a frank epithelioma is more likely when the lesion encroaches upon mucous membrane.

Erythroplasia of Queyrat

Erythroplasia of Queyrat usually involves the glans penis, though it may arise on the

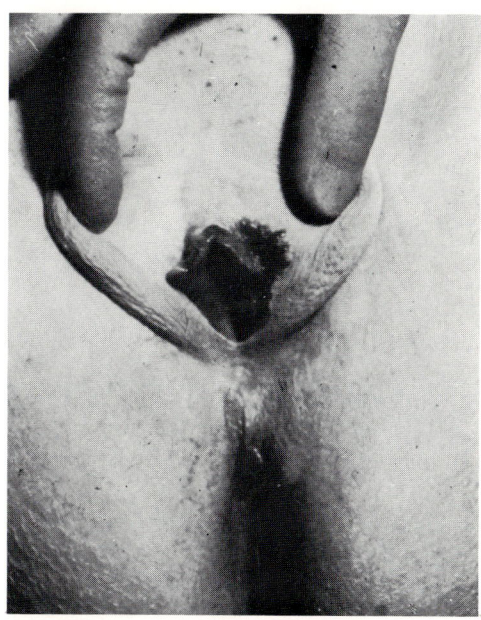

Fig. 10-3. Erythroplasia of Queyrat, exhibited by a well-defined, velvety red lesion. (Courtesy T. N. A. Jeffcoate, Liverpool, England.)

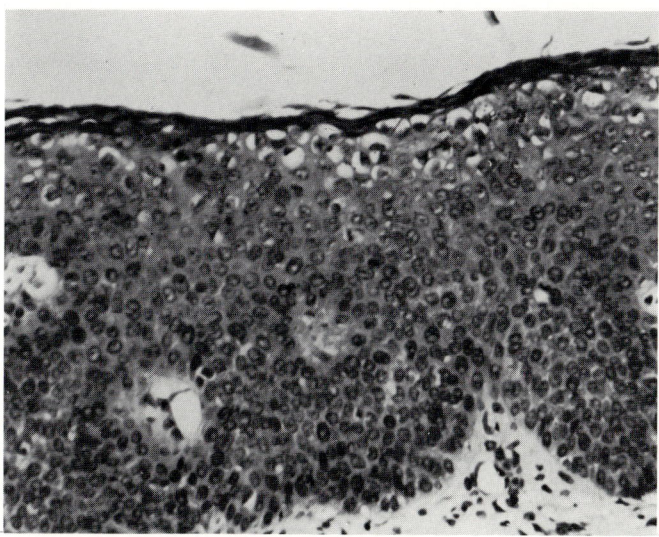

Fig. 10-4. Erythroplasia of Queyrat. The changes are similar to those observed in squamous cell carcinoma in situ. Biopsy from typical velvety red, granular mucosa. (H & E × 180)

mucosa of the vulva. It is an intraepithelial squamous cell carcinoma of the mucous membrane, analogous to Bowen's disease of the skin. The lesion grows slowly and is malignant, eventually invading the underlying corium. Sulzberger and Satenstein have noted a more rapid progression into invasive squamous cell carcinoma than is true of Bowen's disease. Paletta reported one case in which erythroplasia of Queyrat involved the vulva and fourchette and extended into the vagina. One year after its wide local excision, a similar lesion reappeared in the vagina. Paletta believed that the lesion tends to be multicentric and to progress to invasive carcinoma.

Erythroplasia of Queyrat is manifested by a single, well-defined area with a brilliant red, velvety, finely granular surface that exhibits little or no infiltration (Fig. 10-3). Microscopically, erythroplasia demonstrates changes identical to those of squamous cell carcinoma in situ found elsewhere in the body (Fig. 10-4). On the vulva, however, it is distinguished from the latter lesion primarily on the basis of its location and gross appearance.

Squamous cell carcinoma in situ

A third variety of intraepithelial carcinoma, and one that we believe more often arises on the vulva than the two discussed previously, is referred to by Abell and Gosling as "intraepithelial carcinoma simplex." A better term would probably be "squamous cell carcinoma in situ." This lesion, frequently appearing as a thickened white area, is easily confused with other white lesions of the vulva (Fig. 10-5). Only by microscopic evaluation of the tissue can the diagnosis be established.

Histopathology

The microscopic pattern of squamous cell carcinoma in situ (Fig. 10-6) differs from that of Bowen's disease. The features of malignancy are somewhat more subtle; a variation of nuclear size and shape, hyperchromatism, and scattered mitotic figures are observed, although the bizarre nuclear forms

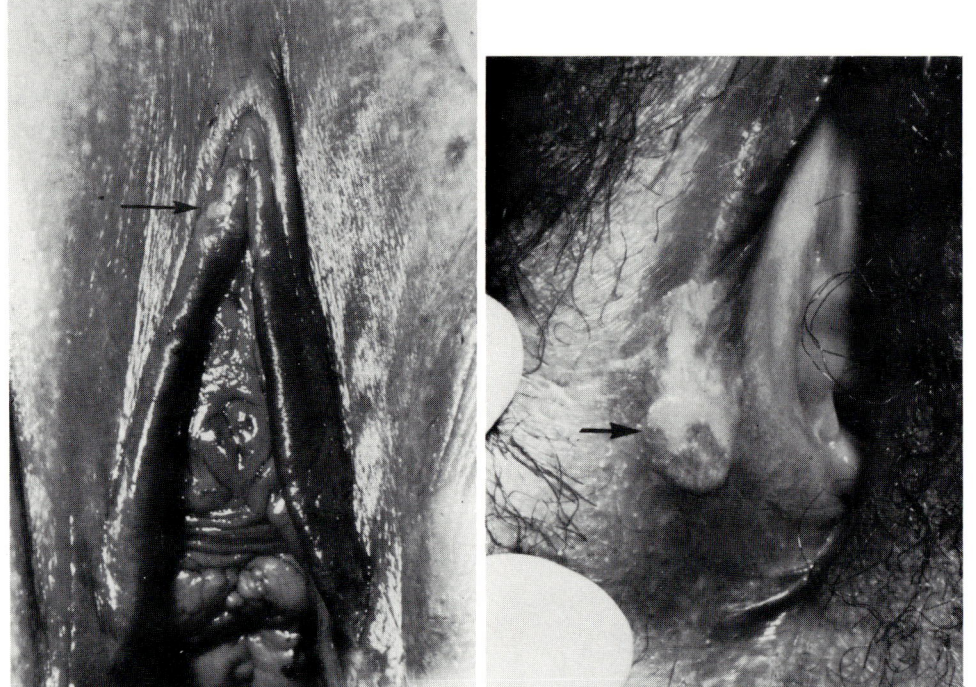

Fig. 10-5. A and B, Squamous cell carcinoma in situ. Single lesions frequently appear as thickened white areas. Also see Fig. 10-9, A and B. A, Kaufman, R. H., and Gardner, H. L.: Clin. Obstet. Gynec. 8:1035, 1965; B, courtesy James A. Friedman, Houston.)

Intraepithelial carcinoma of the vulva 143

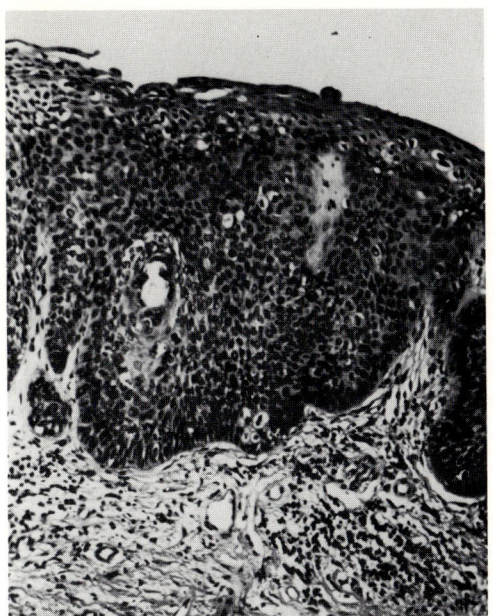

Fig. 10-6. Squamous cell carcinoma in situ. The nuclear changes are less bizarre than those usually found in Bowen's disease. (H & E × 120) (Kaufman, R. H., and Gardner, H. L.: Clin. Obstet. Gynec. 8:1035, 1965.)

and malignant multinucleated giant cells seen in Bowen's disease are lacking. Hyperkeratosis is often a feature and, if present, is responsible for the frequent white appearance of the lesion. The thickness of the epithelium differs widely, but it is usually thicker than normal with a variable elongation of the rete pegs. Frequently, a chronic inflammatory exudate is found within the dermis. The association of this vulvar disease with foci of squamous cell carcinoma in situ involving other areas of the vulva, vagina, and cervix has been reported and will be discussed later in more detail.

Paget's disease

Extramammary Paget's disease is a slowly progressive intraepithelial carcinoma containing the typical vacuolated Paget's cells and is histologically identical to the lesion around the nipple. In contrast to Paget's disease of the nipple, which is considered to be caused by an underlying ductal carcinoma, Paget's disease of the anogenital region is associated with an underlying apocrine carcinoma in 30 to 50 percent of the cases. It may also be associated with a primary carcinoma of the rectum, urethra, and even the breast, especially when it involves the perianal region.

Paget's disease generally develops in postmenopausal women, although it may arise in younger age groups. In view of its frequent association with sweat gland carcinoma of the vulva or some other adjacent internal carcinoma, the prognosis is less favorable than that of the other varieties of intraepithelial carcinoma of the vulva.

Histogenesis

Several theories have been offered regarding the histogenesis of extramammary Paget's disease. It is generally accepted that it affects those areas of the body containing numerous apocrine glands. Several authors are of the opinion that it is probably an intraepithelial metastasis from an underlying glandular or ductal carcinoma. Taki and Janovski have suggested that an underlying sweat gland carcinoma may arise either from a downgrowth of the primary epidermal tumor or from the simultaneous development of an epidermal and sweat gland carcinoma. The theory that Paget's disease has a multicentric and autochthonous origin has been supported by the observations of Helwig and Graham, that is, that the disease may involve the epidermis alone, both the epidermis and underlying adnexal structures, or both the epidermis and adjacent internal organs. Woodruff and Kaufman, Boice, and Knight have concurred in the suggestion that the epidermal disease may arise from epidermal cells having the potential to form apocrine glands. This is plausible when one considers the embryology of the epidermis. The apocrine glands are derived from the primary epithelial germ cells that appear in the third month of fetal life as epithelial buds projecting into the dermis. The primary epithelial germ develops from the inner layer of the epidermis (embryonal stratum germinativum) in the early fetus, which also gives rise eventually to the surface epidermis. It is possible that cell rests from the primary epithelial germ or embryonal stratum germinativum with apocrine gland potential may be left in the surface epidermis and that these cells may be the source of intraepidermal Paget's disease.

Clinical features

The gross appearance of Paget's disease is variable. It is typically described as an ery-

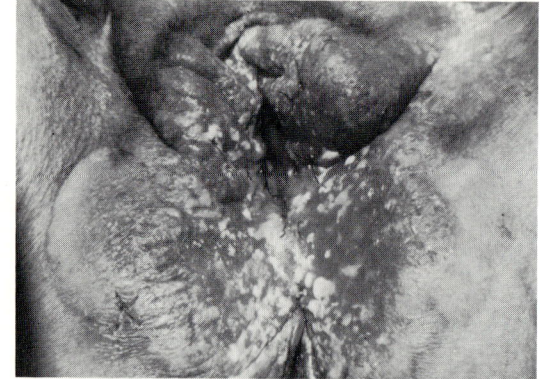
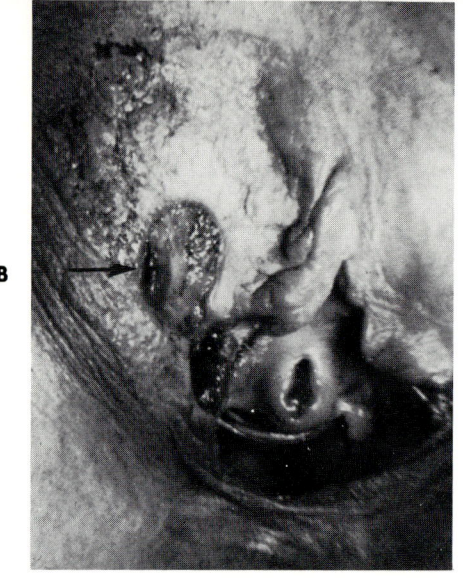

Fig. 10-7. **A**, Paget's disease. An eczematoid lesion covered with scales and crusts. (Courtesy John W. H. Glasser, Fairlawn, N. J.) **B**, Paget's disease. An ulcerated area (arrow) in a crusted white lesion. (Courtesy Felix N. Rutledge, Jr., Houston.)

thematous, eczematoid lesion having scales and crusts scattered over the surface (Fig. 10-7, *A*). Often, however, it may present a whitish-gray appearance. Frequently, the lesions are ulcerated (Fig. 10-7, *B*), moist, and oozing; they may bleed readily on contact. They may involve the perianal area as well as the vulva; among the forty cases reported by Helwig and Graham, the lesions in twenty-nine involved the vulva and/or the perianal region. The diameter of the lesions varied from 0.4 to 12 cm. The clinical diagnosis based on the gross appearance of the disease is usually erroneous, as indicated by the fact that in only two of the cases reported by Helwig and Graham was the lesion recognized prior to biopsy.

Histopathology

Although the microscopic picture of Paget's disease is quite typical, it is often confused with Bowen's disease and, at times, with melanoma. Considerable acanthosis, hyperkeratosis, and parakeratosis of the squamous epithelium are present. The cells are usually large and irregular and contain a clear, vacuolated cytoplasm; this is the identifying feature of the lesion (Fig. 10-8, *A*). In contrast to Bowen's disease, the vacuolated cells do not have prickles, and the malpighian cells between appear normal. The nuclei are vesicular, may vary in size and shape, and may exhibit hyperchromatosis. They rarely contain a mitotic figure. The cells may be separate or in clumps; they are most numerous in the tips and sides of the rete pegs and deep in the epithelium. They may also infiltrate through the full thickness of the epithelium and may be scattered throughout the outer keratinized layer. Many of the Paget's cells lie within the apocrine sweat ducts and around the hair follicles. A chronic inflammatory infiltrate is usually found beneath the epidermis.

Careful histologic study of the excised surgical specimen may reveal that the lesion extends well beyond the grossly visible limits of the disease. This may account for incomplete excision and so-called recurrence of the tumor. Following recurrence of a lesion that had been incompletely removed, Adamson and Reisfield observed intraepidermal migration of Paget's cells across the line of excision of the tumor. Both of these features are important in regard to adequate treatment of this disease and lend support to the necessity for extensive vulvectomy.

The use of histochemical staining techniques will lead to a confirmation of the diagnosis of Paget's disease and will rule out such lesions as melanoma, Bowen's disease, and erythroplasia of Queyrat. The presence of acid or neutral mucopolysaccharides within the cells is pathognomonic of the disease, as shown by Janovski, Taki and Janovski, and Helwig and Graham. These authors demonstrated the histochemical differences between Paget's disease and malignant melanoma, Bowen's disease, and erythroplasia of Queyrat. The most consistent difference ob-

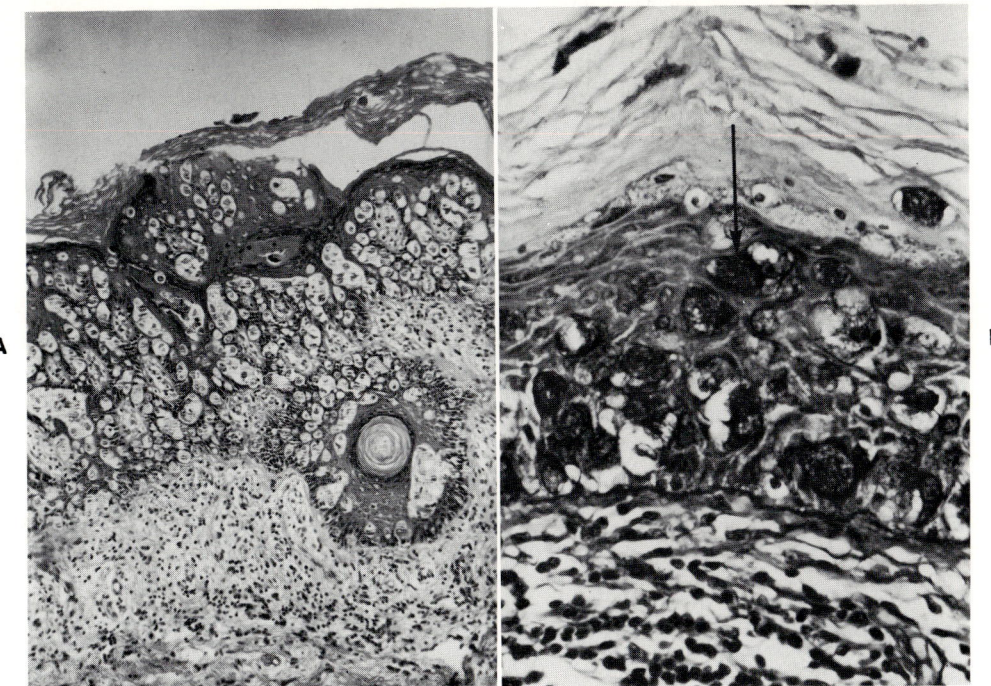

Fig. 10-8. **A**, Paget's disease. Typical pale, vacuolated cells within epidermis and extending around a hair follicle and into outer keratinized layer. (H & E × 120) (Kaufman, R. H., Boice, E. H., and Knight, W. R.: Amer. J. Obstet. Gynec. **79**:451, 1960.) **B**, Paget's disease. PAS-positive material resistant to digestion with diastase, represented by darkly stained areas within cytoplasm (arrow). (PAS × 400) (Kaufman, R. H., Boice, E. H., and Knight, W. R.: Amer. J. Obstet. Gynec. **79**:451, 1960.)

served by Helwig and Graham was the presence of aldehyde-fuchsin and mucicarmine-positive material within the cytoplasm of the Paget's cells, though not within the cells of the other three diseases. The Paget's cells also contained PAS-positive material, which was resistant to digestion with diastase (Fig. 10-8, *B*). All three groups of authors also obtained positive acid mucopolysaccharide stains, resistant to removal with hyaluronidase, and positive alcian blue stains. Helwig and Graham were of the opinion that the Paget's cells probably contain protein, mucoproteins, glycoproteins, acid mucopolysaccharides, neutral polysaccharides, and possibly sulfated acid mucopolysaccharides.

Several authors have observed melanin granules within the cytoplasm of some of the Paget's cells. This is probably attributable to the ability of melanocytes to transfer melanin granules into the cytoplasm of the Paget's cells or possibly to the ability of these cells to phagocytize melanin granules. To help distinguish the Paget's cells from melanoma cells, Woodruff and Williams, using the dopa reaction, tested the Paget's cells for the presence of the enzyme dopa-oxidase. Since this enzyme is necessary for the formation of the melanin complex by a cell, its absence would indicate that a cell is not actively producing melanin. They obtained a negative reaction. Janovski, on the contrary, found a positive dopa reaction in many cells.

Opinion is divided regarding the association of extramammary Paget's disease with an underlying sweat gland carcinoma. Many well-documented cases, both with and without associated sweat gland carcinoma, have been reported. Because of the association of such a malignant tumor within the underlying dermis in 30 to 50 percent of cases, it is mandatory that the surgical specimen be carefully cut and step-sectioned so that a small underlying carcinoma will not be overlooked. Finding such a tumor would certainly influence the subsequent treatment. Helwig and Graham found that eleven of the thirteen patients in their series who had an underlying cutaneous adnexal carcinoma had regional or widespread metastases to the internal organs. All of these eleven patients eventually died of their disease. In contrast, of eighteen patients who had no evidence of adjacent carcinoma, only one died, this death resulting from unknown causes. Helwig and Graham also mentioned the poor prognosis of the patient with perianal Paget's disease: twelve of fourteen patients with lesions of this region had either an underlying adnexal carcinoma or an adenocarcinoma of the rectum or breast. Nine of these twelve patients died of their disease.

General characteristics of intraepithelial carcinoma

Although the gross and microscopic appearance of the various types of intraepithelial carcinoma is variable, the symptoms and the treatment are essentially the same for each lesion. The outstanding symptom is pruritus, having been reported in 63 percent of the patients observed by Abell and Gosling and in more than 50 percent of those in the series of Woodruff and Hildebrandt and of Barclay and Collins. Pain, soreness, and the presence of a tumor are also frequently mentioned. Woodruff and Hildebrandt found that the average age of their patients was 53 years, this being 7 years less than the average age of patients with invasive carcinoma.

The finding of a second squamous cell carcinoma, invasive or in situ, in another area of the vulva, vagina, or cervix is not uncommon. Woodruff and Novak discovered four carcinomata of the cervix in fourteen patients with in situ lesions of the vulva, and Eichner oberved one patient with carcinoma in situ in four noncontiguous areas involving the cervix, right labium minus, left labium minus, and fourchette. Hillemann found a concomitant carcinoma in situ of the ectocervix and intraepithelial carcinoma of the vulva or lower vagina in two patients with Bowen's disease and in one with erythroplasia of Queyrat. We have observed one patient who was found to have an invasive squamous cell carcinoma of the midvaginal region 5 years after a vulvectomy for carcinoma in situ of the vulva, and another woman who was diagnosed as having invasive squamous cell carcinoma, also of the midvagina, 6 years after having had a hysterectomy for carcinoma in situ of the cervix.

Before treatment for intraepithelial carcinoma of the vulva is undertaken, a precise diagnosis is essential. This is best established by biopsy. It is accepted that any white lesion or ulcerated or fissured area of the vulva should be biopsied. Certainly, the presence of one of the varieties of intraepithelial carcinoma should be suspected on the basis of the gross lesions described here. At times, however, the most suitable areas for biopsy pose a problem, since the vulva may well be involved with an extensive white or erythematous lesion. Collins, utilizing a technique used by Richart on the cervix, has recently suggested an excellent means for selecting the sites for biopsy. His technique is also helpful in defining the limits of surgical excision. He has recommended painting the vulva with 1% toluidine blue, then washing the area with 1% acetic acid. Under normal conditions, the toluidine blue will be removed following the application of the acetic acid; in the presence of an in situ or an invasive carcinoma, however, the stain will remain in the area affected. This test was positive in all of thirteen cases of carcinoma he examined. In a comparative study of eighty-one control patients, no retention of the stain was observed. False positive staining was obtained in the presence of some benign ulcers of the vulva. In a limited experience with this test for carcinoma of the vulva, we have found that the stain was retained only in those areas of the vulva where the lesion was located (Fig. 10-9). Also, superficial ulcerations were persistently stained.

Janovski and Clark and others have studied the uptake of parenterally administered radioactive phosphorus in patients with Paget's disease and other vulvar lesions. Janovski reported that the uptake of phosphorus-32 in the region of Paget's disease was three times that in normal skin. Clark and others reported an increased uptake of phosphorus-32 in precancerous lesions and intraepithelial carcinomata of the vulva. This may be of only academic interest in regard to the preoperative diagnosis of these diseases, though it could be of practical value in the follow-up studies of these patients, since areas of increased radioactivity in the vulva would lead

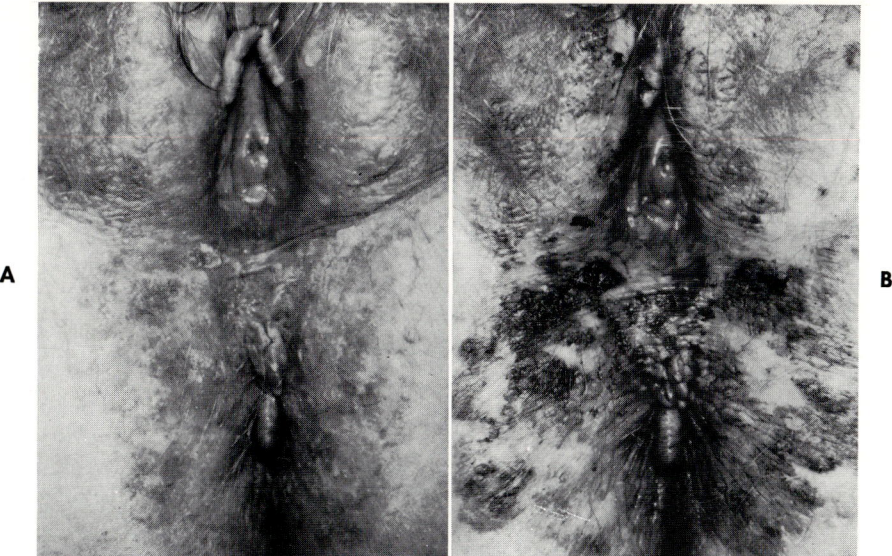

Fig. 10-9. A, Squamous cell carcinoma in situ, multifocal, before being stained with toluidine blue. Extensive red and white plaques. B, Toluidine blue stain (1%) retained by areas of in situ carcinoma after vulva was washed with 1% acetic acid.

one to suspect the presence of persistent or recurrent disease.

Treatment

We are inclined to agree with Barclay and Collins regarding the treatment for intraepithelial carcinoma of the vulva. A complete and extensive vulvectomy should be performed; with the exception of the lymph node dissection, the operation is essentially the same as that for invasive carcinoma. The basis for this procedure is the multicentric origin of the disease in the vulva in many patients and the frequent finding of invasive carcinoma elsewhere in the same vulva. Extensive vulvectomy is especially indicated for squamous cell carcinoma in situ, erythroplasia of Queyrat, or Paget's disease of the vulva. Vulvectomy for true Bowen's disease perhaps need not be so extensive, since the likelihood of associated invasive carcinoma is much less. Abell and Gosling found that ten of twenty patients with carcinoma in situ of the vulva had associated invasive disease. We have observed both lesions in several patients treated primarily for intraepithelial carcinoma of the vulva. It is essential that the vulvectomy specimens be carefully and thoroughly sectioned so that an invasive carcinoma, if present, will be detected. This is also true in Paget's disease, so that an underlying sweat gland carcinoma, if present, will be discovered. In the latter events, a bilateral lymph node dissection should be performed in addition to the vulvectomy.

Even after extensive vulvectomy, Barclay and Collins reported recurrences in two of the twenty-one patients whom they treated. One recurrence appeared 3 years following vulvectomy as an invasive carcinoma that led to the patient's death, and the other recurred as carcinoma in situ 10 years after the initial treatment. Abell and Gosling reported recurrent intraepithelial carcinoma in six of twenty-four patients treated. They felt that the lesions were new carcinomas rather than residual disease. The toluidine blue technique described by Collins would certainly be an excellent method of following patients postoperatively. Areas in which retention of the stain was subsequently demonstrated should be biopsied.

REFERENCES

Abell, M. R., and Gosling, J. R. G.: Intraepithelial and infiltrative carcinoma of the vulva: Bowen's type, Cancer **14**:318, 1961.

Adamson, K., Jr., and Reisfield, D.: Observations on intradermal migration of Paget cells, Amer. J. Obstet. Gynec. **90**:1274, 1964.

Barclay, D. L., and Collins, C. G.: Intraepithelial cancer of the vulva, Amer. J. Obstet. Gynec. **86:** 95, 1963.

Blau, S., and Hyman, A. B.: Erythroplasia of Queyrat, Acta Dermatovener. (Stockholm) **35:** 341, 1955.

Bowen, J. T.: Precancerous dermatoses, J. Cutan. Dis. **30:**241, 1912.

Clark, C. D., Zumoff, B., Brunschweig, A., and Hellman, L.: Preferential uptake of phosphate by premalignant and malignant lesions of the vulva, Cancer **13:**775, 1960.

Collins, C.: In discussion of paper by Woodruff, J. D., and others: Metabolic activity in normal and abnormal vulva epithelia, Amer. J. Obstet. Gynec. **91:**818, 1965.

Dockerty, M. B., and Pratt, J. H.: Extra-mammary Paget's disease, Cancer **5:**1161, 1952.

Eichner, E.: Multiple carcinoma-in-situ, Obstet. Gynec. **8:**508, 1956.

Helwig, E. B., and Graham, J. H.: Anogenital Paget's disease, Cancer **16:**387, 1963.

Hillemann, H. G.: Cervical carcinoma-in-situ as compared with carcinoma-in-situ of other sites, Acta Cytol. **6:**201, 1962.

Huber, C. P., Gardner, S. H., and Michael, A.: Paget's disease of the vulva, Amer. J. Obstet. Gynec. **62:**778, 1951.

Hyman, A. B., and Leider, M.: Erythroplasia of the female genitalia, Arch. Derm. **84:**71, 1961.

Janovski, N. A.: Dopa oxidase and P-32 uptake in extra-mammary Paget's disease of the vulva, Gynaecologia (Basel) **153:**354, 1962.

Janovski, N. A., and Barchet, S.: Multicentric Bowen's disease of the vulva, Obstet. Gynec. **28:**170, 1966.

Jeffcoate, T. N. A., Davie, T. B., and Harrison, C. V.: Intraepidermal carcinoma (Bowen's disease) of the vulva, J. Obstet. Gynaec. Brit. Comm. **51:**377, 1944.

Kaufman, R. H., Boice, E. H., and Knight, W. R., III: Paget's disease of the vulva, Amer. J. Obstet. Gynec. **79:**451, 1960.

Knight, R. van D.: Bowen's disease of the vulva, Amer. J. Obstet. Gynec. **46:**514, 1943.

Lever, W. F.: Histopathology of the skin, Philadelphia, 1967, J. B. Lippincott Co.

McDaniel, W. E., and Mason, L. M.: Malignant dyskeratoses, erythroplasia of Queyrat type, Arch. Derm. (Chicago) **60:**419, 1949.

Paletta, F. X.: Erythroplasia of Queyrat, Plast. Reconstr. Surg. **23:**195, 1959.

Richart, R. M.: A clinical staining test for the in vivo delineation of dysplasia and carcinoma in situ, Amer. J. Obstet. Gynec. **86:**703, 1963.

Sulzberger, M. B., and Satenstein, D. L.: Erythroplasia of Queyrat, Arch. Derm. (Chicago) **28:** 798, 1933.

Taki, I., and Janovski, N. A.: Paget's disease of the vulva: Presentation and histochemical study of four cases, Obstet. Gynec. **18:**385, 1961.

Wiener, H. A.: Paget's disease of the skin and its relation to carcinoma of the apocrine sweat glands, Amer. J. Cancer **31:**373, 1937.

Woodruff, J. D.: Paget's disease of the vulva, Obstet. Gynec. **5:**175, 1955.

Woodruff, J. D., and Hildebrandt, E. E.: Carcinoma-in-situ of the vulva, Obstet. Gynec. **12:** 414, 1958.

Woodruff, J. D., and Novak, E. R.: Pre-malignant lesions of the vulva, Clin. Obstet. Gynec. **5:** 1102, 1962.

Woodruff, J. D., and Williams, T. F., Jr.: Dopa reaction in Paget's disease of the vulva, Obstet. Gynec. **14:**86, 1959.

Chapter 11

Candidiasis (moniliasis)

VULVOVAGINAL CANDIDIASIS

Candidiasis of the vulva and vagina has replaced trichomoniasis as the most prevalent and most obstinate form of "vaginitis." The disease was first described by Wilkinson in 1849, when he related a vaginal fungus to vaginitis. In 1875, Haussman demonstrated the pathogenicity of vaginal fungi by transferring infected material to the normal vagina to produce the disease. Hesseltine, Borts, and Plass, in 1934, further proved the pathogenicity of vaginal *Candida* by repeatedly producing candidiasis in normal patients by inoculation of the cultured organisms.

Genital candidiasis has been variously known as vaginal moniliasis, monilial vaginitis, candidal vulvovaginitis, mycotic vulvovaginitis, yeast vulvovaginitis, vaginal thrush, and numerous other names, including candidosis. It is sometimes incorrectly called a "yeast infection," an error that arose because of the similarity of the conidia of *Candidia* to true yeast cells such as *Saccharomyces*. The latter organisms are not uncommonly recovered from the vagina; they are not vaginal pathogens, however, since they do not produce vulvovaginal disease. The term "yeast-like" infection is an acceptable term.

Failure to agree upon a name is attributable to the taxonomic confusion surrounding the genus of the causative organisms, which have been classified and reclassified many times. According to Wilson, there are 172 synonyms for *Candida albicans*. The terms *Oidium* and *Monilia* survived most others as generic names, until Berkhout, in 1923, proposed the name *Candida* for the medical monilias. Ultimately, *Candida* was officially adopted as a nomen conservandum by the Third International Microbiological Congress in 1939 and by the Eighth Botanical Congress in Paris in 1954. Although the term "moniliasis" is sentimentally preferred, we are impelled to follow the obvious trend and call the disease by its modern name.

Etiology

According to current concepts of mycology, the host factors controlling susceptibility are much more significant in the development of candidiasis than the chance contamination of the vagina by a species of *Candida*. More than the mere presence of *Candida* is necessary for development of the clinical disease.

Etiologic agents. The specific causative agents belong to the genus *Candida*. The organisms are indigenous to practically all human beings and to many animals. Usually, they are commensal, becoming pathogenic when favorable environmental conditions develop in the host. Although reports differ widely, it is probable that less than 50 percent of patients who harbor *Candida* in the vagina have clinical disease. It must be assumed that a limited number of the organisms regularly find entry into the vagina from one or another source and live as transients or produce disease according to the pathogenicity of the organism and host susceptibility.

Candida albicans is the type that most often causes infection, although *C. tropicalis* is a common offender, and *C. pseudotropicalis, C. krusei, C. parakrusei, C. stellatoidea,* and *C. guilliermondi* occasionally give rise to vaginitis. An analysis made in 1957 by Dukes and Gardner of 100 consecutive cases of vaginal candidiasis in both pregnant and nonpregnant patients revealed the following distribution of the different types: *C. albicans,* 67 percent; *C. tropicalis,* 28 percent; *C. pseudotropicalis,* 1 percent; *C. stellatoidea,* 3 percent; and *C. krusei,* 1 percent.

More recently, findings in a group composed entirely of nonpregnant patients with candidiasis showed a far different distribution. *C. stellatoidea, C. tropicalis,* and *C. pseudotropicalis* comprised over 60 percent of the isolations. Two species were often found in the same patient. The change in the distribution of species may be attributable to the change in patient material. The latter series included only gynecologic patients, of whom over 50 percent were taking birth control pills.

The published reports of Carter and associates (1959), Drouhet, Wilson, Dawkins, Edwards, Riddell, Kearns, and Gray, and many others should further dispel any opinion that *C. albicans* is the only pathogenic species. One of us (H. L. G.) has found that *C. tropicalis* is not only a common causative agent but is more likely to be associated with chronicity and recurrences than *C. albicans.*

Sources of infection. Species of *Candida* are recovered frequently from the stools, oral cavity, vagina, and intertriginous areas of normal individuals. De Sousa and van Uden found that of fifty-five women whose vaginal cultures were positive for *C. albicans,* 75 percent harbored the organism in the feces, whereas of 170 women with negative vaginal cultures, only 25 percent had positive fecal cultures. The findings of Rohatiner were similar. Such observations indicate the importance of the intestinal tract as a potential source of vaginal infection. The oral cavity, which yields *Candida* in 20 to 30 percent of normal subjects, could be an important source, depending partly upon the sexual habits of the patient. Animals, vegetables, and inanimate objects have not been proved to be sources of infection. Occasionally, inguinal and mucocutaneous infections of men may be sources. Gilpin found the organisms in the semen of a high percentage of husbands of women with chronic infections.

Predisposing factors. It is probable that predisposing factors exist in every patient with candidiasis, though their identification is not always possible. Host factors that affect vaginal secretions, and thus vaginal environment, appear to play the key role in the causation of this disease.

Pregnancy. Pregnancy is the most common predisposing factor, with the incidence and severity of the infection increasing with the duration of gestation. The high hormone levels in pregnancy lead to a pronounced increase in the glycogen content of the vagina, which constitutes a favorable environment for the growth of candidal oragnisms. Hesseltine (1937) observed that repeated bathing of the vulva with glucose solutions and the instillation of glucose solutions into the vagina frequently precipitated clinical candidiasis in patients previously free of the disease. It is therefore probable that the glycosuria observed in some pregnant patients is also contributory. The reduced glucose tolerance in some pregnant patients and consequent elevation of the blood sugar levels could well further increase the susceptibility of a few women.

After delivery, the precipitous drop of estrogen and progesterone levels is followed by radical changes in vaginal metabolism, chemistry, and cytology and, in most patients, by a rapid disappearance of the clinical signs of candidiasis. Negative cultures are usually obtained within a few days, since the new vaginal environment is extremely unfavorable, if not hostile, to the growth of species of *Candida.* The use of large doses of estrogens to inhibit engorgement of the breasts can alter this postpartum sequence of events.

Menstrual cycle. The intensity of the clinical features of candidiasis tends to coincide with the hormone pattern of the menstrual cycle. Because of available vaginal glycogen, the clinical manifestations are usually more severe before menstruation, with some degree of relief being experienced during and after the menstrual flow.

Contraceptive pills. Statistics compiled from the records of one of us (H. L. G.) reveals an incidence of infection several times higher in patients who are taking cyclic hormones for contraception than in patients of similar age and circumstances who are not taking the pills. For example, of 121 consecutive nonpregnant patients with candidiasis observed in 1964 and 1965, sixty-two (51.4 percent) were taking oral contraceptives. Even more remarkable are the findings of Walsh, Hildebrandt, and Prystowsky in a vaginitis clinic: of thirty-four patients with candidiasis, twenty-two (64.7 percent) were taking the pills. Such effects are understandable, since cylic administration of estrogens and progestogens produces a vaginal environment similar to that present during pregnancy. Gershberg, Javier, and Hulse and Peterson, Steel, and Coyne have shown that the glucose tolerance of many patients who receive norethynodrel and mestranol is diminished, an effect that might also contribute to a predisposition to the disease. Possibly, patients who use the sequential type of hormone contraceptives are less susceptible, since progestogens are taken only during the last five days of the course. Estrogens induce deposition of glycogen, mainly in the intermediate cells, and progestogens cause shedding of these cells into the vaginal pool. Jackson and Spain observed that cultures of vaginal secretions from many patients who changed from cyclic to sequential pills soon became negative; nevertheless, we are still impressed with the incidence of the disease in patients who take the sequential type.

Antibiotics. Since the introduction of antibiotics, the incidence of candidiasis has increased to a degree paralleling their increased usage, whether they are administered systemically or topically. The broad spectrum agents, such as the tetracyclines, are more potent in this respect than penicillin.

The mode of action of antibiotics in precipitating candidiasis remains debatable. According to the most popular opinion, the organisms multiply more rapidly because of the reduction of bacterial competition. Although this explanation seems logical, it is partially discredited by experimental evidence. According to another theory, bacterial organisms secrete an antifungal substance. Direct stimulation of candidal organisms by the antibiotic or a reduction of the defense mechanisms of the host, such as might result from reduction of antibody production, have also been offered as explanations. Regardless of the precise mechanism involved, the use of antibiotics is clearly related to the incidence and severity of the disease. Interested readers are referred to the extensive reports of Seelig (1966 a, b).

Perhaps of more long-range importance is the increased colonization of the host by species of *Candida* after the administration of antibiotics. Loh and Baker reported an increase of 100 to 1,000 times in the intestinal population of *Candida* in patients who were taking chlortetracycline and oxytetracycline. Such heavily colonized sites most surely serve as sources of infection and reinfection, thus favoring perpetuation of the vaginal disease in susceptible patients.

Corticosteroids. That systemically administered corticosteroids reduce resistance to bacterial infection by diminishing inflammatory response is fairly well-established, and many investigators agree that adrenal steroids have an adverse effect on candidal infections. In laboratory studies, the susceptibility of animals to candidal infections after administration of corticosteroids is increased, although the agents seem to have no effect on organisms grown in vitro. Corticosteroids applied topically to the vulvovaginal tissues do not seem to aggravate the disease, a fact worthy of note in the symptomatic treatment for severe candidal infections. The full relationship of systemic corticosteroids to vaginal candidiasis has not yet been fully clarified. Any evaluation of causal relationship involves complexities such as the disorder for which the agent is being used, which might, itself, be a predisposing factor.

Diabetes mellitus. If the glucose tolerance curve can be relied upon to reveal the earliest evidence of diabetes mellitus, then it must be concluded that the disease is of little significance to the gynecologist in the overall picture of vaginal candidiasis. Only a small percentage of patients with candidiasis observed by the gynecologist has sugar in the urine or abnormal glucose tolerance curves. This is not to say, however, that diabetes mellitus is not a potent predisposing factor, since a high percentage of diabetic patients will have obstinate candidiasis. Dobson has suggested that large babies and vaginal candidiasis may be the earliest signs of latent diabetes. So-called diabetic vulvovaginitis is inseparably allied to the increased susceptibility of diabetic patients to candidiasis, this being, as previously stated, seemingly related to increased concentrations of glucose in the tissues, blood, and urine.

Nondiabetic glycosuria. We have found recurrent vaginal candidiasis in several patients with normal glucose tolerance curves who regularly had sugar in the urine because of a low renal threshold. Nondiabetic glycosuria, like diabetes mellitus, fosters the development of candidiasis. We have not, however, observed patients with this condition who presented the classical "diabetic vulvitis."

Diet. Some evidence has been presented of a heavier candidal colonization of the intestinal tract in people who consume large amounts of fruit or sugars. Fruit workers and "sweet lovers" may be predisposed to candidiasis because of the resulting higher-than-average blood sugar levels and possible increased candidal intestinal flora. Perhaps the diet factor deserves consideration in the treatment for resistant infections.

Debilitation. The heightened susceptibility of some debilitated patients to candidal stomatitis or widely disseminated candidiasis is well known. Debilitation as germane to vaginal candidiasis is relatively unimportant, however, because most such patients are postmenopausal and thus are not naturally susceptible to the vaginal infection. The causes of debilitation—including lymphomas, leukemia, and other malignant diseases—should be considered in patients with pronounced cutaneous candidiasis. Generalized candidiasis sometimes follows chemotherapy for carcinoma.

Factor "X." The existence of undefined predisposing factors is apparent to all who are concerned with this disease. Not uncommonly, persistent or recurrent candidiasis is observed in patients who have no demonstrable predisposing factors. The unknown factors are probably multiple, involving both host susceptibility and pathogenicity of the fungus.

The observations of Louria and Brayton point to a natural candidacidal factor in the blood which, when reduced, increases the susceptibility of the patient. Their experiments in growing species of *Candida* in human blood revealed a diminution in the candidacidal property of the serum of those patients with mucocutaneous or systemic candidiasis. This factor appears distinct from agglutinating antibodies, which reportedly do not have a protective action.

Factor "X" could be related to susceptibility of the mucocutaneous tissues of certain patients to allergenic or endotoxic substances derived from the cells of the organisms. Conspicuous reactions of the tissues to minimal infection might perhaps explain "reduced resistance." Rarely, a patient may have a vagina filled with fungus, yet no vulvar erythema or pruritus.

Male factor. Men are more likely to be recipients than donors of candidiasis; nevertheless, men can harbor candidal organisms beneath the foreskin and on the genitocrural tissues and thus constitute a reservoir of infection for women. Gilpin's studies show that the ejaculate of husbands of women with the recurrent disease often yields candidal species. The isolation of species of *Candida* from the male genitals is a simple matter, though the overall importance of this potential source of infection is unknown. Many husbands of infected wives have pruritus and redness of the glans penis, sometimes persistently and sometimes for only a few hours after intercourse. In men, symptoms lasting for several days are suggestive of active infection, whereas an immediate but transient mucocutaneous reaction may be attributed to the allergenic properties of the candidal organisms acquired from the sexual partner. Persistent organisms beneath the prepuce of the clitoris may also be a source of reinfection of women. Scott has expressed the opinion that, unless appropriate attention is given to this concealed area, it may continue to be a potent reservoir of *Candida*.

Incidence

Candidiasis is primarily a disease of the childbearing years, seldom being observed before the menarche or after the menopause. Its presence during either of the latter periods suggests that the patient is diabetic or has recently taken hormones or antibiotics. The reported incidence is as variable as the criteria used by individual investigators in making the diagnosis. For example, the mere recovery of candidal organisms from the vulvovaginal tissues is not proof of clinical disease, although it is frequently so interpreted. Our own experience, as well as that reported by others, indicates that species of *Candida* are recovered during pregnancy about twice as often as clinical infection develops, yet the ratio of active disease to *Candida* is considerably higher in nonpregnant patients. Hildick-Smith, Blank, and Sarkany, in an analysis of thirty-two different studies involving thousands of patients, found that the reported recovery rate of species of *Candida* from the vagina averaged 17.6 percent in nongravid patients and 30.2 percent in obstetric patients.

From an accumulation of all of the data available to us, it would appear that 15 to 20 per cent of patients in late pregnancy have clinical infection, as compared to an estimated 4 to 6 per cent of nonpregnant patients. Such figures could be falsely interpreted to mean that the incidence is three to four times higher during pregnancy, whereas reasonable calculations indicate that it is at least ten to twenty times higher. Any valid comparison of the incidence in the two groups must take into account that only about 2 percent of women are pregnant at a given time, although this group constitutes a high percentage of all patients with candidiasis. Also to be recognized is the fact that many women who become patients have sought attention for the symptoms of candidiasis. In effect, they are a self-screened group of subjects from the general female population.

It is obvious to most physicians that the incidence of candidiasis is on the rise. This is supported by three chronologically separated studies by one of us (H.L.G.). In 1944, before the introduction of antibiotics and birth control pills, clinical candidiasis was found in 2.8 percent of the gynecologic patients in private office practice. In a study of patients from the same practice, Gardner, Dukes, and Damper, in 1957, found candidiasis in 4.3 percent of nonpregnant patients. In a third study (by H. L. G.) of 1,000 consecutive gynecologic patients from the same practice in 1964-1965, this incidence was 5.9 percent. An analysis of 200 consecutive nonpregnant patients with one or the other of the three common vaginitides made in 1966 revealed the following distribution: candidiasis, 95 (47.5 percent); trichomoniasis, 45 (22.0 percent); and *Haemophilus vaginalis* vaginitis, 63 (30.5 percent). Our most recent analysis shows candidiasis to be eight times more frequent than trichomoniasis. From these statistics, the relative importance of candidiasis is obvious. The effects of antibiotics and estrogen-progestogen combinations used for contraception unquestionably account for much of this increased incidence of infection.

Predisposing factors possibly vary according to geographic location and in the practices of different physicians; thus, any assessment of the variables becomes difficult. We do not share the opinion that classical vulvovaginal candidiasis is more common in semitropical climates, as a direct result of the climate, and are unaware of published evidence strongly supporting such a contention. Statistics gathered by Stough and Blank tend to prove that prevalence is essentially the same in the various climatic zones in which Miami, Philadelphia, Chicago, and the Philippines are located. According to this observation, environmental conditions of warmth, moisture, and sugar content of the vagina are little affected by external temperatures and humidity. Primary cutaneous candidiasis of the vulva is relatively rare in all climatic zones of the United States; this special type of infection is probably exceptional and its incidence higher in warm, humid climates where changes in the skin that favor its development are more likely to occur.

Although their effects are difficult to assess, socioeconomic influences that might affect dietary and sexual habits, hygiene, and general health may, to some degree, influence the incidence of candidal infections.

Bacteriology

In his historic treatise published in 1892, Doderlein reported the association of large gram-positive rods (Doderlein bacilli) with fungi and stated that the acid medium that favors the growth of the bacilli was also highly favorable to the yeasts.

In 1951, Young and others reported a symbiosis between *C. albicans* and lactobacilli. They found that some of the essential nutrients for growth of the lactobacillus are produced by *C. albicans*, and from this they concluded that a rational balance exists between lactobacilli and species of *Candida*. In a study of the vaginal flora of 100 patients with candidiasis, Dukes and Gardner found the bacteria listed in Table 1. These were consecutive candidal infections in patients who yielded no other vaginal pathogens, such as *Haemophilus vaginalis* and *Trichomonas vaginalis*. Aciduric rods (lactobacilli or diphtheroids) were the predominant bacterial organisms in all cases. For comparison, the bacteria in normal vaginas of one hundred patients are listed in Table 2. Since the bacteriology of the two groups is essentially identical, it appears that bacterial organisms play no role in determining

Table 1. Bacteriology of candidiasis (Dukes and Gardner) in 100 patients without other specific pathogens

Lactobacilli only	43
Diphtheroids only	6
Lactobacilli + streptococci	11
Diphtheroids + streptococci	18
Diphtheroids or lactobacilli + one or more of *Staphylococcus aureus, Staphylococcus albus, Gaffkya, Proteus, Pseudomonas aeruginosa, Escherichia coli, Torulopsis, Sacchyaromyces*	22

Table 2. Bacteriology of normal vaginas (Dukes and Gardner) of 100 patients

Lactobacilli only	31
Lactobacilli + diphtheroids	5
Diphtheroids only	4
Lactobacilli + alpha streptococci	13
Diphtheroids + alpha streptococci	8
Lactobacilli or diphtheroids + one or more of *Staphylococcus aureus, Staphylococcus albus, Gaffkya, Micrococcus, Streptococcus faecalis,* anaerobic streptococci, *C. albicans, C. Tropicalis, C. krusei*	39

the clinical pattern of candidiasis. Thus, the futility of any attempt to reestablish "normal physiology and bacteriology" as a method of treating patients for the disease becomes obvious.

Clinical features

Since, in the classical vulvovaginal disease, invasion of the tissues by *Candida* cannot be demonstrated in histologic sections, the signs and symptoms cannot be attributed to such process. Local dermatitis can be produced experimentally by applying killed *Candida* or cell-free extracts to the skin under occlusive tape. Presumably, the signs and symptoms could thus be attributable to reactions to allergenic or endotoxic substances produced by the organisms, in a manner similar to the skin reaction to biologic irritants in contact dermatitis. Also, fermentation products, such as acetic aldehyde and acetic and pyruvic acids, are reportedly capable of initiating symptoms.

Symptoms. Vulvar pruritus is the cardinal symptom of candidiasis and is more intense than in the average case of trichomoniasis. The itching varies from slight to intolerable, and it may interfere with normal activities and rest. Many patients complain of vaginal itching, although this probably is vestibular. The existence of true vaginal pruritus is open to question. The intensity of pruritus and the degree of vulvar erythema are closely parallel; pruritus is seldom reported by patients who have no visible vulvar changes. The incidence of pruritus in patients whom we regard as having clinical disease is approximately 90 percent. An occasional patient has thrush or a pseudomembrane involving the entire vagina yet has no subjective symptoms or evidence of vulvitis. Many patients complain of itching and burning immediately after intercourse. This may be an allergic reaction to candidal organisms in the ejaculate.

Burning is a common complaint, particularly upon urination, being most often experienced by patients who have excoriations from scratching. This might be called "vulvar dysuria." Many patients develop reflexogenic urinary urgency and frequency. The combination of dysuria and frequency can be erroneously attributed to cystitis by both the patient and the physician.

Dyspareunia is sometimes a very real symptom, particularly in nulliparas, and it may progress to the point of total intolerance to intercourse. The bride with intractable candidiasis as a result of taking contraceptive pills may have a serious marital problem.

Miscellaneous symptoms of severe infections associated with pronounced vulvar edema include vague generalized vulvar discomfort and even pain on walking and sitting. Worry and apprehension are experienced by some patients with chronic and recurrent disease. At times, it is difficult to convince such patients that their condition is benign.

Leukorrhea is not a classical symptom of candidiasis and is rarely the presenting complaint; however, the majority of patients have a discharge at some stage of the infection. Other patients may complain of a feeling of dryness.

Objective signs. Erythema of the vulva is the sign of candidiasis most often observed. Generally, it is limited to the mucocutaneous surfaces between the labia minora (Plate 1, *A*); the physician who fails to realize that

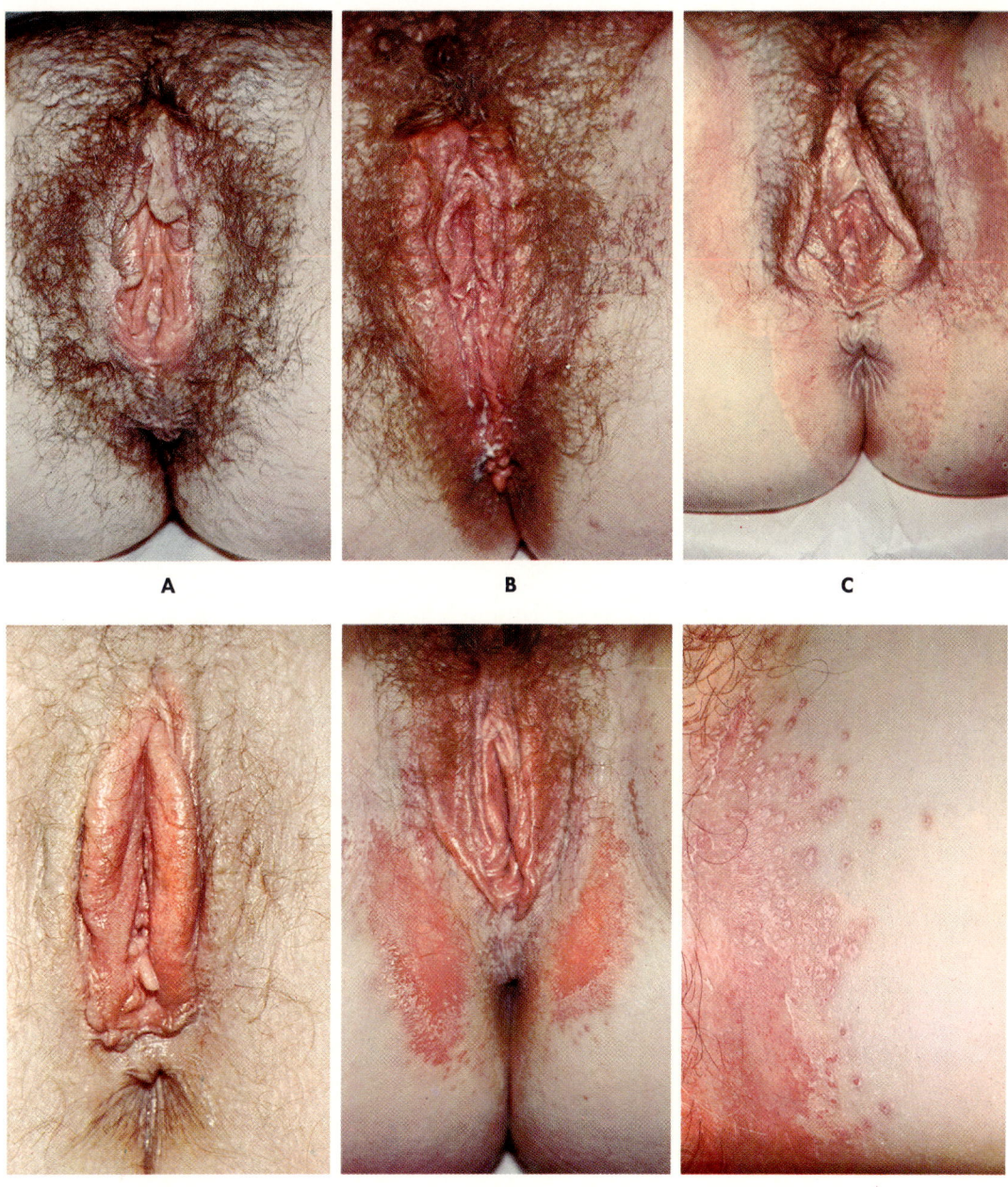

Plate 1. Vulvar manifestations of acute candidiasis. **A**; Classical vulvovaginal candidiasis, exhibited only by redness of the vestibule. **B,** Moderate vulvovaginitis with edema and redness. **C,** Widespread cutaneous changes associated with vaginitis. The cutaneous lesions here are probably an allergic response to candidal organisms from the vagina. **D,** Edema of labia minora, occasionally a prominent sign. **E,** Primary cutaneous candidiasis. Typical, beefy red lesions. **F,** Primary cutaneous candidiasis. A close-up view of lesion in E. Characteristic satellite pustules shown.

erythema is frequently minimal and limited to the vestibule may overlook the true nature of a vulvar pruritus. In other patients, erythema extends to the labia majora (Plate 1, *B*), the perineum, and the perianal tissues and, occasionally, to the mons pubis, genitocrural folds, inner thighs, and even the buttocks (Plate 1, *C*). If widespread, it is more commonly associated with diabetes, pregnancy, or obesity.

Edema of the labia minora is the second most common gross change of the vulva (Plate 1, *D*). Since infection is usually more severe and pelvic congestion greater during pregnancy, edema of the labia is more likely at this time.

Fissuring is an occasional finding and may cause suspicion of a dystrophic disease.

Traumatic excoriations from scratching are often discovered in patients with severe pruritus. Fingernail abrasions, which, if present, are usually found between the small and large labia, may be confused with fissures or herpetic ulcers. Rarely, inguinal adenitis develops from bacterial infection of the excoriations.

Vesicopustules are sometimes regarded by dermatologists as the major clinical feature of vulvovaginal candidiasis, though such lesions are only occasionally observed by the gynecologist. The difference in patient material seen by the dermatologist and gynecologist explains, in part, the differences in lesions observed. Vesicopustules are associated chiefly with primary cutaneous candidiasis, which is discussed elsewhere in this chapter.

The signs of lichen simplex chronicus (localized neurodermatitis) are often observed in patients with chronic candidiasis, especially such as might be associated with diabetes. Because of the scratch-itch reflex, the epidermis may be lichenified and hyperkeratotic and may resemble "leukoplakia." The lesions may be elevated and dull red or brown in color, rather than white.

Candida granuloma (monilial granuloma) constitutes a specific entity which develops mainly in children. Seldom, if ever, does it involve the genitalia. For these reasons, readers are referred to the dermatologic literature for further information.

Eczematoid vulvitis with intense widespread erythema, edema, and ulcerations is sometimes observed in patients who have been overtreated with chemical agents, such as gentian violet, or in those who are hypersensitive to other topically applied agents (Chapter 20). The gynecologist who is referred "difficult" cases of vaginitis frequently sees such patients. The lesions heal within a few days after discontinuance of all therapy or after the use of a drying lotion.

It is often difficult to distinguish between normal vaginal redness and pathologic vaginal erythema. Many patients have an abnormal redness of the vagina, although in our experience it is unmistakably present in only about 20 percent. The mucosa beneath adherent thrush patches is reddened, and,

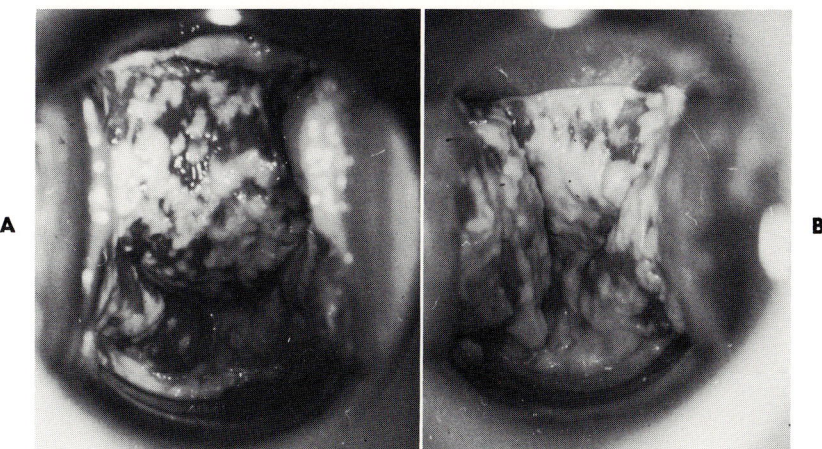

Fig. 11-1. Candidiasis. **A**, Thrush patches of vaginal wall. **B**, Pseudomembrane covering most of vaginal wall.

after their removal, incomplete superficial ulcerations with oozing of blood are sometimes apparent.

Vaginal secretions in most nonpregnant patients with candidiasis are essentially normal in consistency, color, volume, and odor. Failure to suspect candidiasis because of the absence of thrush patches, curds, or caseous masses is a common clinical error. In our experience, thrush patches are present in only 20 percent of nonpregnant patients, as compared with 70 percent of pregnant patients. Thrush patches (Fig. 11-1, *A*) are highly variable in number and physical characteristics. The patches are loosely adherent and usually white, although they are occasionally yellow. Some patients display hundreds of small, thin, discrete patches, whereas others have only a few masses measuring up to 1.0 cm. in thickness. In the occasional patient, a pseudomembrane covers most of the vaginal wall (Fig. 11-1, *B*). The complaint of leukorrhea and the mass of vaginal exudate, as seen through the speculum, do not always correlate. One patient with a measured volume of 22 ml. of curds and epithelial-purulent secretions denied having a discharge. Not infrequently, thin, small thrush patches of the vestibule are observed.

The odor of vaginal secretions in candidiasis is rarely disagreeable unless a *Haemophilus vaginalis* or *Trichomonas* infection is associated. At times, it has the odor of yeast. This may be caused by an associated true yeast, *Saccharomyces*, which is a common nonpathogenic vaginal fungus. The yeast odor is not actually a characteristic of candidiasis.

The acidity of vaginal secretions in candidiasis is usually within the range of pH 4.0 to 4.7, with a pH of 4.5 being the most common reading. On the average, therefore, the secretions are less acid than the normal range of pH 3.8 to 4.2.

Vestibular candidiasis. In a few patients, a candidal infection is limited to the vestibule (Fig. 11-2). The vestibular disease differs from the classical vulvovaginal disease only in that the vagina is free of fungus and signs of infection. Thrush patches (which usually are small) and erythema are present only in the vestibule. In most cases, this particular type of infection eventually spreads to the vagina. It more closely resembles the classical vulvovaginal disease than the primary cutaneous variety.

Histopathology

Our own histologic examinations of vaginal biopsies (Kaufman and Gardner, 1966) taken from many patients with gross clinical disease, subjective symptoms, and positive laboratory findings revealed no evidence of

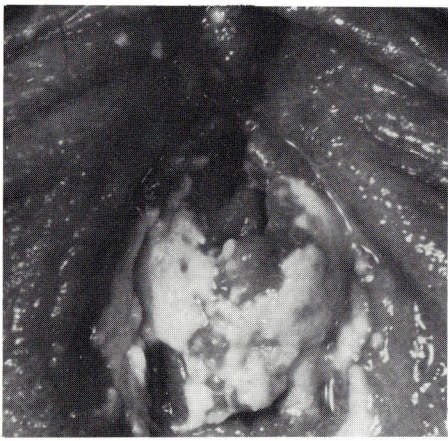

Fig. 11-2. Vestibular candidiasis. Thrush patches in this patient involved only the vestibule. The vagina yielded no candidal organisms.

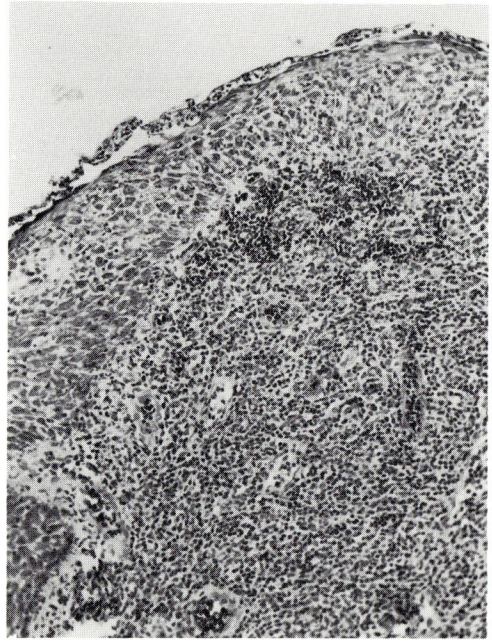

Fig. 11-3. Candidiasis of the vagina, with spongiosis, severe inflammatory infiltrate, and hyperemia. Surface debris is also present. (H & E × 88)

invasion of the vaginal tissues by the organism. Adair and Hesseltine and Taubert and Smith came to the same conclusion after studying biopsies of infected patients. The changes induced in the tissues by acute candidiasis are similar to those found in acute trichomoniasis, though they are less pronounced. A moderate acanthosis with elongation of the epithelial folds is observed (Fig. 11-3). The latter seem to adhere to one another in the deeper dermis, apparently "trapping" stroma and vessels within the epithelium. A mild spongiosis and intracellular edema, a mild to moderate degree of edema of the papillae, and hyperemia of the lamina propria are also associated. A chronic inflammatory infiltrate, consisting primarily of lymphocytes, a few plasma cells, and an occasional neutrophil, involves the superficial lamina propria. In focal areas, this infiltrate extends into the epidermis. The surface of the epithelium may exhibit derbris consisting of degenerated squamous cells, neutrophils, and, frequently, buds and hyphae of *Candida*.

In the presence of chronic candidiasis, biopsies of vaginal mucosa exhibit a less severe reaction. The usual features are mild to moderate infiltration of lymphocytes into the epidermis.

Diagnosis

Regardless of the clinician's diagnostic abilities, the distinction of candidiasis from other types of vaginitis is not always possible from clinical evidence alone. The diagnosis of candidiasis depends upon both the demonstration of a species of *Candida* and the presence of clinical features compatible with the disease. Recovery of a species of *Candida* is not in itself proof of candidiasis.

Clinical diagnosis. Any patient with pruritis, redness, or thrush-like patches of the vagina must be suspected of having candidiasis. Various dermatoses, most of which cause both pruritus and gross changes in the skin, may occasionally be confusing. Unmistakable thrush patches of the vestibule or vagina should perhaps be considered pathognomonic. At times, masses of epithelial cells from a physiologic increase in desquamation are mistaken for thrush patches (Fig. 11-4). Leukoplakia of the cervix is seldom confused with thrush patches, since the hyperkeratotic epithelial patches do not wipe off as readily

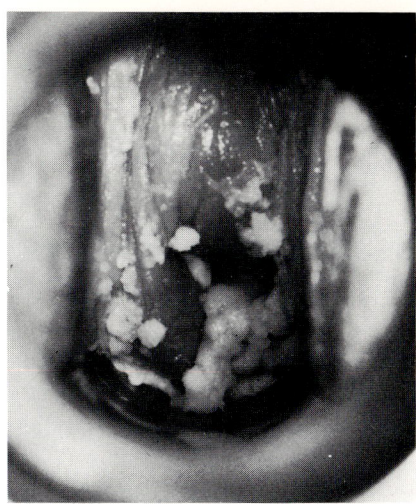

Fig. 11-4. Masses of desquamated epithelial cells forming "pseudo" thrush patches in a normal vagina. This finding could be mistaken for candidiasis.

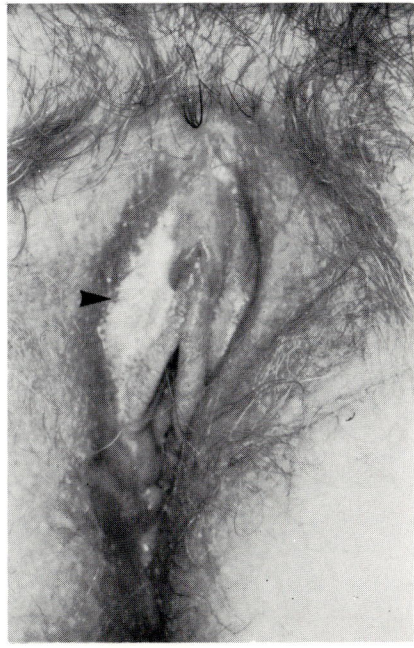

Fig. 11-5. Smegma of interlabial fold. This may be confused with candidiasis.

as do thrush patches. A rare patient with trichomoniasis may have a splotchy, thin pseudomembrane of the vaginal epithelium (Plate 2), which can be mistaken for thin thrush patches. Herpes genitalis of the vestibule, vagina, or ectocervix is sometimes associated with a white membranous lesion. A thin pseudomembrane of the vagina may also be observed in patients who have recently used a strong vinegar or medicated douche (Chapter 20); to the experienced eye, however, this should be easily recognizable. Smegma of the vulva may be mistaken for thrush patches (Fig. 11-5).

Laboratory studies. Regardless of the microscopic methods employed in suspected cases of candidiasis, the identification of *Candida* depends upon the finding of filamentous forms (pseudohyphae) of the organisms. All vaginal fungi that produce filaments belong to the genus *Candida*. The mere demonstration of ovoid forms, variously called "yeast cells," buds, conidia, or spores, is not proof of the presence of *Candida,* since the vagina may contain such nonpathogenic fungi as *Saccharomyces* and *Cryptococcus,* both of which have yeast cells but no filaments. *Torulopsis glabrata,* a fungus of low pathogenicity, also has budding forms though no filaments. The individual species of *Candida* allegedly exhibit minor morphologic variations, yet these differences are too slight for routine species identification.

Potassium hydroxide preparation. Microscopic examination of vaginal material mixed in 10 to 20% potassium hydroxide is the most efficient method for rapid identification of *Candida*. In this solution, pus cells and red blood cells undergo immediate dissolution. The vaginal epithelial cells, unlike skin scrapings with a high keratin content, rapidly clear from translucent to transparent and for a time continue to appear as a type of "ghost" cell. The conidia, as well as the filaments of *Candida,* stand out distinctly under both low and high power magnifications (Fig. 11-6).

Wet mount preparation. Microscopic examination of vaginal material, mixed with physiologic saline and viewed under both low and high power magnifications, provides the most valuable single method for the differential diagnosis of vaginitis, although the inexperienced examiner may have difficulty in identifying the two elements of *Candida* (Fig. 11-7). The wet mount preparation should be relatively thin, and this can be ensured by a greater dilution or by firm pressure upon the cover slip. Conidia may be confused with the nuclei of epithelial and pus cells, powder granules, and other artifacts. The filaments may be confused with cotton fibers, rolled edges of epithelial cells, leptothrix, and scratches on the slide. The number of pus cells is usually moderate. The lactobacillus is the bacterial organism most often associated; it is usually identifiable in the wet mount when viewed under the high power objective. The predominance of lactobacilli in a case of vulvovaginitis with pruritus is strong evidence of candidiasis.

Stained smears. Under the high power or oil immersion lens of the microscope, smears that have been fixed and stained with gentian violet or other simple stains vividly reveal both the conidia and filaments of *Candida*. In the gram-stained smear, conidia are

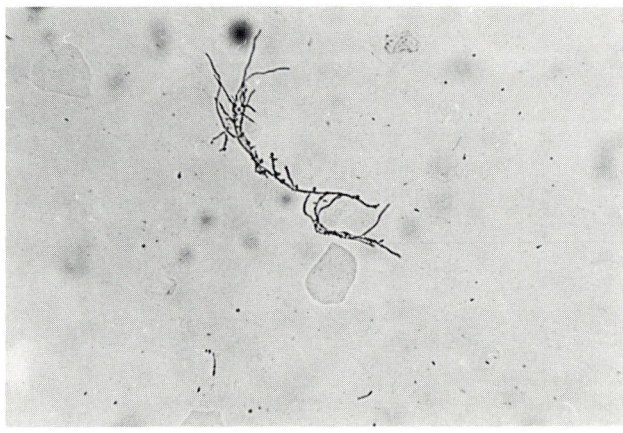

Fig. 11-6. Candidal organisms in vaginal secretions following treatment with 20% potassium hydroxide solution. (Low power)

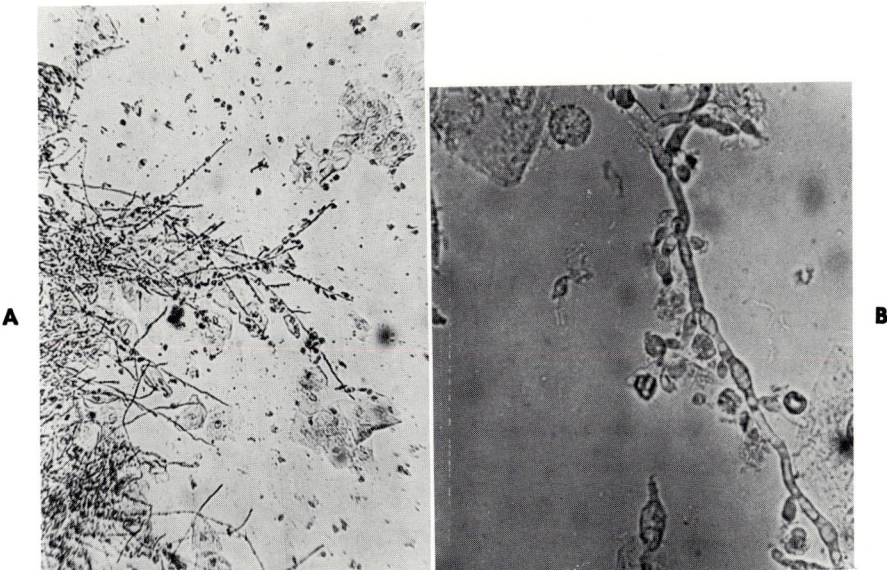

Fig. 11-7. Candidal organisms in wet mount preparation. Hyphae and conidia are clearly demonstrated. (**A**, Low power; **B**, high power)

strongly gram-positive, and the filaments are uniformly gram-positive or have large gram-positive granules. In the Papanicolaou smear, the organisms stain rather poorly.

Culture techniques. Both Sabouraud's (or modified Sabouraud's–Difco mycobiotic) and Nickerson's media are satisfactory for growing *Candida* in an incubator or at room temperature, although they do not permit identification of the species. The most reliable differentiation of the species is provided by sugar fermentation reactions. Formerly, the demonstration of chlamydospores in certain culture media was regarded as diagnostic of *C. albicans;* this structure, however, is sometimes observed in cultures of other species and thus cannot always be considered as species specific.

Treatment

The simple discovery of candidal organisms in the absence of signs and symptoms of vaginitis does not constitute an indication for treatment. When the diagnosis is established, the primary object of therapy is to effect a cure through destruction of all organisms by whatever method is least injurious to the vulvovaginal tissues. Currently, this can be accomplished only by the topical application of candidacidal agents. Many failures can be attributed to the short period of therapy prescribed by the physician or to the fact that many patients immediately discontinue therapy upon relief of symptoms. Irregular and erratic treatment, such as the omission of medications during menstruation, must account for additional failures. Instructions to the patient should be specific and, preferably, should be given in writing. Patients want quick and easy cures, and long courses of treatment will be interrupted often unless the instructions are meticulously detailed.

Gentian violet is one of the oldest and most reliable of all forms of treatment. The symptoms are rapidly controlled by topical applications of a 0.25 to 2.0% aqueous solution to the vulvovaginal tissues. This method, however, has three disadvantages: (1) clothing and linens are stained; (2) it must be applied in the physician's office; and (3) chemical vulvovaginitis often develops. The chemical vulvovaginitis is induced by solutions that are too strong or by their too frequent use. When solutions of 1 to 2% are applied at intervals of less than 2 to 3 days, chemical reactions may be anticipated. Such a response may be misinterpreted as an exacerbation of the disease.

Gentian violet in convenient form is also

available in special suppositories, tampons, creams, and foams under a number of trade names—Gentersal cream, G. V. S. Aerosol Foam, G. V. S. cream, Gentia Jel, and Genepax tampons. Some of these preparations are claimed to be stainless, which means that they are easily removed by washing. Occasionally, any of the group give rise to a chemical reaction. Instructions for their use vary slightly, although the duration of treatment should generally be extended beyond the period recommended by the distributors.

Nystatin (Mycostatin cream, vaginal tablets, and ointment) is an antifungal antibiotic obtained from cultures of *Streptomyces noursei*. Its in vitro and in vivo potency has been well-substantiated. The agent was discovered in 1950 by Hazen and Brown, and its vaginal use as a treatment for candidiasis was reported by Sloane in 1955. At this time, we are not aware of a more effective candidacidal agent, and its continued widespread use attests its efficacy and the low incidence of its side reactions. The vaginal tablets should be inserted high into the vagina twice daily for 7 to 14 days, then nightly for an additional 2 to 3 weeks.

Candicidin, which was discovered in *Streptomyces griseus* by Lechevalier and his co-workers in 1953, is an antifungal antibiotic agent. It is marketed as Candeptin ointment and vaginal tablets. According to in vitro studies, it is more potent than nystatin, although it has not proved to be superior in clinical practice. In our experience, its effectiveness approaches that of nystatin. The instructions for its use are essentially the same—insertion of the vaginal tablet or ointment twice daily for 7 to 14 days, followed by nightly insertions for an additional 2 to 3 weeks.

Chlordantoin, a synthetic organic fungicide, was reported by Kittleson in 1952. For gynecologic use, it is marketed under the name of Sporastacin cream. In our experience, this preparation is somewhat less effective than either nystatin or candicidin; further, it seems to elicit more local reactions. The instructions for its use are essentially identical to those recommended for the other preparations.

Amphotericin B, discovered in 1955 by Gold and his co-workers, is also an antibiotic substance derived from *Streptomyces nodosus*. Although it can be given intravenously for serious systemic candidiasis, its administration by this route to patients with vulvovaginal disease would rarely, if ever, be justified because of its frequent toxic reactions. No form of amphotericin B is at present available for intravaginal use. As a topical agent, it is reportedly effective in the cutaneous vulvar disease. For this purpose, it is available as a 3% lotion, cream, or ointment. All are marketed as Fungizone. The medication is rubbed well into the infected areas of the skin two to four times daily for 2 to 4 weeks. Our results with the use of this antibiotic have been somewhat disappointing.

Proprionic acids—a combination of proprionic acid and its calcium and sodium salts (Proprion gel)—was found to be moderately efficacious as a treatment for candidiasis, by Alter, Jones, and Carter. This preparation has been used and endorsed since 1949. It should be instilled into the vagina twice daily for 7 to 14 days and at bedtime for an additional 2 to 3 weeks. In our experience, it is somewhat less effective than the antifungal antibiotics, nystatin and candicidin.

Topical anesthetics for the relief of itching, even on a temporary basis, have no place in the therapy for this disease. The danger of adverse reactions far outweighs any possible benefits.

Corticosteroids, applied topically, are occasionally justified to reduce inflammatory reactions and relieve itching until a candidacidal agent has time to take effect. Local application of corticosteroids does not appear to stimulate the growth of *Candida*, as might be true of systemic agents. Two convenient forms are 1% hydrocortisone acetate ointment (Cortef) and 0.025% fluocinolone acetonide cream (Synalar). These agents may be particularly useful in long-standing chronic cases such as diabetic vulvovaginitis in which chronic inflammatory reactions such as lichen simplex chronicus have developed.

Treatment for chronic and recurrent candidiasis

In view of the several predisposing and perpetuating factors, chronic and recurrent candidiasis are increasingly troublesome. Most cases are probably caused by autogenous reinfections. No uniformly successful approach to this vexing problem has been found. Obviously, not only must the vulvovaginal organisms be destroyed, but every effort must be made to remove foci of infection and to correct all predisposing factors. Reassurance of the patient also frequently becomes an important part of the treatment. Until more information is available concerning the host factors, problem cases will continue to appear in large numbers. One or more of the following suggestions may be useful in difficult cases.

1. The period of continuous therapy should be increased beyond the recommended 3 or 4 weeks, without interruption during the menstrual flow.

2. After control of the active disease, intravaginal candidacides may be used at bedtime for 7 to 10 days before each menstrual period, the time of greatest susceptibility.

3. Intravaginal candidacides should be used during and for several days after any course of antibiotic therapy.

4. When tetracycline or its congeners are indicated for patients susceptible to *Candida*, the medication should perhaps be combined with nystatin or amphotericin B to inhibit the growth of intestinal organisms.

5. After control of the active disease, the daily use of a douche containing an agent such as sodium perborate, borax, Stomaseptin douche powder, or Betadine solution frequently controls the symptoms of the "incurable" patient.

6. Theoretically, the daily application of a candidacidal cream or ointment to the vulva could prevent entry of large numbers of new organisms into the vagina. The actual value of this procedure in preventing reinfection is unproved.

7. The oral candidacides (chiefly nystatin and amphotericin B) are not absorbed appreciably from the intestinal tract and, consequently, have no direct beneficial effect upon vulvovaginal candidiasis. On the assumption that the majority of vaginal reinfections arise from the intestinal tract, oral nystatin (500,000 U. t.i.d. for 10 days) or amphotericin B (100 mg. t.i.d. for 10 days) might be worth a trial in an attempt to destroy or reduce the candidal population of the intestinal tract.

8. Some investigators, including Scott, believe that antiseptic soaps containing such agents as hexachlorophene destroy bacteria on the skin that are normally protective against *Candida*. Perhaps patients subject to the chronic and recurrent disease should not use bactericidal soaps.

9. Frequently, control of diabetes is necessary before a cure of candidiasis is possible. Patients with chronic or recurrent candidal infections should be investigated for either active or latent diabetes.

10. The potentiating nature of the estrogen-progestogen preparations used for contraception has been well-documented. In many cases, it is necessary to discontinue these agents before control is possible.

11. The patient's intake of carbohydrates and fruit should be reduced. In this disease, the patient needs the benefit of all doubt, and a change in dietary habits may well be beneficial.

12. The preputial folds should be considered as a possible source of reinfection. Smegma should be carefully removed from beneath the foreskin and a candidacide, such as gentian violet solution, should then be applied. Repeated use of candidacidal ointments by the patient may accomplish the same result.

13. The husband, particularly if uncircumcised, should be considered a possible source of reinfection. Such preparations as Candeptin, Fungizone, or Mycostatin ointment may be applied to the penis two to three times daily for 7 to 10 days. Genitocrural candidiasis in the husband should be ruled out. Gilpin's experiences in correlating frequent recurrence with infected ejaculate shows the need for protective sheaths during intercourse.

14. Species of *Candida* are recovered from the oral cavities of about 30 per cent of patients. Thus, the presence of cunnilingus as a factor in reinfection might be considered.

15. The less likely but still possible sources of reinfection should be eliminated. In this respect, the role of contaminated douche nozzles, wet bathing suits, and bathtubs is unknown. On theoretical grounds, perhaps the douche apparatus should be sterilized and the shower substituted for the tub.

16. The disease frequently recurs even after all known predisposing factors have been eliminated and all precautions taken against reinfection. The patient with such obstinate disease must use a vaginal candidacide upon the slightest suggestion of pru-

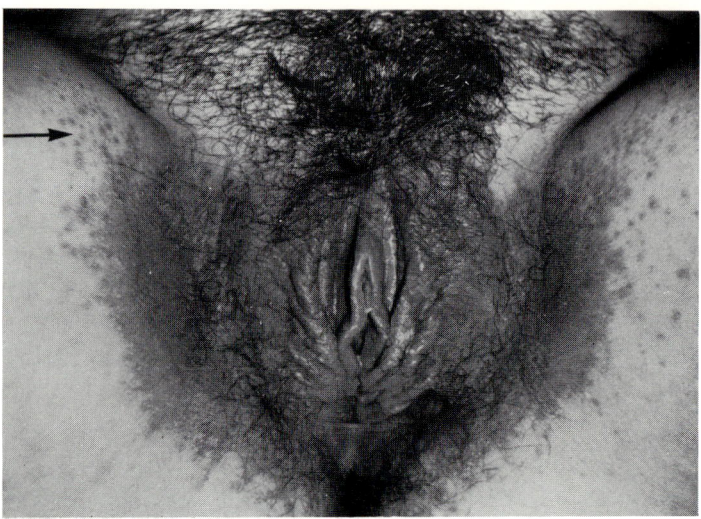

Fig. 11-8. Primary cutaneous candidiasis. Diffuse involvement of vulva and inner thighs. Satellite lesions indicated by arrow.

ritus, or every 2 to 3 days for an indefinite period.

17. Since cure during pregnancy is often next to impossible, control of symptoms may be all that can be accomplished. The use of intravaginal agents several times weekly throughout pregnancy is sometimes necessary for this half goal. Since the effect of such long-term treatment upon the patient is unknown, the medication should, perhaps, be changed from time to time.

PRIMARY CUTANEOUS CANDIDIASIS OF THE VULVA

Primary cutaneous candidiasis of the vulva, as compared to the vulvovaginal disease, is relatively rare in the United States. The majority of the patients with the skin infection also harbor vaginal organisms. As a rule, they have, or give a history of having had, predisposing conditions such as recent antibiotic therapy, diabetes, or debilitation. Cutaneous candidiasis of the vulva is favored by warm, humid climates in which maceration or other changes in the skin provide a good environment for fungus growth. Perhaps maceration from prolonged exposure to moisture, such as from sweating, is a necessary prelude to development of the vulvar cutaneous disease. Obese patients seem particularly susceptible.

Clinical features

Primary cutaneous candidiasis is not to be confused with the usual vulvovaginal dis-

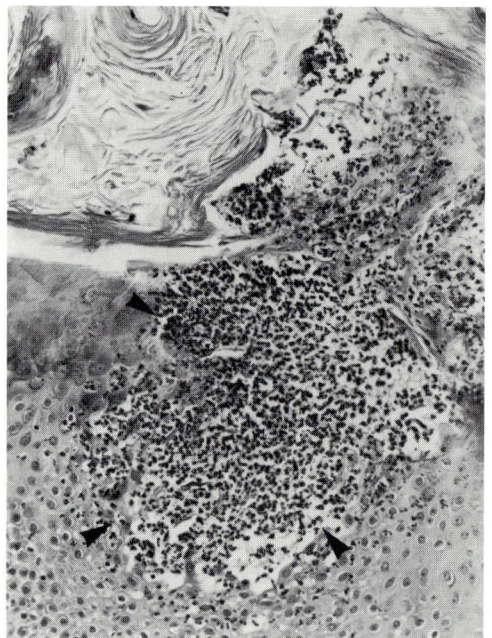

Fig. 11-9. Primary cutaneous candidiasis. Collection of acute inflammatory cells within epidermis forms a small pustule (arrows). (H & E × 375)

ease in which the symptoms and most prominent gross changes in the vulvar tissues are reactions to the allergenic and endotoxic substances of the vaginal organisms. As a rule, primary cutaneous lesions involve the labia majora and the genitocrural folds (Fig. 11-8 and Plate 1, *E*) and, not infre-

Candidiasis (moniliasis)

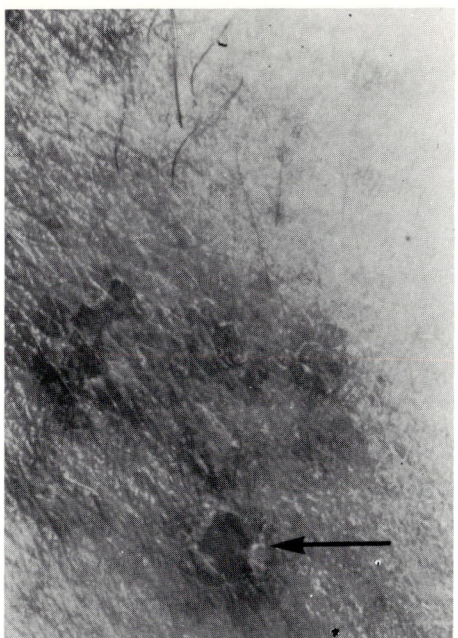

Fig. 11-10. Primary cutaneous candidiasis. Superficial ulcerated area resulting from ruptured vesicopustule.

quently, the mons pubis, the perianal region, and the inner thighs. Large vulvar lesions tend to be beefy red and weeping (Plate 1, *E*), with precisely defined, scalloped edges. Older, larger lesions are characteristically associated with smaller, discrete, satellite lesions (Plate 1, *F* and Fig. 11-8); the latter individually pass through the same developmental stages, also becoming large and tending to coalesce. All cutaneous lesions begin as small papules on a red base and rapidly progress to a well-defined bullus, then to flaccid vesicopustules (Fig. 11-9), and finally, to ulceration (Fig. 11-10). The symptoms include severe pruritus, burning, irritation, and, occasionally, pain. The individual larger primary lesions with typical satellites provide a strong clue to the diagnosis.

Diagnosis

The budding forms and pseudohyphae of candidal organisms can be demonstrated in skin scrapings treated with 20% potassium hydroxide. Culture techniques are identical to those employed in vulvovaginal disease. The mere isolation of candidal organisms from the vulvar skin does not prove that the patient has cutaneous candidiasis, since almost any necrotizing lesion can be secondarily infected with *Candida*. The diagnosis is justified only after a careful correlation of clinical and laboratory findings.

The cutaneous disease must be differentiated from almost all of the dermatoses that develop in the vulvar area, the most important of which are psoriasis, seborrheic dermatitis, and eczematoid dermatitis from any cause. Further, candidiasis should be distinguished from tinea cruris. It is not always practical, on the basis of microscopic morphology, to distinguish between the two; however, the presence of both spores and filaments in smear preparations indicates candidal infection, whereas hyphae alone suggest a tineal infection. Unless the clinical appearance of the lesions is characteristic, cultures may be required for generic identification. Occasionally, most of the venereal diseases and some ulcerative conditions, including herpes genitalis, also must be differentiated.

Treatment

The treatment includes improvement of general health (if the patient is debilitated) and control of all obvious predisposing factors—stabilization of diabetes, weight loss if the patient is obese, and avoidance of excessive moisture.

For active treatment, topical applications of amphotericin B (Fungizone) or nystatin (Mycostatin) are recommended. In the moist, weeping stage of the disease, a lotion is preferable by far to creams or ointments. The preparation used should be massaged into the lesions several times daily for 14 or more days. Engel published evidence that a drying lotion is as effective as amphotericin B lotion, though the majority of investigators have found that a lotion containing the antifungal agent affords better results. In our experience, nystatin is superior to amphotericin B. Castellani's paint and 1 to 2% gentian violet solution afford rapid relief. Vaginal fungicides should be used concurrently.

DIABETIC VULVITIS

Only since the concept of "diabetic vulvitis" was advanced by Hesseltine in 1933 has its relationship to candidiasis become widely recognized. Diabetes mellitus, although a powerful predisposing factor to candidiasis, is of little importance to the overall problem of these infections, since only 1 to 2 percent of the population has diabetes. Vulvovaginal candidiasis does, however, become a major problem to women with diabetes; more than half of these patients develop a chronic vulvitis, which is prone to be severe and extensive. The possibility of diabetes, therefore, should be considered in any patient with recurrent or chronic candidiasis or if the infection is acquired before puberty or after the menopause.

Published papers exclusively concerned with diabetic vulvitis are relatively scarce, and most authors are content to think of the disease only as candidiasis in a predisposed patient. The term "diabetic vulvitis" is, in our opinion, both acceptable and desirable for the special variety of chronic vulvar dermatitis that develops only in diabetics. In addition to its distinctive features, it frequently persists long after the fungus that initiated its development has been eradicated.

Etiology and pathogenesis

The species of *Candida* found in diabetic vulvitis are also recovered from nondiabetics. Since patients with reduced glucose tolerance, even without glycosuria, are more likely than normal subjects to have candidiasis, it must be assumed that elevated glucose levels in body fluids and tissues contribute to the growth of *Candida*. Bathing of vulvar tissues with glucose-laden urine further stimulates candidal growth. It is Parks' opinion that diabetes causes not only inadequate metabolism of carbohydrates and fats but also depletion of nicotinic acid and riboflavin. He believes that these deficiencies contribute to vulvar pruritus and edema. Obesity contributes to intertriginous eruptions including cutaneous candidiasis, an essential part of diabetic vulvitis. In uncontrolled diabetes, the presence of abnormal amounts of metabolites, such as acetone, B-hydroxybutyrate, and urea, in the urine might well have an aggravating effect upon the overall picture of the problem. Low-grade secondary bacterial infections frequently develop in excoriated vulvar skin, although whether such infections are an essential component of the ultimate clinicopathologic entity is unknown.

Obviously, the widespread chronic vulvitis in diabetics develops from a multiplicity of factors, some only indirectly related to the diabetes. The chronologic stages in its development may well be diabetes, vulvovaginal candidiasis, pruritus, scratching, traumatic dermatitis, cutaneous candidiasis, further scratching and spread of candidal infection, bacterial dermatitis, lichen simplex chronicus, and, finally, classic diabetic vulvitis. Stress, tension, anxiety, and frustration may play a perpetuating role. The severity and extent of the infection depend to some degree upon the duration of poorly controlled diabetes and pruritus, the duration of

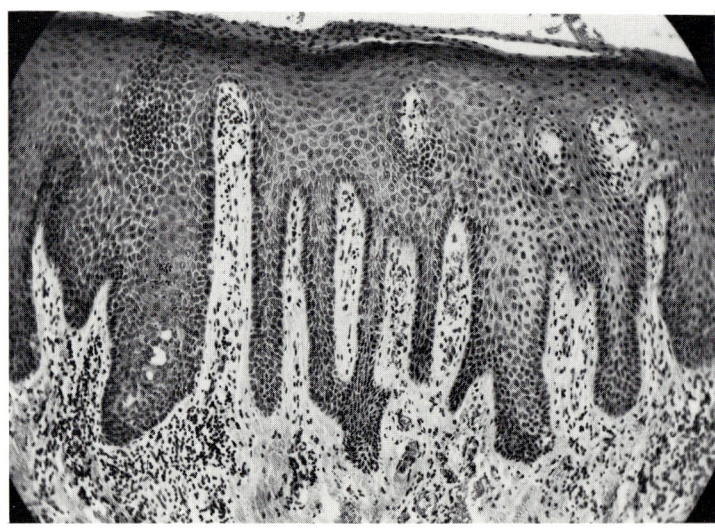

Fig. 11-11. Diabetic vulvovaginitis. Biopsy from vulva in patient with long-standing vulvitis. Some of the changes are consistent with lichen simplex chronicus. (H & E × 148)

untreated candidal and bacterial infections, the vigor of the scratching, and the patient's individual response to the allergenic and endotoxic substances produced by the fungi and bacteria. Persistent infection, obstinate pruritus, and continued scratching eventually result in a chronic dermatitis compatible with lichen simplex chronicus (neurodermatitis) (Fig. 11-11). It is improbable that candidal infection without chronicity and aggravating factors would lead to "diabetic vulvitis." Fully developed vulvitis may persist in some degree for months or years after control of the diabetes and after all fungi have been eradicated. This is explained partially, perhaps, on the basis of well-developed, widespread chronic neurodermatitis perpetuated by an uncontrolled scratch-itch reflex.

Clinical features

Symptoms. The symptoms generally reported include chronic pruritus, irritation, burning, dysuria, and dyspareunia, all of which tend to persist in varying degrees after treatment for the diabetes and candidiasis.

Objective signs. Gross clinical features of the vulva and surrounding skin are determined by many factors, among them the stage and duration of the candidal infection, obesity, sensitivity to responsible agents, hygienic measures, and previous therapy. The clinical variability of the disease is evidenced by the many terms used to describe the appearance of involved tissues. Descriptions always include several of the following characteristics.

Extensive involvement, not only of the vulvovaginal tissues, but also of the inner thighs, mons pubis, lower abdomen, perianal skin, and inner side of the buttocks is commonly present (Fig. 11-12).

Edema of the involved tissues is practically always observed. It is sometimes designated simply as swollen, thickened, galled, or elevated.

Erythema is exhibited by typical livid color of the tissues and is variously described as beefy, bright, diffusely or intensely red.

Thrush patches appear in the vestibule and vagina and, occasionally, on the labia majora.

A superficial grayish-white film is frequently observed, particularly in patients who neglect careful cleansing. A "boiled" or "cooked" appearance has been described. The reddish-blue hue is usually visible beneath any surface film.

A glazed or shiny appearance of the involved skin surface is common. It is probably attributable to removal by cleansing of dead, adherent epithelial cells.

Satellite vesicopustules characteristic of cutaneous candidiasis often are present.

Excoriations from scratching and fissuring in the natural skin folds are frequently associated.

Pigmentary changes such as hyperpig-

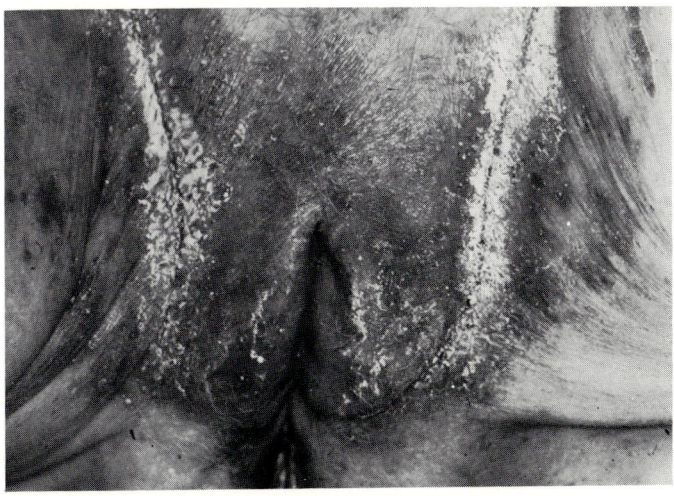

Fig. 11-12. Diabetic vulvovaginitis. Extensive skin lesions usually present. Candidal organisms isolated from both vulva and vagina.

mentation in light-complexioned persons and hypopigmentation or bleaching in Negroes and other dark-complexioned patients may appear.

Furunculosis of the vulvar skin is also sometimes observed, since diabetes predisposes to pyogenic infection.

Treatment

Control of diabetes by weight loss, dietary measures, and the use of insulin or oral hypoglycemic agents is essential in the case of patients with diabetic vulvitis. The patient should be placed under the care of a physician experienced in this field. Treatment for the diabetes alone, however, is unlikely to immediately effect significant changes.

Treatment of associated candidiasis should be initiated. In our experience, the most reliable candidacidal agent for temporary use in diabetic vulvitis is 1% aqueous gentian violet applied two or three times weekly to all affected areas, including the vagina. Other fungicides include nystatin cream, amphotericin B lotion, and candicidin (Candeptin) ointment. Antifungal medications must be used over a period of many weeks or even months, and a change from one agent to another is sometimes beneficial.

Control of pruritus is important, although it is not always accomplished by control of the candidiasis. Topical corticosteroid preparations are often invaluable for this purpose; 0.025% fluocinolone acetonide cream (Synalar), 0.05% flurandrenolone cream (Cordran), and 1% hydrocortisone cream (Cortef) are highly effective in most cases. Shake lotions, such as calamine lotion with 0.25% menthol, with or without 0.5% phenol, are protective, soothing, and often antipruritic.

Systemic corticosteroids, such as oral prednisone, have been found effective for dermatitis and pruritus that respond poorly to other measures. Since oral corticosteroids frequently have an unfavorable effect on diabetes, they must be administered with caution. The danger may be partially circumvented by use of hydrocortisone sodium succinate (Solu-Cortef) intravenously or triamcinolone-acetonide (Kenalog) intramuscularly. Corticosteroids often facilitate resolution of chronic inflammatory reactions and other slowly reversible changes in the involved tissues. When dermatitis and pruritus persist after control of the diabetes and candidiasis, the presence of a complicating neurodermatitis must be presumed. In addition to the anti-inflammatory and antipruritic agents, tranquilizers are sometimes helpful in breaking the scratch-itch reflex, a commonly acquired nervous habit. The lightest scratch in these patients can initiate a severe episode of pruritus.

Control of any associated bacterial infection is necessary. Topical applications of antibiotics are usually effective. Since antibiotics by any route tend to potentiate candidiasis, however, they should be used only in combination with an antifungal agent. Mycolog cream contains nystatin, neomycin sulfate, and gramicidin with triamcinolone-acetonide. Topical sulfonamides may also be helpful.

Supplemental vitamins, especially the B complex group, have been advocated by Parks as beneficial, the assumption being that vitamin deficiency is often associated with diabetes and contributes to the development of diabetic vulvitis.

REFERENCES

Adair, F. L., and Hesseltine, H. C.: Histopathology and treatment of vaginitis, Amer. Obstet. Gynec. **32**:1, 1936.

Alter, R. L., Jones, C. P., and Carter, B.: The treatment of mycotic vulvovaginitis with propionate vaginal jelly, Amer. J. Obstet. Gynec. **53**:241, 1947.

Berkhout, C. M.: De schimmelgeschlachten Monilia, Oidium, Oospora, en Torula, Dissertation, University of Utrecht, 1923.

Bernstine, J. B., and Rakoff, A. E.: Vaginal infections, infestations, and discharges, New York, 1953, McGraw-Hill Book Co.

Carter, B., Jones, C. P., Creadick, R. N., Parker, R. T., and Turner, V.: The vaginal fungi, Ann. N. Y. Acad. Sci. **83**:265, 1959.

Carter, B., Jones, C. P., Ross, R. A., and Thomas, W. L.: Vulvovaginal mycoses in pregnancy, Amer. J. Obstet. Gynec. **39**:213, 1940.

Dawkins, S. M., Edwards, J. M. B., and Riddell, R. W.: Yeasts in the vaginal flora: Their incidence and importance, Lancet **2**:1230, 1953.

deSousa, H. M., and van Uden, N.: The mode of infection and reinfection in yeast vulvovaginitis, Amer. J. Obstet. Gynec. **80**:1096, 1960.

Dobson, H. L.: Personal communication, 1966.

Döderlein, A.: Das Scheidenseknet und seine Bedeutung für das Puerperafiehen, Leipzig, 1892.

Drouhet, E.: Biologie des infections à Candide II. Sur les manifestations pathologiques de 175 cas de candidase, Sem. Hôp. **33**:807, 1957.

Dukes, C. D., and Gardner, H. L.: Bacteriology of moniliasis, Unpublished data.

Engel, M. F.: Amphotericin B lotion in monilial intertrigo, Arch. Derm. 92:687, 1965.

Gardner, H. L.: Unpublished data.

Gardner, H. L.: Vaginal infections. In Conn, H., editor: Current Therapy, Philadelphia, 1963, W. B. Saunders Co.

Gardner, H. L.: Vaginal thrush, Texas J. Med. 40:333, 1944.

Gardner, H. L., Dukes, C. D., and Damper, T. K.: The prevalence of vaginitis, Amer. J. Obstet. Gynec. 73:1080, 1957.

Gershberg, H., Javier, Z., and Hulse, M.: Glucose tolerance in women receiving an ovulatory suppressant, Diabetes 13:378, 1964.

Gilpin, C. A.: Resistant monilial vaginitis: The male aspect, Florida State Med. J. 54:337, 1967.

Gold, W., Stout, H. A., Pagano, J. F., and Donovick, R.: Amphotericins A and B, antifungal antibiotics produced by a streptomycete: In vitro studies, Antibiotics Annual, New York, 1956, Medical Encyclopedia, Inc.

Haussman, D., cited by Bernstine, J. B., and Rakoff, A. E.: Vaginal infections, infestations, and discharges, New York, 1953, McGraw-Hill Book Co.

Hazen, E. L., and Brown, R.: Two antifungal agents produced by a soil actinomycete, Science 112:423, 1950.

Hesseltine, H. C.: Biologic and clinical import of vulvovaginal mycoses, Amer. J. Obstet. Gynec. 34:855, 1937.

Hesseltine, H. C.: Diabetic of mycotic vulvovaginitis: Preliminary report, J.A.M.A. 100:177, 1933.

Hesseltine, H. C.: Factors relating to mycotic and trichomonal infections, Ann. N. Y. Acad. Sci. 83:245, 1959.

Hesseltine, H. C., Borts, I. C., and Plass, E. D.: Pathogenicity of the Monilia (Castellani) vaginitis and oral thrush, Amer. J. Obstet. Gynec. 27:112, 1934.

Hesseltine, H. C., and Campbell, L. K.: Diabetic or mycotic vulvovaginitis, Amer. J. Obtet. Gynec. 35:272, 1938.

Hildick-Smith, G., Blank, H., and Sarkany, I.: Fungus diseases and their treatment, Boston, 1964, Little, Brown and Co.

Jackson, J. L., and Spain, W. T.: A comparative study of combined and sequential anovulatory therapy on vaginal moniliasis: Scientific Exhibit, Amer. Col. Obstet. Gynec., Chicago, May 2-5, 1966.

Kaufman, R., and Gardner, H. L.: Unpublished data on histopathology of vaginitis, 1966.

Kearns, P. R., and Gray, J. E.: Mycotic vulvovaginitis: incidence and persistence of specific yeast species during infection, Obstet. Gynec. 22:621, 1963.

Kittleson, A. R.: A new class of organic fungicides, Science 115:84, 1952.

Lechevalier, H., Acker, R. F., Corke, C. T., Haenseler, C. M., and Waksman, S. A.: Candicidin, a new antifungal antibiotic, Mycologia 45:155, 1953.

Loh, W. P., and Baker, E. E.: Fecal flora of man after oral administration of chlortetracycline or oxytetracycline, Arch. Intern. Med. 95:74, 1955.

Louria, D. B., and Brayton, R. G.: A substance in blood lethal for *Candida albicans,* Nature 201:309, 1964.

Maibach, H. I., and Rees, R. B.: How we treat cutaneous candidiasis, Postgrad. Med. 42:A75, 1967.

Parks, J.: Diagnosis and management of vulvar lesions, Med. Ann. D. C. 30:582, 1961.

Peterson, W. F., Steel, M. W., and Coyne, R. V.: Analysis of the effect of ovulatory suppressants on glucose tolerance, Amer. J. Obstet. Gynec. 95:484, 1966.

Rohatiner, J. J.: Relationship of *Candida albicans* to the genital and anorectal tracts, Brit. J. Vener. Dis. 42:197, 1966.

Scott, J. S.: Personal communication, 1966.

Seelig, M. S.: Mechanism by which antibiotics increase the incidence and severity of candidiasis and alter the immunological defenses, Bact. Rev. 30:442, 1966.

Seelig, M. S.: The role of antibiotics in pathogenesis of *Candida* infections, Amer. J. Med. 40:887, 1966.

Sloane, M. D.: A new antifungal antibiotic, Mycostatin (nystatin) for the treatment of moniliasis: A preliminary report, J. Invest. Derm. 24:569, 1955.

Stone, O. J., and Mullins, J. F.: Role of *Candida albicans* in chronic disease, Arch. Derm. 91:70, 1965.

Stough, W. V., and Blank, H.: Vaginal candidiasis in South Florida, Obst. Gynec. 12:338, 1958.

Taubert, H. D., and Smith, A. G., cited by Smith, A. G., Taubert, H. D., and Martin, C. W.: The use of Trichomycin in the treatment of vulvovaginal mycosis in pregnant women, Amer. J. Obstet. Gynec. 87:455, 1963.

Walsh, H., Hildebrandt, R. J., and Prystowsky, H.: Candidal vaginitis associated with the use of oral progestational agents, Amer. J. Obstet. Gynec. 93:904, 1965.

Wilkinson, J. S.: Some remarks upon the development of epiphytes, Lancet 2:448, 1849.

Wilson, D. G.: Vaginal candidiasis during pregnancy, Western J. Surg. Obst. Gynec. 64:180, 1956.

Young, G., Resca, H. G., and Sullivan, M. T.: Interactions of oral strains of *Candida albicans* and lactobacilli, J. Dent. Res. 30:426, 1951.

Chapter 12
Trichomoniasis

In 1836, Donne reported his observations of "animalcules" in purulent discharges from the genital tracts of men and women and called the organisms *Trico-monas vaginale*. Ehrenberg, in 1838, suggested the term *Trichomonas vaginalis*. In 1916, Hoehne correlated a characteristic clinical vaginal disease with the presence of trichomonads. For decades, scientists interested in trichomoniasis have acknowledged that it is not an infection of the vagina alone but also of Skene's ducts and the lower urinary tract, as well as the lower genitourinary tract of men.

The isolation of *T. vaginalis* in pure culture by Trussell and Plass, in 1940, was a major milestone in the study of this disease; previously, the effects of bacteria-free cultures on the vagina could not be determined. The extensive efforts of Karnaky in the 1930's and 1940's were, to a considerable extent, responsible for the awakening of the medical profession to the prevalence and problems of trichomoniasis. Before the introduction of metronidazole (Flagyl) by Durel in 1959, the treatment for the disease was easily more perplexing than that for any of the other vaginal infections.

Considering the physical discomfort and esthetic revulsion experienced by millions of women because of trichomoniasis, its true medical importance cannot be overemphasized. Moreover, evidence has been published that trichomoniasis may predispose to cervical cancer.

CLASSIFICATION

According to the severity of infection, trichomoniasis may be classified as asymptomatic, chronic, or acute.

Asymptomatic trichomoniasis

Living trichomonads in small numbers are sometimes observed in patients with a vaginal pH 3.8 to 4.2 and with vaginal flora in which lactobacilli predominate. These patients usually have no clinical, bacteriologic, or histologic signs of the disease. This is the asymptomatic or carrier stage of the infection. It is unknown whether the vaginal organisms present in such small numbers are capable of inciting infection in the male urethra. The majority of patients with asymptomatic infections give a clear-cut history of past clinical disease and almost all later experience exacerbations.

Chronic trichomoniasis

Patients without distinct gross changes in the vulvar or vaginal tissues, yet whose vaginal secretions are of abnormal volume, odor, consistency, pH, and bacteriology, are considered to have the chronic type of trichomoniasis—the most common variety. Irritative subjective symptoms may or may not be present. Probably the chronic stage is maintained (and the acute stage prevented) in some patients by the frequent use of acid or medicated douches. Although the criteria do not include distinct gross tissue reactions, varying degrees of inflammatory infiltration may be observed in histologic sections of the vagina.

Acute trichomoniasis

Acute infection is characterized by an abnormal vaginal discharge, gross tissue reactions of the vagina or vulva, or both, and, generally, irritative symptoms, particularly pruritus. Edema and erythema are the common gross abnormalities of the vulva, and the vagina usually exhibits one or more of the following signs: erythema, swollen papillae, petechiae, or ecchymoses. Rarely, a thin, splotchy pseudomembrane is present. As in the chronic stage, the vaginal flora is essentially devoid of lactobacilli and the pH is elevated. The histologic appearance of the vagina is that of acute inflammation.

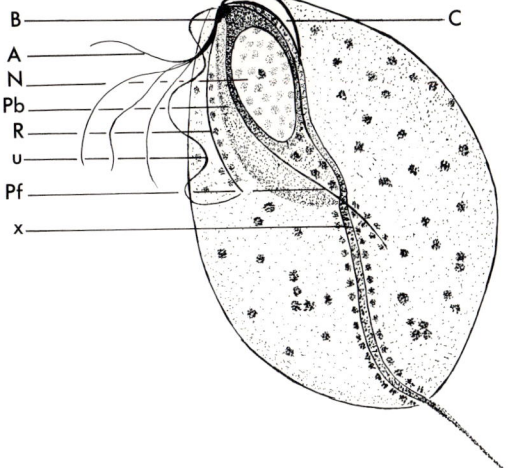

Fig. 12-1. Drawing of detailed morphology of *Trichomonas vaginalis*. *A,* Four anterior flagella (usually one to two times the length of the organism); *B,* blepharoplast; *C,* cytosome; *N,* nucleus; *R,* chromatic basal rod; *u,* undulating membrane; *X,* axostyle; *Pb,* parabasal body; *Pf,* parabasal fibril.

GENERAL DISCUSSION
Etiology

Causative agent. The organism *Trichomonas vaginalis,* according to the consensus and in fulfillment of the demands of Koch's postulates, is the sole cause of trichomoniasis in human beings, even though an occasional observer still finds reason to question the relationship of the organism and the clinical entity. The evidence supporting its pathogenicity is so overwhelming that further debate on this point is unwarranted. According to Manwell and Hegner and Ratcliffe, *T. vaginalis* may possibly be found in certain Macaca species and chimpanzees, though there is no evidence that it exists in other animals. The rectal and oral organisms *Trichomonas hominis* and *Trichomonas buccalis,* when implanted into the vagina, are transient and fail to produce vaginitis. So far as is known, *Trichomonas bovis (T. foetus),* pathogenic in cattle, does not give rise to disease in the human subject.

T. vaginalis is a unicellular protozoan flagellate (Figs. 12-1 and 12-2). When actively motile, *T. vaginalis* is fusiform in shape, similar to a grain of wheat. The organisms are usually larger than polymorphonuclear leukocytes, though smaller than mature epithelial cells. The length varies from 7 to 30 μ, the majority being 15 to 20 μ long. The factors that influence cellular size are unknown; in some patients the organisms are

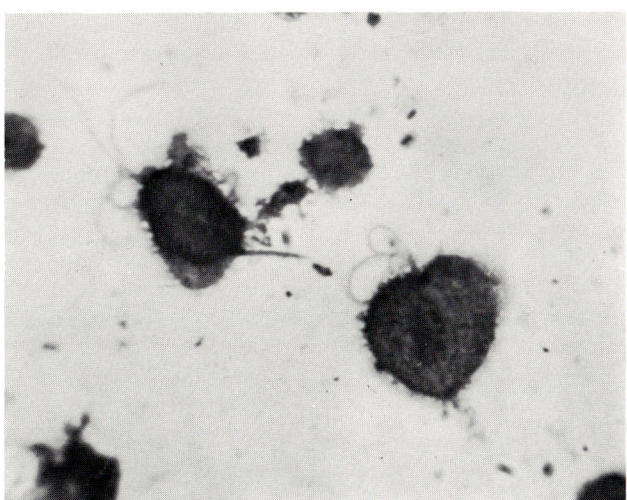

Fig. 12-2. Trichomonads in a wet mount preparation containing pinacyanole **vital** stain. Morphology of individual trichomonads well demonstrated. (Courtesy Robert B. Greenblatt, Augusta, Ga.)

consistently small, whereas in others they are above average size.

Four flagella of approximately equal length (from one to two times the length of the organism itself) protrude from the forward end of the trichomonad. An undulating membrane extends from the blepharoplast (where the flagella are attached) to about half-way down one side of the organism. Also arising from this point is a rod-like structure, the *axostyle,* which traverses the organism lengthwise, curving around the nucleus and projecting through the end of the cell to resemble a short, stiff tail. The axostyle, which is one-half to one-third the length of the organism, seems to function as an organ of attachment; particulate matter, including other trichomonads, is frequently adherent to it, as though a sticky substance were present on its surface. The nucleus, in the anterior half of the organism, is spindle shaped and is approximately one-third the length of the body.

Healthy trichomonads in vaginal secretions or physiologic saline are actively motile, usually moving in the direction of the flagella. Their motions are jerky and, in addition to the forward movement, they frequently rotate on their long axis. When entrapped in particulate vaginal matter, they sometimes send out pseudopodia-like extensions in an amoeboid fashion.

In an unhealthy environment, trichomonads frequently assume a spherical (balled-up) shape (Fig. 12-10, *B*) and are difficult to distinguish from cellular elements of the host. Such forms may be seen in urinary sediment, in vaginal material after medicinal douches, in the more acid vaginal content of asymptomatic patients, or in any adverse environment. The rounded forms have been referred to as *pseudocysts,* although trichomonads do not form true cysts under any circumstance. Individual trichomonads are extremely fragile and succumb to almost any strong chemical agent with which they come in contact. The balled-up organisms are usually extremely sluggish. To be recognized in this form, they must often be observed under a high microscopic magnification; even then, the only motion observed may be that of the undulating membrane or the flagella.

Several investigators have demonstrated that agglutinating antibodies can be produced in some animals, particularly rabbits, by injections of both living and killed organisms. Specific antibodies can be produced in human beings, yet no influence upon the course of the disease has been demonstrated.

Trichomonads multiply by binary division. The division process seems to be initiated at the blepharoplast. The nucleus then divides and the organism separates longitudinally into two daughter cells. Since the organisms do not form cysts, they are adapted for transfer from one host to another only in a moist environment.

Sources of infection.

Venereal disease. Trichomoniasis is no less a venereal disease than gonorrhea and syphilis. With the exception of an infinitesimally small percentage of cases, it is transmitted by sexual intercourse. Reluctance to accept trichomoniasis as a venereal disease in the past was perhaps based upon timidity, fear of implications, and disregard of medical logic. Actually, it is axiomatic that the majority of sexual consorts of infected women or men harbor the organisms and offer a potential source of infection for other sexual partners. With respect to the disease in anatomic virgins, careful inquiry will usually establish previous heterosexual contact without intromission.

Homosexual contact. Undoubtedly, vulvar contact between homosexuals is also a mode of transfer of the disease. Circumstantial evidence of such transfer has been observed on several occasions; for example, it has occurred in homosexual roommates, both with intact hymens and both with trichomoniasis.

Communal fomites. Vulvovaginal contamination from inanimate objects, such as douche nozzles, bath towels, and wet bathing suits, may explain an occasional infection. Burch, Rees, and Reardon demonstrated that trichomonads could be cultured from washcloths used to cleanse the external genitalia of infected women after the cloth had remained at room temperature for as long as 23 hours thereafter.

Swimming pools and bathtubs. It is improbable that a sufficient number of organisms to incite an infection could survive in a chlorinated swimming pool. Transmission by communal bathtubs is possible, though unlikely. The incidence of infection in sexually mature virginal daughters of infected mothers is extremely low. According to experimental evidence, several thousand organisms must be implanted into the vagina before infection can be established.

Toilet seats and toilet splash. Trichomoniasis, like gonorrhea, can be contracted from a contaminated toilet seat or from a toilet splash, yet the danger of infection by this means is surely minimal. Trichomonads can survive in water closets for several hours, and Kessel and Thompson have shown that they can survive in a semi-dry state for as long as 6 hours. It has been suggested that the mucus of vaginal secretions might encase trichomonads and retard their desiccation.

Gloves and instruments. Gloves and instruments could be an occasional source of infection in the office of a physician careless about asepsis.

Oral cavity and intestinal tract. Neither the oral cavity nor the intestinal tract has been proved to be a source of infection. *Trichomonas buccalis* is not a vaginal pathogen, and there is no evidence that *T. vaginalis* can survive in the mouth to become a source of vaginal infection. *Trichomonas hominis* of the intestinal tract is not a vaginal pathogen; *T. vaginalis* lives in the colon for only a short time. Thus, precaution to prevent fecal contamination of the vaginal orifice, although a laudable habit, is of doubtful value in the prevention of recurrent trichomoniasis.

Maternal birth canal. Some female infants acquire infection from their mothers during birth, though such infections usually are transitory. Maternal hormones in the infant soon disappear and allow the vagina of the newborn to revert to an immature state. This is an unfavorable environment for the trichomonad.

Autogenous sources. Patients who have apparently been cured of the infection by topical applications often are reinfected by trichomonads in the urethra and Skene's ducts. The cervical canal is a dubious source of reinfection; the organisms can seldom, if ever, be recovered from the cervical canal after their complete eradication from the vagina. On an extremely rare occasion, an infected Bartholin's duct or Bartholin's gland sinus may be a focus of infection. We have discovered an infection in the Bartholin system in only one patient; she had a chronic Bartholin's sinus, which is itself an unusual lesion.

Predisposing factors.
Estrogens. Trichomoniasis is primarily a disease of women with relatively high estrogen levels. The occasionally expressed opinion that it is a sign of hypoestrinism would seem to be unfounded. The idea that low estrogen levels predispose patients to trichomoniasis probably arose from the observation that wet smears from patients with active infection exhibit a high percentage of parabasal epithelial cells (Fig. 12-11), as is also true in the presence of estrogen deficiency. The hyperestrinism of pregnancy appears to promote the development of severe infection, while the vaginas of premenarchal girls and postmenopausal women have the opposite effect. At times, postmenopausal women with atrophic vaginas and quiescent infections have acute exacerbations of trichomoniasis soon after the administration of systemic estrogens.

Hypoacidity of the vagina. Allegedly, a highly acid vaginal secretion (pH 3.8 to 4.0) in which the lactobacillus predominates affords some protection against the development of trichomoniasis; nevertheless, the neutralizing effects of a large ejaculum of semen containing numerous trichomonal organisms might permit infection in an otherwise resistant environment. Although the full importance of low vaginal acidity in predisposing to *T. vaginalis* infection is unknown, available evidence strongly suggests that hypoacidity from causes such as menstrual blood, cervical mucorrhea, and *Haemophilus vaginalis* vaginitis encourages establishment of *T. vaginalis*. The exacerbations of infection that frequently take place in the vagina after menstruation illustrate this point. Although the postmenopausal vagina is also of low acidity and thus would theoretically favor the growth of trichomonads, the lack of other nutritional requirements at this time offsets any possible favorable effect of the elevated pH.

Bacterial flora. Whether pre-existing abnormalities of the vaginal flora predispose to trichomoniasis is unclear; undoubtedly, however, certain bacterial organisms, such as gram-positive cocci and gram-negative bacilli, function symbiotically with trichomonads to intensify the clinical pattern of the disease. A vaginal flora in which lactobacilli predominate, yet which contains trichomonads, seldom gives rise to clinical manifestations. An inoculation with trichomonads sufficient to produce clinical vaginitis is followed by an essential disappearance of lactobacilli and a predominance of such organisms as diphtheroids, streptococci, and staphylococci. The altered vaginal environment that follows trichomonal infection is unfavorable to the lactobacillus, although it seems to stimulate rapid multiplication of other bacteria usually already present in small numbers. We have been able to demonstrate that destruction of most abnormal bacterial content in the vagina with systemically administered broad spectrum antibiotics reduces the severity of trichomoniasis. As this destruction proceeds, the vaginal tissues rapidly improve, the purulent nature of the discharge diminishes, and the foul odor tends to disappear, even though trichomonads persist in profusion.

Emotionalism. Moore and Simpson regard *T. vaginalis* as the specific infectious agent of trichomoniasis, though they believe that the organism is incapable of producing symptoms unless the vagina is conditioned by the effects of disturbed emotions. They state: "We believe that trichomonas vaginitis is a psychosomatic symptom [sic] which occurs as a result of changes in vaginal physiology which are produced by emotional stress."

Melody proposed that the common denominator in women with refractory trichomoniasis is depression. McEwen attempted to show that emotional tension was the most important factor of recurrence of the disease in seventy of ninety-two patients. An analysis of his report revealed that most of the patients fell within one of these categories: unmarried mothers, the emotionally unstable, patients of known moral laxity who had a reactive anxiety to fornication, women who were frigid or complained of dyspareunia, those with a history of divorce, separation, or "chronic domestic strife," and those who reported "social dissatisfaction." Seemingly, the problems with which McEwen's patients were plagued are the ones commonly reported by sexually promiscuous women. As a group, emotionally disturbed wives also have husbands who are likely to have extramarital relations and thus to be exposed to repeated infections.

In our opinion, emotional instability alone cannot explain the fact that the incidence of trichomoniasis in Negro charity patients is five times higher than in Caucasian patients in private practice. Undeniably, many patients with trichomoniasis have emotional problems, but it would appear that they are the ones most likely to acquire infections from promiscuity and more likely to complain of the symptoms, giving the impression of a causal relationship between emotionalism and exacerbations. Conversely, many patients experience emotional reactions from prolonged trichomoniasis, just as many patients acquire greater emotional stability after cure of the infection.

Emotionalism as a precipitating cause of trichomoniasis is a vulnerable thesis in view of the immeasurables with which its advocamust deal. The fact is, after microbiologically proved cure of the disease, sexually abstinent patients do not have recurrences.

Prevalence

Trichomoniasis is chiefly a disease of the reproductive years. Seldom is a patient with clinical manifestations of the infection observed before the menarche or after the menopause, although fairly often trichomonads are recoverable from postmenopausal women. Before the introduction of metronidazole (Flagyl), it was commonly estimated that 20 to 25 percent of women in the United States harbored trichomonads, although 15 percent was perhaps a more realistic figure. Since availability of Flagyl, prevalence has shown a precipitous drop. Most reported studies are from institutional populations, such as teaching clinics, in which the incidence is several times higher than that in private practice—which, after all, is the largest group of patients in this country. Naguib, Comstock, and Davis, in 1966, recovered trichomonads from 14.5 percent of a large number of subjects who represented a fair sampling of the general population.

The reported prevalence of this disease is as variable as the patient material utilized by individual investigators. The highest incidence is always reported among the less fortunately situated groups. The prevalence among prostitutes is reportedly as high as 90 percent and among female inmates of penal institutions it is often 75 percent. Of all socioeconomic groups, the fewest infections are found in Caucasian patients observed in a private practice; according to numerous investigators, 6 to 12 percent of this group is infected. Gardner, Dampeer, and Dukes (1957) discovered that only 8.1 percent of 2,251 consecutive Caucasian private patients harbored trichomonads, while among 993 unselected patients in charity clinics in Houston, trichomonads were found in 29.5 percent of Caucasian women and 45.3 percent of Negro women attending the same clinic. The highest prevalence—53.5 percent was in nonpregnant Negro patients.

In summary, the incidence of trichomoniasis increases with indigency. Trichomoniasis is more prevalent in "patients" than in the total female population and in gynecologic than in obstetric patients of the same age group. It is more common in the Negro race, in divorcees and women separated from their husbands, and in those with promiscuous sexual habits or with poor genital hygiene. It is extremely prevalent among patients with other venereal diseases. Of the few women with intact hymens who have the disease, the majority admit heterosexual contact without intromission or homosexual contact. Since the availability of metronidazole, the prevalence of trichomoniasis has diminished precipitously.

Pathogenesis

Trichomonads are always present in the classical case of trichomoniasis. Their eradication is accompanied by clinical healing of the vaginitis, although it reappears if the patient is reinoculated with the organism. Once active infection is established, the glycogen content of the vaginal cells is reduced; the many-layered vaginal lining becomes thinner, and at times foci of true ulceration may develop. The vaginal pH rises; lactobacilli practically disappear, while the bacterial flora becomes mixed (Fig. 12-3). Numerous pus cells appear in the vaginal secretion, and the number of parabasal and intermediate epithelial cells increases (Fig. 12-11). Gross abnormalities of the vulva and vagina may appear, and vaginal secretions lose their curdy or crumbly texture, becoming homogeneous in consistency.

The mode of action of the organism in effecting these many vaginal changes remains speculative. We have examined microscopically many slides of vaginal tissues removed from thirty-five patients with acute infection. The tissues were stained with hematoxylin-eosin, iron hematoxylin, and Giemsa stains, yet we have been unable to identify a single organism within a cell or tissue space. Frost found a single trichomonad within the cytoplasm of an endocervical cell on histologic study of tissue taken from the squamocolumnar junction. Turner and Riva, with the use of acridine orange stains and variable depth focusing, demonstrated trichomonads within desquamated vaginal epithelial cells. The significance of these isolated discoveries has not been established.

Attempts have been made to explain the cytopathology of the infection on the basis of toxic substances rather than mechanical damage. Kotcher and Hoogasian were unable to demonstrate a toxic factor when filtrates from *Trichomonas* cultures were

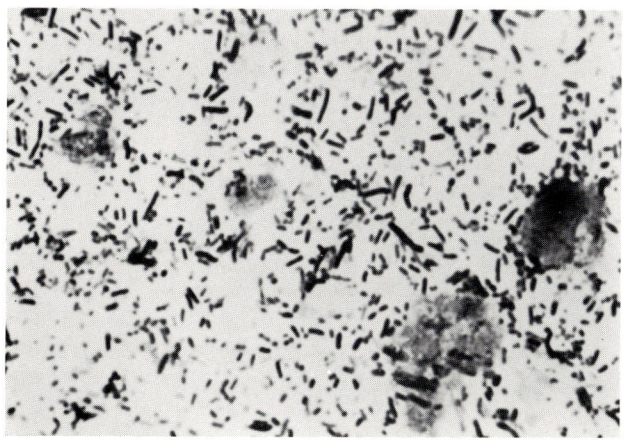

Fig. 12-3. Gram-stained smear of vaginal secretions of patient with acute trichomoniasis. Note large variety of bacterial organisms, the usual finding.

placed on chick embryo explants or human synovial cells. Christian and others could not detect a toxin in a filtrate prepared from HeLa cells destroyed by trichomonads on fresh uninfected HeLa cultures. After watching movies of infected cell cultures, they expressed the opinion that strenuous mechanical action by trichomonads could possibly be a factor in cell destruction; however, they were unable to exclude an extremely labile toxin as the cause of tissue damage. Although their findings were inconclusive, the basic research performed by these investigators seems to be significant to future studies of the mode of action of trichomonads. They conclusively demonstrated that trichomonads grew, divided, and destroyed HeLa cells in bacteria-free cell cultures and that the cytopathology observed in the test tube was similar in many respects to that in the human vagina. Further, the inoculation of the HeLa cell cultures with a small number of trichomonads failed to produce an infection in the test tube and destruction of the HeLa cell tissues, although the organisms persisted in a "carrier" state. Hesseltine, Wolters, and Campbell had previously demonstrated that a large inoculum was usually necessary to produce clinical disease.

From these observations, it might be postulated that an enzyme system can be produced by a sufficient number of organisms to cause destruction of intracellular bridges, subsequent cellular shedding, and, thus, reduction in the thickness of the layers of epithelial cells. Many of the cytologic and gross vaginal changes in acute infections could well be explained by such a mechanism. The susceptibility to bacterial infection of a vaginal mucosa only a few cell layers in thickness might explain the apparently symbiotic role of bacteria. Despite such theories, the exact mechanism that provokes the clinical patterns of trichomoniasis remains unproved.

Bacteriology

The altered vaginal environment induced by a *Trichomonas* invasion favors establishment and rapid growth of a large variety of "abnormal" bacterial agents (Fig. 12-3). Aciduric rods (lactobacilli and diphtheroids) predominate in most normal vaginal environments and possibly contribute to a condition somewhat hostile to other bacteria. For this reason, most "abnormal bacteria" seem to have only a transitory existence in normal vaginas. The chief difference in the flora of the normal vagina and the vagina in trichomoniasis is the relative numbers of the various bacteria. If an investigator is determined to isolate lactobacilli, it is probable that he will find insignificant numbers in most cases of trichomoniasis, even if gram-stained smears from the vagina appear to be free of the organisms. We believe that the notable alteration in flora is a direct result of the ability

Table 3. Bacteriology of active trichomoniasis (Dukes and Gardner)

	Acute (39)	Chronic (28)	Total (67)
Lactobacilli	6 (15%)	6 (21%)	12 (18%)
Diphtheroids	23 (59%)	18 (64%)	41 (61%)
Alpha streptococci	29 (74%)	21 (75%)	50 (75%)
Anaerobic streptococci	2 (5%)	2 (7%)	4 (6%)
Streptococcus pyogenes		1	1
Staphylococcus aureus	7 (18%)	5 (18%)	12 (18%)
Staphylococcus albus	2 (5%)	1	3 (4%)
Micrococcus species		1	1
Gaffkya	2 (5%)		2 (3%)
Aerobacter aerogenes	2 (5%)		2 (3%)
Alkaligenes faecalis	1		1
Escherichia coli	1	1	2 (3%)
Proteus mirabilis	1		1
Proteus vulgaris		1	1
Pseudomonas aeruginosa	1		1

of trichomonads to produce an environment favorable to abnormal bacteria and unfavorable or hostile to aciduric rods. Bacteriologic study of the vagina of a patient with a Grade III flora and with trichomoniasis who has been treated with metronidazole will prove this point; within a few days, the aciduric rods become re-established and predominant. The only explanation for the radical change is the elimination of trichomonads.

Table 3 is a summary of the bacteriologic findings in sixty-seven patients with active trichomoniasis from whom no other vaginal pathogens were elicited. The incidence of the various organisms differs slightly in acute and chronic disease. Although it is universally agreed that bacterial organisms contribute appreciably to the clinical disease, the similarity of the findings in the acute and chronic varieties, as shown in this table, seems to suggest that factors other than the associated bacterial flora must influence the severity of infection.

Table 4 shows the comparative bacteriologic findings in thirty-three patients with asymptomatic trichomoniasis and in 100 patients with normal vaginas. For all practical purposes, both groups of patients had normal vaginas with normal secretions, and, aside from the presence of rare trichomonads in the group with asymptomatic trichomoniasis, all smears were normal and essentially identical.

The aspect of vaginal bacteriology that has been almost completely ignored is that of quantitation. To the urologist, quantitation of bacteria is of vital importance. This has not been true of gynecologists with reference to vaginitis. Because of the large variety of bacteria usually recovered from the vagina and their varied multiplication rates in transport media, relative numbers by colony count can be misleading and difficult to interpret. In the experience of Dukes and Gardner, a correlation of culture identification with findings on stained smears provides a more practical method of estimating relative numbers of various species. Investigators who report that vaginal bacteriology is essentially identical in active trichomoniasis and in normal vaginas may be qualitatively correct, though quantitatively they could not be further from the truth. A lactobacillus versus alpha hemolytic streptococcus ratio of 100:1 is a decidedly different bacteriologic

Table 4. Comparative bacteriology of normal vaginas and asymptomatic trichomoniasis (Dukes and Gardner)

	100 normal vaginas (percent)	33 cases asymptomatic trichomoniasis (percent)
Lactobacilli	78	76
Diphtheroids	42	36
Alpha streptococci	41	48
Streptococcus faecalis	1	
Anaerobic streptococci	1	
Gaffyka	5	
Staphylococcus aureus	3	6
Staphylococcus albus	5	
Micrococcus species	2	
Candida species	17	
Torulopsis glabrata		3

balance than a lactobacillus versus alpha hemolytic streptococcus ratio of 1:100.

Cytology

The Papanicolaou stained smear of vaginal secretions in patients with active trichomoniasis frequently exhibits characteristic features. At first glance, one usually observes a dirty or smudgy background, an increased number of pus cells, and a "spread" in the maturation index as a result of a relative increase in the parabasal and intermediate cells. Hypes and Ladewig discovered clusters of pus cells on epithelial cells in the Papanicolaou smears of 85 percent of patients. They did not consider this finding diagnostic, although they thought it highly suggestive. Such a high percentage of leukocytic clusters has not been reported by the majority of investigators.

The cytotoxic effects of trichomonads upon the epithelial cells sometimes produce changes that may be confused with those of neoplasia—for example, perinuclear halo, vacuolation of cytoplasm, hyperchromatic nuclei, and an increased nuclear-cytoplasmic ratio. A not uncommon finding is a thick nuclear membrane, incident to condensation of chromatin against the inner side of the nuclear membrane. Almost without exception, however, these changes can be distinguished from those of carcinoma.

As a rule, only minor morphologic changes are apparent in smears, and extreme aber-

176 Benign diseases of the vulva and vagina

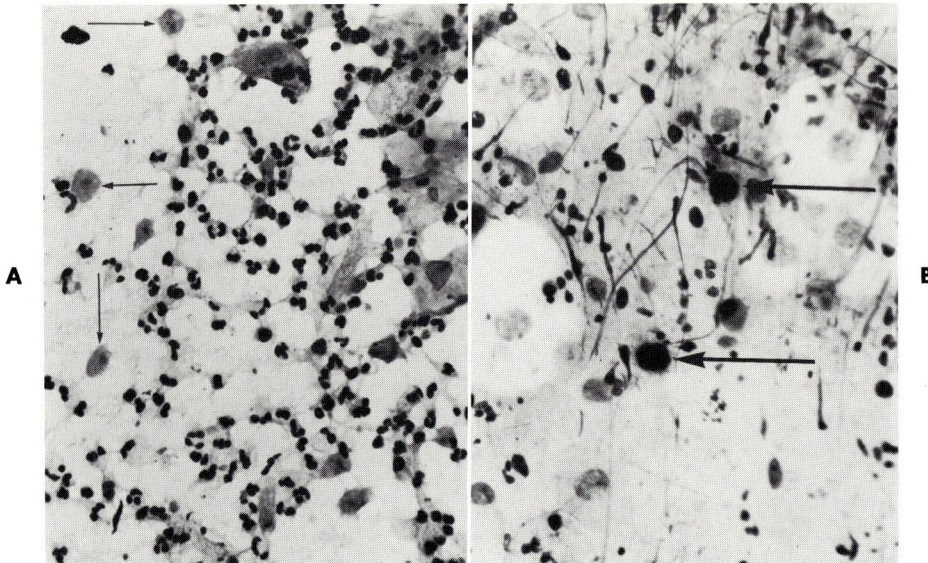

Fig. 12-4. Trichomoniasis. **A,** Cervicovaginal smear containing numerous trichomonads (arrows). (Papanicolaou × 494) **B,** Vaginal smear from postmenopausal patient. Arrows point to "purple blobs." These should not be confused with malignant nuclei. (Papanicolaou × 780)

rations are rare. Nevertheless, it may be necessary to reinterpret Papanicolaou smears after eradication of the trichomonal infection. The importance of atypical changes in the presence of trichomonads is not to be discounted because of the possibility of a concurrent carcinoma.

Frequently, trichomonads can be identified on the Papanicolaou smear (Fig. 12-4). They are oval to pear shaped, grayish-pink blobs. A more deeply staining centrosome may be detected within the substance of the cell. As a rule, the flagella are not identifiable on this type of smear. Extreme caution is necessary to avoid confusion of "naked nuclei" or fragments of cytoplasm from epithelial cells with trichomonads. Often the inexperienced cytologist makes the error of an "overcall."

Clinical features

Trichomoniasis exhibits a wider variety of clinical patterns than does any other vaginal infection. Generally, the course of the disease tends to be one of chronicity and acute relapses, although an occasional patient denies ever having had signs or symptoms. Infections are prone to be slightly worse immediately after menstruation and are sometimes most acute during pregnancy. Proved cases of spontaneous microbiologic cure must be extremely rare. We have observed a number of patients who harbored the organisms continuously for more than 20 years.

The characteristic manifestations are a malodorous discharge and pruritus. Many patients who deny having an abnormal discharge readily admit the necessity of frequent douching to prevent odor and soiling and acknowledge favorable changes following treatment. Vaginal trichomonicides, medicated douches, and other intravaginal agents, although seldom if ever curative, materially influence the clinical course of the disease.

The factors that determine the degree of tissue response to *T. vaginalis* are poorly understood. Since the clinical and laboratory patterns are so varied in different patients infected with the same strain of trichomonad, host factors, rather than strain virulence, must be the major determinants. Whereas variations in antigenicity of different strains have been demonstrated in experimental animals, the results have been inconclusive in human beings.

Symptoms. A *discharge* is the cardinal symptom of trichomoniasis. It is considered a subjective symptom when offered by the patient as a complaint. From a study of many reports, it is estimated that approxi-

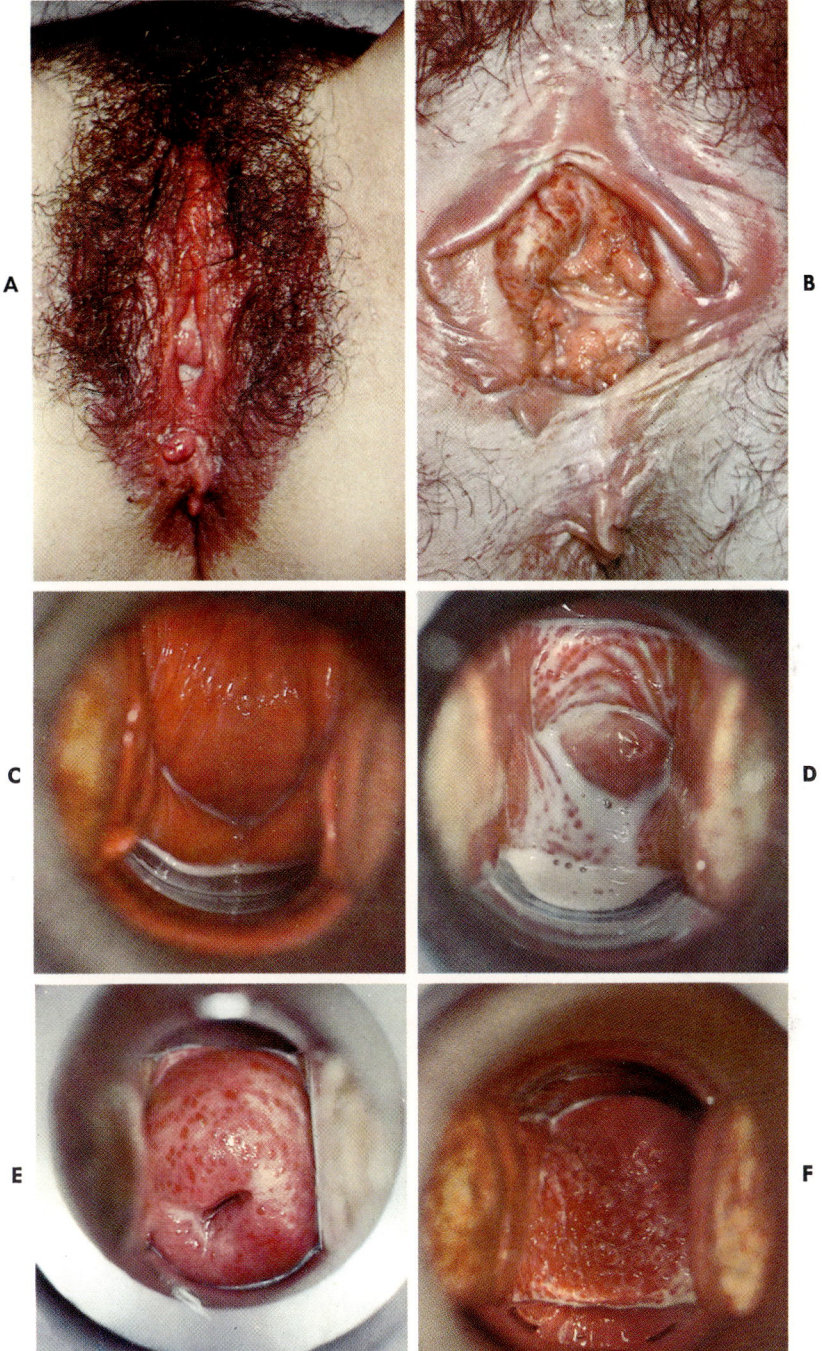

Plate 2. Acute trichomoniasis. **A,** Vulvitis with symmetrical erythema. Most patients do not display acute vulvitis. **B,** Redness of vestibule and ecchymoses of lower vagina. Patient had dyspareunia and the unusual symptom of bleeding with intercourse attributable to the vaginitis. **C,** Diffuse redness of the vagina, the most common gross feature of acute trichomoniasis. **D,** Swollen papillae with petechiae and a greenish, homogeneous vaginal discharge. These features are diagnostic, although present in only a small percentage of patients. **E,** Petechiae and swollen papillae of ectocervix, evidence of acute trichomoniasis. **F,** Pseudomembrane, present in a small but definite percentage of patients with acute trichomoniasis.

mately half of patients who complain of a discharge have trichomoniasis. In contrast, the majority of patients with candidiasis complain chiefly of pruritus. Many patients are also aware of a disagreeable odor; others are habituated to a personal odor. Patients who deny having a discharge often admit taking douches at frequent intervals for cleanliness or for hygienic reasons.

Pruritus, or itching of the vulva, the second most common manifestation, can become intolerable, although it is usually less intense than in candidiasis. Practically all patients give a history of pruritus, yet less than half have the symptom on the day of the initial examination. The complaint of "vaginal itch" usually means itching of the vestibule. It is doubtful whether true vaginal itching ever exists.

Tenderness and burning are reported by many patients. The descriptive terms applied to any type of vulvar irritation are necessarily dependent upon the patient's interpretation and use of words.

Chafing, according to Karnaky (1937), is almost pathognomonic of trichomoniasis. It is caused by rubbing and friction between moist upper thighs, though it is aggravated by the chemical irritants in the trichomonal discharge.

Dyspareunia from trichomoniasis arises from superficial tenderness incident to edema and erythema of the vulvovaginal tissues. The importance of dyspareunia in some cases becomes impressive only after treatment with metronidazole brings relief.

Urinary symptoms may be reported by the patient. Urethrocystitis solely from the effects of a *T. vaginalis* infection is occasionally observed in patients with or without vulvovaginal trichomoniasis. Mild abacteriuric pyuria associated with demonstrable trichomonads in the clean voided or catheterized urinary specimen is generally attributable to the organism. The true nature of a previously persistent pyuria is assured if the pus and trichomonads immediately disappear upon the administration of metronidazole, an agent ineffective against bacterial infections.

As a rule, the symptoms from trichomonal urethrocystitis are mild. Burning on urination is likely to be associated with severe vulvitis, particularly in the presence of excoriations. Urinary frequency can be the result of trichomonal urethrocystitis or it can be a reflex response induced by the vulvitis.

Emotional symptoms are more often a manifestation of trichomoniasis than a factor that predisposes to exacerbations and relapses. Curative treatment, in removing the emotional and physical burdens of a malodorous discharge, vulvar irritation, and dyspareunia, is frequently followed by improved marital relations and better emotional health.

Objective vulvar signs. An analysis of case records of one of us (H. L. G.) revealed that approximately 40 percent of patients with trichomoniasis had some evidence of gross organic disease of the vulva at the time of the initial examination. Patients who seek medical attention naturally have a higher incidence of gross changes in the tissues than the total number of women who harbor trichomonads.

Erythema of the vulva is usually limited to the vestibule and the labia minora, although redness occasionally spreads to and beyond the labia majora (Plate 2, *A*). Obvious vulvar erythema is more characteristic of candidiasis than of trichomoniasis; nevertheless, a distinction between the two is usually impossible solely from the gross appearance of the vulva.

Edema of the vulva indicates acute infection. As a rule, it is limited to the labia minora, although it can involve the labia majora as well.

Intertrigo may result from a profuse discharge that may spread to the outer labia majora, genitocrural folds, and inner thighs, producing reactions in the skin. Rubbing and friction between the inner thighs contribute to the dermatitis. Long-standing irritation and friction eventually lead to thickening of the skin, hyperkeratosis, and pigmentary changes.

Excoriations or superficial abrasions from scratching are frequently observed in the acute disease. They are usually narrow, superficial linear ulcerations in the area of the interlabial sulci and perineum. Fissuring or linear excoriations in the natural folds of the skin are caused by chronic moisture and irritation. They are less common in this condition than in candidiasis or the primary vulvar dermatoses.

Abnormal secretions can occasionally be milked from the urethra (Fig. 12-5). This is rarely an impressive finding, however, since

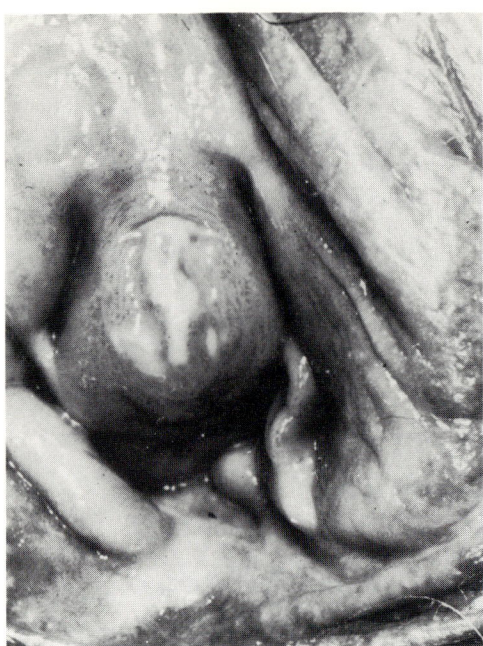

Fig. 12-5. Trichomoniasis. Purulent material, loaded with trichomonads, expressed from urethra and Skene's ducts. This is not an uncommon finding.

urethral discharges are continuously being washed away by the urinary system.

Discharge from Skene's ducts is a fairly common objective sign. Trichomonads often can be demonstrated in droplets of purulent material expressed from these ducts (Fig. 12-5). Such a finding readily explains the incurability of trichomoniasis by vaginal medications alone.

Infection of Bartholin's glands and ducts by trichomonads is seldom evident. Over many years, our attempts to recover trichomonads from the ducts have been uniformly unsuccessful. One patient had a chronic sinus from a Bartholin's gland that yielded trichomonads, though this does not, of course, prove glandular involvement. Murrell and Scott-Gray reported finding trichomonads in the pus of abscessed Bartholin's glands.

Objective vaginal signs in acute trichomoniasis. The squamous epithelial linings of the vagina and portio vaginalis of the cervix are essentially identical histologically and respond similarly to vaginal infection. Thus the ectocervix can be considered a part of the vaginal lining and its involvement as a part of vaginitis, rather than cervicitis. The vagina is seldom, if ever, grossly altered by only a few trichomonads in a flora composed predominantly of lactobacilli. In our opinion, chronic trichomoniasis is an infection with an abnormal discharge but without gross changes in the tissue. According to this definition, gross changes are observed only in acute infections. A review of our records disclosed that only 30 percent of patients yielding trichomonads displayed gross abnormalities of the vaginal mucosa.

Generalized erythema (Plate 2, *C*) is the only gross change in the vaginal tissue of approximately two-thirds of patients with acute trichomoniasis. The remainder have erythema in addition to other changes.

In the highly acute infection, edema and inflammatory infiltration of the vaginal papillae often cause grossly visible lesions resembling small papules (Plate 2, *D* and *E*). Probably the appearance of these swollen papillae projecting through a layer of discharge has caused such a vagina to be compared to the surface of a strawberry and thus to be described as "strawberry vagina."

Granular vaginitis is a condition in which the swollen papillae are numerous and large; on digital examination, they give the sensation of sandpaper or granules. Although this granular characteristic is occasionally detected in other types of vaginitis, trichomoniasis is, with few exceptions, responsible. A few of the patients with this sign also have vaginitis emphysematosa (Chapter 17).

Vaginal ecchymoses and petechiae are small hemorrhagic spots that follow increased vascularity combined with patchy thinning of the vaginal epithelium (Plate 2, *B, D,* and *E*). They are commonly associated with swollen papillae. Similar lesions are observed in other varieties of vaginitis, such as atrophic vaginitis from estrogen deficiency and in certain rare streptococcal infections. Hemorrhagic spots in conjunction with swollen papillae are always indicative of trichomoniasis. Trauma subjects the vagina with petechiae and ecchymoses to minimal bleeding. The patient demonstrated in Plate 2, *B* had pain and bleeding with intercourse.

Pseudomembrane formation is occasionally observed. During a 13 year period, one of us (H. L. G.) has personally found a pseudomembrane in the vagina of twelve patients in whom *T. vaginalis* was the only pathogen (Plate 2, *F*). Whether other investigators have reported this lesion in association with trichomoniasis is unknown to us. The pseudomembrane is usually spottily distributed, thin, and gray; it cannot be wiped away. Small individual lesions are round and closely grouped. In other cases, an uninterrupted membrane is present without intervening uninvolved mucosa. Most patients with the pseudomembrane have visible swollen papillae.

Leukorrhea in trichomoniasis. The characteristics of vaginal discharge in trichomoniasis are highly variable; however, a profuse, extremely frothy discharge, greenish in color and foul smelling (Plate 2, *D* and Fig. 12-6), when associated with swollen vaginal papillae, is pathognomonic of the disease. Only a small percentage of patients exhibits such a combination of objective signs, although some writers on the subject imply that they are usual. Frequently, a discharge is the only gross objective sign of trichomoniasis. The nature of the discharge may be altered by the number and strength of medicated douches used by the patient; in fact, the discharge itself may account for the habit of frequent douching.

The volume of the discharge is more abundant in acute trichomoniasis than in almost any other vaginal infection. In the chronic case, the discharge is usually moderately profuse, although the volume is often influenced by "hygienic" measures. The patient's account sometimes bears little relation to the examiner's findings.

The consistency of discharge varies. In active trichomoniasis, the discharge is homogeneous and has been described as creamy, purulent, fluid, thin, or watery (Fig. 12-6 and Plate 2, *D*). In contrast, the vaginal secretions in normal, mature women are curdy or crumbly, incident to the mixture of epithelial particulate matter with serous secretions, without appreciable pus and mucus (Fig. 13-6).

In our experience, at the time of their initial visit, frothiness of the discharge has been found in less than 10 percent of a large number of patients with trichomoniasis. Murrell and Scott-Gray, however, reported frothiness of the discharge of 42 percent of such patients. This discrepancy is probably attributable to differences in patient material and methods. For example, patients with symptoms who seek medical

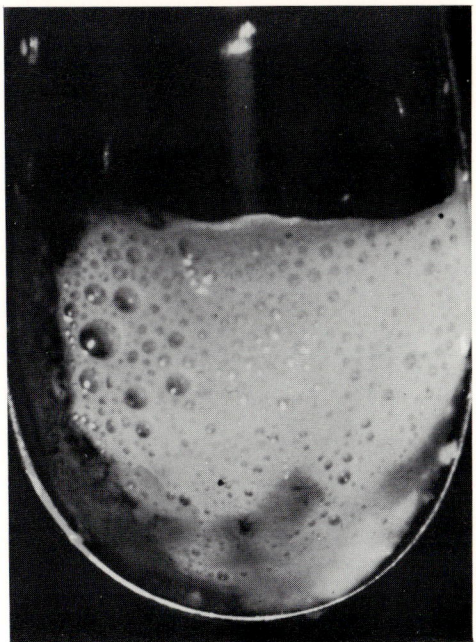

Fig. 12-6. Acute trichomoniasis. Abundant discharge with marked frothiness, shown on speculum, is indicative of the disease.

attention without having taken douches have a frothy discharge several times more often than those whose infections are discovered by routine screening methods. Frothiness is not a pathognomonic sign of trichomoniasis although, if pronounced, it is strongly suggestive (Fig. 12-6). Occasionally, *Haemophilus vaginalis* vaginitis is accompanied by frothiness, usually of minimal degree. The gas responsible for the frothiness is probably produced by both trichomonads and associated bacteria, since each is capable of fermentation.

The color of the discharge in acute trichomoniasis often is light green (Plate 2, *D*) or yellow, although in chronic infections it is practically always gray. Any discharge with a greenish tint points to trichomoniasis. The color distribution of discharges in our patients with acute and chronic infections was as follows: gray, 74 percent; greenish-gray, 10 percent; greenish-yellow, 5 percent; yellow, 2 percent; and yellow-gray, 4 percent. Thus, approximately three-fourths of the discharges were gray in color. Since the discharges of approximately 90 percent of patients with *H. vaginalis* vaginitis are also gray in color and homogeneous in consistency, the distinction is usually dependent upon laboratory studies.

The acidity of the discharge, as determined by the simple use of Hydrion Paper (Micro Essential Laboratory, Inc., Brooklyn, N. Y.) and a color chart, is a valuable tool in the differential diagnosis of vaginitis. Of the women of childbearing age with a vaginal pH 5.0 or higher, more than 95 percent have either trichomoniasis or *H. vaginalis* vaginitis. In practically all patients with chronic or acute trichomonal infection, the pH ranges from 5.2 to 5.5. A pH of less than 5.0 essentially eliminates trichomoniasis as a cause of leukorrhea.

The odor of the discharge in trichomoniasis is usually more offensive than in *H. vaginalis* vaginitis. Other than conditions in which fusospirochetal organisms are rapidly multiplying, trichomoniasis produces the most offensive odor of any vulvovaginal infection. Apparent loss of libido in some husbands can be traced to the unpleasant odors from trichomoniasis.

Histopathology

Although acute trichomoniasis can be divided into several gross categories, depending upon the visible changes of diffuse hyperemia, swollen papillae, petechiae, and pseudomembrane formation in the vagina, the histopathology in each case is quite similar. Each of these gross features may be explained by microscopic changes in the tissue, yet the differences are variable and not pathognomonic. The histopathologic changes in the tissue in the presence of acute trichomoniasis are striking (Figs. 12-7 and 12-8); they include epithelial hyperplasia secondary to acanthosis, spongiosis, and intracellular edema. At times the intracellular edema is pronounced, leading to vacuolation within and marked swelling of individual cells. Also, at times it may cause considerable separation of the cells and lead to the appearance of small vesicles. The nuclei are vesicular and contain prominent nucleoli. The epithelial folds are elongated, blunted, and frequently club shaped. If markedly elongated, the folds appear to adhere to one another, "trapping" dermis containing congested vessels between strands of the epithelium. Edema of the papillae is often pronounced, being described as "swollen papillae." This gives rise to considerable thinning of the suprapapillary epithelium;

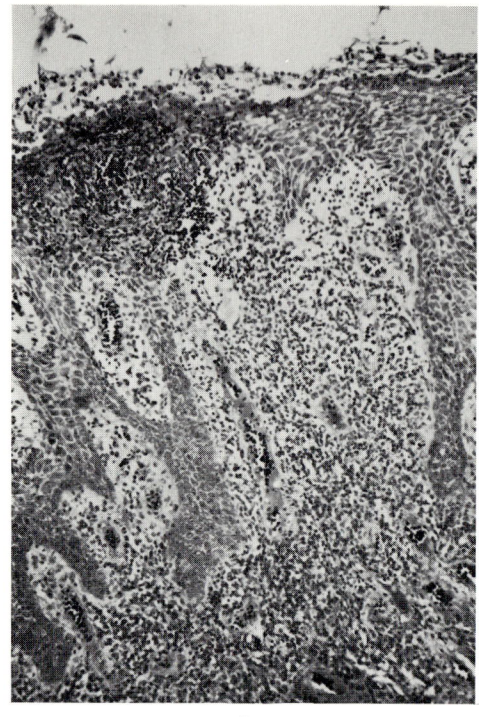

A

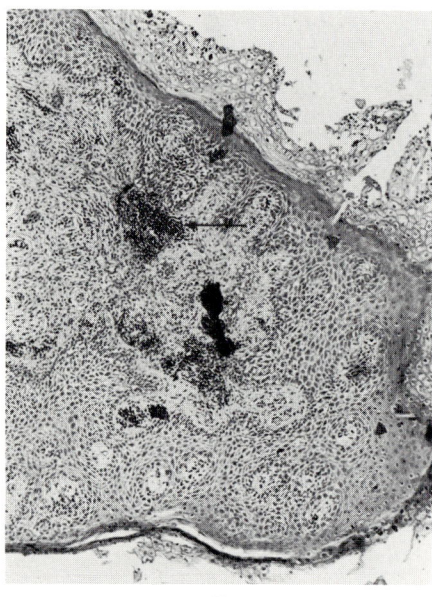

B

Fig. 12-7. A, Acute trichomoniasis. Focal area of ulceration and hemorrhage producing gross appearance of a petechia. Elongation of epithelial folds and marked inflammatory infiltration. (H & E × 162) B, Acute trichomoniasis. From patient with diffuse redness of vagina. Arrow indicates area of stromal hemorrhage. (H & E × 100)

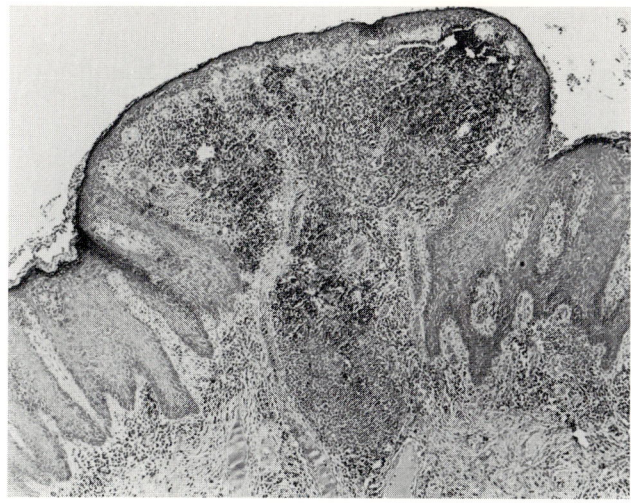

Fig. 12-8. Acute trichomoniasis from patient with swollen papillae. Small pseudoabscess within mucosa. (H & E × 60)

in fact, focally, the suprapapillary plate may be so thin as to become ulcerated (Fig. 12-7, *A*). Frequently, the vessels in the papillary region are congested, and areas of the stroma are hemorrhagic, both presenting the gross appearance of petechiae. At times, rather diffuse hyperemia or extravasation of blood into the dermis, or both, is observed (Fig. 12-7, *B*).

Inflammatory infiltration of the dermis is striking and consists primarily of lymphocytes, plasma cells, and smaller numbers of neutrophils. Occasionally, this inflammatory exudate extends into the epidermis. In patients with gross "swollen papillae," small pseudoabscess formations may often be seen beneath the vaginal epithelium (Fig. 12-8). In many cases, necrotic debris heavily infiltrated with neutrophils and with some lymphocytes lies on the epithelial surface of the vagina. If a pseudomembrane has formed, the surface of the epidermis is diffusely coated with inflammatory cells.

The changes associated with chronic trichomoniasis (Fig. 12-9) are much less pronounced than those observed in acute infection, such as mild to moderate acanthosis with some elongation and blunting of the epithelial folds, mild spongiosis, slight intracellular edema, mild to moderate edema of the papillae, and some dilation and congestation of the vascular channels. The inflammatory infiltrate in the lamina propria

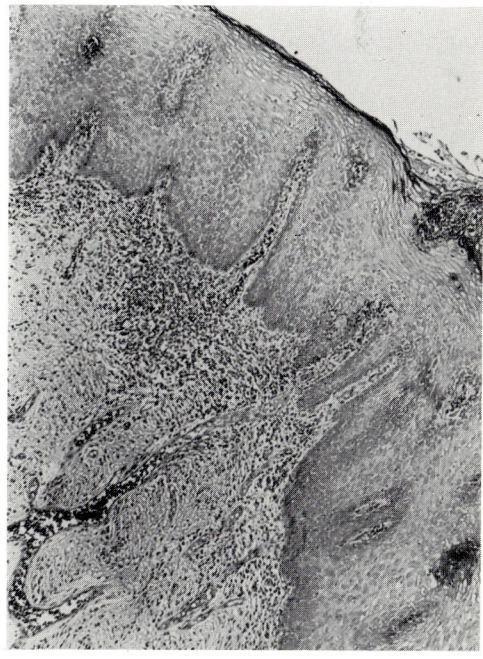

Fig. 12-9. Chronic trichomoniasis. Acanthosis and mild inflammatory infiltrate beneath vaginal epithelium. (H & E × 80)

consists primarily of lymphocytes and plasma cells.

Biopsy specimens from the vagina of a patient with asymptomatic trichomoniasis usually reveal no abnormal microscopic changes of the epithelium. Occasionally, the dermal vessels are slightly dilated and congested.

Diagnosis

Clinical findings. A profuse, homogeneous discharge with pronounced frothiness, offensive odor, and greenish color that is associated with vaginal petechiae and swollen papillae is pathognomonic of trichomoniasis. In most patients, however, this combination of diagnostic signs is lacking. Instead, they have only a moderate amount of gray, malodorous discharge and no gross organic changes. To repeat, since patients with *H. vaginalis* vaginitis also display a gray, homogeneous, malodorous discharge, these entities must often be distinguished by laboratory methods.

Vaginal erythema, petechiae, and swollen papillae are indicative of trichomoniasis. Gross pathologic changes in the vagina are observed in not more than a third of patients harboring trichomonads, and the majority deny irritative symptoms.

Frothiness of the vaginal discharge has long been considered almost pathognomonic of the disease, although in reality this sign is apparent in only a few patients. Further, some frothiness is present in the discharge of a significant number of patients with *H. vaginalis* vaginitis.

Any patient in the childbearing age with a vaginal pH of 5.0 or higher who has pruritus is likely to have trichomoniasis. In the absence of pruritus, the infection is as likely to be *H. vaginalis* vaginitis.

Laboratory findings. Because of its simplicity, expediency, and accuracy, the *wet mount preparation,* with the use of physiologic saline, is the laboratory method of choice for the diagnosis of trichomoniasis. Medical technicians with widely diverse responsibilities tend to be less accurate than the dedicated, specially trained technician who accepts each smear as a challenge. In many laboratories, including our own, the accuracy of wet mount preparations approaches that of cultures, while others report that they are even more accurate than the culture method.

On examination, actively motile organisms are seen moving about in their characteristic fashion (Fig. 12-10, *A*). In thick smears, the organisms can usually be detected by the disturbance which they cause among clumps of particulate matter. Sluggish, rounded organisms (Fig. 12-10, *B*) are more easily discernible under the high power objective.

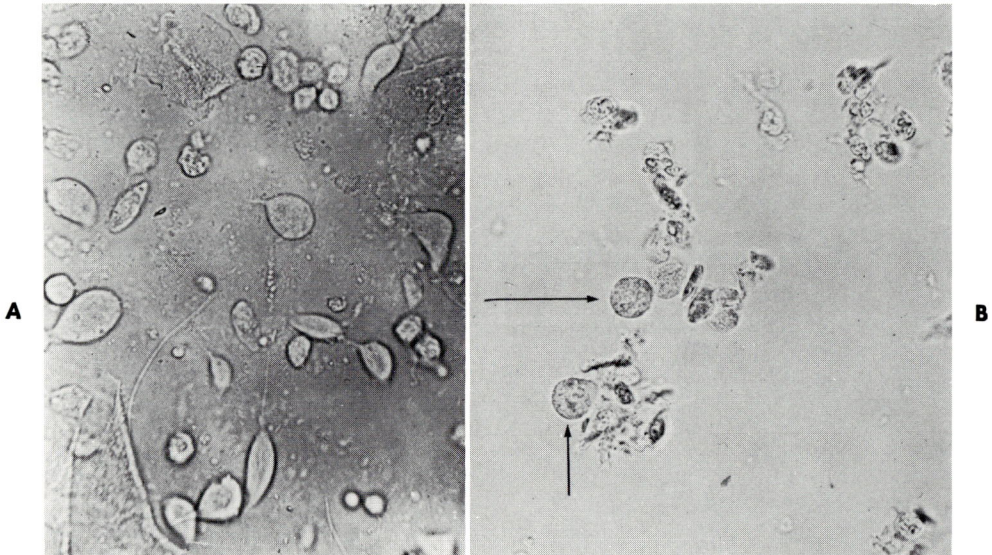

Fig. 12-10. Trichomoniasis. **A**, Numerous trichomonads in wet mount prepared with physiologic saline. Usually, more pus and immature epithelial cells are found in the secretions of active trichomoniasis. (High power) **B**, Balled-up trichomonads in urinary sediment. Similar organs found in male urethra.

In the later morphologic state, the organisms do not move as a body, though under the high power objective the flagella and undulating membrane can usually be seen moving, at least in a sluggish fashion. In suspected cases, smears should never be considered negative until examined under high power. The smears of patients with asymptomatic disease or of those who have recently taken a douche may exhibit only the rounded, relatively immotile forms. The degree of accuracy in such cases parallels the experience and sleuthing ability of the technician.

If a patient who has had a severe vaginitis for only a day or so is suspected of having trichomoniasis, yet no trichomonads are detected on the wet mount preparation, a reexamination is in order. Occasionally, in the early stage of infection no trichomonads will be apparent in the ordinary wet mount preparation. Many investigators have made this observation. Further, Christian and others found the same phenomenon in tissue cultures. They theorized that the trichomonads were too inactive to be distinguished from dead or exfoliated cells, or that they were too intimately associated with the host cells to be independently visible. A prominent finding in practically all patients with acute trichomoniasis is a large number of pus cells and immature epithelial cells, mainly parabasal (Fig. 12-11).

Trichomonas diluent (Ortho) is a special diluent which, when mixed with vaginal secretions, stains pus cells and epithelial cells a light pink while leaving the trichomonads unstained. In testing this preparation, it was found that maximum staining of the cells is usually delayed for a few minutes. Since trichomonads are identified chiefly by their motility, use of the diluent can hardly influence the diagnostic accuracy of a well-trained technician.

Stained smears can also be problematic. The typical morphologic characteristics of trichomonads are largely destroyed by fixation and staining techniques, the cells often being totally disrupted and impossible to identify. They are particularly difficult to distinguish on most stained smears unless the flagella also stain. The dirty background of stained smears caused by increased mucus, disintegrated epithelial and pus cells, a large variety of bacteria (Fig. 12-3) and disrupted trichomonads, however, offers a clue to the diagnosis. Gram's stain is essentially useless for the demonstration of trichomonads. Giemsa's stain, when properly applied, reveals the organisms clearly; the body stains blue and the flagella, red. Thoroughly experienced technicians may have difficulty in obtaining consistently good results even with this staining technique. Iron hematoxylin stain is among the best for displaying the individual morphologic characteristics of the organism, although the technique of preparation is fairly complex and time-consuming, and the slides are not uniformly reliable. Acridine orange smears clearly reveal tricho-

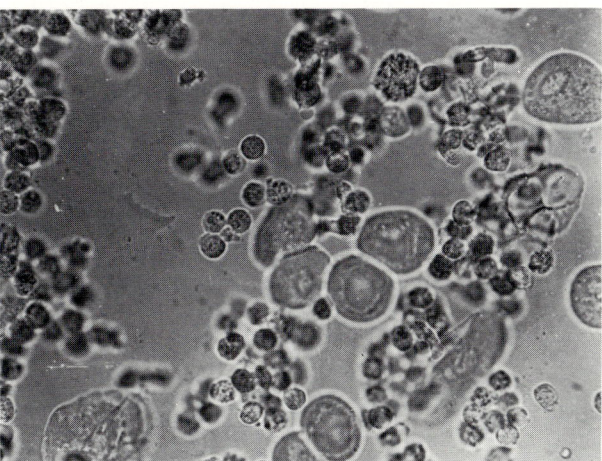

Fig. 12-11. Wet mount preparation of vaginal secretions, showing typical features of acute trichomoniasis—a large quantity of pus and immature vaginal epithelial cells. (High power)

monads, the nucleus and axostyle being readily identified. The cytoplasm stains a bright red and the nucleus a golden yellow, in contrast to the pale green and pale yellow staining of the other cellular elements.

The *Papanicolaou smear* (Fig. 12-4) for diagnosis of trichomoniasis is subject to a high degree of error, whether reported as positive or negative. In comparison to the wet mount and culture techniques, the Papanicolaou smear is the least satisfactory of the three, and its use for this purpose alone is hardly justified. Recognition of the organisms depends mainly upon finding intact structures of appropriate size and shape, with characteristic nuclei. The cytoplasm of trichomonads appears in almost any color; usually, however, it is stained gray or pink. The organisms are pale, as are the nuclei. The flagella rarely stain; when apparent, they confirm the diagnosis.

Trichomonads in the Papanicolaou smear must be differentiated from bare epithelial nuclei, distorted neutrophils, histiocytes, parabasal cells with small nuclei, and mucous blobs. This is one of the aspects of cytology in which the experience and interest of the cytologist count a great deal.

Trichomonas *cultures* for diagnosis and determination of cure of trichomoniasis are seldom warranted; with few exceptions, if the patient has clinical evidence of the disease, wet mounts yield positive findings. Although trichomonas cultures possibly offer the most reliable laboratory method for diagnosis, they must be painstakingly performed if the results are to surpass or even to equal the accuracy of wet mount preparations. Ordinarily, the several days required for a final culture reading mean a needless delay in diagnosis. Cultures are valuable in isolating the organisms from men, from the urinary tracts of women, and from the exceptional patient with repeated negative smears who is still suspect.

Numerous trichomonas culture media have been tested and found satisfactory. We consider the Simplified Trypticase Serum of Kupferberg to be highly suitable. Its use requires the addition of human serum containing essential growth factors, as well as penicillin and streptomycin for inhibition of bacterial organisms. In our hands, the Wittington-Feinburg medium has also been satisfactory.

Colposcopic examination has been suggested as a diagnostic aid in trichomonal vaginitis. Lang and Ludmir have described a colposcopic sign which they consider pathognomonic—a minute red point, approximately 0.1 mm. in diameter, surrounded by white areola having a total diameter of approximately 0.5 mm. In their opinion, the absence of the sign is not a sure indication that trichomonads are absent. Bergsjo, Koller, and Kolstad, in a colpophotographic study, correlated the presence of "double-crested capillaries" with the finding of *T. vaginalis*. They believe such a correlation could be of practical value in diagnosis. Colposcopic findings in trichomoniasis are still largely of only academic interest, yet their incidental finding by the colposcopist should incite further investigation.

Treatment

The many unsuccessful treatment methods employed for trichomoniasis exemplify a glaring lack in gynecologic therapeusis. The expounded virtues of the numerous topical trichomonacidal agents available have been attributed to many different modes of action, including acidification, alkalinization, desication, and digestion. Other essentially useless measures include supersonics, ultraviolet irradiation, vaccines, and a host of systemically administered chemotherapeutic agents.

Studies of the efficacy of therapy, based upon temporary symptomatic relief and temporary eradication of only the vaginal organisms, have largely accounted for the proclaimed high cure rates obtained with almost any agent investigated. The real test, however, the vade mecum for cure, is the eradication of every trichomonad from the host and not from the vagina alone. This proof of cure is seldom obtained solely by the use of topical applications.

Metronidazole. The development and proof of the therapeutic value of systemically administered metronidazole (Flagyl) must be regarded as one of the significant discoveries in gynecology. Although trichomoniasis is not a killer, any physician who is familiar with the fear, physical dsicomfort, esthetic revulsion, emotional disturbances, and sometimes shame suffered by affected women realizes the value of this drug. Durel and others first reported the clinically successful results with metronidazole at a meeting of the French Gynecological Society in January, 1959. The drug, a derivative of nitroimidazole, had been developed only a short time before by Cosar and Julou. Previously, another derivative of nitroimidazole had been marketed in this country under the name Tritheon. Gardner and Dukes, in 1956, reported forty-two consecutive failures of treatment with the latter preparation, although the clinical effect was often temporarily favorable.

The limited value of topical medicaments for eradicating trichomonads from the host, and the necessity of a systemic agent for reaching inaccessible foci in the urinary tracts of both sexes, has long been recognized. Thus far, metronidazole is the only effective agent available for this purpose. Its success has been confirmed by hundreds of investigators, and the opinion is essentially unanimous that, if properly administered, it affords a cure rate approaching 100 percent. Since the concurrent use of Flagyl suppositories does not enhance the cure rate, their use is not justified.

The dosage schedule of metronidazole most widely employed has been 250 mg. three times daily for 10 days, or a total dosage of 7.5 gm. The schedule we recommend is 500 mg. (2 tablets) every 12 hours for 5 days, or a total of 5 gm. This schedule is more acceptable to patients and is more likely to be completed than a program covering 10 days. Our results in over 500 patients have been comparable to any reported; not a single serious reaction has developed. The relative safety of metronidazole has been demonstrated by reports of unsuccessful attempts of patients to commit suicide by taking a single dose of as much as 12 gm.

Since the majority of men with infected sexual partners also harbor trichomonads and are, therefore, a continuous source of reinfection for the woman, medical logic dictates that these men should receive treatment simultaneously. In a study by Gardner and Dukes in 1964, reinfection rate was two and a half times higher in patients whose sexual partners were not treated. Two years after publication of this study, the reinfection rate had climbed to 27 percent in those women whose sexual partners were untreated, whereas in the group in which both were treated simultaneously, the long-term reinfection rate was only 8.4 percent.

The dosage schedule of metronidazole for men recommended by the distributors in this country is 250 mg. twice daily for 10 days. We advocate simultaneous and identical treatment of both sexual partners with 500 mg. every 12 hours for 5 days. To give a smaller dosage to a larger person, the man, as has been advocated, seems incongruous. Strains resistant to metronidazole will surely be encouraged by inadequate dosage schedules. We have no knowledge of reports describing ill effects on semen.

Side effects for metronidazole are, as a rule, of minor degree, rarely necessitating discontinuance of treatment (Table 5). The gastrointestinal tract is most often involved. In our experience, posttherapy moniliasis has not been a problem. Evidence is meager that the agent either suppresses or stimulates the growth of *Candida*. The darkened urine sometimes described is probably caused by a metabolite of metronidazole and is considered insignificant.

Contraindications to metronidazole reportedly include signs of blood dyscrasia and disease of the central nervous system. It has also been suggested that the drug be withheld during pregnancy, although no detrimental effect upon either mother or unborn child has been observed. No teratogenic in-

Table 5. The order of frequency of side effects from Flagyl in 4,148 consecutive patients (Tabulations by Searle Products, June 15, 1966)

Side effect	Number reported	Percent of total patients
Nausea	219	5.28
Taste	157	3.78
Furry tongue	111	2.68
Headache	44	1.06
Diarrhea	33	0.80
Dizziness	27	0.65
Vaginal burning	21	0.51
Dry mouth	18	0.43
Rash	16	0.39
Vaginal dryness	12	0.29
Gastritis	11	0.27
Drowsiness	11	0.27
Pruritus	11	0.27
Sore tongue	9	0.22
All others*	82	1.97

*None more than 0.2 percent.

186 Benign diseases of the vulva and vagina

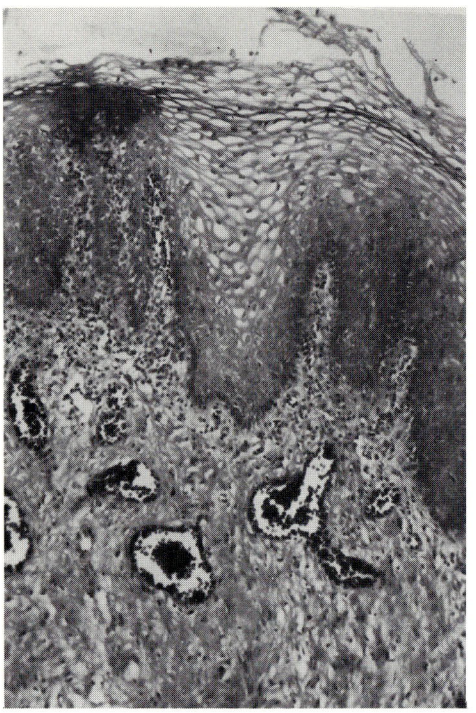

Fig. 12-12. Trichomoniasis. Biopsy of vagina 2 weeks after initiation of treatment with metronidazole (Flagyl). Vascularity is still increased. From patient whose biopsy is shown in Fig. 12-7, *A*.

fluence upon human beings has been reported. The experiences of Scott-Gray, Perl, Peterson, Stauch, and Ryder, and Sands with the treatment of several hundred women in all stages of pregnancy attest to its safety during this time. Sands obtained a high cure rate of pregnant patients with the use of 250 mg. three times daily for 3 days. Until more is known about its effects, the agent should probably be avoided during the first trimester.

Clinical and laboratory changes after metronidazole are impressive. Subjective symptoms and gross evidence of trichomonal vaginitis disappear within 7 days from the institution of treatment. The cellular elements and flora of the vagina usually become normal within this time. The histologic appearance of the vagina largely returns to normal within 2 weeks (Fig. 12-12). As a rule, minor degrees of atypism from inflammation, apparent on cytologic smears, disappear within 2 weeks.

Topical agents. Treatment with topical agents has been largely unrewarding. The possible microbiologic cure rate from their use is probably less than 20 percent. Although local therapy is not dependable for curative purposes, it must still be used for an occasional patient who is extremely sensitive to drugs, perhaps during pregnancy, and in patients with blood dyscrasias or disease of the central nervous system until Flagyl has been accepted as safe in all these conditions.

Some of the more effective topical agents include Neosporin vaginal suppositories containing polymyxin B; Devegan tablets, the active principal of which is acetarsone; Trichofuron suppositories, which contain the trichomonacide furazolidone; metronidazole suppositories; and Floraquin, which contains the trichomonacidal agent, diiodohydroxyquin. Whatever the topical agent used, it should be continued for 30 days or longer, including the period of menstrual flow. No vaginal medicament will eradicate organisms from Skene's ducts and the urinary tract, and urethral installations are largely ineffective in destroying organisms in the urethra.

Adjunctive therapeutic considerations. Perhaps mechanical cleansing of the vagina of menstrual blood, semen, desquamated debris, and mucus might protect the patient to some degree against reinfections, though it is highly improbable that vaginal douches ever have a curative effect. Douches can temporarily remove malodorous secretions and relieve subjective symptoms. Before the discovery of an effective systemic agent for the treatment of trichomoniasis, the long-term use of acid or medicated douches once or twice daily was almost essential to afford the patient comfort and prevent recurrence of symptomatic vaginitis.

Reassurance should be given to the patient. The relation between emotionalism and clinical trichomoniasis has already been discussed in some detail. Unquestionably, emotional stability frequently improves with effective treatment; psychotherapy, however, apparently has no direct influence upon the organic disease and cannot be considered a part of the essential therapy. This does not mean that some patients with trichomoniasis do not require considerable reassurance.

Estrogens can potentiate a quiescent, asymptomatic infection in a patient with an atrophic vagina to become active and symptomatic. Since hypoestrinism is more inhibitory than stimulative, estrogens, except perhaps occasionally when used concurrently with Flagyl in an estrogen deficient patient, have no place in treatment for trichomoniasis. Some evidence exists that the effects of Flagyl are sometimes enhanced by the use of estrogens in such patients.

Lactobacilli, commercially grown, have been instilled into the vagina for therapeutic purposes. From personal experience and from published reports, this measure seems to be of no value. Aciduric rods naturally become reestablished after destruction of the trichomonads, yet instilled lactobacilli rarely, if ever, become established as a new flora, much less effect a cure of trichomoniasis.

Prophylaxis. Postcoital douching with a strongly acid or medicated preparation soon after intercourse with an infected man probably affords considerable protection against trichomoniasis. The number of vaginal trichomonads would surely be reduced and, according to clinical and laboratory evidence, a large number of organisms is necessary to incite an infection.

Contraceptive creams, jellies, and foams usually have trichomonacidal properties. If used before or after intercourse, it is likely that they provide a degree of protection against trichomoniasis.

Condoms and similar protectives naturally are safeguards against infection of both sexual partners.

Prophylactic use of metronidazole after intercourse would afford protection from the disease, although the prophylactic systemic dosage has not been established.

Epidemiologic measures have received insufficient attention. Some of the same methods of controlling other venereal diseases should perhaps be applied in trichomoniasis. The admission of venereal transmission by one sex partner should not necessarily have tragic consequences, since the physician can always explain other possibilities. Even with the new wonder drug, metronidazole, trichomoniasis will remain one of the most widespread and recurrent infections unless the sexual partner of each patient is treated, and unless appropriate community and educational control measures are applied. The control of trichomoniasis should be less formidable than that of other venereal diseases since it is considerably less contagious. In view of the fact that the disease affects the general health of the patient to a relatively mild degree, health authorities have little interest in community projects directed against its eradication.

TRICHOMONIASIS OF THE LOWER URINARY TRACT

Trichomoniasis is a disease not only of the vagina but of the lower urinary tract as well. The affected sites include Skene's ducts, the urethra, the many paraurethral glands, and, occasionally, the bladder. Isolated reports describe the finding of organisms in the ureters and kidney pelves; however, infection of these structures is so rare that, clinically, it is insignificant.

According to our observations, the majority of patients who are treated for trichomoniasis by topical vaginal agents continue to harbor trichomonads from the lower urinary tract or Skene's ducts after all vaginal organisms have been eradicated. It was perhaps these autogenous sources of vaginal reinfection that largely accounted for the low cure rates before the introduction of metronidazole.

Kean, in a significant study, found trichomonads as often in the urethra as in the vagina. He also related recurrent cystitis from *Escherichia coli* and other bacteria to trichomoniasis. According to his theory, the bacterial organisms reach the bladder on "the backs" of *T. vaginalis*. Riba, in cystoscopies of forty women with resistant or recurrent trichomoniasis, found a high incidence of gross reaction in the bladder or urethra. Bernstine and Rakoff, as well as other investigators, have mentioned trichomonal cystitis. Gardner and Dukes (1964) reported the disappearance of abacteriuric pyuria in fourteen of seventeen patients with urinary trichomonads after they were given metronidazole.

A catheterized urinary specimen that yields trichomonads is not necessarily proof of bladder infection, since the catheter can collect organisms from the urethra during its introduction. A positive specimen collected by slowly introducing a catheter and discarding the first portion of urine would be evidence of invasion of the bladder. Infection of Skene's duct is easily proved by examination of expressed material, either directly or mixed with a drop of physiologic saline solution. Demonstration of urethral organisms can be more difficult because of the repeated irrigations of the urethra by the urinary stream. This also partially explains the difficulty of finding trichomonads in the urethras of men. Organisms in the lower urinary tract of either sex are frequently balled-up (Fig. 12-10, B) and relatively immotile, thus identification is difficult. For this reason, sedimented urine and secretions from Skene's duct and the urethra often must be examined under high power magnification for detection of movement of the flagella and undulating membrane. Culture techniques are valuable as a means of studying the disease in the urinary tract.

Symptoms

Since most patients with trichomonal infection of the lower urinary tract also have vulvovaginitis, it may be difficult to attribute specific urinary symptoms to the infection of the urinary tract, particularly since urinary frequency may be a reflex response to the vulvar disease. We have evaluated a number of patients with normal, trichomonas-free vaginas whose voided urinary specimens contained trichomonads. Almost half of these patients admitted having urinary frequency, nocturia, and mild dysuria. Other patients who denied urinary symptoms before treatment found that metronidazole afforded relief of mild symptoms of which they were not previously aware. An occasional patient is found to have trichomonal pyuria, with or without mild symptoms. Also, the incidence of bacterial urethrocystitis appears to be higher in patients with trichomoniasis.

Treatment

Eradication of organisms from the urinary system depends upon the administration of a systemic agent, and metronidazole is the only such agent presently available. Installation of topical trichomonacidal agents into the urethra and bladder of either sex is ineffective. Transurethral operative procedures for women, as reported by Riba, currently have no place in the treatment for this disease.

TRICHOMONIASIS IN MEN

A denial that men also have trichomonal infections would be contrary to the findings of many careful investigators who are equipped to recover the organisms from the male urethra. This does not necessarily mean that symptomatic trichomoniasis is as prevalent in men as it is in women, although Teokharov found the same incidence of urogenital trichomoniasis in both sexes. Keutel discovered trichomonads in 79 percent of the sexual partners of infected women, Watt and Jennison in 60 percent, Bedoya, Rico, and Rios in 78 percent, and Block in 61.5 percent. We have been able to recover trichomonads from the urethras of the majority of husbands of infected wives, generally without resort to culture techniques. Many failures to detect trichomonads in men can be attributed to technical difficulties rather than to freedom from infection.

Most men harboring trichomonads are unaware of having the infection; probably fewer than 20 percent have signs or symptoms of the disease. Most often, any discharge, such as "the morning drop," is minimal; reportedly, however, in the rare patient it is abundant and purulent. Block found that 21 percent of ninety-one patients had either a discharge, dysuria, a burning and irritation after coitus or a combination of these manifestations. It is Keutel's opinion that more than 90 percent of infected male patients have symptoms of prostatitis and that infection of the seminal vesicles can be assumed. Obviously, the majority of urologists would not agree with this opinion.

Interestingly, Coutts and others, in a study of 2,482 men with nongonococcal urethritis, found trichomonads in the urethras of 1,690 (68 percent). Catterall and Nicol demonstrated *T. vaginalis* in all female sexual partners of fifty-six men with *T. vaginalis* urethritis. This would seem to be highly suggestive evidence that *T. vaginalis* is transmitted during sexual intercourse. The epidemiologic implications cannot be ignored. Perhaps the time has come when urologists should recognize the potential importance of trichomoniasis in men.

Diagnosis

The diagnosis of trichomoniasis in men is much more difficult than in women because of the difficulty of isolating trichomonads from the male urethra. Discharges containing the organism are usually scant, being flushed away by the urinary stream; also, organisms are frequently balled-up (Fig. 12-10, *B*) and relatively immotile. Failure to demonstrate the organisms on one or two microscopic or even culture examinations is not proof that the male is not a carrier. They can usually be detected in a drop of secretion that has been removed from the urethra after the patient has not voided for several hours. The secretion is placed on a glass slide, firmly pressed with a cover-slip, and examined under the high microscopic power. If the secretion is profuse and purulent, dilution with physiologic saline may be necessary. The first ounce of an early morning voided specimen of urine is also a useful source of the organisms. The specimen must be centrifuged and the sediment examined under the high power objective. Some investigators find that the organisms are more easily isolated in prostatic secretions after massage. If trichomonads cannot be demonstrated by slide techniques, cultures are necessary; however, we have observed many positive smears of material that failed to yield positive cultures. Recovery of trichomonads from fluid from the prostate gland or seminal vesicles after massage is not proof of infection of these structures, since the fluid could have picked up the organisms from the urethra.

Treatment

Metronidazole is as effective against trichomoniasis in men as in women. Urethral instillations are of no value. Massage to eradicate *T. vaginalis* from the prostate or seminal vesicles may have been laudable in past years, but it would be difficult to justify today.

RELATIONSHIP OF TRICHOMONIASIS TO CARCINOMA

The cytotoxic effect of trichomonads in some patients so alters the squamous epithelium of the cervix and vagina that the cells resemble the changes of early neoplastic lesions. Other observers have reported an unusually high incidence of trichomoniasis in patients with squamous cell carcinoma in situ of the cervix. The majority of patients with carcinoma in situ have an abnormal bacterial flora that cannot be attributed to the cervical lesion itself, yet which might be secondary to trichomoniasis. From available information, it appears that although trichomoniasis in itself may not predispose to carcinoma, patients with the disease, as a group, have a higher incidence of cervical carcinoma. Possibly this may be explained by the presence of the same predisposing factors in both diseases.

REFERENCES

Bedoya, J. M., Rico, L. R., and Rios, G.: Trichomoniasis der menschlichen Genitalien; venerische Erkrankung II, Geburtsch. Frauenheilk. 18: 994, 1958.

Bedoya, J. M., Rios, G., and Rico, L. R.: Trichomonadenbefall der Genitalien; venerische Erkrankung I, Geburtsch. Frauenheilk. 18:989, 1958.

Bergsjo, P., Koller, D., and Kolstad, P.: The vascular pattern of trichomonas vaginalis cervicitis, Acta Cytol. 7:292, 1963.

Bernstine, J. B., and Rakoff, A. E.: Vaginal infections, infestations, and discharges, New York, 1953, McGraw-Hill Book Co.

Block, E.: Occurrence of trichomonas in sexual partners of women with trichomoniasis, Acta Obstet. Gynec. Scandinav. 38:398, 1959.

Burch, T. A., Rees, C. W., and Reardon, L. V.: Epidemiological studies on human trichomoniasis, Amer. J. Trop. Med. 8:312, 1959.

Catterall, R. D., and Nicol, C. S.: Is trichomonal infestation a venereal disease?, Brit. Med. J. 1:1177, 1960.

Christian, R. T., Miller, N. F., Luddvici, P. P., and Riley, G. M.: A study of Trichomonas vaginalis in human cell culture, Amer. J. Obstet. Gynec. 85:947, 1963.

Cosar, C., and Julou, L.: Activité de 1′(hydroxy-2″ ethyl)-1 methyl-2 nitro-5 imidazole (8.823 R. P.) vis-à-vis des infections expérimentales à trichomonas vaginalis, Ann. Inst. Pasteur 96: 238, 1959.

Coutts, W. E., Vargas-Salazar, R., Silva-Inzunza, E., Olmedo, R., Turteltaub, R., and Saavedra, J.: Trichomonas vaginalis infection in the male, Brit. Med. J. 2:885, 1955.

Donne, A.: Animalcules observés dans les metières purulentes et la produit des secretions des organes génitaux de l'homme et de la femme, Compt. Rend. Acad. Sci. 3:383, 1836.

Dukes, C. D., and Gardner, H. L.: Unpublished data.

Durel, P., Couture, J., Collart, P., and Girot, C.: Flagyl (metronidazole), Brit. J. Vener. Dis. 36:154, 1960.

Durel, P., Rioron, V., Siboulet, A., and Borel, L. J.: Essai d'un antitrichomonas dérivé de l'imidazole (8823 R.P.), C. R. Soc. Franc. Gynec. 29:36, 1959.

Durel, P., Rioron, V., Siboulet, A., and Borel, L. J.: Systemic treatment of human trichomoniasis with a derivative of nitro-imidazole 8823 R.P., Brit. J. Ven. Dis. 36:21, 1960.

Ehrenberg, C. G.: Die Infusionsthierchen als volkommene Organismen, Leipzig, 1838, L. Voss.

Frost, J. K.: Intracellular *Trichomonas vaginalis* and *Trichomonas gallinae* in natural and experimental infections, J. Parasit. 47:302, 1961.

Gardner, H. L.: Trichomoniasis, Obstet. Gynec. 19:279, 1962.

Gardner, H. L.: Vaginal infections. In Conn, H., editor: Current therapy, Philadelphia, 1963, W. B. Saunders Co.

Gardner, H. L., Dampeer, T. K., and Dukes, C. D.: The prevalence of vaginitis, Amer. J. Obstet. Gynec. 73:1080, 1957.

Gardner, H. L., and Dukes, C. D.: Clinical and laboratory effects of metronidazole, Amer. J. Obstet. Gynec. 89:990, 1964.

Gardner, H. L., and Dukes, C. D.: Tritheon in Trichomonas vaginitis, Obstet. Gynec. 8:591, 1956.

Hegner, R. W.: The protozoa of wild monkeys, Science 70:539, 1929.

Hegner, R. W., and Ratcliffe, H. L.: Trichomonads from the vagina of the monkey, J. Parasit. 14:27, 1928.

Hesseltine, H. C., Wolters, S. L., and Campbell, A. J.: Experimental human vaginal trichomoniasis, J. Infect. Dis. 71:127, 1942.

Hoehne, O.: Trichomonas Vaginalis also Haufiger Erreger einer Typischen Colpitis Purulenta, Zbl. Gynaek. 40:4, 1916.

Huffman, J. W.: The detailed anatomy of the paraurethral ducts in the adult human female, Amer. J. Obstet. Gynec. 55:86, 1948.

Hypes, R. A., and Ladewig, P. P.: Leukocytic clusters on epithelial cells in cervico-vaginal smears: A presumptive test for trichomonas infection, Amer. J. Clin. Path. 26:94, 1956.

Karnaky, K. J.: Trichomonas vaginalis vaginitis pathognomonic lesion and pathologic findings in 4000 cases, Texas J. Med. 32:803, 1937.

Karnaky, K. J.: Trichomoniasis, Western J. Surg. 54:61, 1946.

Kaufman, R. H., and Gardner, H. L.: Histopathology of the common vaginitides. In preparation.

Kean, B. H.: Urethral trichomoniasis in the female, Amer. J. Obstet. Gynec. 70:397, 1955.

Kessel, J. F., and Thompson, C. F.: Survival of Trichomonas vaginalis in vaginal discharge, Proc. Soc. Exp. Biol. Med. 74:755, 1950.

Keutel, H. J.: Trichomonadenerkrankung des Mannes, Verh. Deutsch. Ges. Urol. 7:159, 1959.

Kotcher, E., and Hoogasian, A. C.: Cultivation of *Trichomonas vaginalis*; by Donne, 1837, in association with tissue cultures (abstract), J. Parasit. 43:39, 1957.

Lanceley, F.: Serological aspects of trichomonas vaginalis, Brit. J. Ven. Dis. 34:4, 1958.

Lang, W. R., and Ludmir, A.: A pathognomonic colposcopic sign of trichomonas vaginalis vaginitis, Acta Cytol. 5:390, 1961.

Manwell, R. D.: Introduction to protozoology, New York, 1961, St. Martin's Press.

McEwen, D. C.: Common factors in trichomonas vaginitis, J. Obstet. Gynaec. Brit. Comm. 66:482, 1959.

Melody, G. F.: Trichomonas vaginitis in depressed women, Amer. J. Obstet. Gynec. 82:521, 1961.

Moore, S. F., Jr., and Simpson, J. W.: The emotional component in trichomonas vaginitis, Amer. J. Obstet. Gynec. 68:974, 1954.

Murrell, M., and Scott-Gray, M.: The treatment of trichomonal vaginitis, Practitioner 181:611, 1958.

Naguib, S. M., Comstock, G. W., and Davis, H. J.: Epidemiologic study of trichomoniasis in normal women, Obstet. Gynec. 27:607, 1966.

Perl, G.: Metronidazole treatment of trichomoniasis in pregnancy, Obstet. Gynec. 25:273, 1965.

Peterson, W. F., Stauch, J. E., and Ryder, C. D.: Metronidazole in pregnancy, Amer. J. Obstet. Gynec. 94:343, 1966.

Riba, L. W.: Resistant trichomoniasis in the female, Amer. J. Obstet. Gynec. 73:174, 1957.

Sands, R. X.: Pregnancy, trichomoniasis, and metronidazole, Amer. J. Obstet. Gynec. 94:350, 1966.

Scott-Gray, M.: Metronidazole in obstetric practice, J. Obst. Gynaec. Brit. Comm. 71:82, 1964.

Teokharov, B. A.: Sources of trichomonas vaginalis and routes of infestation therewith (translation of title), Akush. Ginek. 38:85, 1962.

Trussell, R. E.: Trichomonas vaginalis and trichomoniasis, Springfield, Ill., 1947, Charles C Thomas, Publisher.

Trussell, R. E., and Plass, E. D.: The pathogenicity and physiology of a pure culture of Trichomonas vaginalis, Amer. J. Obstet. Gynec. 40:883, 1940.

Turner, T. R., and Riva, H. L.: Personal communication, 1966.

Watt, L., and Jennison, R. F.: Incidence of *Trichomonas vaginalis* in marital partners, Brit. J. Ven. Dis. 36:163, 1960.

Chapter 13
Haemophilus vaginalis vaginitis

Any patient whose ovarian activity is normal and who has a gray, homogeneous, malodorous vaginal discharge with a pH 5.0 to 5.5 that yields no trichomonads is likely to have *Haemophilus vaginalis* (H. V.) vaginitis. A wet smear preparation from the vagina of such a patient will contain the "clue cells" of *Haemophilus vaginalis;* in the stained smear the bacterial flora will consist predominately of heavy fields of short, gram-negative bacilli.

Probably more than 90 percent of vaginitides previously classified as "nonspecific" are caused by *H. vaginalis.* The clinical and laboratory patterns of H. V. vaginitis are more consistent than those of either trichomoniasis or candidiasis, although the clinical significance of H. V. vaginitis is hardly comparable. Following eradication of *H. vaginalis,* the clinical findings of the disease disappear and the vaginal secretions and bacterial flora revert to normal.

This vaginal infection was first described by Gardner and Dukes in 1954. In 1955, the same authors published a more detailed clinical and laboratory report, in which the name *Haemophilus vaginalis* was proposed for the bacterial agent. Previously, species of *Haemophilus* had been isolated from the vagina by a number of workers; none, however, had suggested a relationship of the organisms to vaginitis and leukorrhea. Judging from the biochemical activities of the hemophilic organisms previously described, the majority were of a species other than *H. vaginalis.* In 1949, Blinik, Steinberg, and Merendino reported the bacteriologic findings in "nonspecific leukorrhea" of forty-five patients in whom neither trichomonads nor species of *Candida* could be demonstrated. Species of *Haemophilus* were isolated from fifteen of the forty-five patients, although the authors did not attribute the leukorrhea to these organisms. In 1953, Leopold reported a "heretofore undescribed organism isolated from the genito-urinary system," which he believed to be closely related to *Haemophilus.* He recovered the organism from the urethras of men with prostatitis, with or without urethritis, and from the cervices of women with signs of cervicitis. Like earlier workers, Leopold did not associate the organism with vaginitis or with leukorrhea of vaginal origin. Lutz and Wurch, in 1954, reported the finding of small gram-negative bacilli in vaginal discharges, and in 1956 Lutz, Grootten, and Wurch published a report in which the organism was called *Haemophilus vaginalis hemolyticus.* The independent investigations of Gardner and Dukes, Lutz and Wurch, and Lutz, Grootten, and Wurch yielded essentially identical clinical and laboratory findings. Since the original description of *H. vaginalis* vaginitis in 1954, numerous confirmatory reports have appeared in the literature.

Etiology

Causative agent. *Haemophilus vaginalis* (Figs. 13-1 and 13-12, *A*) is the sole etiologic agent of *H. vaginalis* vaginitis. The minute, rod shaped, gram-negative bacillus is nonmotile and nonencapsulated and does not form endospores. It is a true parasite that grows only in the presence of serum and other accessory growth factors. *H. vaginalis* is a distinct species and can be separated from the other members of the genus *Haemophilus* serologically and biochemically, and, to a certain extent, by its growth and nutritional characteristics.

Sources of infection.

Veneral disease. Aside from an infinitesimally small percentage of cases, sexual inter-

192 Benign diseases of the vulva and vagina

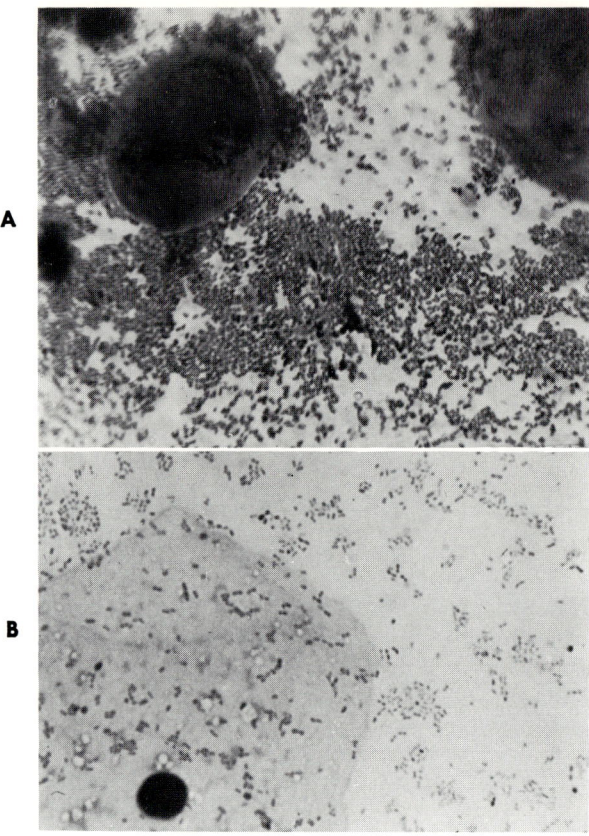

Fig. 13-1. **A** and **B**, *Haemophilus vaginalis,* a short gram-negative bacillus usually observed in heavy fields. (Gram's stain × 1200)

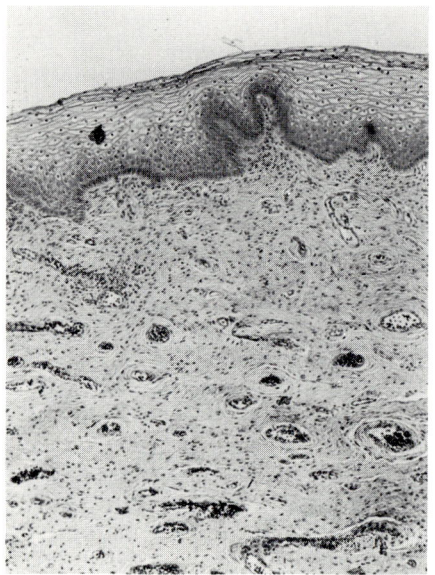

Fig. 13-2. Biopsy from vagina of patient with *H. vaginalis* vaginitis. Findings are usually identical to those of a normal vagina.

course is surely the method of transmission. The high rate of reinfection in patients whose husbands remain untreated and the recovery of the organism from the majority of husbands of infected wives are evidence of its venereal transmission. *H. vaginalis* is essentially nonexistent in premenarchal subjects. Practically all patients with intact hymens with this disease give a history of heterosexual contact without intromission or admit to homosexual contact. The incidence of infection immediately following marriage is too high to be attributed to coincidence alone. The large majority of workers who have expressed opinions agree upon the venereal nature of the disease.

Communal fomites. Transmission by inanimate objects, such as douche nozzles, bath towels, and wet bathing suits, may explain an occasional case; however, no reports of infection by these routes have appeared. Bath tubs and swimming pools are improbable sources, as are toilet seats and toilet splash.

In a carelessly managed physician's office, gloves and instruments could be sources of infection.

Since the viability of *H. vaginalis* depends upon the presence of moisture, the organism is extremely susceptible to drying. Edmunds (1960) found that drying in a desiccator for 2 hours resulted in 99.9 percent reduction in viable organisms. He also observed that viability was reduced by 99.99 percent upon their exposure to room temperature for 24 hours, even under moist conditions.

Oral cavity. Deming suggested cunnilingus as a source of infection, although his circumstantial evidence has not been substantiated. In fact, isolation of *H. vaginalis* from the oral cavity has not been reported.

Autogenous sources. Whereas autogenous reinfection with trichomonads from the urethra and Skene's ducts is common, apparently autogenous reinfection with *H. vaginalis* is exceptional. The female urethra probably harbors the organism after treatment, yet its constant irrigation by the urinary stream probably prevents a sufficiently large accumulation of bacteria to cause reinfection.

Predisposing factors.

Estrogens. Natural or exogenous estrogens stimulate the vagina to produce the nutrients that support a luxuriant growth of *H. vaginalis*. Edmunds (1962) after observing the ability of *H. vaginalis* to ferment glycogen and to grow well at pH 4.5, stated: "It thus seems well equipped for establishment in the vagina during the reproductive age, when glycogen is present in the epithelial cells and a low pH prevails." Although the vagina in a postmenopausal patient will support the organism, the glycogen and epithelial content are inadequate to foster rapid bacterial growth. Since the leukorrhea in H. V. vaginitis consists primarily of bacteria and affected epithelial cells, failure of these cells to proliferate may explain why estrogen-deficient women seldom have the classical disease. The clinical features of H. V. vaginitis are largely dependent upon the availability of estrogens, whether from ovarian activity, pregnancy, or an exogenous source. Postmenopausal patients who harbor the organisms asymptomatically frequently exhibit classical signs of the infection following estrogen replacement therapy.

Leukorrhea from other causes. Whether establishment of *H. vaginalis* infection is facilitated by cervical leukorrhea, trichomoniasis, blood, or grade III flora from any cause has not been determined. It has been demonstrated, however, that infections are easily established in normal vaginas, a fact that indicates that a low vaginal pH and the presence of lactobacilli are not strong deterrents.

Prevalence

H. V. vaginitis is primarily a disease of the reproductive years. At present, an estimated 10 to 20 percent of women in this period of life harbor *H. vaginalis*. Postmenopausal patients also harbor the organism, though it is seldom manifested clinically unless they are receiving estrogen replacement therapy. To our knowledge, the only case of premenarchal infection thus far reported was that of de la Fuente, Rico, and Soria, who discovered it in a child of 3 years.

As is true of trichomoniasis, the prevalence of H. V. vaginitis is as variable as the population groups screened. For example, Gardner, Dampeer, and Dukes (1957) reported the disease in 10.1 percent of unselected private Caucasian obstetric patients and in 40.9 percent of unselected nonpregnant Negro charity patients. In the majority of controlled clinical investigations, approximately 40 percent (Table 6) of patients with leukorrhea or vaginitis yield *H. vaginalis*. The ratio of H. V. vaginitis to trichomoniasis will surely rise as more patients with trichomoniasis are cured with metronidazole.

Approximately 25 percent of patients with trichomoniasis seen in an average private office practice have an associated *H. vaginalis* infection. In this group, the persistence of a gray, homogeneous, malodorous discharge after treatment with metronidazole may well lead clinicians and patients to draw the false conclusion that the trichomoniasis has not been cured.

Pathogenicity

H. V. vaginitis is a distinct disease of the vagina in which very uniform clinical and laboratory patterns are displayed. Further, the disease disappears abruptly upon eradication of *H. vaginalis,* the only organism consistently isolated from the vagina of patients with the entity.

To our knowledge, in only three or four

Table 6. Acceptance or rejection of H. vaginalis vaginitis as a clinical entity by various investigators

Investigators	Country	Year	Accept	Reject	Prevalence of H. vaginalis in all patients with vaginitis or leukorrhea	Prevalence of H. V. vaginitis in population groups
Amies and Jones	Canada	1957	+		—	—
Bergman, Lundgren, and Lundstrom	Sweden	1965	+		40%	19%
Bray	Belgium	1963	+		—*	21
Bret and Cohen-Debray	France	1959	+		—	6
Brewer, Halpern, and Thomas	U.S.A.	1957	+		42	—
de la Fuenta, Rico, and Soria	Spain	1959	+		—	36
Delaha and others	U.S.A.	1964	+		—	22
Deming	U.S.A.	1955	+		—	—
Döll	Germany	1958		+	0	0
Dunkelberg and Bosman	Germany-U.S.A.	1961	+		34	—
Edmunds	Scotland	1959	+		43	—
Frampton and Lee	England	1964		+	(25)†	(23)†
Gardner and Dukes (private patients)	U.S.A.	1954-1955	+		47	12
Gardner, Dampeer, and Dukes (clinic patients)	U.S.A.	1957	+		40	29.1
Gray and Barnes	U.S.A.	1965	+		37	—
Heltai and Taleghany	U.S.A.	1959		+	(24)	—
Kummel and Ritzerfeld	Germany	1961	+		33	—
Lapage	Denmark	1960		+	—	—
Muller, Pech, and Walch	Germany	1962	+		—	—
Pinter, Csorba, and Zekany	Hungary	1962	+		51	—
Ray and Maughan	U.S.A.	1956	+		39	16
Rico	Spain	1959	+		40	16
Sbrocca	Spain	1962	+		23	—
Stewart	U.S.A.	1961	+		35	—
Tarlington and D'Abrera	Australia	1966	+		18	—
Tarulis, Jensen, and Lake	U.S.A.	1963	+		53	—
Wauters	Belgium	1963	+		13	—
Wu and Lee	Formosa	1962	+		15	—
Wurch and Lutz	France	1955	+		22	—
			25	4		

*—Information not given.
†( ) H. vaginalis isolated but given no significance.

reports has the pathogenicity of H. vaginalis or the existence of H. V. vaginitis as a clinical entity been seriously questioned. Döll's dissent was based upon his inability to culture H. vaginalis. The other investigators, Lapage, Heltai and Taleghany, and Frampton and Lee, were able to demonstrate the organisms in association with vaginitis or leukorrhea; according to their special methods of correlation, however, they were unable to prove its pathogenic role.

Brewer, Halpern, and Thomas state: "Clinical evidence of pathogenicity is suggested by the frequency with which the organism is the predominant one in the vaginal flora of patients with bacterial vaginitis and by the fact that reports, including ours, note that the leukorrhea and vaginitis disappear when H. vaginalis disappears from the flora." They added: "In our study, the flora varied considerably in individual patients over the year and one-half that cultures were made. No one organism was consistently found in association with H. vaginalis which might be considered capable of producing infection and leukorrhea. These bacteria appeared and disappeared from the flora without any rhyme or reason as far as leukorrhea was concerned. As a cause of leukorrhea in the patients studied the bacteria other than *H. vaginalis* were obviously unrelated to vaginitis."

Infection by direct inoculation. Gardner and Dukes (1955) successfully inoculated disease-free vaginas with material from the vaginas of patients who exhibited the classical signs of *H. vaginalis* infection. The inoculated patients were not only free of all clinical evidence of vaginal infection, but their vaginal flora consisted predominantly of lactobacilli. The vaginal pH of each patient was normal and contained no *Haemophilus* organisms. The donor material yielded *H. vaginalis* in pure culture or as the predominant bacterial agent. Of the fifteen normal patients inoculated, eleven had the classical disease within 7 to 14 days, *H. vaginalis* being the predominant bacterium in the vaginal material from all of the eleven. The experimentally induced infections persisted for years in several patients, one of whom was followed for 14 years.

Infection by inoculation from cultures. Criswell and others demonstrated the infectivity of *H. vaginalis* by inoculating normal women with organisms taken from cultures. Successful inoculations were exhibited by clinical evidence of vaginal disease within 2 weeks. The vaginal secretions of every patient who had such changes were examined by five laboratory tests, all of which were positive for *H. vaginalis*. None of the organisms were found in the secretions of the women whose vaginas remained normal. These authors interpreted their findings as proof of the pathogenicity of *H. vaginalis*.

Infection in husbands. In a study reported by Gardner and Dukes (1959), the predominant organism in the urethras of ninety-one husbands of 101 infected wives was *H. vaginalis*. In contrast, in a study of urethral cultures obtained from thirty-eight male medical students, only one was found to harbor the organism. Numerous other investigators have reported a high recovery rate of *H. vaginalis* from the urethras of husbands of infected wives. Moreover, it has been repeatedly observed that the majority of successfully treated patients have recurrences of the disease if their husbands are not treated simultaneously and successfully with appropriate systemic antibiotics.

Animal experiments. Attempts to establish infections in the vaginas of experimental animals have largely failed. Inoculations into subcutaneous tissues, the peritoneal cavities, and bloodstreams of animals have yielded variable and inconclusive results. Such experimentation neither proves nor disproves the pathogenicity of the organism in the human vagina.

Pathogenesis

In their first major communication on *H. vaginalis* in 1955, Gardner and Dukes expressed their opinion that the organism is a parasite that does not produce gross disease of the tissues. Kaufman and Gardner, after examining many specimens of vaginal tissue from infected patients, further concluded that the organism does not invade viable tissues of the vagina (Fig. 13-2). Such observations explain the paucity of pus cells in the vaginal discharge and the lack of inflammation of the tissues. According to the evidence, the organism is a surface parasite that creates an abnormal vaginal status by altering the consistency and biochemical reactions of the vaginal secretions.

It is probable that undetached surfaces of epithelial cells remain uninvolved; however, the findings of Tarlington and D'Abrera suggest that desquamation is accelerated incident to attack by the organisms upon the glycogen-laden intermediate cells. Indeed, these investigators offer strong evidence that *H. vaginalis* acts as a true parasite on individual epithelial cells by demonstrating a distinct reduction in the glycogen content of the affected cells. The large number of organisms floating in the cell-free vaginal secretions indicates that multiplication also takes place in this medium.

The incubation period of the infection is probably 5 to 10 days; the majority of patients inoculated with infected material develop clinical and laboratory signs of the disease within this time. As a rule, within 1 week after inoculation, the color, consistency, odor, pH, and bacteriology of vaginal secretions change from normal to abnormal.

Some observers have reported a higher incidence of puerperal infection in patients who yield *H. vaginalis* on culture. We have made no statistical survey to confirm these findings, though we suspect that, as a group, patients with H. V. vaginitis are affected by socioeconomic factors that favor puerperal morbidity and that *H. vaginalis* is not the causative organism. One of us (H.L.G.) has observed one pregnant patient at term who had uterine signs of premature placental separation and evidence of gas in the uterine wall. The latter sign was indicated by an apparent crepitation of the uterine wall on palpation of the uterus through the abdomen. At the time of cesarean section, gas was found between the chorion and uterus, and possibly between the chorion and amnion. Bacterial cultures were made from the fetal membranes, and large numbers of *H. vaginalis* were recovered in pure culture. The patient subsequently was proved to have H. V. vaginitis. Her course following the cesarean section was uneventful.

Bacteriology

Once *H. vaginalis* has been established in the vagina, it soon becomes the prevailing organism. Lactobacilli are largely eliminated during the first week of infection. A high vaginal acidity and abundance of lactobacilli do not protect the vagina against infection.

Other bacterial organisms frequently found in the flora of patients with H. V. vaginitis are shown in Table 7. These findings were from consecutive patients who had no cervicitis, estrogen deficiency, or bleeding; who had not recently douched, had coitus, or used vaginal medicaments or contraceptives; and who harbored no other specific vaginal pathogens. Institutionalized and charity patients were not included; as groups they are poor subjects for most bacteriologic investigations of vaginal flora. Bacteria other than *H. vaginalis* were usually transient and their numbers were inconsequential; they appeared and disappeared without demonstrable reason or significance and without altering the clinical pattern of the disease. That pure cultures of *H. vaginalis* were obtained in 19.2 percent would seem remarkable had the patients not been highly selected.

As may be observed in Table 8, *H. vaginalis* was the causative agent of bacterial vaginitis in 94 percent of 100 consecutive cases. The other organisms listed were only possible vaginal pathogens. They were usually transient, arising in an imbalanced flora

Table 7. Bacterial organisms associated with *H. vaginalis* in ninety-four patients

Haemophilus vaginalis — pure culture	18 (19.2%)
Haemophilus vaginalis + diphtheroids	5 (5.3%)
Haemophilus vaginalis + streptococci	26 (27.6%)
Haemophilus vaginalis + streptococci + diphtheroids	26 (27.6%)
Haemophilus vaginalis + one or more other organisms*	19 (20.3%)
	94

Staphylococcus albus, Staphylococcus aureus, Gaffkya, Vibrio species, anaerobic streptococci.

Table 8. Etiologic agents isolated from 100 consecutive cases of bacterial vaginitis (Gardner and Dukes, 1960)

Haemophilus vaginalis	94
Proteus vulgaris	1
Proteus mirabilis	1
Escherichia coli	1
Staphylococcus aureus	1
Streptococcus pyogenes	1
Mixed	1
	100

incident to an altered vaginal physiology. In the majority of cases, such organisms as *Pseudomonas, Proteus,* and *Staphylococcus,* when associated with leukorrhea or "vaginitis," were observed after the patients had received antibiotics.

Clinical features

H. V. vaginitis is the most benign of the common infectious vaginitides. In fact, the signs and symptoms are usually so mild that many clinicians fail to recognize it as a clinical entity and the majority of patients do not complain of its manifestations. Often, however, those who deny having symptoms admit the necessity of frequent douches for cleanliness or for hygienic reasons. After successful treatment, many patients without complaints immediately realize that an abnormal vaginal secretion and disagreeable odor had been problems. Other patients, of course, are conscious of symptoms from the onset of the infection. Most investigators

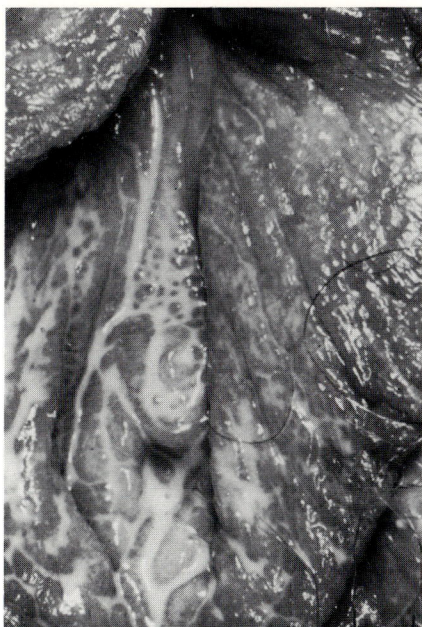

Fig. 13-3. *H. vaginalis* vaginitis. A gray, homogeneous, malodorous discharge is present in the vestibule of this patient who had not recently douched or bathed.

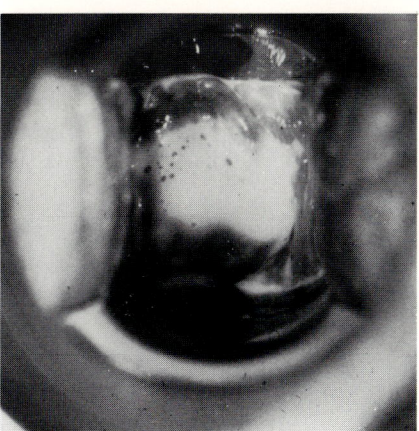

Fig. 13-4. *H. vaginalis* vaginitis. A gray homogeneous discharge with slight frothiness is apparent in this undouched patient.

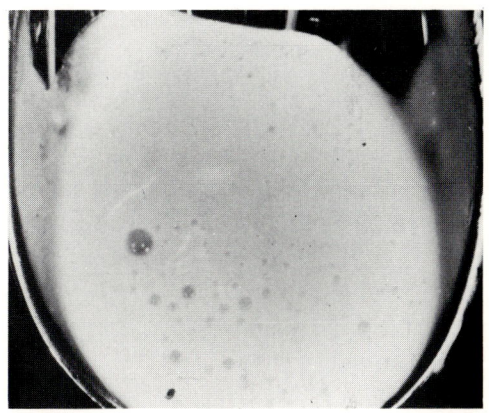

Fig. 13-5. Discharge of *H. vaginalis* on a speculum. Slight frothiness, as shown here, is found in a small percentage of patients. Few patients exhibit this amount of discharge. Compare with normal vaginal secretions in Fig. 13-6.

agree with respect to the clinical features of this disease and concede that the manifestations are those of "nonspecific" vaginitis.

Symptoms. Leukorrhea (Figs. 13-3 to 13-5), or excessive vaginal secretion, is considered a subjective symptom when the patient voluntarily complains of discharge or admits its presence. Probably fewer than 25 percent of patients with *H. vaginalis* vaginitis mention this problem, although the majority report a discharge and soiling of the underwear upon direct questioning. Many other patients comment on the necessity for frequent douches and the appearance of a discharge when douches are discontinued.

Malodor is described by many patients as the most disagreeable symptom of the infection. Others are oblivious to any odor and deny its presence. Many husbands are acutely conscious of the unpleasant odor, a fact that has resulted in marital problems.

Pruritus and burning of mild degree were reported by forty-four of 141 patients with H. V. vaginitis observed by Gardner and Dukes (1955). Of these forty-four patients, nineteen had associated *Candida* or trichomonads to which the symptoms probably were attributable. In a subsequent and more extensive study by the same authors, these symptoms were recorded in only 13 percent of 940 separate observations.

Although a number of authors have reported the association of mild pruritus, burning, and other irritations in a much higher percentage of patients with this infection, it is probable that, in reality, these symptoms are rarely manifestations of the disease. Theoretically, this should be true, since the organism does not invade living tissues and since allergenic or toxic metabolic substances have not been demonstrated. Further, a significant number of patients with clinically and bacteriologically normal vaginas answer affirmatively when directly questioned concerning vulvovaginal irritations, indicating that these symptoms are not always dependent upon the presence of vulvovaginal infection.

Objective signs. Leukorrhea is the most familiar objective sign of the disease. When vaginal secretions are referred to as a discharge or leukorrhea, the usual connotation is increased volume or pronounced alteration of its physical characteristics such as consistency and odor. The discharge of H. V. vaginitis varies from scant to profuse, although it is usually much less abundant than in the average case of trichomoniasis.

The consistency of the discharge is approximately the same as that of the discharge associated with trichomoniasis. It resembles a thin flour paste, being turbid and uniformly homogeneous, and has a tendency to adhere to the vaginal wall in a thin film rather than to pool in the posterior fornix. Brewer, Halpern, and Thomas described the discharge as "smooth," whereas others have used the word "creamy." Although the discharge is rarely, if ever, of a normal curdy consistency, it is slightly so in approximately 5 percent of infected patients. The rapid return of the consistency to normal upon eradication of *H. vaginalis* is striking.

The color of the discharge, as recorded by Gardner and Dukes (1959) in 940 independent clinical observations, was gray in 94.9 percent, white in 2.0 percent, and yellowish or greenish in 3.1 percent. Brewer, Halpern, and Thomas described the discharge as white or gray in 89.2 percent, yellow in 6.4 percent, green in 2.2 percent, and clear in 2.2 percent. Normal vaginal secretions are usually white or slate colored.

The odor of the discharge on a withdrawn speculum is characteristic. Usually it is less offensive than that of trichomoniasis. Gardner and Dukes (1955) recorded the odor as disagreeable in 82 percent and as offensive in 18 percent. Brewer, Halpern, and Thomas described it as "uniformly disagreeable." Most patients when questioned directly will admit being aware of a disagreeable odor. Upon eradication of the organisms, the odor disappears.

Frothiness of the discharge (Figs. 13-4 and 13-5) is apparent in 10 to 15 percent of cases. This is usually minimal, consisting only of small bubbles. The discharge of an occasional patient, however, is extremely frothy. The degree of frothiness varies from day to day, apparently being influenced by douches or any vaginal medicament.

The pH of the vaginal discharge as determined by Gardner and Dukes (1959) in 940 separate clinical observations of 371 private patients was as follows: 82 percent (771) within the range of 5.0 to 5.5; 71 percent (669) within the narrow range of 5.0 to 5.2; and 18 percent (169) less than 5.0. Of the last groups only 3.4 percent (32) fell below an estimated pH 4.7. Brewer, Halpern, and Thomas reported an average pH of 5.2 in their series. Practically all investigators agree that most patients with H. V. vaginitis have a discharge within the range of pH 5.0 to 5.5. In contrast, the pH of normal vaginal secretions of practically all patients is within the range of pH 3.8 to 4.5. More than 90 percent of patients in the childbearing age with vaginal secretions of pH 5.0 or higher who have no trichomonads have H. V. vaginitis. The

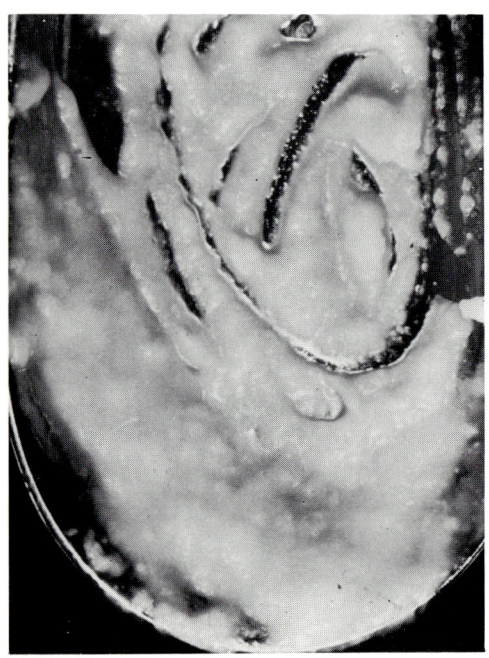

Fig. 13-6. Normal, curd-like vaginal secretions from a patient with a normal microbial flora. Compare with the discharge of H.V. vaginitis in Fig. 13-5.

vaginal acidity returns to normal upon eradication of *H. vaginalis.*

Gross changes in the tissues of the vulva and vagina were found by Gardner and Dukes only sixty-eight (7.2 percent) times in 940 separate observations. Ray and Maughan reported that only five of sixty-eight patients had redness or edema, though Brewer, Halpern, and Thomas and others have reported a higher incidence of organic changes. Theoretically, gross vulvitis and vaginitis should not be a part of the disease, since the organisms do not invade living tissues or elaborate substances that are toxic to the tissues. It can only be concluded that gross organic changes are rarely attributable to this infection alone and, when present, are extremely mild.

Since *H. vaginalis* rarely produces gross or microscopic signs of inflammation, a question occasionally arises as to whether the infection should be considered vaginitis. The term "vaginitis" has a broad interpretation and its use is not limited to vaginal disorders associated with gross changes in the tissues. H. V. vaginitis is an infection, and it gives rise to distinctly abnormal vaginal secretions. The disease must be accepted for what it is and the criteria set forth in this chapter should be the sole basis for its diagnosis.

Histopathology

H. vaginalis, being a surface parasite, does not invade the vaginal tissues or provoke an inflammatory reaction. A review of biopsies of the vagina from a large group of women with H. V. vaginitis revealed epithelium identical with that removed from normal vaginas (Fig. 13-2). Various staining techniques failed to demonstrate the organism within the tissues. A minimal dilation and congestion of capillaries within the dermis was observed in several cases. No inflammatory infiltrate was apparent within the dermis or within the epithelium; microscopically, the epithelium was completely normal.

Diagnosis

If H. V. vaginitis is suspected, a careful correlation of clinical and microscopic findings affords a degree of diagnostic accuracy that ordinarily obviates the need for cultures.

Clinical findings. As previously stated, any woman in the childbearing age who has a gray, homogeneous, somewhat malodorous vaginal discharge with a pH 5.0 to 5.5 that is not associated with gross changes in the tissues is likely to have H. V. vaginitis. Since many patients with trichomoniasis have a similar or identical type of discharge and no visible tissue changes, the distinction between the two diseases frequently requires the use of laboratory methods. Being fairly characteristic, the odor of the discharge as evaluated on the withdrawn speculum offers a clue to diagnosis.

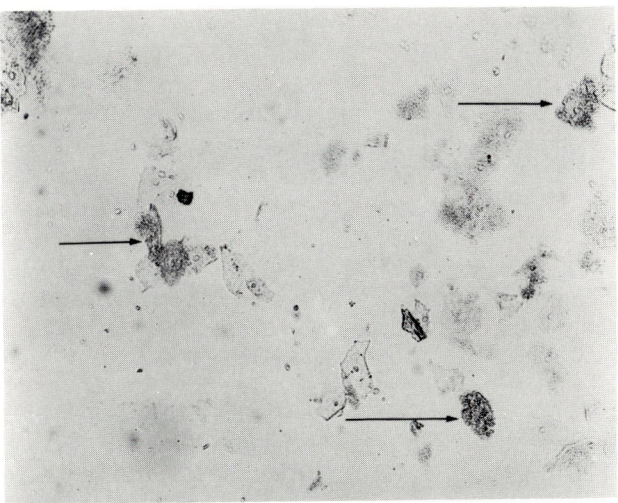

Fig. 13-7. Wet mount preparation of vaginal secretions from patient with *H. vaginalis* vaginitis. The "clue cells" appear as darker stippled epithelial cells (arrows). (Low power)

200 Benign diseases of the vulva and vagina

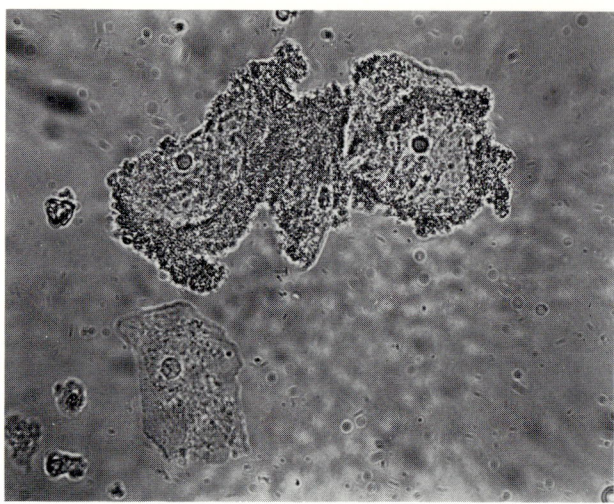

Fig. 13-8. "Clue cells" of *H. vaginalis* vaginitis. Normal epithelial cell in lower left. Pus cells are few and lactobacilli are lacking. (Wet mount preparation) (Gardner, H. L., and Dukes, C. D.: Amer. J. Obstet. Gynec. **69:**962, 1955.)

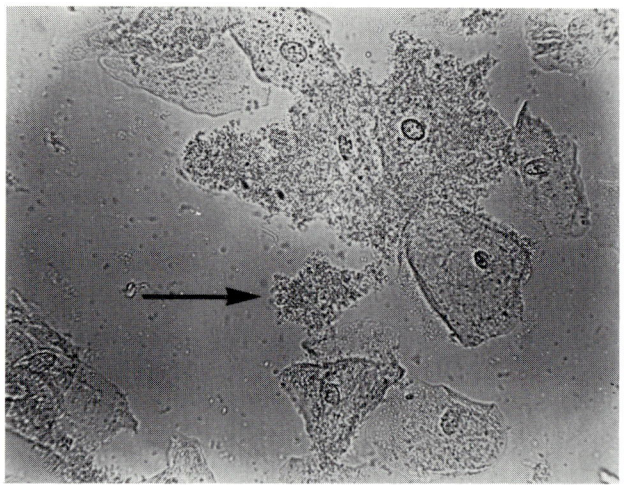

Fig. 13-9. "Clue cells" of *H. vaginalis* vaginitis. Clumps of *H. vaginalis* float free in fluid (arrow). (Wet mount preparation) Compare with scattered lactobacilli in Fig. 13-10.

Laboratory findings.

Wet mount preparations. Wet mount preparations should be examined under low power and high power objectives. Vaginal material from patients with H. V. vaginitis, when mixed with physiologic saline on a glass slide, exhibits a characteristic microscopic picture of the utmost diagnostic value (Figs. 13-7 to 13-9). Pus cells are few unless a concomitant vaginal infection or incidental cervicitis is present. Lactobacilli are conspicuously absent. The appearance of many of the epithelial cells provides the strongest evidence of H. V. vaginitis—they appear to be stippled or granulated. Gardner and Dukes (1955) have referred to such cells as "clue cells." Their appearance is incident to adherent and uniformly spaced *H. vaginalis* upon their surfaces. Some of the cells are only partially involved; others, not at all. Although occasionally bacterial organisms such as diphtheroids and cocci will adhere to epithelial cells, mimicking the clue cells of H. V. vaginitis (Fig. 13-

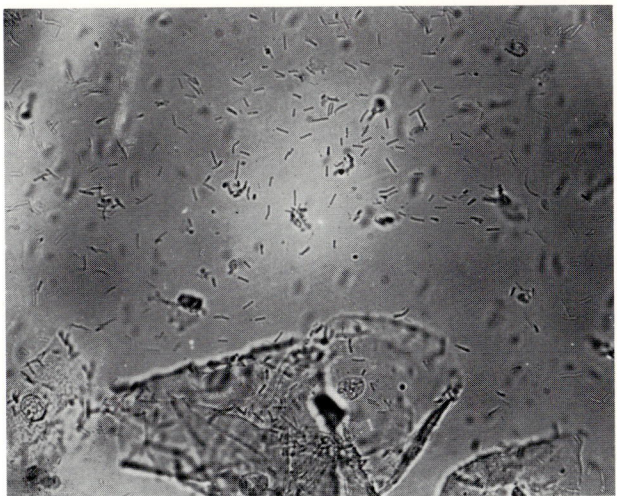

Fig. 13-10. Lactobacilli in wet mount preparation made from normal vaginal secretions. Compare epithelial cells with those parasitized by *H. vaginalis* in Figs. 13-7, 13-8, and 13-9.

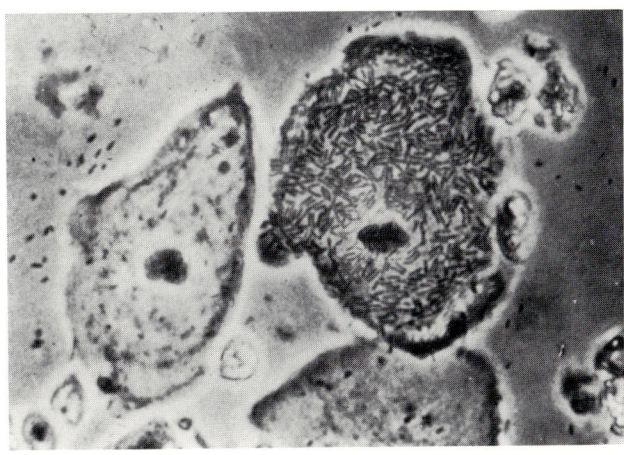

Fig. 13-11. "False" clue cell, incident to adherence of larger bacilli to surface of an epithelial cell. Small diphtheroids on epithelial cells are often confused with true clue cells of *H. vaginalis*. (Courtesy Peter Stroll, Germany.)

11), as a rule the distinction is not difficult. Clumps of *H. vaginalis* organisms are usually attached to the edges of some epithelial cells or float free in the surrounding fluid. These floating clumps of small bacteria (Fig. 13-9) are characteristic and of additional diagnostic value. The outlines of some of the epithelial cells may be obscured by the masses of *H. vaginalis*. A motile organism, not yet identified, but which appears to be a vibrio, if often associated with *H. vaginalis*.

Medical technologists experienced with wet mount preparations can recognize more that 90 percent of cases of H. V. vaginitis. If trichomoniasis is associated, the accuracy of the diagnosis by this method falls to about 50 percent. The several possible reasons for this precipitous drop in accuracy are purely theoretical.

Stained smears. The most striking feature of the gram-stained smear is the tremendous number of *H. vaginalis* organisms (Figs. 13-1 and 13-12, *A*), represented by small gram-

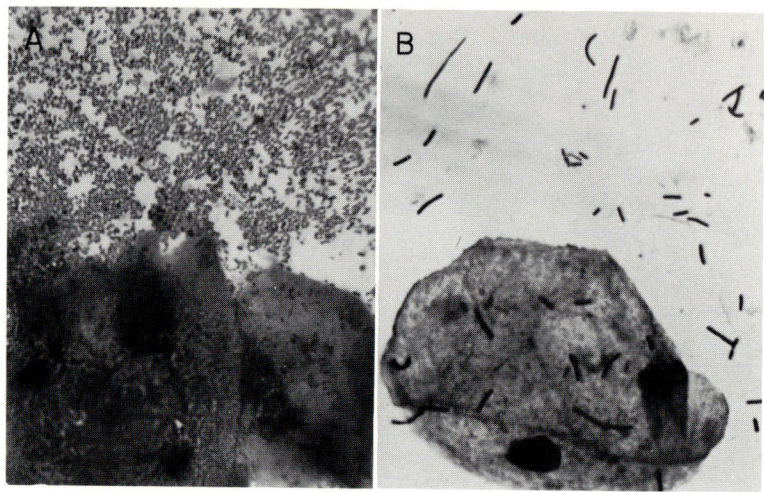

Fig. 13-12. **A,** *H. vaginalis* from vaginal secretions, Gram-stained smear. Compare with **B. B,** Lactobacilli, large gram-positive bacilli from normal vaginal secretions. (Gardner, H. L., and Dukes, C. D.: Ann. N. Y. Acad. Sci. **83:**280, 1959.)

negative bacilli 0.3 to 0.6 micron wide and 1.0 to 2.0 micron long, with rounded ends. Most stained smears also contain other types of bacteria, although their numbers are usually relatively insignificant. As in the wet mount, lactobacilli are conspicuously rare or absent.

For general use, the grain-stained smear is probably the most reliable laboratory method for diagnosis of this disease. Dunkelberg (1965), for example, examined 300 unmarked smears from patients with proved diagnoses —comprising seventy-two without disease, forty-six with candidiasis, forty-two with trichomoniasis, eight with candidiasis-trichomoniasis, and 132 with H. V. vaginitis—and identified *H. vaginalis* on each of the 132 slides containing *H. vaginalis*. He made an erroneous diagnosis of H. V. vaginitis on fifteen additional slides, the overall gross error thus being 12.8 percent. Diphtheroids are chiefly responsible for confusion of the diagnosis from the gram-stained smear; like *H. vaginalis,* they are also often present in large numbers and sometimes appear to be gram-negative. Dunkelberg concluded, after restudying the diphtheroid slides falsely interpreted as *H. vaginalis,* that they are morphologically different and should not cause confusion. No other small gram-negative bacillus appears in sufficient numbers in the vagina to be mistaken for *H. vaginalis.*

When stained by the Giemsa method, the organism exhibits either uniform or bipolar staining. It does not form endospores, and capsules have not been demonstrated by the India ink, Anthony, Liefson, or Hiss techniques. Dukes has found the acridine orange stain useful for establishing the diagnosis.

The Papanicolaou smear of secretions from patients with H. V. vaginitis reveals, as a rule, a few pus cells, a lack of lactobacilli, and a background of myriads of small bacteria. Together, these findings provide a strong clue to the presence of *H. vaginalis.* The organism is not cytotoxic and thus does not produce atypical changes of the squamous epithelial cells, as may *Trichomonas vaginalis.* Cytologists in the Houston area almost routinely report *H. vaginalis* when it is present in the Papanicolaou smear, although the morphology of the organism is far less distinct than on the gram-stained smear.

Fluorescent antibody technique. In direct smears from the vagina or from cultures, *H. vaginalis* stains specifically with fluorescent antibody prepared from sera of rabbits immunized with the organism. *H. vaginalis* is the only bacterium that will absorb the specifically tagged antibody. Redmond and Kotcher were the first to prepare and describe this species specific fluorescent antibody stain.

Culture identification. Cultures are seldom required for differential diagnosis of vag-

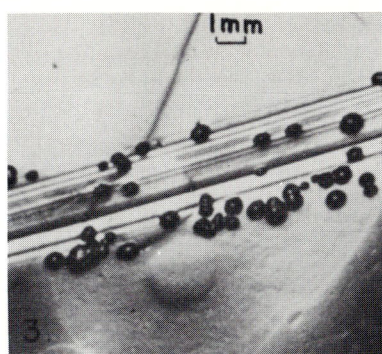 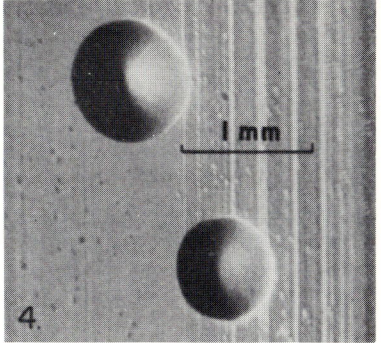

Fig. 13-13. Colonies of *H. vaginalis* on Casman's blood agar after 60 hours of incubation. (Dukes, C. D., and Gardner, H. L.: J. Bact. 81:277, 1961.)

initis. Material for culture is obtained from the vaginal vault ahead of a bivalve speculum. The material is emulsified in 1.0 ml. of thioglycollate broth, Brewer-modified without indicator (BBL), and this is used as the transport medium. The emulsified material, stored at room temperature or in the refrigerator (not in the freezing compartment), is transferred within 3 to 4 hours to solid media by means of a sterile cotton swab. The swab is rolled over the diameter of the plate and the deposited material distributed by streaking at right angles with a wire loop.

Thus far, the most efficient medium for the isolation and maintenance of *H. vaginalis* is Casman's blood agar base (Difco), adjusted to pH 7.5 before autoclaving and containing 5 percent fresh defibrinated rabbit blood. Isolation of *H. vaginalis* is more consistent if the cultures are incubated under increased CO_2 tension (candle jar) for 24 hours at 37° C.

By direct and transmitted light, the surface of the plates frequently seems to be devoid of bacterial growth. When oblique lighting is employed, however, the myriads of minute colonies can be detected by reflection. Under low power stereoscopic magnification (×-36) by reflected light, the colonies appear to be smooth, glistening, convex, transparent, circular, entire-edged, and of the dewdrop type; they tend to coalesce when in proximity (Fig. 13-13). *H. vaginalis* is oxidase-negative, and in CTA medium (cystine trypticase agar, BBL) produces acid from glucose, maltose, dextrin, glycogen, and starch. The organism exhibits no effect upon lactose, sucrose, mannitol, trehalose, glycerol, raffinose, salicin, or dulcitol and yields slow and weak acid in xylose, anabinose, rhamnose, and levulose.

Treatment

Many patients with H. V. vaginitis are unaware of the infection until they experience the favorable changes that follow its cure. Patients who have the habit of frequent douching and those habituated to their own odors are unlikely to complain and seek treatment. While most patients should be treated upon diagnosis of the infection, certain asymptomatic patients should, perhaps, be allowed to continue in ignorance if cooperation between husband and wife is likely to be difficult. A lasting cure is often difficult to accomplish because of the very real problem of reinfection.

Topical agents. Oxytetracycline (Terramycin) vaginal suppositories, when inserted into the vagina at bedtime for 10 days, are highly effective. The method is often successful after other topical agents and oral tetracyclines have proved worthless. A frequent unfavorable aftermath of intravaginal Terramycin is the development of vulvovaginal candidiasis. Concurrent use of vaginal nystatin (Mycostatin) tablets or other fungicidal agents, however, will usually protect the patient against this complication. Occasionally, bacterial vaginal infections caused by proteus, pseudomonas, or staphylococci also follow the use of intravaginal Terramycin. As a rule, they are mild and transient and the patient requires no specific treatment.

Intravaginal sulfonamides are somewhat less effective than intravaginal Terramycin, though they are advantageous in that they do not tend to promote secondary candidal or bacterial infections. Sulfonamides available for intravaginal use include triple sulfa (Sultrin) cream and tablets, sulfisoxazole (Gantrisin) cream, and sulfadiazine (Gynben) vaginal suppositories and cream. These preparations should be inserted twice daily for a minimum of 10 days.

Furacin vaginal suppositories and cream contain the antibacterial agent nitrofurazone. The cream, which is probably superior to the suppositories, should be instilled into the vagina morning and night for a minimum of 10 days. This agent gives results comparable to the sulfonamides.

Systemic agents. Ampicillin, 500 mg. administered every 6 hours for 5 days, has proved to be the most effective systemic agent used by us to date, but even so, many strains are resistant to it.

Oral tetracyclines are partially effective, some strains responding rapidly and others not at all. No statistical evidence to prove the superiority of any one of these drugs has been published. Karnaky, however, has found oxytetracycline (Terramycin) effective. The tetracyclines should be administered in a minimum dose of 250 mg. every 6 hours for 5 days. Some resistant infections have responded to Panalba capsules containing tetracycline phosphate complex equivalent to 250 mg. of tetracycline hydrochloride and 125 mg. of albamycin (Sodium Novobiocin).

Oral sulfonamides in the usual dosage have been almost uniformly unsuccessful as a treatment for H.V. vaginitis.

Penicillin, although reportedly effective, is of little value, most strains of H. vaginalis being highly resistant to the drug. A number of our patients have received no benefit from injections of 1,000,000 U. of penicillin per day for 10 days.

Miscellaneous measures. Douches temporarily remove malodorous secretions, though they contribute nothing toward cure of the patient.

Estrogens, used locally or systemically, have no place in treatment. The vaginal nutrients necessary for rapid propagation of the organism depend upon estrogenic activity. Hyperestrinism potentiates and hypoestrinism inhibits the disease.

Lactobacilli, which have been commercially grown, have been instilled into the vagina in the hope of reestablishing flora antagonistic to *H. vaginalis*. As a therapeutic measure, this procedure, in our experience, has been uniformly unsuccessful. The fallacy of the method is suggested by the ease with which H.V. vaginitis can be established in vaginas with a predominantly lactobacillus flora.

Prophylaxis. According to the experiences of Gardner and Dukes (1955) and Criswell and others with vaginal inoculations, a large number of organisms is necessary to establish infection. For this reason, it might be assumed that immediate postcoital douching, particularly when a bactericidal douche solution is used, would afford some protection. The routine use of contraceptive creams, jellies, and foams, the majority of which are bactericidal, might also afford protection. The intravaginal use of tetracyclines and sulfonamides and the oral use of tetracyclines theoretically should be protective to a high degree, although the prophylactic dosage of these agents has not been determined. The use of protective sheaths by the male partner should also serve as a safeguard against infection.

HAEMOPHILUS VAGINALIS INFECTION IN MEN

It is probable that Leopold was the first to isolate from men the species of *Haemophilus* that subsequently became known as *H. vaginalis*. In his report he stated that all men from whom this organism was isolated showed signs of moderate prostatitis, with or without urethritis. Perhaps his patient material consisted chiefly of men with such symptoms. De la Fuente, Rico, and Soria found *H. vaginalis* in the urethras of thirty-seven of forty-four men whose wives had H.V. vaginitis. Gardner and Dukes (1959) found that *H. vaginalis* was the predominant bacterial organism of the urethra in ninety-one of 101 men whose wives were infected. Since these men were not examined for evidence of clinical disease, the effects of *H. vaginalis* were not determined; nevertheless, the failure of most of this group to report the symptoms of urethritis voluntarily might suggest that they suffered no such discomforts.

Dunkelberg and Woolvin found that *H. vaginalis* was the predominant bacterial organism in the urethral discharges of five males suspected of having gonorrhea, yet who did not yield gonococci. The microscopic and cultural findings were identical to those seen in H.V. vaginitis. Hughes and Carpenter discovered an unidentified, small, gram-negative bacillus in some of the discharges of 216 male patients with urethritis, all of whom had received a clinical diagnosis of penicillin-resistant gonorrhea. Dunkelberg and Woolvin suggested that many of these may actually have been cases of H.V. urethritis. Whether *H. vaginalis* is a primary cause of symptomatic genitourinary infection in men has not been determined, although it has been fairly well-established that many men with "nonspecific" urethritis harbor *H. vaginalis*.

Treatment

Since more than 90 percent of men whose sexual partners are infected with *H. vaginalis* also yield the organism, they constitute a continuous source of reinfection. For this reason, the male sexual partner must be treated simultaneously with the patient if reinfections are to be prevented. The reinfection rate in women whose sexual partners are not treated far exceeds the rate in those whose consorts are successfully treated. In fact, reinfection is predictable if the consort is not treated. Treatment schedules which have proved most successful in men are: ampicillin, 500 mg. every 6 hours for 5 days; Panalba, 250 mg. every 6 hours for a minimum of 5 days; and Terrastatin, 250 mg. every 6 hours for a minimum of 5 days. These schedules, however, are not uniformly successful.

REFERENCES

Amies, C. R., and Jones, S. A.: A description of Haemophilus vaginalis and its L forms, Canad. J. Microbiol. **3**:579, 1957.

Bergman, S., Lundgren, K. M., and Lundstrom, P.: Haemophilus vaginalis in vaginitis, Acta Obstet. Gynec. Scand. **44**:8, 1965.

Blinick, G., Steinberg, P., and Merendino, J. V.: Effect of sulfonamide cream on the bacterial flora of the infected vagina and cervix, Amer. J. Obstet. Gynec. **58**:176, 1949.

Bray, G.: Hemophilus vaginalis, Acta Clin. Belg. **18**:248, 1963.

Bret, A. J., and Cohen-Debray: Vaginites à "Haemophilus vaginalis," Presse Med. **67**:1611, 1959.

Brewer, J. I., Halpern, B., and Thomas, G.: Hemophilus vaginalis vaginitis, Amer. J. Obstet. Gyenc. **74**:834, 1957.

Criswell, B. S., Ladwig, C. L., Gardner, H. L., and Dukes, C. D.: *Haemophilus vaginalis* vaginitis by inoculation from culture, Obstet. Gynec. **33**:195, 1969.

de la Fuente, F., Rico, L. R., and Soria, F.: Hemofilasis urogenital afeccion venerea?, Rev. Esp. Obstet. Ginec. **18**:252, 1959.

de la Fuente, F., and Salcedo, J.: Lesividad del "Hemophilus vaginalis," Rev. Esp. Obstet. Ginec. **19**:22, 1960.

Delaha, E. C., Curtin, J. A., Stevens, G., and Osborne, H. J.: Incidence and significance of Hemophilus vaginalis in nonspecific vaginitis, Amer. J. Obstet. Gynec. **89**:996, 1964.

Deming, J. E.: Haemophilus influenzae vaginitis, Northwest Med. **54**:992, 1955.

Döll, W.: Vorkommen von Haemophilus vaginalis bei unspezifischer Vaginitis?, Zbl. Bakt. **171**:372, 1958.

Dukes, C. D.: Unpublished data, 1967.

Dukes, C. D., and Gardner, H. L.: Identification of *Haemophilus vaginalis*, J. Bact. **81**:277, 1961.

Dukes, C. D., and Gardner, H. L.: Unpublished data, 1957.

Dunkelberg, W. E., Jr.: Diagnosis of Hemophilus vaginalis vaginitis by Gram stained smears, Amer. J. Obstet. Gynec. **91**:998, 1965.

Dunkelberg, W. E., Jr.: Haemophilus vaginalis determination in clinical laboratories, read at the Laboratory Officers Conference, WRGH, Washington, D. C., October, 1963.

Dunkelberg, W. E., Jr., and Bosman, R. I.: Haemophilus vaginalis: Incidence among 431 specimens examined, Milit. Med. **126**:920, 1961.

Dunkelberg, W. E., Jr., Hefner, J. D., Patow, W. E., Wyman, F. J., Jr., and Orup, H. I.: Hemophilus vaginalis among asymptomatic women, Obstet Gynec. **20**:629, 1962.

Dunkelberg, W. E., Jr., and Woolvin, S. C.: Haemophilus vaginalis relative to gonorrhea and male urethritis, Milit. Med. **128**:1098, 1963.

Edmunds, P. N.: The biochemical, serological, and haemagglutinating reactions of *"Haemophilus vaginalis,"* J. Path. Bact. **83**:411, 1962.

Edmunds, P. N.: The growth requirements of *Haemophilus vaginalis,* J. Path. Bact. **80**:325, 1960.

Edmunds, P. N.: *Haemophilus vaginalis,* J. Obstet. Gynaec. Brit. Comm. **66**:917, 1959.

Edmunds, P. N.: *Haemophilus vaginalis:* Morphology, cultural characteristics and viability, J. Path. Bact. **79**:273, 1960.

Frampton, J., and Lee Y.: Is *Haemophilus vaginalis* a pathogen in the female genital tract?, J. Obstet. Gynaec. Brit. Comm. **71**:436, 1964.

Gardner, H. L., Dampeer, T. K., and Dukes, C.

D.: The prevalence of vaginitis, Amer. J. Obstet. Gynec. **73**:1080, 1957.

Gardner, H. L., and Dukes, C. D.: Haemophilus vaginalis vaginitis, Amer. J. Obstet Gynec. **69**: 962, 1955.

Gardner, H. L., and Dukes, C. D.: Haemophilus vaginalis vaginitis, Ann. N. Y. Acad. Sci. **83**: 280, 1959.

Gardner, H. L., and Dukes, C. D.: New etiologic agent in nonspecific bacterial vaginitis, Science **19**:853, 1954.

Gardner, H. L., and Dukes, C. D.: Unpublished data, 1960.

Gray, L. A., and Barnes, M. L.: Vaginitis in women, diagnosis and treatment, Amer. J. Obstet. Gynec. **92**:125, 1965.

Heltai, A., and Taleghany, P.: Nonspecific vaginal infections, Amer. J. Obstet. Gynec. **77**:144, 1959.

Hughes, R. P., and Carpenter, C. M.: Alleged penicillin-resistant gonorrhea, Amer. J. Syph. Gonor. Ven. Dis. **32**:265, 1948.

Karnaky, K. J.: Do trichomonas vaginalis, candida albicans, hemophilus vaginalis, and nonspecific infections of the vagina produce a vaginitis often?, Med. Rec. Ann. **51**:750, 1958.

Karnaky, K. J.: Personal communications, 1966.

Kaufman, R. H., and Gardner, H. L.: Histopathology of the common vaginitides. Unpublished data.

Kummel, J.: Die unspezifische kolpitis in neurer Sicht, Vortrag Med. Ges. Munster **19**:50, 1961.

Kummel, J.: Klinische und bakteriologische Untersuchungen über die unspezifische Scheidenentzundung, Arch. Gynaek. **199**:42, 1963.

Kummel, J., and Ritzerfeld, W.: Untersuchungen uber die klinische Bedeutung von "Haemophilus vaginalis," Geburtsch. Frauenheilk. **21**:249, 1961.

Lapage, S. P.: Haemophilus vaginalis and its role in vaginitis, Acta Path. Microbiol. Scand. **52**: 34, 1961.

Leopold, S.: Heretofore undescribed organism isolated from the genitourinary system, U. S. Armed Forces Med. J. **4**:263, 1953.

Lutz, A., Grootten, O., and Wurch, T.: Etude des caractères culturaux et biochimiques de bacilles du type *Hemophilus hemolyticus vaginalis*, Rev. Immunol. **20**:132, 1956.

Lutz, A., and Wurch, T.: Recherches sur la sensibilité aux antibiotiques d'élèments de la flora vaginale au cours de la gestation, Bull. Fed. Soc. Gynec. Obstet. France. **6**:115, 1954.

Lutz, A., Wurch, T., and Grootten, O.: Quelques donnes sur les "petits bacilles gram négatif" agents d'une leucorrhée individualisée, Gynec. Obstet **55**:75, 1956.

Maggiora-Vergano, T.: L'associazione furazolidone-antifurossima nella terapia delle vaginiti da trichomonas vaginalis, monilia ed hemophylus vaginalis, Clin. Obstet. Ginec. **64**:537, 1962.

Mulla, N., and McDonough, J. J.: Local therapy in vaginitis, Ann. N. Y. Acad. Sci. **82**:182, 1959.

Muller, H., Pech, H., and Walch, E.: Untersuchungen zur Frage der pathogenetischen bedeutung des Haemophilus vaginalis für die menschliche Vagina, Geburtsch. Frauenheilke. **22**:350, 1962.

Pederson, C. S.: Symposium on problems in taxonomy, Bact. Rev. **20**:274, 1956.

Pinter, M., Csorba, L., and Zekany, G.: Haemophilus vaginalis in the etiology of colpitis (translated title), Orv. Hetil. **103**:585, 1962.

Ray, J. L., and Maughan, G. M.: Hemophilus vaginalis as an etiological agent in vaginitis, Western J. Surg. **64**:581, 1956.

Redmond, D. L., and Kotcher, E.: Comparison of cultural and immunofluorescent procedures in the identification of *Haemophilus vaginalis*, J. Gen. Microbiol. **33**:89, 1963.

Redmond, D. L., and Kotcher, E.: Cultural and serological studies on *Haemophilus vaginalis*, J. Gen. Microbiol. **33**:77, 1963.

Ritzerfeld, W.: Verschiebungen in der Kiembesiedlung der Vagina, Zbl. Bakt. **184**:84, 1962.

Ritzerfeld, W., and Kummel, J.: Untersuchungen zur bakteriologischen Diagnostik von "Haemophilus vaginalis," Zbl. Bakt. **180**:334, 1960.

Ritzerfeld, W., Kummel, J., and Weis, M.: Zur Keimbesiedlung von Vagina und Cervix, Arch. Hyg. Bakt. **148**:505, 1964.

Rodriguez Rico, J.: Valoracion del frotis vaginal bacteriologico, Bol. Soc. Ginec. Espan. **9**:17, 1959.

Sbrocca, L.: Contributo allo studio delle vaginiti da Haemophilus vaginale nella gravida, Minerva Ginec. **14**:721, 1962.

Stewart, R. H.: Nongonococcal vulvovaginitis, Amer. J. Obstet. Gynec. **82**:525, 1961.

Stoll, P.: Die Schnelldiagnose mittels Phasenkontrastmikroskopie in der gynäkologischen Sprechstunde, Sonderdruck aus Zeiss. Mitt. **2**:33, 1960.

Tarlinton, M. N., and D'Abrera, V. St. E.: Identity of a disputed pathogenic, Haemophiluslike organism in "nonspecific" vaginitis, J. Path. Bact. **93**:109, 1967.

Tarulis, S. A., Jensen, R. L., and Lake, J.: Hemophilus vaginalis in leukorrhea: incidence, diagnosis, and treatment, J. Amer. Osteopath. Ass. **62**:522, 1963.

Teckharov, B. A.: Classification of diseases contracted sexually (translated title), Vestn. Derm. Vener. **38**:55, 1964.

Thiery, M.: Fluor vaginalis, Belg. T. Geneesk. **18**: 743, 1962.

Wauters, G.: Hemophilus vaginalis, Acta Clin. Belg. **18**:246, 1963.

Weill, G., and Lutz, A.: De quelques aspects microscopiques de leucorrhées, Strasbourg Med. No. 9, p. 649, 1960.

Wu, C-C., and Lee, T-Y.: Hemophilus vaginalis, J. Formosa Med. Ass. **61**:251, 1962.

Wurch, T., and Lutz, A.: Etude du contenu vaginal dans 500 cas de leucorrhées, Rev. Franc. Gynec. Obstet. **50**:289, 1955.

Zinnemann, K.: Haemophilus influenzae and its pathogenicity, Ergeb. Mikrobiol. **33**:307, 1960.

Zinnemann, K., and Turner, G. C.: The taxonomic position of "Haemophilus vaginalis" (Corynebacterium vaginale), J. Path. Bact. **85**:213, 1963.

Zinnemann, K., and Turner, G. C.: Taxonomy of Haemophilus vaginalis, Nature **195**:203, 1962.

Chapter 14

Nonvenereal bacterial vulvovaginitides

The isolation of a predominant bacterial organism from the vagina of a patient who has vaginitis or leukorrhea does not prove an etiologic relationship between that bacterium and the disease condition present. Various types of bacteria are recoverable from the vaginas of any population group of women, not only those with gross evidence of vaginitis or an abnormal discharge but also those who are clinically normal. The organisms are almost as heterogeneous in the normal as in the abnormal vagina. Quantitatively, however, there is often a wide difference in vaginal organisms found in the two groups.

Allegedly, vaginitis is sometimes caused by one or more of several types of bacteria, including streptococci, staphylococci, *Escherichia coli, Haemophilus* species, pseudomonas, proteus, bacterioids, mycoplasma, and others. However, with the exception of *Haemophilus vaginalis* and perhaps, occasionally, beta hemolytic streptococci and *Mycobacterium tuberculosis,* no characteristic clinical patterns of infection have ever been attributed individually to the organisms so often mentioned. In other words, the gross tissue changes, the nature of the discharge, the symptoms experienced, and the microscopic features of the vaginal secretions resulting from infection by such organisms have never been definitively described and corroborated. This is especially true in connection with so-called nonspecific vaginitis.

An unnatural predominance of a vaginal bacterium most often means that the flora is temporarily imbalanced incident to antibiotic therapy or overzealous topical use of medications present in douche preparations, contraceptives, and therapeutic agents. Aside from these factors, debilitating diseases, nutritional deficiencies, leukemia, and carcinomatosis may occasionally play an important role in an apparent bacterial vaginitis. Not infrequently, one observes patients who, supposedly, have intractable vaginitis from one or more isolated bacterial agents, yet evidence nothing more than the *over-treatment syndrome*—the more she was treated, the worse she became.

Despite the difficulty in proving the etiologic relationship between the unnatural predominance of a bacterium and vaginitis, authentic examples of such infections must occasionally develop. Even so, the vast majority are associated with predisposing conditions, which themselves should perhaps be considered the primary cause of the condition present.

DIAGNOSIS

Vaginitis should not be attributed to the presence of unusual bacteria until every effort has been made to exclude the common, readily recognized pathogens—trichomonads, *H. vaginalis,* and *Candida* species—as the causative agent. After one becomes convinced that none of these is present, a thorough study of the patient for evidence of serious systemic disease is indicated. The patient should be questioned regarding her general health, recent treatment with antibiotics, hygienic practices, and use of vaginal contraceptives.

A search for the cause of an obscure vaginitis should always include wet mount preparations, stained smears, and bacteriologic cultures performed by a microbiologist known to be reliable. The presence of large numbers of parabasal vaginal epithelial cells and pus cells in the secretions of a patient in the reproductive years of life is indicative of vaginitis, whether of bacterial, trichomonal, or other origin. The wet mount preparations of vaginal secretions from an occasional patient with trichomoniasis may contain no discernible trichomonads, yet cultures may be positive. Cultures for *Candida* species should perhaps be included in the study, although a candidal infection with sufficient organisms to induce vulvovaginitis will, almost without exception, be exhibited by conidia and hyphae in the potassium hydroxide preparation. The probability that agents such as schistosomes and *Entamoeba histolytica* are responsible is extremely remote in this country, yet it should not be overlooked. Special tests for their identification should be performed, especially in the presence of otherwise unexplained ulcerative lesions.

Before bacteriologic cultures of the vagina are performed, the patient should have abstained from sexual relations and the use of vaginal medicaments of any type, including contraceptives and douches, for several days. Almost any chemical agent instilled into the vagina will be selectively bactericidal and may disturb the quantitative bacteriologic findings. Should the patient with severe vulvar irritation demand treatment during the period of waiting, applications of a corticosteroid cream (without antibiotics) to the vulva will often afford relief. Also, the external applications of an innocuous agent such as boric acid ointment should partially relieve the patient, yet not materially affect the vaginal flora. Following this essentially "hands off" regimen for a few days before undertaking the bacteriologic investigation, the tissues and vaginal flora often return to normal and the patient may become totally asymptomatic.

Since the vaginal flora of subjects in the reproductive years is decidedly different from that of premenarchal and postmenopausal subjects, knowledge of the ovarian activity of a patient with vaginitis becomes mandatory. As a rule, the normal vagina of a woman in the reproductive years of life contains a predominance of lactobacilli and mature vaginal epithelial cells, whereas women with hypoestrogenism have thin vaginas with a low glycogen content, many immature epithelial cells, and a flora composed of a wide variety of bacterial organisms. An occasional patient in the reproductive years with an entirely normal vagina and secretions yields a variety of bacterial agents that predominate over lactobacilli; for example, a combination of diphtheroids and streptococci often constitute the vaginal flora of patients with no demonstrable vaginal disease. Such a temporary imbalance or "abnormal" flora is not to be interpreted as infection or vaginitis.

The acidity of the vagina is often a better indicator of vaginal health than is the flora. In the reproductive years, unless the patient has candidiasis, pH 4.2 or less indicates vaginal health, whereas pH 5.0 or higher usually is a sign of vaginal disease.

The point at which the volume of vaginal secretions becomes sufficient to warrant a diagnosis of disease is difficult to determine. Many patients complain of an abnormal discharge when the cervix, vagina, and vulva, as well as the physical characteristics of the vaginal secretions, are normal in every respect. Perhaps many such patients are merely overly fastidious, have emotional problems, or are simply misinformed.

Streptococcal vaginitis

Streptococci are widely distributed in nature. With the exception of lactobacilli and diphtheroids, they are the most common bacteria in the normal vagina. Alpha and gamma types of streptococci, although frequently a part of the flora in trichomoniasis, rarely, if ever, act as independent pathogens. Even beta type streptococci, which can be highly pathogenic in other tissues, are usually no more than harmless commensals in the vagina. In our experience, *Streptococcus pyogenes,* a member of the pyogenic species, is the only streptococcal organism that produces a vaginitis with a recognizable clinical pattern. We have observed five patients with vulvovaginitis attributable to this organism, all of whom have had low estrogen levels; one was a premenarchal patient, two were postmenopausal, and two were postpartal.

Grossly, the vagina infected with hemolytic (beta) streptococci is fiery red and thin. The vulva, particularly the vestibule, often has a mottled erythematous appearance (Fig. 14-1). The secretions are usually of a seropurulent nature. The symptoms consist chiefly of burning, pruritus, and a discharge.

All of the five patients observed with beta type streptococcal vaginitis responded rapidly to treatment. Both postmenopausal patients received a combination of vaginal estrogens and sulfonamides, the premenarchial patient was treated with vaginal applications of estrogens, and the two postpartum patients were given systemic tetracyclines.

Staphylococcal vaginitis

Although pyodermas of the vulva are not unusual, few proven examples of staphylococcal vaginitis have been reported. Lang, Israel, and Fritz reported two cases of staphylococcal vulvovaginitis, both following the administration of antibiotics and both with accompanying skin infections, one of which was associated with vulvar folliculitis. On one or more occasions, cultures from the vagina of both patients yielded *Staphylococcus aureus*.

Practically every patient whom we have observed with a predominately staphylococcal flora (Fig. 14-2) had recently been treated intensely with antibiotics or had been over-treated with topical medications. For this reason, we can only conclude that a predominance of staphylococci in the vagina is usually related to their opportunistic tendency, the organism multiplying rapidly in an environment that is favorable to them yet perhaps antagonistic to lactobacilli.

With few exceptions, a predominance of staphylococci, with or without evidence of vaginitis or leukorrhea, requires no treatment other than the removal of factors that initiated the change in flora. This failing,

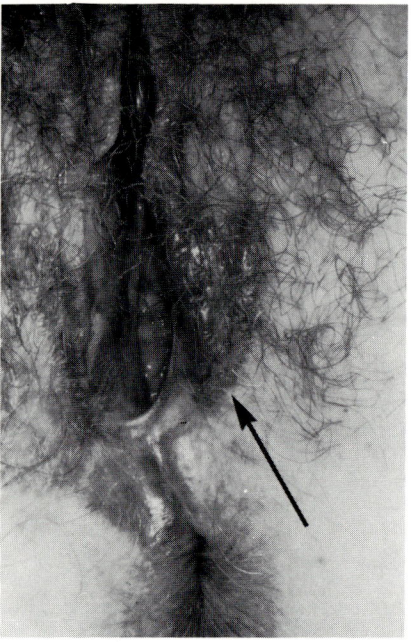

Fig. 14-1. Streptococcal vulvitis. In this case, sharply demarcated, red, elevated, erythematous areas were present. The patient also had a fiery red vagina.

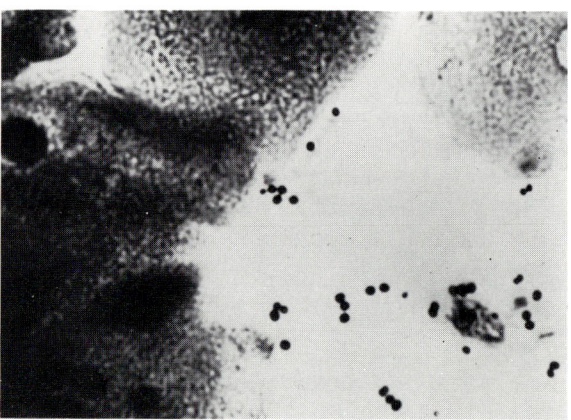

Fig. 14-2. Staphylococcal vaginitis. Smear showing staphylococci as predominant organism appeared following antibiotic therapy. (Gram-stained smear)

sensitivity tests and treatment of the patient with appropriate antibiotics may be necessary.

Infection with *Escherichia coli*

Escherichia coli, a normal inhabitant of the intestinal tract and frequently pathogenic in the urinary tract, can seldom be proved responsible for vulvovaginitis, even though the organism is commonly isolated in the vaginal secretions. We have observed a few patients with an abnormal vaginal discharge in which *E. coli* seemed to play a part; however, in only two or three patients have gross tissue changes appeared that were believed attributable to the organism. Nevertheless, if any patient has a persistent abnormal vaginal discharge in which *E. coli* is the predominant bacterial organism, whether or not gross tissue changes are associated, a cause and effect relationship should be considered.

Of more than 600 patients with vaginitis, Perez-Miravete and Jaramillo found only two whose secretions yielded pure cultures of the organism; these patients had "infections associated with a discharge of clearly inflammatory origin." The same authors also found *E. coli* in about 15 percent of patients with "nonspecific vaginitis," in a similar number of patients with trichomoniasis, and in a smaller number with candidiasis.

Theoretically, local applications of sulfonamides would be effective against the organism. In our experience, most patients with an abnormal discharge in which *E. coli* predominates have not required treatment. Here, again, it seems likely that, in most instances, the organism is an opportunistic one that grows rapidly in an altered environment brought about by factors previously mentioned. Their correction often effects a cure.

Vincent's infection (fusospirochetosis)

Borrelia vincentii and *Fusobacterium fusiforme* are the etiologic agents in Vincent's infection (fusospirochetosis). The evidence that they ever become primary pathogens in the normal vagina of a healthy woman is inconclusive.

Almost without exception, Vincent's infection is preceded by malnutrition, debilitating disease, or gross organic lesions. It is most often associated with lesions involving tissue necrosis and retained secretions, which means that the organisms are usually saprophytic, living primarily on dead tissue and exudate. Callomon and Wilson believe that spirochetosis is the most common cause of genital gangrene. Examples of sexual transmission of Vincent's infection of the genitalia have been reported, as well as vulvar ulcers following orogenital contact. We have never observed primary lesions of Vincent's infection of the vulvovaginal tissues. Fusospirochetosis, however, is frequently found in patients with necrotic lesions arising from such causes as the ulcerative venereal diseases, extensive condylomata acuminata, and carcinoma, as well as other conditions associated with tissue proliferation, destruction, and ulceration. In most cases, the fetid odor of these lesions is probably the result of

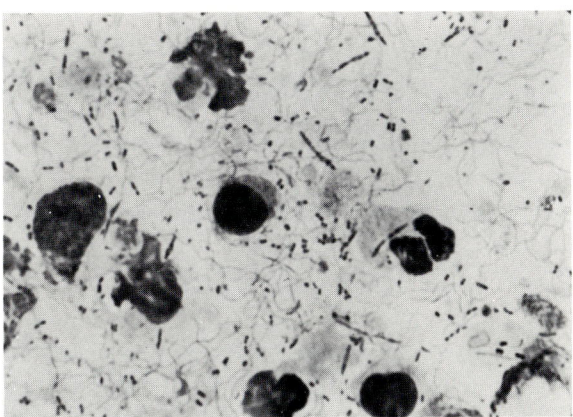

Fig. 14-3. Vincent's infection. Vaginal smears containing a predominance of fusospirochetal organisms. (Gram-stained smear)

secondary infection with Vincent's organisms. It is our conclusion that fusopirochetosis is important as a genital infection only insofar as it involves the crevices and devitalized tissues of other lesions, producing odors and possibly additional necrosis and pain.

The organisms are difficult to isolate in pure cultures; usually the diagnosis must be based upon their abundance in smears (Fig. 14-3). They stain well with carbolfuchsin. Experienced technicians can easily distinguish between *Treponema pallidum* and the spirochetes of Vincent's infection.

Treatment is directed toward eradication of the primary disease. It is often advisable, however, to administer penicillin to patients with severe secondary fusospirochetosis before surgical treatment for ulcerated proliferative processes is undertaken.

Pseudomonas and proteus infections

We are unaware of primary vulvovaginal infections caused by either pseudomonas or proteus organisms, other than those related to an occasional wound infection of the lower genital area. At times, the organisms are recovered in significant numbers from the vagina, usually following intensive antibiotic therapy. Because of their exuberant growth on culture plates (especially by proteus), they frequently overgrow all other organisms; in such cases, cultural identification of the true offending pathogen may be difficult. During a period of observation after factors influencing the flora of the vagina have been corrected, these organisms tend to disappear, or their numbers become too insignificant to require active therapeutic attention. They are resistant to the sulfonamides and to the majority of antibiotics.

Infection with *Mycoplasma*

Members of the genus *Mycoplasma*, also known as pleuropneumonia-like organisms (PPLO), are tiny pleomorphic organisms without rigid cellular walls. They differ from viruses in that they can be cultivated in cell-free media and are visible under the light microscope. Isolated examples of urinary infection and septic abortion have been ascribed to organisms belonging to this genus, yet little convincing evidence has been offered that they are responsible for primary infections of the vulvovaginal tissues. Although obviously commensal in many normal women, they are found more often in patients with trichomoniasis, candidiasis, and so-called nonspecific vaginitis. Bercovici and others found *Mycoplasma* in 60 percent of patients with trichomoniasis, 33 percent of those with "nonspecific" vaginitis, and in only 7 percent of patients with normal vaginas. The association of *Mycoplasma* with vaginitis induced by other agents hardly suggests that this organism plays a causal or even a symbiotic role.

Corynebacterium in vulvovaginitis

The genus *Corynebacterium* owes its name to the club shaped swellings at the ends of the bacilli. Various nonpathogenic corynebacteria, known as *diphtheroids*, are normal inhabitants of the human vagina. In fact, aside from the lactobacillus, we consider diphtheroids the most normal bacterial component of a normal vaginal flora. The only proved species of pathogenic corynebacterium of the vulvovaginal tissues are *Corynebacterium diphtheriae* (Klebs-Loeffler bacillus), which gives rise to diphtheritic vaginitis (Chapter 19), and *Corynebacterium minutissimum,* which causes vulvar erythrasma (Chapter 17).

Laufe reported thirty-two cases of self-limiting acute ulcerative vulvovaginitis, eleven of which he ascribed to "*Corynebacterium pyogenes*." As stated many times in this book, the isolation of a predominant bacterium does not prove its etiologic relationship to the vaginitis observed. The fact that corynebacteria inhabit a high percentage of normal vaginas throws even further doubt upon their possible pathogenic role.

Anaerobic bacterial vaginitis

Little attention has been given to the possible role of anaerobic organisms in vaginitis. Jones and others found anaerobic bacteria predominating in cases of "nonspecific" vaginitis in premenarchial patients whose vaginal secretions contained no specific agents such as foreign bodies or gonococci. These authors expressed the opinion that so-called nonspore-forming anaerobic bacteria of the human vagina form a large group of gram-positive, gram-negative, and gram-variable cocci and bacilli concerning which we have too little information to permit species identification.

The mere discovery of anaerobic bacteria would be, at most, only slight evidence of a relationship of these organisms to vaginitis. Since practically all vaginal infections can now be attributed to other identifiable agents, we believe that anaerobic bacteria play little, if any, role as primary pathogens in vaginitis. Certainly, a recognizable clinical entity for such infections has not been described, and even a symbiotic relationship with other vaginal pathogens has not been proved.

Leptothrix vulvovaginitis

Although most gynecologists have heard references to vaginal *Leptothrix*, these references have been mainly through conversation. Only a few reports concerning *Leptothrix* infection of the vagina have appeared in medical literature. Most authors fail to agree on the morphologic and biochemical identification of such an organism; almost without exception, they have not attempted to relate *Leptothrix* to a well-defined clinical pattern of disease.

Organisms usually referred to as *Leptothrix* or "leptotrichia" are described as large filamentous bacteria (Fig. 14-4) that are larger than lactobacilli yet smaller than the filaments of *Candida*. They are most often described as nonbranching, segmented, narrow, thin, filamentous forms. Because of their cultural characteristics and biochemical properties, Feo and Dellette placed such agents in the family of the lactobacillus. These authors related the organism to a mild vaginitis characterized by diffuse erythema and by discrete white areas the size of a pinhead scattered over the vagina. They also detected minute ulcerations but stated that these were more often present when the bacteria were associated with candidal infections.

We have often found *Leptothrix* in clinic patients with trichomoniasis. The vaginal flora of one private patient with trichomoniasis contained predominant and persistent *Leptothrix*, and the vagina exhibited the gross characteristics of candidiasis. We have never observed a patient with vulvovaginitis associated with a predominance of *Leptothrix* in the absence of other pathogens. Although we do not deny the possible existence of such a specific vulvovaginal infection, it can be stated unequivocally that if vaginal infection is ever induced by the *Leptothrix*, its incidence is extremely rare and it poses no problem to the gynecologist.

Tuberculosis of the vulva and vagina

The incidence of tuberculosis of the vulvovaginal tissues is so low that the average gynecologist never recognizes a single case. While microscopic evidence of tuberculosis of the cervix is demonstrable in 3 to 10 percent of patients with the pelvic disease, gross tuberculous lesions of the vagina and vulva are even more exceptional.

Almost all lower genital lesions develop in subjects who have pelvic, pulmonary, or generalized tuberculosis. Authentic primary infections, however, have been reported in women following intercourse with men suffering from tuberculous epididymitis or open lesions of the genitalia. Apparently, therefore, inoculation may take place either directly or via the bloodstream. Leone observed a patient with primary tuberculous lesions of the vulva that developed 3 weeks after her marriage to a man with contagious pulmonary tuberculosis and urine containing Koch's bacilli. The initial ulcerative lesions of the patient were rapidly followed by "caseified bacilliferous adenopathy."

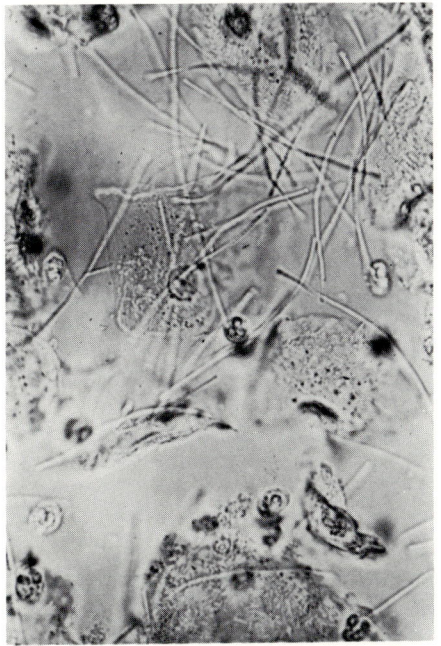

Fig. 14-4. *Leptothrix*. Wet mount preparation demonstrating *Leptothrix*, a questionable pathogen.

Reportedly, the lesions are grossly of three general types: tuberculous ulcers, lupus vulgaris, and scrofuloderma. In each type the inguinal and pelvic glands are often affected. Tuberculosis should be suspected in any patient with lesions of the vulva such as chronic ulcerations, draining sinuses, and adenopathy; their tuberculous nature should be particularly suspected in patients who have pulmonary tuberculosis or in whose family it exists. Schaefer has found that a firm, painless swelling in the region of a Bartholin's gland may be the first indication of the lower genital disease.

Histologic examination of the affected tissues usually reveals central caseation, epithelioid cells, round cell infiltration, and tuberculous giant cells. At times, a distinction from syphilis, chancroid, chronic venereal granulomata, carcinoma, the deep mycoses, and other disease may be necessary.

The acid-fast bacillus *Mycobacterium tuberculosis* may be found in material obtained from exudate or from scrapings of the lesion. Since *M. tuberculosis* may be confused with *Mycobacterium smegmatis* or *Nocardia asteroides,* cultures may be required. Both the American Trudeau Society medium and the Lowenstein-Jensen medium are considered excellent.

Essentially the same principles apply to the treatment for vulvovaginal tuberculosis as apply to that for tuberculosis elsewhere in the body. While treatment must be highly individualized, tuberculostatic drugs play an extremely important therapeutic role. Schaefer recommends antimicrobial therapy for at least 1 year when the diagnosis is based upon an excised lesion. If the diagnosis is made preoperatively, he believes that the patient should be given chemotherapeutic agents for several months before operation, should it be indicated.

Lipschütz ulcers (ulcus vulvae acutum)

Lipschütz, in 1918, reported a type of recurrent ulcerative lesion of the vulva to which he assigned the term "ulcus vulvae acutum." He found it most frequently in virgins from 14 to 20 years of age. The lesion has been attributed to the *Bacillus crassus,* a large gram-positive bacillus closely resembling, if not identical to, the lactobacillus.

Several varieties of ulcerative lesions carrying the designation of Lipschütz ulcers have been described. These include a gangrenous form with extensive tissue destruction, a "venereal" form resembling multiple chancroids, and a variety exhibited by multiple minute ulcerations. The disease is supposedly associated with fever at the onset, pain, and a clinical course of 3 to 4 weeks duration.

Lipschütz believed that he had described a distinct entity. Such ulcers are mentioned in all gynecologic texts, as well as in all treatises dealing with vulvar diseases. At this time we are unconvinced of the existence of a specific entity carrying the designation "Lipschütz ulcer." For example, *B. crassus* has never been taxonomically placed; most likely it belongs to the group of bacteria classified as lactobacilli. Such organisms are probably never pathogenic and most surely have never been demonstrated to infect and cause ulcerations in humans. Also, the described clinical features of the lesions alluded to are highly varied. Ephraim and Phillips and Scott (Chapter 16) expressed the opinion that the lesions were essentially identical to those of Behçet's syndrome. Instead of accepting unexplained ulcerations of the vulva as "Lipschütz ulcers," we are more inclined to believe that the majority are manifestations of other diseases, such as Behçet's syndrome, erythema nodosum, and herpes genitalis. Perhaps the term "Lipschütz ulcer" could be a wastebasket diagnosis for ulcerative lesions of the vulva, being used when the exact cause is undetermined.

REFERENCES

Bercovici, B., Persky, S., Rozansky, R., and Razin, S.: Mycoplasma (pleuropneumonia-like organisms) in vaginitis, Amer. J. Obstet. Gynec. **84:**687, 1962.

Bernstine, J. B., and Rakoff, A. E.: Vaginal infections, infestations, and discharges, New York, 1953, McGraw-Hill Book Co.

Callomon, F. T., and Wilson, J. L.: The nonvenereal diseases of the genitals, Springfield, Ill., 1956, Charles C Thomas, Publisher.

Carter, B., Jones, C. P., Alter, R. L., Creadick, R. N., and Thomas, W. L.: Bacteriodes infections in obstetrics and gynecology, Obstet. Gynec. **1:**491, 1953.

Ephraim, H.: Triple symptom complex of Behçet: Report of a case, Arch. Derm. Syph. **50:**37, 1944.

Feo, L. G., and Dellette, E. R.: Leptotrichia (leptothrix) vaginalis, Amer. J. Obstet. Gynec. 64:382, 1952.

Harwick, H. J., Iuppa, J. B., Purcell, R. H., and Fekety, F. R., Jr.: Mycoplasma hominis septicemia associated with abortion, Amer. J. Obstet. Gynec. 99:725, 1967.

Hite, K. E., Hesseltine, H. C., and Goldstein, L.: A study of the bacterial flora of the normal and pathologic vagina and uterus, Amer. J. Obstet. Gynec. 53:233, 1947.

Hunter, C. A., Jr., and Long, K. R.: A study of the microbiological flora of the vagina, Amer. J. Obstet. Gynec. 75:865, 1958.

Jones, C. P., Carter, F. B., Thomas, W. L., Peete, C. H., and Cherny, W. L.: Nonspore-forming anaerobic bacteria of the vagina, Ann. N. Y. Acad. Sci. 83:259, 1959.

Kotcher, E.: Microbiology of the human uterine cervix, Clin. Obstet. Gynec. 6:316, 1963.

Lang, W. R., Israel, S. L., and Fritz, M. A.: Staphylococcal vulvovaginitis: A report of two cases following antibiotic therapy, Obstet. Gynec. 11:352, 1958.

Laufe, L. E.: Acute ulcerative vulvovaginitis, Obstet. Gynec. 3:46, 1954.

Leone, R.: Complesso primario tuberculare vulvare da contagio coniugale, Minerva Derm. 38:94, 1963.

Lipschütz, B.: Über ulcus Vulvae acutum, Wien. Klin. Wschr. 31:461, 1918.

Malkani, P. K., and Bannerjee, A.: Tuberculosis of the cervix, J. Obstet. Gynec. India 8:1, 1957.

Perez-Miravete, A., and Jaramillo, H.: Studies on vaginal flora, Amer. J. Obstet. Gynec. 80:80, 1960.

Phillips, D. L., and Scott, J. S.: Recurrent genital and oral ulceration with associated eye lesions—Behçet's syndrome, Lancet 1:366, 1955.

Rakoff, A. E., Feo, L. G., and Goldstein, L.: Biologic characteristics of normal vaginas, Amer. J. Obstet. Gynec. 47:467, 1944.

Rippmann, E. T.: The clinical aspects of female genital tuberculosis today, Gynaecologia 157:77, 1964.

Rubin, A., and Morton, H. E.: The incidence and clinical significance of pleuropneumonia-like organisms in the genital tract of the human female, Ann. N. Y. Acad. Sci. 79:642, 1960.

Schaefer, G.: Diagnosis and treatment of female genital tuberculosis, Clin. Obstet. Gynec. 2:530, 1959.

Turk, D. C., and Porter, I. A.: A short textbook of microbiology, Philadelphia, 1965, W. B. Saunders Co.

Chapter 15

Atrophic vulvovaginitis

Vaginal atrophy, a prerequisite to atrophic vulvovaginitis, ensues when the estrogens available to the vagina fall below certain physiologic levels. Such atrophy ultimately develops in practically every postmenopausal woman, though it is not to be implied that all postmenopausal women have "senile vaginitis." The postirradiation type of atrophic vulvovaginitis, being materially different from that which follows natural menopause, is discussed as a separate entity in this chapter.

Postmenopausal type

The stage at which atrophy becomes "atrophic vulvovaginitis" is often designated most arbitrarily, since the criteria for diagnosis followed by different clinicians are highly variable. Atrophy begins in all patients with the beginning of estrogen withdrawal, and the stages range from the slightest shift of the maturation index to an almost total loss of vaginal epithelium. Also, the rapidity of development of atrophy varies widely in different patients. Some women of menopausal age have visible thinning of the vaginal mucosa and a high percentage of intermediate vaginal cells, or even parabasal cells, in the cytologic smear before missing the first menstrual period. Other women well into the menopause have a sufficient amount of ovarian or adrenal estrogens to preserve a grossly normal, mature condition of the vulvovaginal tissues. Folsome, Napp, and Tanz reported senile vaginitis in 95.8 percent of a group of elderly patients; our observations, however, do not correspond with these figures. In most patients, even the senile, the vaginal changes are too mild to warrant the diagnosis of atrophic vulvovaginitis. Whether the entity should include all cases of extreme atrophy or only those of atrophy with associated subjective symptoms remains unanswered.

Advanced vaginal atrophy is commonly called "senile vaginitis." This term is, perhaps, entirely appropriate if the patient is senile, yet it is hardly suitable for the young woman with atrophy incident to surgical castration or premature ovarian failure. The word "atrophic" more clearly defines the condition than does "senile." Since the term "atrophic vaginitis" might apply to atrophy of the vaginal epithelium alone, "vulvovaginal atrophism" is possibly a more inclusive and appropriate designation.

Etiology

Loss of estrogens, whether from natural menopause, castration, ovarian destruction from disease processes, or functional ovarian failure for any reason, is followed by varying degrees of atrophy of all vulvovaginal and uterine tissues. Natural menopause, of course, accounts for most vulvovaginal atrophism. A point of current debate is whether ovarian failure, with its consequent anatomic changes, is physiologic or pathologic. Women are apparently the only females who outlive their period of reproduction and upon whom nature regularly imposes such changes.

Atrophic changes incident to surgical castration, aside from the rapidity with which they appear, are identical to those that follow the natural menopause. The ovaries of some postmenopausal women probably secrete estrogens in diminishing amounts for several years. Also, the adrenal cortex is believed to be a limited source of estrogens in some women. These uncertain sources of hormones, combined with the variations in genital response to estrogens, partially explain the widely varying degrees of vulvovaginal atrophism in different patients. The fact remains that advanced degrees of atrophism develop in many women immediately after the menopause, whereas others in their sixties have only minimal atrophy.

A great deal has been written about the increased susceptibility of the atrophic vagina to infection, yet clinical candidiasis, trichomoniasis, and *H. vaginalis* vaginitis do not conform to this thesis, being rarely observed in the extremely atrophic vagina. It is apparent that the bacterial flora affects the symptoms of this disease, though it is not clear whether bacterial effects are essential to clinical manifestations in all cases. Most types of bacteria in the atrophic vagina are contaminants unrelated to the clinical disease. Their usual and immediate disappearance after the institution of treatment with estrogens proves that they are not primary factors. The most logical explanation, however, for the sudden onset of a discharge and subjective irritative symptoms in a patient with otherwise stable atrophism is bacterial infection of the tissues or tissue reaction to bacterial metabolites. Although a relation between specific bacterial organisms and signs and symptoms in atrophic vulvovaginitis has not been authenticated, we have observed several examples of acute vaginitis attributable to various types of streptococci, particularly beta streptococci and *Streptococcus faecalis*.

Bacteriology

The availability of the intravaginal nutrients necessary for rapid multiplication and maintenance of lactobacilli depends upon the proliferation of a glycogen-laden vaginal mucosa. In estrogen deficiency, the vagina atrophies, glycogen diminishes, and the pH rises. The consequent changes discourage the growth of lactobacilli and promote the growth of various contaminating organisms. Establishment and multiplication of contaminants result not only from the altered vaginal physiology incident to ovarian depletion but also from the extinction of competitive lactobacilli, sometimes referred to as the "policemen" of the vagina. The new flora is usually highly mixed, often including numerous types of streptococci, staphylococci, coliform bacteria, and diphtheroids. Some bacteria incite superficial infection (particularly of the denuded areas), alter the character of the vaginal secretions, and thus contribute to the clinical picture. The types most likely to precipitate symptoms have not been determined, and the mere isolation of a predominant bacterial organism does not prove its etiologic relationship to the vaginal processes observed.

Not infrequently, *T. vaginalis* and *Candida* are recoverable from the postmenopausal vagina. Clinical infections from these pathogens are unusual, however, unless potentiating or predisposing factors are present. If a postmenopausal patient reports an irritating discharge, however, infections from these pathogens should be excluded before the signs and symptoms are attributed to atrophic vaginitis.

Cytology

The earliest demonstrable changes that follow diminution of circulating estrogens are apparent in the vaginal cytologic specimen. Depending upon the extent and rapidity of estrogen withdrawal, the maturation index of the cells gradually shifts to the left, with the number of intermediate and parabasal cells progressively increasing (Figs. 15-5 and 15-6). In some women, the vagina continues to shed superficial and intermediate cells almost idefinitely. In others, teleatrophy (100/0/0) rapidly develops. Since the response of the vaginal epithelium varies from patient to patient following the administration of estrogens, use of the vaginal cytogram alone as a barometer of the patient's estrogen needs is inadequate. Occasionally, squamous cell atypism is observed in the patient with a pronounced degree of atrophy. The intravaginal use of estrogens for 10 to 14 days will bring about a rapid maturation of cells and help to distinguish the atypism from that associated with cervical dysplasia or carcinoma.

Glycogen in epithelial cells progressively diminishes from the beginning of estrogen withdrawal. In advanced atrophy, a large number of red blood cells and leukocytes and a highly mixed bacterial flora with numerous cocci are present. Free nuclei of cytolyzed intermediate cells are found in some smears. The smear background is often "dirty," being similar in some respects to that of trichomoniasis. Occasionally the vaginal smear of postmenopausal women contains trichomonads. These are often associated with well-defined, amorphous "purple blobs" (Fig. 12-4, *B*).

Clinical features

The signs and symptoms of vulvovaginal atrophism usually develop insidiously. The changes that follow surgical castration and natural menopause vary only in the rapidity of their development. This cannot be accurately predetermined in any particular patient.

Symptoms. The majority of postmenopausal patients, even those with pronounced vaginal atrophy, deny having symptoms. Vaginal spotting, which is probably most commonly reported, may be spontaneous or may follow slight trauma. As a rule, bleeding results from a break in the thin vaginal mucosa, yet occasionally it arises from an associated urethral caruncle. The bleeding is rarely enough to be alarming, although all postmenopausal bleeding is a matter of concern until the source has been determined. The most meticulous examination sometimes fails to distinguish between vaginal and uterine bleeding; in this event, a diagnostic curettage is necessary to rule out endometrial disease.

Irritative symptoms include dysuria, external burning, pruritus, tenderness, and dyspareunia. The sudden appearance of these symptoms is probably related to bacterial effects upon the atrophic vagina. Dyspareunia may result from fissuring and ulceration of the vulvovaginal epithelium or from stretching of the deeper inelastic tissues surrounding a stenotic introitus or narrow, shortened vagina. Dyspareunia is more common in nulliparous women or in those who have had snug repair of episiotomies or vaginoplasty.

Symptoms of bladder irritability (frequency, urgency, and burning) are often reported by the elderly patients, since the bladder and urethral mucosa share in the postmenopausal atrophic processes. Fortunately, estrogen therapy will control many mild urinary symptoms in the postmenopausal patient, including incontinence.

Objective signs. The earliest observable signs of vulvovaginal atrophism are exhibited by the vaginal mucosa. As a rule, they precede gross vulvar changes by months and sometimes years.

As the blood supply diminishes, the vagina often loses some of its normal pink color and assumes a pale or pasty appearance. As the mucosa becomes thinner, diffuse redness may appear. The patient who develops a sudden onset of a discharge and

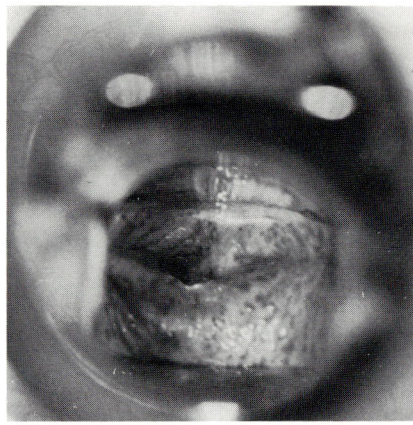

Fig. 15-1. Atrophic vaginitis. Petechial spots are often apparent. Vagina is subject to trauma and bleeding.

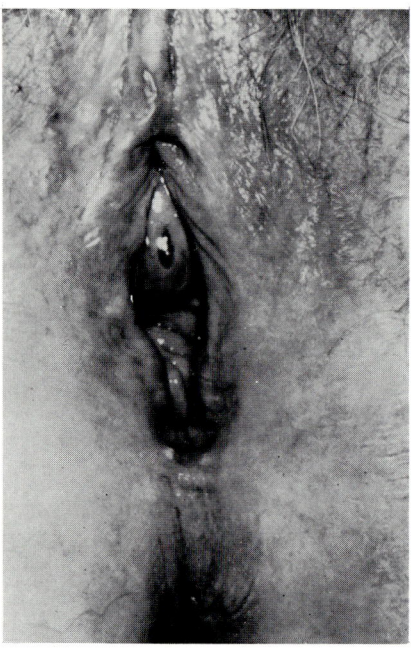

Fig. 15-2. Advanced postmenopausal atrophy of the vulva in a woman 72 years old. The skin is thin, hair sparse, and labia minora markedly atrophic. Most of these changes probably are a part of generalized wasting.

irritative symptoms usually has vaginal erythema. Because of atrophy of the papillae and general shrinkage of tissues, the vaginal folds and rugae largely disappear, and the vaginal wall becomes smoother and tubular. Petechial (Fig. 15-1) and ecchymotic spots may develop from exposure of the subepithelial capillaries beneath areas of advanced mucosal thinning. The mucosa then becomes vulnerable to trauma from intercourse and digital or speculum examination, either of which can cause spotty bleeding. Also, at this stage, minute ulcerations and areas of granulation may be observed.

In advanced vaginal atrophy, after the mucosa has lost most of its epithelium, opposed denuded surfaces may agglutinate to produce *adhesive vaginitis*. This is seldom a natural process; more often it develops after surgical trauma or irradiation (Fig. 15-11). Adhesions that form spontaneously or after abrasion can usually be separated; however, if left undisturbed for a long time, they may become inseparable, resulting in permanent vaginal atresia. Fortunately, aside from adhesions incident to irradiation effects, this condition is extremely uncommon. The possibility of postoperative vaginal adhesions might justify the administration of estrogens to elderly patients before and after vaginal operations.

An unusual change after complete estrogen withdrawal is the formation of gross masses of granulations of the vagina, especially of the lower half, and sometimes of the vestibule (Fig. 15-4, *A*). Thin sheets of granulation tissue, 2 or 3 cm. long, were present in the demonstrated case.

Shrinkage of the vaginal mucosa and the paravaginal tissues leads to some degree of stenosis. The earliest contractions involve the fornices, normally the most voluminous part of the vagina. All patients with long-standing depletion of estrogens exhibit this change. Annular constrictions may be produced by localized contractions at varying distances below the cervix, though a degree of stenosis of the entire vagina is more likely. Sexual intercourse is usually unaffected.

The discharge associated with advanced senile vaginal atrophy is highly variable, yet seldom profuse. The discharge may be purulent, serosanguineous, "gluey," thick and viscid, or watery. The color may be gray, yellow, or, rarely, greenish or chartreuse. Acidity of the vaginal secretions is always diminished, often reaching pH 7.5; as a rule, it is in the range of pH 5.5 to 7.0. Occasionally, a patient with symptomatic atrophy will have a relatively dry vagina.

Vulvar changes, chiefly in the nonhirsute areas, are usually apparent only some

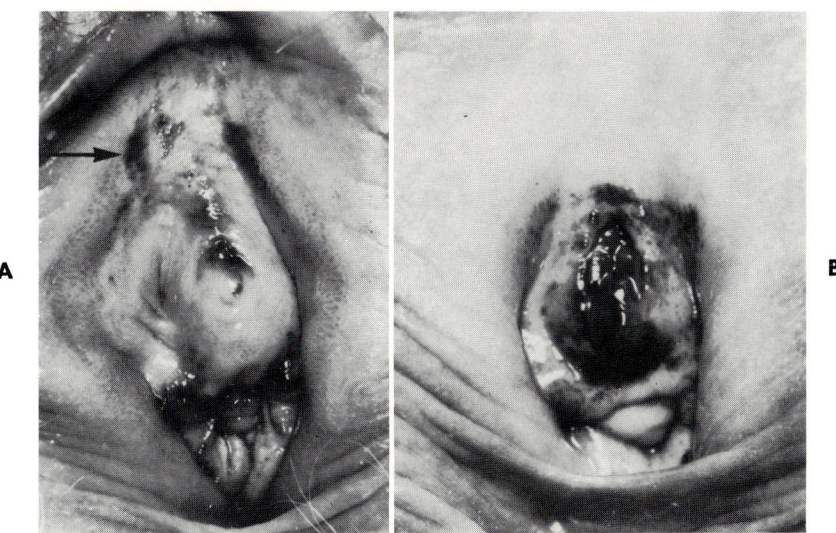

Fig. 15-3. Atrophic vulvovaginitis. **A** and **B**, Ecchymoses of vulva and vagina present. Both patients had advanced introital stenosis and severe dyspareunia. Both had bleeding following intercourse.

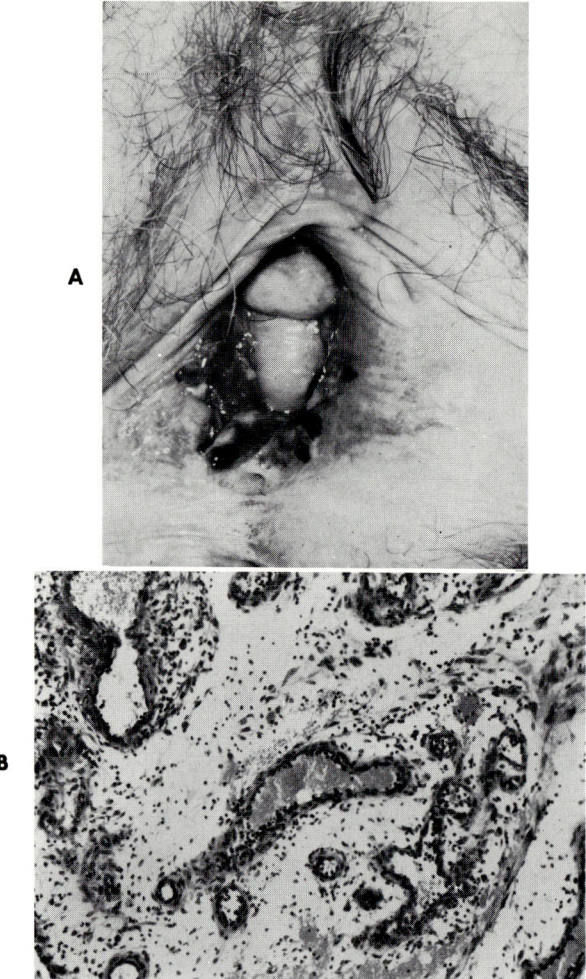

Fig. 15-4. **A,** Granulations of vestibule and lower half of vagina in a senile patient, an unusual lesion occasionally accompanying advanced atrophism. Note scanty hair. **B,** Microscopic section of lesion in **A** demonstrating granulation tissue. (H & E × 100)

months or perhaps years after vaginal atrophy. The skin and mucosal surfaces tend to become thin and eventually almost translucent (Fig. 15-2). They are easily traumatized (Fig. 15-3) and in severe atrophism areas of excoriation and fissuring are sometimes present. Distribution of hair over the labia majora and mons pubis becomes sparse, and the hairs become brittle and coarse (Figs. 15-2 and 15-4, *A*). The labia majora are frequently flabby and wrinkled, partly because of the loss of subcutaneous fat. The labia minora shrink in thickness and length and may almost disappear (Fig. 15-2). The glans of the clitoris may atrophy and disappear beneath the prepuce. The vaginal introitus may become so narrowed, tender, and rigid that intercourse is almost impossible, especially in the nulliparous patient (Fig. 15-3). With extreme shrinkage and retraction of the vagina, the urethral mucosa may evert at the meatus, constituting a variety of caruncle (Fig. 4-32).

Histopathology

During estrogen withdrawal, the vaginal papillae flatten relatively early, often before other gross signs of atrophy appear. Eventually the rugae almost disappear, leaving the vagina relatively smooth. The mucosa progressively becomes thinner and within months or years may be only a few layers of

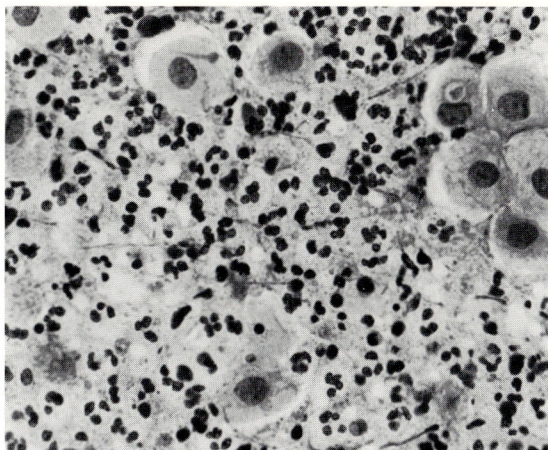

Fig. 15-5. Atrophic vaginitis. Cervicovaginal smear exhibiting parabasal cells within a background of numerous polymorphonuclear leukocytes. (Papanicolaou × 630)

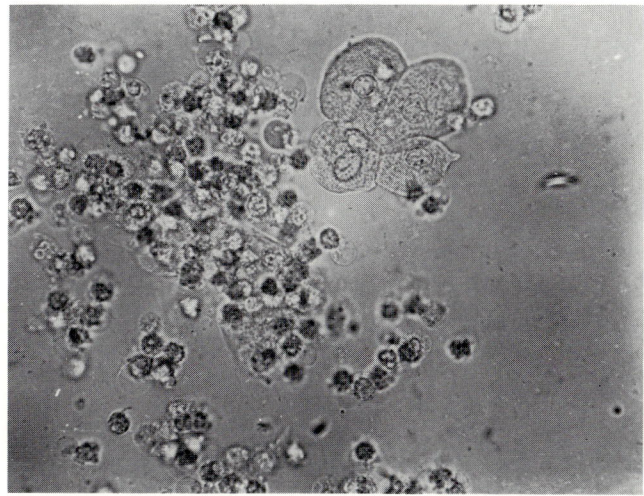

Fig. 15-6. Atrophic vaginitis. Parabasal cells predominate. An abundance of polymorphonuclear leukocytes are usually present. (Wet mount preparation, high power)

cells in thickness. A moderately thick layer of intermediate cells may be present in some areas, and only a row of basement cells in others. Ultimately, in some areas the vagina may become almost denuded of epithelium, leading to small ulcerations and patches of granulation. The cytologic smear at this time would show numerous parabasal, if not basal, cells (Figs. 15-5 and 15-6). The subepithelial connective tissue of most atrophic vaginas shows infiltration with round cells and plasma cells. When bacteria cause superficial infection of unprotected areas of submucosa, acute inflammatory reactions can be expected.

The blood supply to the vulvovaginal tissues is reduced, and some vessels become sclerotic. As elastic and muscle tissues atrophy and fibrous connective tissues contract, the diameter and length of the vagina are reduced. These changes are most conspicuous in the fornices. Advanced vaginal stenosis and gynatresia from inseparable vaginal adhesions might be considered final stages of atrophic vaginitis. Fortunately, both are exceptional.

Involutional changes in the vulva (Fig. 15-2) appear simultaneously with the vaginal changes, although less rapidly. Atrophy of the vulva is probably more closely related to the general bodily wasting processes than to estrogen deficiency per se. The changes include reduction of subcutaneous fat and elastic tissues, shrinkage of the labia majora and minora, and thinning and coarsening of pudendal hair. The glands of the skin and Bartholin's glands undergo partial atrophy and loss of function. The epithelium becomes thinner and the dermis atrophies. Minimal hyperkeratosis and a mild subepithelial inflammatory reaction may be present. Severe vulvar atrophy may be accompanied by secondary infection, inflammatory reactions, and superficial ulceration.

Diagnosis

Clinical diagnosis. Slight vaginal discharge, slight to moderate vulvar irritation, and dyspareunia in the postmenopausal patient are usually attributable to vulvovaginal atrophism and, rarely, to trichomoniasis or candidiasis. The typical clinical features leave little doubt as to the correct diagnosis.

Laboratory diagnosis. According to the stage of atrophy, wet mount preparations (Fig. 15-6) or stained smears will include intermediate cells, parabasal cells (Fig. 15-5), and, in extreme atrophy, basal cells. Pus cells easily migrate through the thin vaginal epithelium and pour through ulcerations into the vaginal secretions. The flora is usually grade III and consists of numerous types of bacteria. In stained smears the background is dirty, as in trichomoniasis.

Differential diagnosis. Widespread superficial vaginal and cervical endometriosis or adenosis, both of which are subject to minimal bleeding upon traumatization, might conceivably be mistaken for atrophic vaginitis. The distinction can be established by vaginal biopsy.

Grossly and microscopically, the vagina in acute trichomoniasis closely resembles the atrophic vagina after advanced estrogen deficiency. Findings common to both include ecchymoses and petechiae, redness and thinning of the mucosa, a mixed bacterial flora, and immature epithelial cells. The presence or absence of trichomonads in the wet smear would clarify the question.

Scant bleeding from an atrophic vagina or endometrial carcinoma is sometimes distinguished with difficulty. The doubt may often be removed by the administration of vaginal estrogens.

Desquamative inflammatory vaginitis, a rare condition of unknown etiology, develops in women with normal ovarian activity. The microscopic findings are almost identical with those in atrophic vaginitis; for example, the secretions contain many pus and parabasal cells. We have observed several such cases, as have Gray and Barnes. The latter believe that infection causes dissolution of the superficial cornified cells or prevents their maturation. This disease shows little or no cytologic response to estrogens (see Chapter 17).

Pruritus from other causes must be differentiated from atrophic vulvovaginitis. Lichen sclerosis et atrophicus, "leukoplakia," and neurodermatitis might cause diagnostic confusion. Histologic examination of the vulvar epithelium is frequently required for differentiation.

Treatment

As life expectancy is increased, more and more women reach the age when true senile vulvovaginitis develops and requires treatment. Should the philosophy of "estrogens forever" be universally adopted, however, the incidence of atrophic vaginitis might well diminish.

All postmenopausal women have some vulvovaginal atrophism, though few have such an advanced degree as to produce symptoms or warrant a diagnosis of atrophic vulvovaginitis. If the disease is of slight degree and the patient has no symptoms, no treatment is required.

Estrogens. Estrogens given systemically or intravaginally are highly effective. Administered by injections, they usually provide erratic hormone levels, whereas by the oral method a relatively uniform level can be maintained. Within a few days after institution of estrogen therapy by whatever route, the vaginal epithelium thickens; the hemorrhagic spots, excoriations, and minute ulcerations disappear; normal flora and acidity return; and, as a rule, subjective symptoms are relieved.

If the signs and symptoms are limited to the vulvovaginal mucosa, application of estrogens to the vagina will prove effective. Many preparations for topical use are available, including conjugated estrogens (equine) in the form of Premarin cream (0.625 mg/gm. of cream), dienestrol cream (0.01%), and diethylstilbestrol (Stilbestrol) suppositories (0.1 mg. to 0.5 mg.). The estrogenic creams (2 to 4 gm.) may be instilled into the vagina nightly for a week or 10 days, or until symptoms are relieved and the desired vaginal cornification is obtained. A normal, well-cornified vaginal mucosa is usually maintained by instillation of the cream once or twice weekly. Stilbestrol or other estrogenic suppositories can be used according to a similar schedule. Vaginal absorption of estrogens in overdosage can produce systemic effects that include nausea, vomiting, mastalgia, and uterine bleeding.

Although the use of bactericidal agents with topical estrogens in the early part of therapy has been advocated to control associated infection, it is our opinion that the combination therapy is rarely needed. Almost without exception, the flora reverts to normal within a few days after estrogen therapy alone. If such pathogens as trichomonads or *Candida* are present, specific therapy is required, particularly since vaginitis from these agents is potentiated by estrogens.

Among the effective systemic agents are conjugated estrogens (equine) available as Premarin tablets (0.625 mg., 1.25 mg., and 2.5 mg.), ethinyl estradiol tablets, available as Estinyl tablets (0.02 mg., 0.05 mg., and 0.5 mg.), and diethylstilbestrol tablets (0.1 mg., 0.5 mg., and 1.0 mg.). The smallest effective dosage is the one recommended, and the smallest dose of the foregoing preparations is probably adequate in the majority of cases. Quinlivan reported optimal results with 0.1 mg. of diethylstilbestrol daily. As is true of the topical agents, after the desired results have been obtained, the dosage may be reduced.

Contraindications. Patients with effective estrogen levels tend to retain electrolytes and fluid. For this reason, systemic estrogens should, perhaps, be withheld from certain patients with severe cardiovascular disease, such as congestive heart failure. Minimal dosages applied vaginally, however, should do no harm.

As a group, women who have been treated for carcinoma of the endometrium or breast should not receive estrogens. There may be exceptions, and some respected physicians do not follow the estrogen withholding policy in such cases. Subbleeding levels of estrogens probably have little influence upon the growth of leiomyomata.

Treatment for dyspareunia

When dyspareunia follows introital and vaginal constriction, systemic therapy is probably more beneficial because of the effects of circulating estrogens on the deeper tissues. An extremely valuable and almost essential adjunctive procedure in overcoming postmenopausal dyspareunia is digital stretching or "ironing out" of the perineum and lower vagina with well-lubricated gloved fingers. This should be done gently in the beginning, and only after estrogens have effected good vaginal cornification. Several treatments may be necessary. Advanced postmenopausal shrinkage of the introitus occasionally requires perineotomy. This can be performed under local anesthesia.

Treatment for atrophic urethrocystitis

Since the urethral and trigonal mucosae are also affected by the atrophic processes of the postmenopause, a type of urethrocystitis unrelated to bacterial infection may develop. The symptoms are similar to those of mild infection, including frequency, urgency, and minor incontinence. This abacterial, atrophic condition usually responds satisfactorily to systemic estrogens. Estrogen replacement may also be beneficial in recurrent bacterial cystitis. Caruncles usually respond to estrogens (see Chapter 4); rarely do they require surgical treatment. Urethral dilations, if necessary to relieve atrophic stenosis, can be accomplished after instillation of an anesthetic lubricant into the urethra.

Postirradiation vulvovaginitis

The vaginal effects that often follow radiotherapy for carcinoma of the cervix, and occasionally of the endometrium, may constitute a distressing problem for the patient. The changes arise from physical trauma to the vagina produced by radium applicators and packs, from the irradiation per se of the vagina, and from irradiation castration.

Varying degrees of *physical damage* to the vaginal mucosa are sustained during placement of radium applicators and packing materials used for distance screening and for securing the radium applicators in the proper position. The vaginas of older women, already atrophic and thus more vulnerable, are often partially denuded of mucosa from the trauma caused by placement of the applicators and packing. Also, varying degrees of necrosis of the mucosa may be sustained from the associated prolonged pressure.

The *direct effects of irradiation* upon the vagina accounts for the most serious changes. Damage to mucosa and submucosal tissues is particularly pronounced when the applicators and packing are not designed to effect good distance screening. For example, the use of Ernst applicators in a narrow vagina is associated with more destruction of tissue by hot spots of irradiation than the use of large ovoids in a voluminous vagina.

Radiotherapy, in a dosage sufficient to destroy cervical carcinoma, also destroys ovarian function, resulting in *irradiation castration*. The effects of the ovarian destruction are not fully manifested in the vagina for several weeks. Many patients treated for carcinoma of the cervix by irradiation already have postmenopausal vaginal atrophy; thus, destruction of ovarian function is less important to this group than to premenopausal women. The ultimate changes, however, are often more pronounced in the older group.

Cytology

Radiation changes take place in otherwise normal squamous cells even after a small amount of radiation has been delivered to the vaginal tissues. These changes consist primarily of cellular and nuclear enlargement, multinucleation (Fig. 15-7), nuclear wrinkling, and cytoplasmic vacuolation. Graham has attempted to use these changes in prognosticating results to be expected from irradiation therapy for carcinoma of the cervix.

It is well known that in the vagina subjected to intense irradiation for cancer, basal and parabasal epithelial cells predominate in the Papanicolaou smear or the wet mount preparation. Pitkin and Bradbury, in their sequential studies of the cytologic effects of irradiation, found that, for a period of weeks or even months, epithelial cells were essentially lacking in the smear. They found that basal cells were the predominant epithelial element during the following several months. The time of appearance of parabasal cells varied, although intermediate and precornified cells usually were observed only after months or years (Fig. 15-8).

One of us (R. H. K.), in a study of a large number of patients from 6 months to 25 years after irradiation, found that basal and parabasal cells usually predominated in a relatively clean background. Clumping of cells was prominent, the cellular borders in these

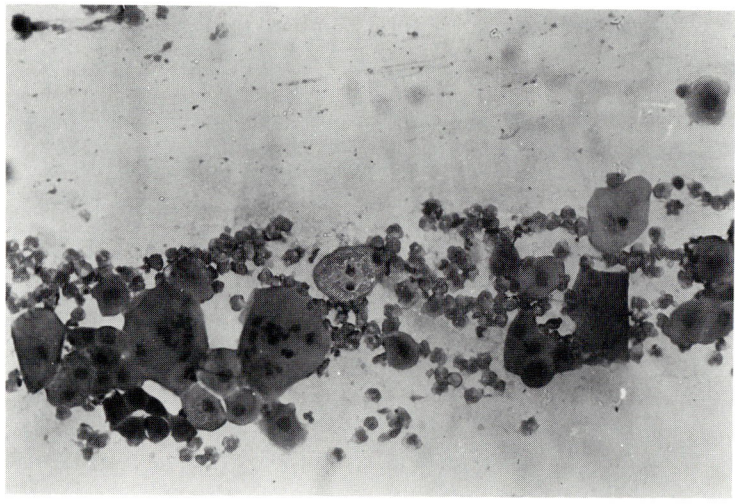

Fig. 15-7. Vaginal smear 8 months after irradiation. Red blood cells and multinucleated giant cells are prominent. (Pitkin, R. M., and Bradbury, J. T.: Amer. J. Obstet. Gynec. **92:** 175, 1965.)

clumps being indistinct and the nuclei being somewhat enlarged and irregular and having a homogeneous appearance without chromatin clumping. The cells within the clumps were frequently fusiform in shape and contained spindle shaped nuclei (Fig. 15-9). In smears exhibiting more pronounced late radiation changes, the nuclei were larger and frequently the normal cytoplasmic-nuclear ratio was lost. Many of the nuclei assumed

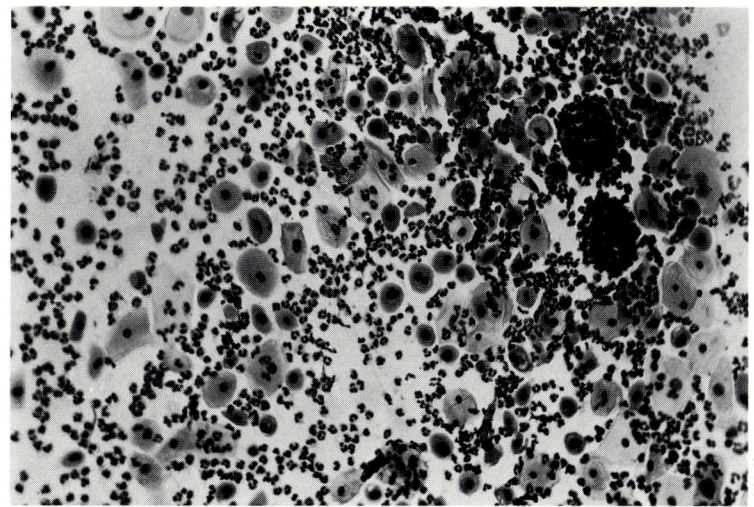

Fig. 15-8. Vaginal changes 24 months after irradiation. Parabasal cells and many white blood cells are present. (Pitkin, R. M., and Bradbury, J. T.: Amer. J. Obstet. Gynec. 92:175, 1965.)

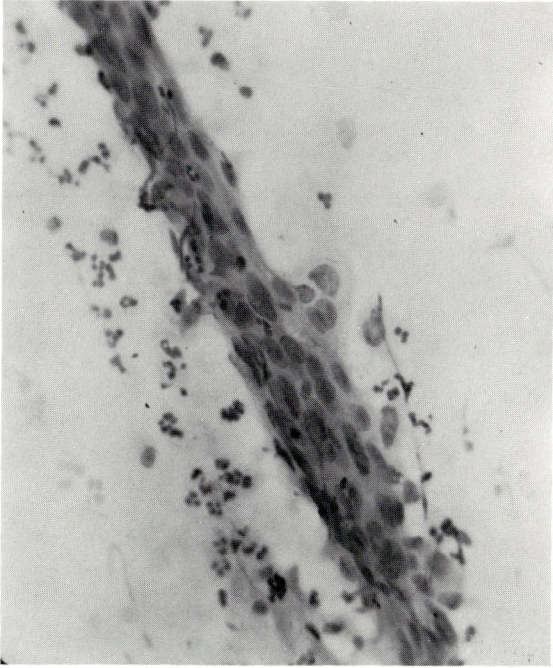

Fig. 15-9. Postirradiation vaginal changes. Clump of cells with indistinct borders and large homogeneous, slightly irregular nuclei, some of which are spindle-shaped. (Papanicolaou × 300) (Kaufman, R. H., Topek, N. H., and Wall, J. A.: Amer. J. Obstet. Gynec. 81:859, 1961.)

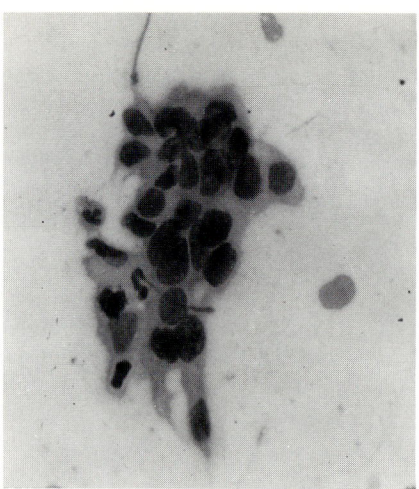

Fig. 15-10. Postirradiation vaginal changes. Clump of cells containing enlarged bizarre shaped, hyperchromatic nuclei. (Papanicolaou × 300) (Kaufman, R. H., Topek, N. H., and Wall, J. A.: Amer. J. Obstet. Gynec. 81:859, 1961.)

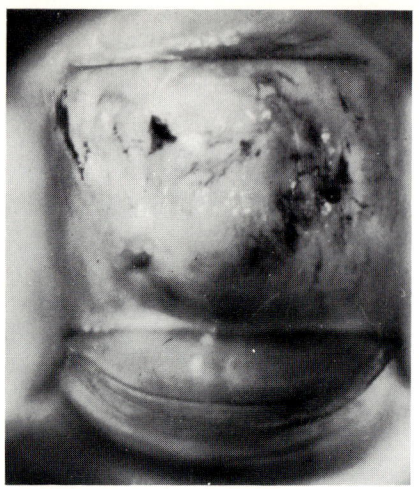

Fig. 15-11. Vaginal atrophy 6 years after radiotherapy. Pale, thin mucosa with telangiectases. The vaginal vault was completely obliterated.

bizarre shapes and were hyperchromatic (Fig. 15-10); little chromatin clumping was observed. Multinucleated cells were fairly numerous. It was believed that swelling of the cells, loss of cytoplasmic-nuclear ratio, and cellular clumping could not be specifically identified as late radiation changes. The relative degree of late radiation change was not significantly altered with the elapse of time.

Clinical features

Symptoms. A vaginal discharge usually appears within a week after the initiation of radium therapy. The discharge results from the effects of trauma and pressure necrosis incident to the radium applicators and gauze packs, from transudation and slough incident to the direct effects of the radiotherapy, and from the altered vaginal physiology and bacteriology. Following a reduction of vaginal glycogen, increased transudation, and altered flora, vaginal acidity soon approaches a pH of 6.0 to 8.0. The degree and frequency with which bacterial organisms influence the characteristics of the vaginal discharge are unknown, although it is probable that superficial bacterial infection increases the intensity of the reaction of the mucous membrane. The discharge may diminish after reparative processes begin, usually several weeks or months following treatment. The resultant atrophic vagina is subject to the same changes and symptoms as the "senile vagina"; however, they are usually more pronounced.

Contact and spontaneous bleeding, minimal as a rule, is experienced by many patients at any time after removal of the radium and may continue indefinitely. Spotting may result from the extremely atrophic vagina, from abrasions, or from the telangiectases that so often develop. Many patients report dyspareunia; this is easily explained on the basis of a vulnerable mucosa, a shortened, constricted vagina, and a stenotic introitus. Irritative symptoms such as pruritus and burning are fairly common.

Objective signs. Abrasions and erythema of the vaginal vault are often the immediate traumatic effects of the radium applicators and packs. The effects of irradiation soon appear, with the vagina remaining erythematous for weeks or months; during this time, it is usually tender and subject to trauma. Frequently a white "radiation membrane" covers the cervical portio and areas of the upper vaginal mucosa. Over a period of months, the mucosa assumes a pale or bleached appearance, and telangiectases develop (Fig. 15-11). Adhesions tend to form at the sites of maximum irradiation—between the ectocervix and the mucosa of the vaginal vault, as well as the anterior and posterior surfaces of the upper third of the

Atrophic vulvovaginitis 227

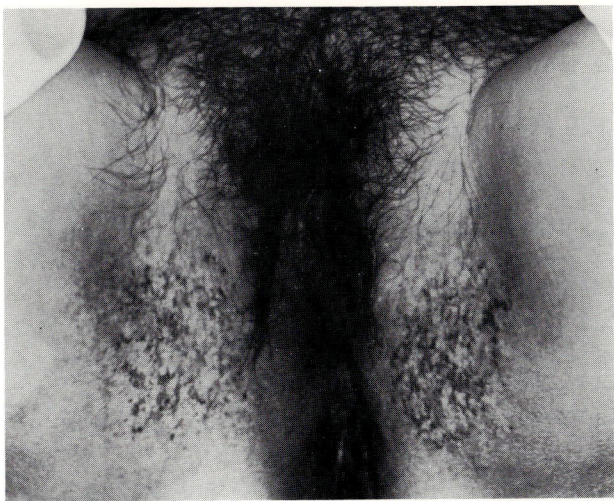

Fig. 15-12. Postirradiation (x-ray) changes of skin of vulva (poikeloderma).

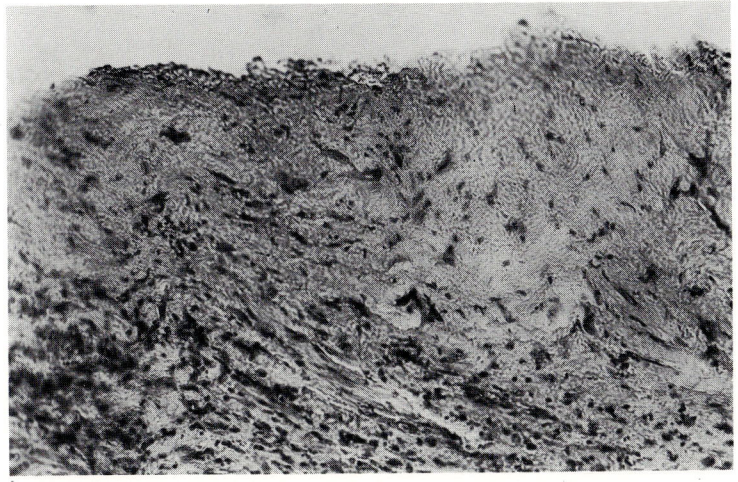

Fig. 15-13. Postirradiation changes. Vaginal biopsy taken 6 months after therapy for carcinoma of the cervix, showing lack of viable epithelium. (Pitkin, R. M., and Bradbury, J. T.: Amer. J. Obstet. Gynec. 92:175, 1965.)

vagina. These adhesions, if not broken up soon after their formation, often become permanent, causing occlusion of the vault and pronounced shortening of the vagina. The mechanism of occlusion of the vaginal vault is easily understood when one realizes that most of the surface epithelium in the upper vagina is lost following irradiation, as pointed out by Pitkin and Bradbury (Fig. 15-13).

Since the vulva is rarely subjected to intense irradiation, dermatitis from this cause is seldom observed. An example of postirradiation vulvitis (poikeloderma) is shown in Fig. 15-12.

Histopathology

As a result of the effects of irradiation and the destruction of ovarian activity, extreme vaginal atrophy can be anticipated in all patients who are adequately treated for cervical carcinoma. The sequential changes in the vagina have been described by Pitkin and Bradbury as follows:

. . . as a direct and immediate response to radiation, there was a loss of virtually all epithelium

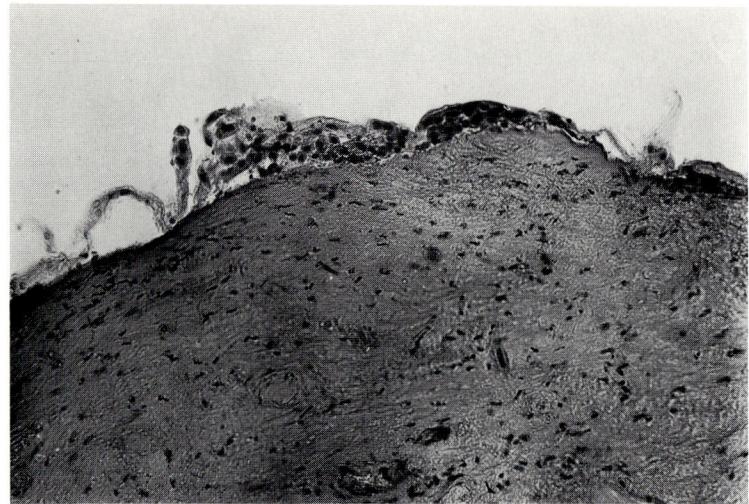

Fig. 15-14. Postirradiation changes. Vaginal biopsy taken 12 months after therapy. Only an incomplete layer of basal cells is present. (Pitkin, R. M., and Bradbury, J. T.: Amer. J. Obstet. Gynec. 92:175, 1965.)

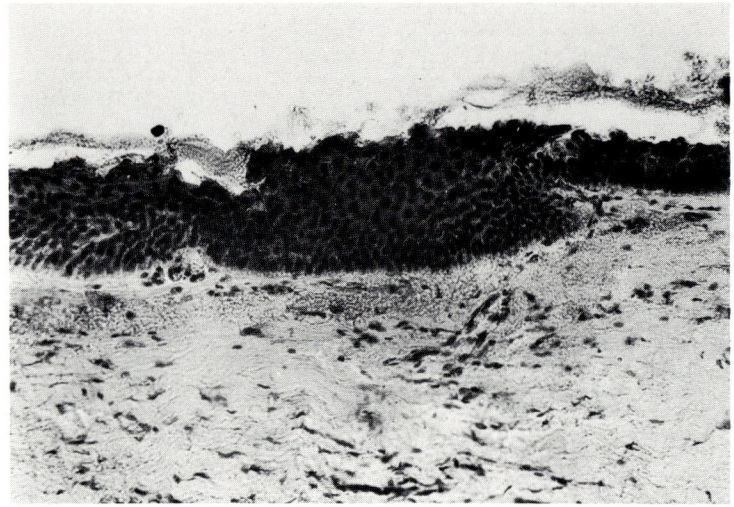

Fig. 15-15. Postirradiation changes. Vaginal biopsy taken 36 months after therapy. The entire epithelial layer has matured into an intermediate layer. (Pitkin, R. M., and Bradbury, J. T.: Amer. J. Obstet. Gynec. 92:175, 1965.)

[Fig. 15-13] in the areas receiving the maximal surface radiation and this loss persisted through the first 3 to 6 months after radiation. Following this period there was a beginning epithelialization consisting initially of a thin and incomplete layer of basal cells [Fig. 15-14]. The epithelial covering becomes progressively more complete during the second year after irradiation. There was maturation into the intermediate epithelial layer [Fig. 15-15]. When two years had elapsed after radiation the epithelium assumed a more nearly normal structure, although in no instance was a fully developed, stratified squamous epithelium observed. Inflammatory changes in the stroma gradually diminished in a manner roughly reciprocal to the epithelial changes.

Treatment

Since little evidence is available that cervical carcinoma is estrogen-dependent or that estrogens are carcinogenic in human

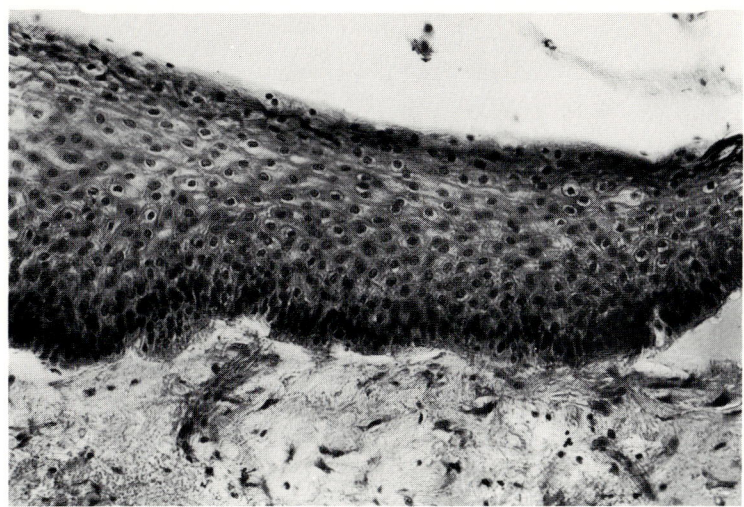

Fig. 15-16. Biopsy from vagina of patient in Fig. 15-14 after 3 months of vaginally applied estrogens. Mature epithelium. (Pitkin, R. M., and Bradbury, J. T.: Amer. J. Obstet. Gynec. 92:175, 1965.)

beings when administered in physiologic dosages, there appears to be no valid argument against their use following irradiation for carcinoma. Topical applications of estrogens to the postirradiated vagina accelerate regeneration of the epithelium, as may be demonstrated both cytologically and histologically (Fig. 15-16); however, the response is less rapid and less complete than is observed in the usual case of postmenopausal atrophy.

Grossly, reversion toward normal epithelium is less dramatic than the microscopic changes. Even under continuous topical estrogenic therapy, the cytologic findings may never indicate a return to the preirradiated status of the vagina. The majority of postirradiated vaginas retain their smooth, tubular appearance. The pallid vagina may assume a pinker color than before estrogen therapy, yet this, too, is incomplete. The telangiectases so often observed after irradiation usually persist to some degree. Neglected occlusive adhesions of the vault are largely unaffected by vaginal estrogens.

Some investigators, including Schwartz, Lynbrook, and Nardiello, have recommended the immediate use of antibacterial agents, such as nitrofurazone (Furacin), to reduce the amount and odor of the vaginal discharge.

Pitkin and Bradbury believe that vaginal narrowing and agglutination between vaginal surfaces may be prevented by encouraging continuation of sexual intercourse, although dyspareunia and vaginal spotting may be anticipated during this time. It seems obvious that vaginal estrogens and a continuance of sexual intercourse following irradiation may contribute materially to the maintenance of a healthy, functional vagina.

REFERENCES

Folsome, C. E., Napp, E., and Tanz, A.: Pelvic findings in the elderly institutionalized female patient, J.A.M.A. 161:1447, 1956.

Graham, R. M.: The effect of radiation on vaginal cells in cervical carcinoma: The prognostic significance, Surg. Gynec. Obstet. 84:165, 1947.

Gray, L. A., and Barnes, M. L.: Vaginitis in women, diagnosis and treatment, Amer. J. Obstet. Gynec. 92:125, 1965.

Kaufman, R. H., Topek, N. H., and Wall, J. A.: Late irradiation changes in vaginal cytology, Amer. J. Obstet. Gynec. 81:859, 1961.

Pitkin, R. M.: Personal communication, 1967.

Pitkin, R. M., and Bradbury, J. T.: The effect of topical estrogen on irradiated vaginal epithelium, Amer. J. Obstet. Gynec. 92:175, 1965.

Quinlivan, L. G.: The treatment of senile vaginitis with low doses of synthetic estrogens, Amer. J. Obstet. Gynec. 92:172, 1965.

Schwartz, J., Lynbrook, N. Y., and Nardiello, V.: Furacin vaginal suppositories: Their use with radiation therapy for malignant pelvic neoplasms, Amer. J. Obstet. Gynec. 65:1069, 1953.

Chapter 16

Viral infections

Specifically, *virus* is a term applied to a group of minute infectious agents, the majority of which individually pass through filters that are impenetrable by other microorganisms, and which are too small to be seen by light microscopy. Viruses are believed to be organisms or complex chemical bodies of the nature of nucleoproteins with an outer protein coat. They seem to occupy a position in nature between the living and the nonliving. True viruses have a core of nucleic acid, either ribonucleic (RNA) or deoxyribonucleic (DNA), through never both. The psittacosis-lymphogranuloma group and trachoma agents are not considered to be true viruses, since they contain both RNA and DNA. No criteria have been generally accepted as a basis for classification of viruses; it is probable, however, that an ultimate agreement will be influenced by their DNA or RNA content.

Viruses found in human beings can be grown in the laboratory only inside living animal cells, including tissue cultures, corneas of rabbits, chick embryos, monkey kidneys, and others. Because of an almost complete lack of independent metabolic activities, viruses are incapable of growth or multiplication (replication) apart from living cells. This means that they multiply at the expense of the host cell and only with the assistance of its enzymes. Since the enzyme systems of true viruses are primitive or lacking, they are immune to the effects of antibiotics. The psittacosis-lymphogranuloma group of agents, having a more complex structure than true viruses, is affected by antibiotics.

Viruses are adsorbed to susceptible cells, and individual types have an affinity for certain types of tissue. The cytoplasm or nucleus of some cells infected with viruses contains microscopically visible clumps of foreign material, which probably represent aggregates of virus particles. These collections of viruses, called "inclusion bodies," offer a clue to the viral nature of the disease (Fig. 16-1). Viruses infect all tissues of the body, though the gynecologist is mainly concerned with those that infect primarily the skin and mucosa. Viral diseases that involve the female genitalia are listed below somewhat in the order of their importance to the gynecologist:

1. Condyloma acuminatum
2. Herpes genitalis
3. Lymphogranuloma venereum (Chapter 22)
4. Molluscum contagiosum
5. Herpes zoster
6. Vaccinia
7. Behçet's syndrome
8. TRIC virus infection
9. Vulvar manifestations of systemic viral infections

Condylomata acuminata

Basically, condylomata acuminata or acuminate condylomata, also called venereal or genital warts, are wart-like papillomata of the genitalia. They consist of a fibrous tissue overgrowth from the dermis, covered with extremely thick epithelium (Fig. 16-7).

Etiology

Although absolute proof is perhaps still lacking, condylomata acuminata are believed to be caused by the same epidermatrophic virus that causes the common wart *verruca vulgaris*. Aside from minor morphologic differences, which probably are caused by local environmental conditions, the two lesions are similar.

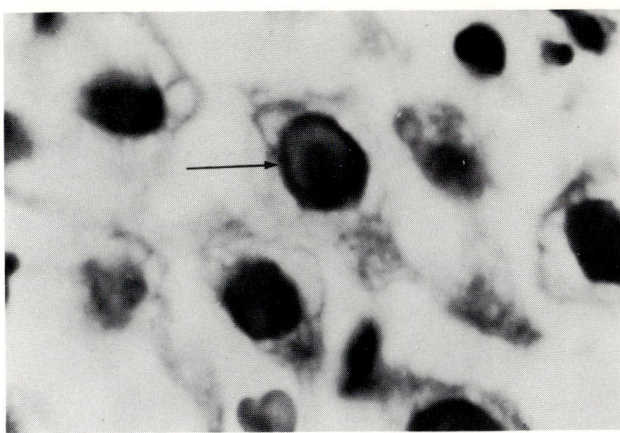

Fig. 16-1. Intranuclear viral inclusion body with clearing around the inclusion. Nuclear chromatin displaced peripherally. Tissue from patient with herpes genitalis. (H & E × 1020)

Women in the childbearing age are the most susceptible to condylomata acuminata, the growths being only occasionally observed before puberty or after the menopause. This fact might suggest a venereal transmission or a relative hormone dependency. Formerly, these excrescences were called venereal warts on the assumption that they were contracted only by sexual contact, particularly in association with gonorrhea. The most common method of transmission is still unknown, though it would be more than naive to assume that they are never transmitted by coitus. The frequency with which a sexual consort has a "wart" of the penis is more than coincidental. The sexually promiscuous and the patient whose vulva and vagina are bathed in leukorrheic discharges are more subject to the disease. Although such infections as gonorrhea, trichomoniasis, and candidiasis produce a favorable environment for establishment and rapid growth of the warts, they are by no means essential. Condylomata acuminata are also observed in patients without other demonstrable pathogens, leukorrhea, or habits of uncleanliness. They develop more often during pregnancy; at that time, the tissues not only afford a more fertile nidus for establishment of the lesion, but they also provide an environment that promotes almost uncontrollable growth.

Clinical features

Symptoms. Few symptoms are produced by the uncomplicated tumor per se, although they are often a source of chronic

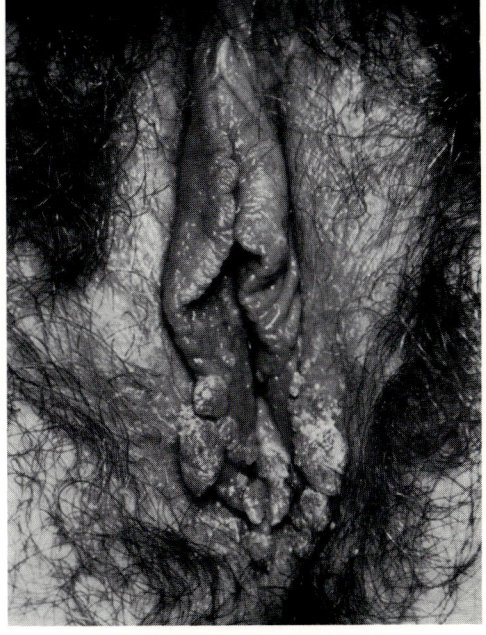

Fig. 16-2. Multiple, discrete, papillary lesions of condylomata acuminata. (Gardner, H. L., and Kaufman, R. H.: Clin. Obstet. Gynec. 8:938, 1965.)

annoyance to the patient. Associated infections such as trichomoniasis may produce a discharge, odor, and irritative symptoms. Infection with fusospirochetal organisms often involves the crevices of the larger lesions, causing a foul discharge and irritative symptoms. At times, the deeper tissues become infected and painful. Extensive lesions of the vagina, particularly during pregnancy, can give rise to severe pain and exquisite vaginal tenderness.

Objective signs. The vulva, particularly the vestibule and the labial folds (Figs. 16-2 and 16-10, *A*), is the most common site of this disease. Not infrequently, the lesions arise on the perianal skin, the mons pubis, the vagina (Fig. 16-4), and the cervix (Fig. 16-5), and rarely, on the mucosa of the lower half of the anal canal. The patient shown in Fig. 16-9 also had numerous warts of the anal mucosa. Pommerening, Hill, and Hammer reported eight patients with lesions at this site.

The early warts are small, discrete, papil-

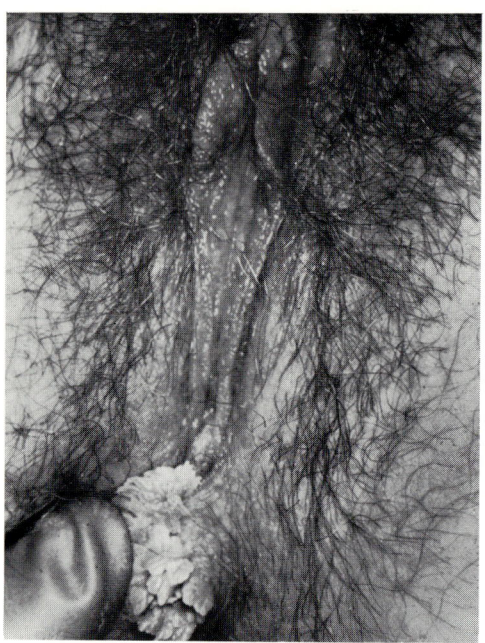

Fig. 16-3. Condyloma acuminatum of perineum resembling verruca vulgaris.

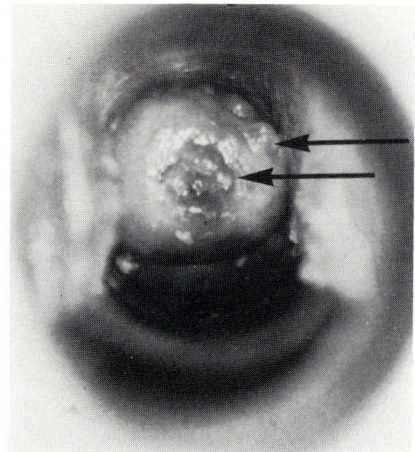

Fig. 16-5. Condylomata acuminata of cervix exhibited by flat, often white, papules.

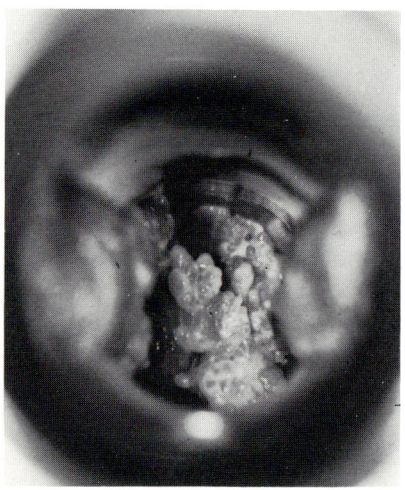

Fig. 16-4. Multiple condylomata acuminata of vagina in a pregnant patient.

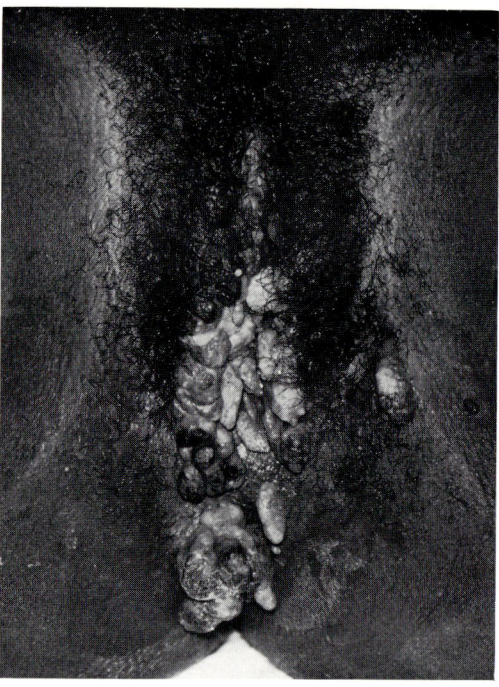

Fig. 16-6. Condylomata acuminata, present and untreated for many years.

lary, and usually multiple (Fig. 16-2). As they spread and enlarge, they may coalesce, forming large cauliflower-like masses with broad bases (Figs. 16-9 and 16-10, *A*). Many of these large lesions become ulcerated and infected and exude a foul odor. The color of the growths varies from pink to brown, depending somewhat upon their age and environment.

A variant of the usual condyloma is the condyloma of Bueschke. This is a large, single, sessile, frequently cauliflower lesion which, microscopically, may be mistaken for carcinoma. It arises more often on the penis than on the vulva.

Histopathology

The basic microscopic appearance is that of a markedly thickened epithelium forming numerous folds around stalks of connective tissue (Fig. 16-7). Prominent features include pronounced acanthosis, elongation of epithelial folds, papillomatosis, little or no hyperkeratosis, a variable degree of parakeratosis, and an inflammatory reaction within the dermis. Mitotic figures may be observed. The chief difference between the common wart and a condyloma acuminatum is the hyperkeratosis of the former. Usually, the corneum in condylomata is only slightly thickened and is composed largely of parakeratotic cells. The rete malpighii are narrow and elongated. Cytoplasmic vacuolation of individual cells in the upper half of the epithelium may be conspicuous. The cells are large, their arrangement is orderly, and their nuclei are uniform. These cellular characteristics and the sharp border between the epidermis and corium are useful in the distinction of benign warts from carcinoma. Although intranuclear inclusion bodies have been described, they are not consistently present and thus are not dependable diagnostic signs.

Malignant potential

Reportedly, vulvar carcinoma and condylomata are seldom associated, yet we have recently observed three patients with both lesions and have knowledge of a fourth in the Houston area. Others have made similar observations. The incidence of these combined diseases is too high to be explained by mere coincidence. Since many patients with condylomata who develop carcinoma have been treated repeatedly with podophyllin, a causal relationship is suggested.

Treatment

The first step in the treatment for condylomata acuminata should be the eradication of any associated infection that may serve as an independent source of leukorrhea. Specific therapeutic agents are currently available for most vulvovaginal infections—metronidazole for trichomoniasis; penicillin for syphilis, gonorrhea, and secondary saprophytic infection; the tetracyclines or ampicillin for *Haemophilus vaginalis* vaginitis; and nystatin, applied locally, for candidiasis.

Kaplan's discovery, in 1942, of the effectiveness of podophyllin as a treatment for condylomata acuminata was a significant accomplishment. Like Graber, Barber, and O'Rourke, however, we believe this agent is highly overrated. For small lesions, a 20% solution of podophyllin in tincture of benzoin and a 25% ointment have been equally

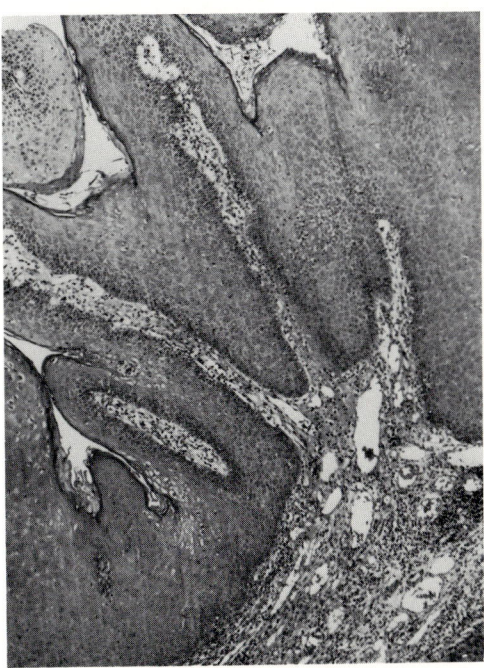

Fig. 16-7. Condyloma acuminatum with pronounced acanthosis, minimal hyperkeratosis, cellular vacuolation, and dermal infiltration with inflammatory cells. (H & E × 40) (Gardner, H. L., and Kaufman, R. H.: Clin. Obstet. Gynec. 8: 938, 1965.)

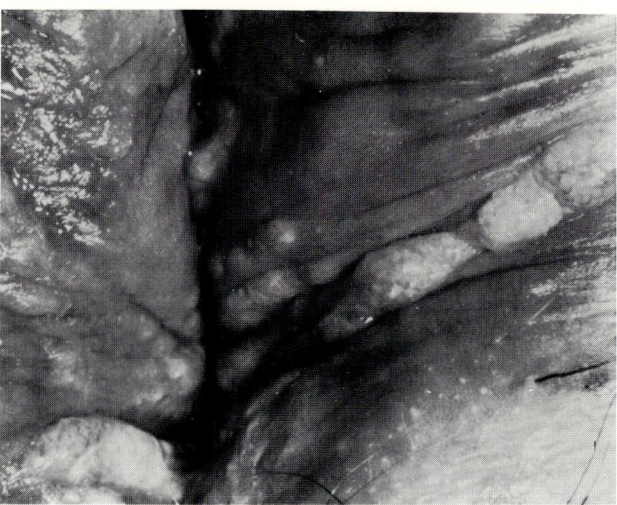

Fig. 16-8. Low, smooth papules of condylomata acuminata, refractory to further treatment with podophyllin.

effective. Local application will usually cause blanching of the lesions within a few hours and sloughing within 2 to 4 days. These effects have been attributed to arteriolar spasm and ischemic necrosis, although a cytotoxic affect may be the explanation. No scarring follows this treatment; the tissues largely return to normal within 1 week. Adjacent normal skin, although frequently exposed to the medication, is affected to a lesser degree than the warts; nevertheless, the surrounding skin should, perhaps, be covered with a layer of petroleum jelly. Complete eradication of the disease from a single application of podophyllin is unlikely; new lesions commonly arise within a few days, requiring further applications. Occasionally, the lesions slough incompletely, leaving a type of quiescent wart resembling a small, low papule with a smooth surface (Fig. 16-8). This is often refractory to further treatment with podophyllin; instead, desiccation or the use of escharotics, such as bichloracetic or trichloracetic acid, is required.

We are convinced that podophyllin should be reserved for lesions under 2 cm. in diameter. This does not apply to widespread, closely grouped smaller lesions. Frequently, podophyllin does not destroy large cauliflower lesions, and it can provoke undesirable complications. Incomplete necrosis and sloughing of large lesions may lead to the formation of craters (Fig. 16-9). A

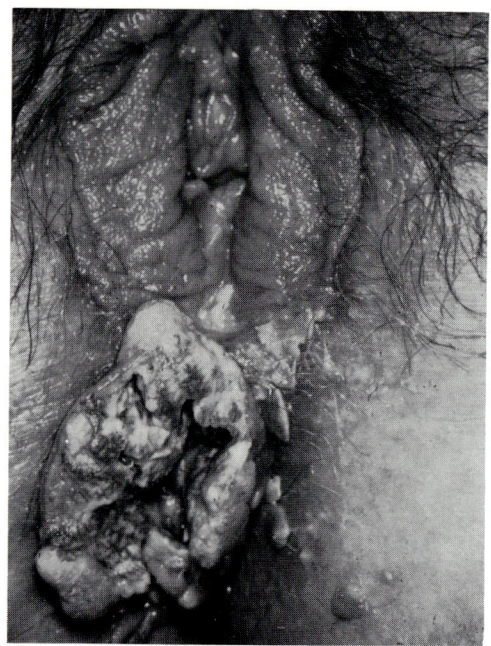

Fig. 16-9. Partial necrosis and deep ulceration of a large condyloma, following repeated and unwise applications of podophyllin.

saprophytic infection of the partial slough is extremely malodorous, and a low grade cellulitis about the base of the partially devitalized lesion may give rise to severe pain and tenderness. Large numbers of lesions within the vagina or on the cervix should not be treated with podophyllin at the same

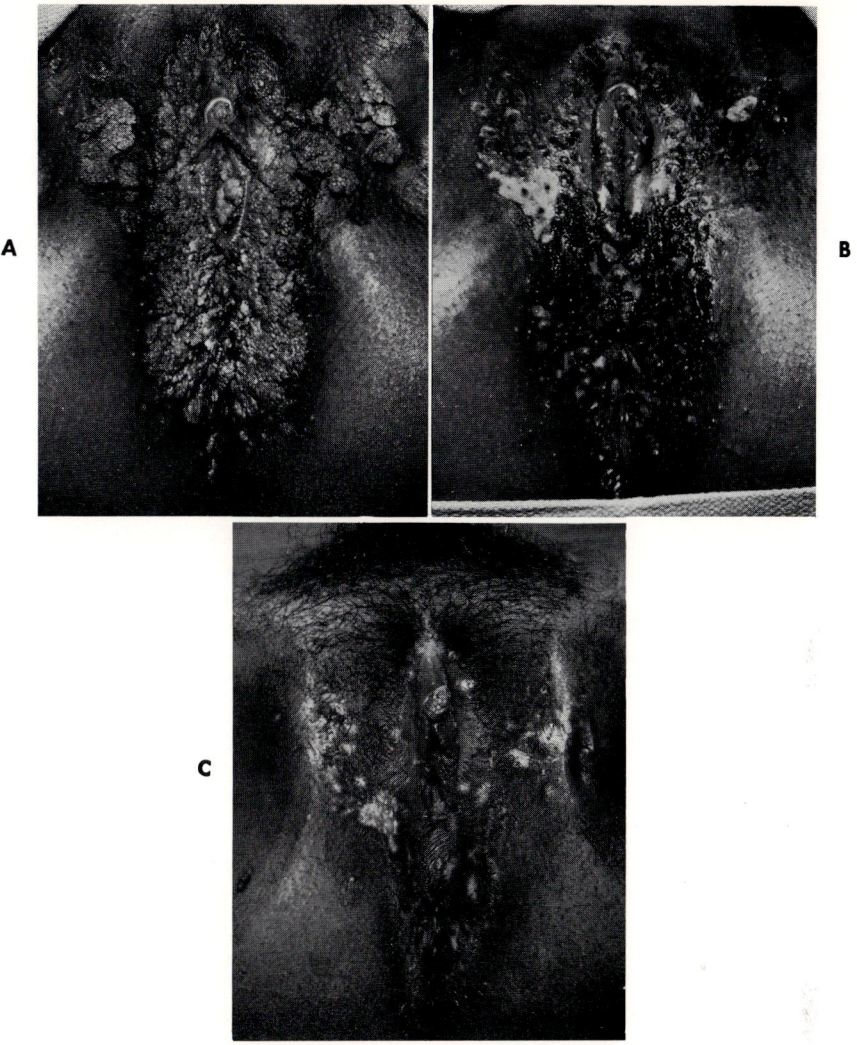

Fig. 16-10. Extensive condylomata acuminata in a pregnant patient. **A,** Before treatment. **B,** Immediately after hospital electrodesiccation and curettement. **C,** Two weeks following treatment. Several small new lesions present.

time because of the possibility of intolerable pain or a systemic reaction. The pain is experienced within 4 to 6 hours after application of the agent and may persist for hours, necessitating the use of narcotics. When practicable, the lesion treated with podophyllin should be washed with soap and water 4 to 6 hours after the application for removal of any residual podophyllin. The patient should return every 7 days for further treatment of refractory lesions and for treatment of any new ones that may have developed.

Large lesions are best removed by the *electric loop* or by *knife excision.* Sutures are often required after excision. For years, *electrodesiccation* followed by curettage of the condylomata has been effectively used by dermatologists (Fig. 16-10). The recurrence rate is low and scarring is negligible. We have found this method highly satisfactory as either a hospital or an office procedure. Desiccation in the office should be preceded by injection of the base of the lesion with an anesthetic solution through a 27 gauge needle. After desiccation, the lesions are scraped away with a skin curette or a small curved Bard-Parker blade. Graber, Barber, and O'Rourke have also found desiccation and curettage highly satisfactory;

they recently described the method in an excellent manner. The freezing of lesions with liquid nitrogen (cryocautery) has been effective in the hands of dermatologists and is perhaps a method with which the gynecologist should become more familiar.

Neglected lesions can spread and proliferate so rapidly during pregnancy that they may completely fill the vagina (Fig. 16-4) and produce massive vulvar tumors, occasionally obstructing labor. Vigorous attacks on vaginal lesions in late pregnancy can be hazardous to the patient because of the danger of serious bleeding, either immediate or delayed, and infection. Postpartum sepsis is also a possibility. If the patient with massive vaginal lesions is in the last month or two of pregnancy, postponement of active treatment until after delivery by cesarean section might be wise. Reportedly, the application of large amounts of podophyllin to lesions during pregnancy has led to abortion, premature labor, and death of the fetus. Gorthy and Krembs attributed a death in utero to arteriolar spasm of the decidua basalis, incident to the systemic absorption of the drug. During the puerperium, such lesions may shrink materially or even disappear.

Baker, in 1957, reported a 99 percent cure rate from the introduction of triple sulfa cream into the vagina twice daily. The lesions disappeared within 4 weeks after the institution of treatment. Although our experience with this measure has been less extensive, the results obtained from its use according to Baker's instructions have been disappointing. In 1966, Baker reported a revision of the treatment schedule. In addition to the twice daily intravaginal applications, he advised a 5 minute massage of the cream into all external warts five times or more daily for 6 weeks to 6 months. He reported that this regimen was 100 percent effective. His results await corroboration by other investigators.

Undoubtedly, many more patients have recurrent and refractory condylomata than is generally appreciated. For these women, discouragement must be avoided and conservative treatment diligently pursued. Powell and associates have reported uniformly successful results from the use of an autogenous vaccine prepared by extracting serum from the patient's own ground-up warts. Veterinarians have for years successfully used a vaccine for cattle warts, so it is reasonable to assume that a therapeutic vaccine for the human wart virus will ultimately be available.

For lesions that have failed to respond to all other methods, Sherman suggests external delivery to the vulva of 400 to 600 roentgens of radiation in divided doses. We have used the method with disappointing results. Barclay has reported the occasional need for vulvectomy for extensive and persistent lesions.

Herpes genitalis

Herpes genitalis is an acute herpetic inflammatory disease of the genitalia caused by the herpes simplex virus, type 2. Justifiably, the term "herpes progenitalis" has been largely abandoned, since the vagina and cervix frequently are affected, either independently or in association with the vulvar disease. The first case report of this disease, according to Unna, is credited to Duparque, in 1837. Slavin and Gavett were the first to isolate the herpes virus from herpetic vulvovaginitis. Recurrent herpes genitalis is the important variety of this disease, being relatively common. It affects only those individuals with partial immunity from previous primary infection. Probably the vast majority of primary genital infections are mild and unrecognized; the skin and mucous membrane usually exhibit no obvious signs. Many of the primary infections in which outward signs are apparent are observed in children between the ages of 5 months and 6 years, although we have observed such a case in a postmenopausal woman.

That neutralizing antibodies to herpesvirus type 2 are often demonstrable in adults indicates a high incidence (approximately 20 percent) of previous primary infection in the general population. Allegedly, all who have had the infection possess an antibody titer. Since the immune response is generally incomplete, the virus is probably seldom eradicated from the host; instead, it may be harbored in a dormant state in the tissues of the lower genitalia to subject the susceptible patient to repeated recrudescences of the active disease.

Etiology

Herpes simplex virus, sometimes called *Herpesvirus hominis,* is the pathogen responsible for herpes genitalis. Until recently, herpesviruses causing herpes labialis and herpes genitalis were considered to be of a single type. Several investigators, including Josey, Nahmias, and Naib and Rawls and others have shown that herpesvirus may be divided into two antigenic types, *type 1,* the primary agent of nongenital herpes lesions, and *type 2,* the primary agent of herpes genitalis in both sexes. Type 1 is occasionally isolated from the genital lesions of children. Nahmias and Dowdle (1968) have recently given a thorough review of the antigenic and biologic characteristics of the strains.

Recurrent attacks represent flare-ups of latent infection, whereas primary infections represent inoculation from an exogenous source—for example, direct or indirect transmission from a person with an active infection. Epidemics of cutaneous lesions have developed among persons, such as wrestlers, who have considerable bodily contact. Occasional transmission by sexual contact is unquestioned; however, the number of primary vulvar inoculations by this means as compared to inoculation through other routes is unknown. Nahmias, Josey, and Naib feel that most are from venereal contact. Reagan, however, is of the opinion that venereal transmission is most unusual. That herpes infections are frequently associated with other venereally transmitted diseases would seem to carry significant implications. Lazar traced the source of primary infections in two women to one male consort who had recurrent herpes of the penis. The site of a primary infection probably reflects the portal of entry of the virus.

Recurrences are often provoked by specific physical or emotional factors, particularly the premenstrum. The exact mechanism of this is unknown, though it is suspected of being associated with the premenstrual tension syndrome. Other triggering factors are respiratory infections, including colds, fever of any origin, digestive disturbances, trauma, exposure to ultraviolet rays, and emotional upsets from any cause. One of our patients frequently had flare-ups after extramarital sexual relations.

Incidence

The small space in gynecologic literature allotted to recurrent herpes genitalis is not commensurate with its incidence and importance. The underestimates of its incidence are perhaps explained in part by the delay of patients in seeking attention before the herpetic lesions have ruptured, and by the physician's reluctance to make a diagnosis solely upon the basis of superficial ulcerations. The incidence increases as clinicians become more aware of the infection and cytologists more accurate in their reports. Nahmias and others discovered numerous examples of this virus infection through use of the Papanicolaou smear. Rawls, Tompkins, and Figuero, utilizing serologic methods, found herpesvirus type 2 antibodies in approximately 20 percent of a control group of patients. The late Dr. Hunt, a widely experienced dermatologist in England, observed no patients with recurrent herpes genitalis among several hundred with vulvar diseases. This is surely a difference in patient material rather than a geographic difference, since other workers in that country have reported the disease. To describe herpes genitalis as extremely rare is erroneous, as it applies to most areas of the United States. One of us (H. L. G.) has observed over forty-five patients with the recurrent disease in private practice over a period of 14 years. Only five patients were observed with primary infections during this period; two were children under 4 years of age, and one, a 61-year-old adult.

Clinical features

Symptoms. The chief symptoms are hyperesthesia, burning, itching, burning and pain on urination, and, frequently, exquisite tenderness. These symptoms are less severe and of shorter duration than the symptoms of herpes zoster; usually, they persist from 7 to 10 days. Vulvar dyspareunia sometimes makes intercourse unbearable. Occasionally, some degree of urinary retention is experienced. We have found it necessary to place retention catheters in a number of patients. The inconvenience and discomfort suffered by patients who have frequent recurrences for a period of years can be emotionally disturbing.

When externally manifested, the severity and duration of symptoms of primary vulvar infections usually far exceed those of the recurrent disease. A sudden, unexplained burning leukorrhea is a common symptom of primary infection, but less so of recurrent dis-

238 Benign diseases of the vulva and vagina

ease. Another difference between the primary and recurrent forms lies in the fact that primary infection is accompanied by constitutional symptoms. These often include fever, malaise, headache, indigestion, and anorexia.

Objective signs. In view of its higher incidence, the recurrent form of the disease is the most important variety. The sites most often showing gross lesions are the vestibule, the labia minora and majora, and the skin about the clitoris (Fig. 16-11). Nahmias, Josey, and Naib (1967), their opinion influenced by the findings on Papanicolaou smears, feel that the cervix is the principal site of genital herpetic infection. The lesions of herpes appear as small grouped vesicles, similar to "fever blisters," filled with a clear serum that becomes turbid within 24 to 36 hours. Individual vesicles vary from 1 to 5 mm. in diameter. The epithelium about the vesicles is usually erythematous and edematous. The vesicles rupture within 24 to 72 hours, particularly if located in the moist areas of the vestibule. The overlying thin epithelium in these moist areas may assume the appearance of a gray membrane. On the dry areas, such as the outer sides of the labia majora, where the corneum is thicker and less subject to maceration, the vesicles persist longer, often drying and healing before ulceration develops. Lesions in the skin give rise to fewer symptoms and their bases are less erythematous. After rupture of the vesicles, superficial ulcers (Figs. 16-11, *B* and 16-12) persist for 7 to 10 days; in this stage, the lesions are difficult to visualize and may not be noticed. The bases of the erosions or superficial ulcers remain erythematous and are often covered with a yellowish exudate. They may coalesce, forming larger

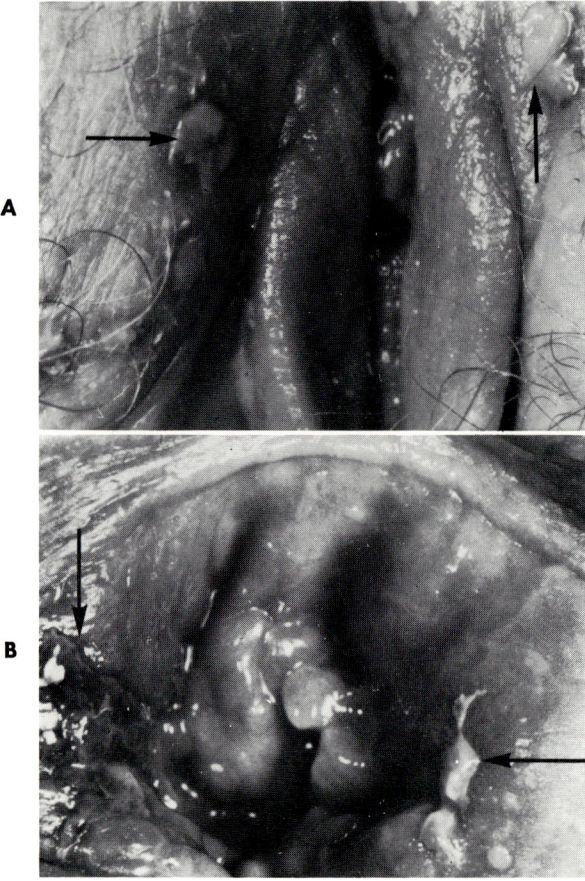

Fig. 16-11. **A,** Herpes genitalis. Unruptured vesicles of both labia majora. **B,** Herpes genitalis. Unruptured vesicles of vestibular mucosa on right. Superficial ulcerations on left.

vesicles and ulcers. Secondary bacterial infection can prolong healing and give rise to varying degrees of inguinal lymphadenitis. In the absence of severe bacterial infection, healing takes place spontaneously, without scar formation.

The typical vesicle is less commonly observed on the vaginal wall (Fig. 16-13, *A*) and cervix (Fig. 16-13, *B*). On these surfaces, the lesions often resemble a thin membrane or mucous-like patch. At times, diffuse redness of the cervix and vagina is associated. Reportedly, severe infection may cause a necrotizing lesion of the cervix that may be confused with carcinoma, although such lesions must be extremely rare. The primary infection, found mainly in children and young adults, when grossly manifested, sometimes spreads over wide areas of the skin and mucosa (Fig. 16-14). For example, extensive herpetic and ulcerative lesions may affect the entire vulva, the upper inner thighs, the mons pubis, the vagina, and the cervix. Our observations suggest that the lesions of the primary infection are associated with a greater inflammatory induration, often giving the impression of a flat papule. Primary vulvovaginal infections persist longer than the recurrent lesions, usually for 2 or 3 weeks or even longer. Also, a rather profuse thin vaginal discharge is often present, as is generalized erythema and edema of the vulva. Lymphadenopathy is more pronounced than in the recurrent disease.

Histopathology

The microscopic pictures of the primary and recurrent varieties of herpes genitalis are essentially identical and are similar to those of herpes zoster and varicella. The most prominent microscopic finding is the intraepithelial vesicle caused by degen-

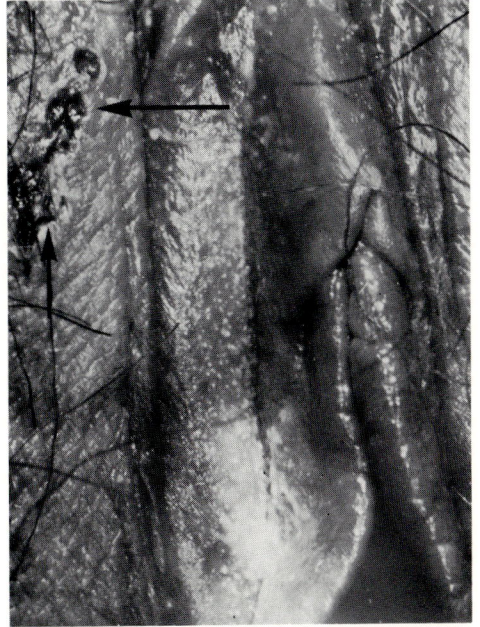

Fig. 16-12. Herpes genitalis. Superficial ulcers after rupture of vesicular lesions on labial skin.

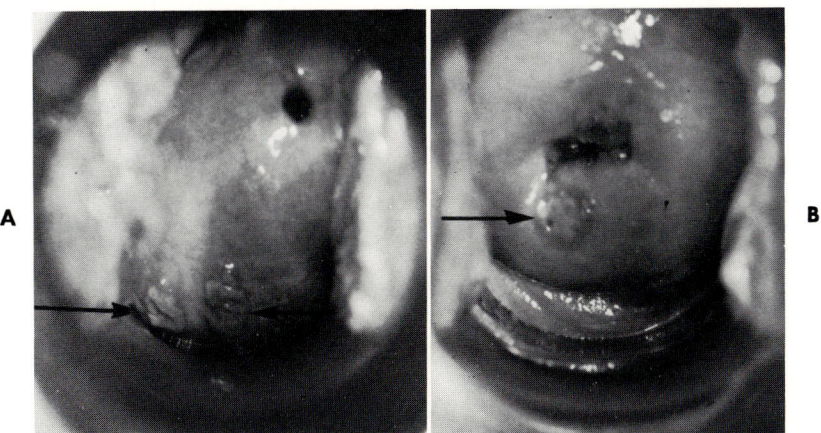

Fig. 16-13. Herpes genitalis. **A,** Lesions of posterior vaginal vault. **B,** Lesions of cervix. These sites are frequently affected.

eration of the epithelium, particularly acantholysis, and accumulation of serum beneath the stratum corneum (Fig. 16-15). Intense epidermal and dermal leukocytic infiltrations soon follow. If degenerative processes involve the deepest layers of the epithelium, a true superficial ulcer develops after rupture of the vesicle. Ballooning degeneration of epithelial cells is a characteristic of viral infection and is found more often than reticular degeneration, which is occasionally observed in other dermatitides. Degenerating cells frequently enlarge, become multinucleated from amitotic nuclear division, and give rise to the viral type of giant cells (Fig. 16-16). These giant cells are most pronounced at the edges of the lesion. Intranuclear inclusion bodies are often present, filling most of the nucleus of some cells (Fig. 16-1).

Diagnosis

Herpes genitalis should always be suspected in the presence of a herpetic or superficial ulcerative condition of the vulvovaginal tissue. If the lesions are recurrent, the diagnosis is even more certain.

Laboratory studies.

Cytologic findings. Cytologic studies offer confirmatory evidence of herpes simplex infection and afford a screening method for the detection of unsuspected cases. During the acute phase of the primary or recurrent infection, a correlation between the characteristic clinical and cytologic findings is virtual proof of the disease. The cytologic changes are most pronounced in the nuclei. Early in the course of the infection, the nuclei enlarge and the chromatin is displaced against the nuclear membrane, giving the nuclei a glassy appearance. This finding is observed in both mononucleated

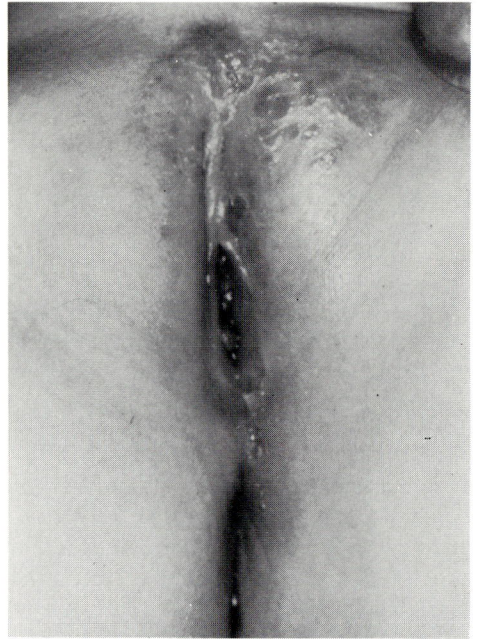

Fig. 16-14. Primary herpes genitalis in child 4 years old. Primary lesions are more extensive and persistent than recurrent lesions.

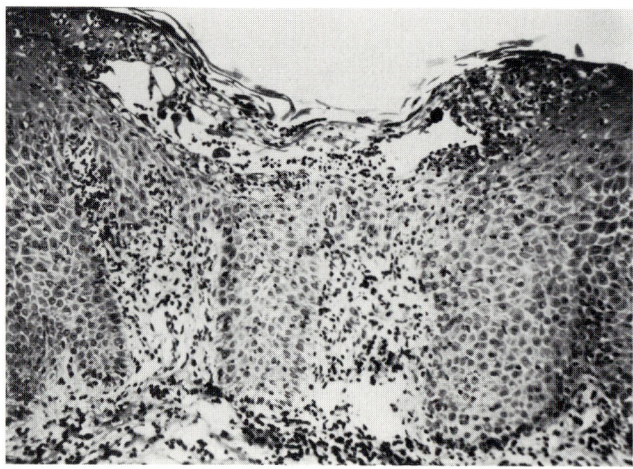

Fig. 16-15. Herpes genitalis. Collapsed intraepithelial vesicle. Dermal and epidermal leukocytic infiltration. (H & E × 100)

and multinucleated cells. Many of the epithelial cells contain a distinct acidophilic intranuclear body surrounded by a clear zone. Multinucleated giant cells are usually observed; their presence in any vaginal smear should always suggest this disease (Fig. 16-17). The cytoplasm of the epithelial cells is often vacuolated and occasionally fragmented. At times, bizarre nuclear changes, such as enlargement, irregularity, and hyperchromatism, may be seen. These changes should not be confused with those associated with a malignant lesion.

Rabbit cornea inoculation. The causative virus, when inoculated onto the scarified cornea of a rabbit, causes a keratoconjunctivitis in which the epithelial cells contain characteristic type A intranuclear inclusion bodies. The herpes zoster virus does not infect the cornea of rabbits.

Tissue cultures. The virus grows on the chorioallantoic membrane of chick embryos

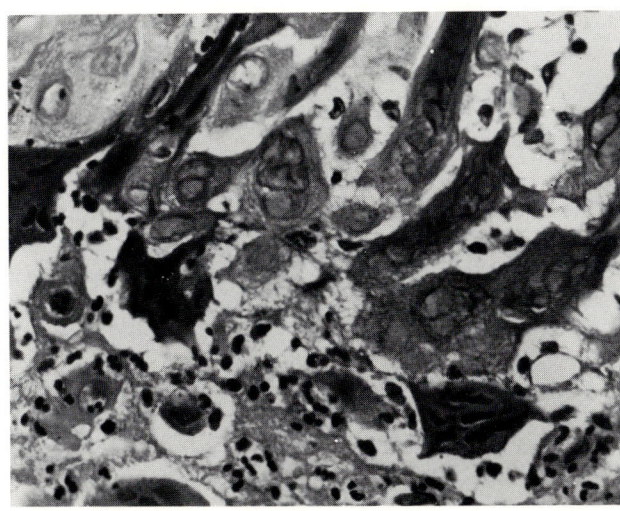

Fig. 16-16. Herpes genitalis. Multinucleated giant cells in biopsy from herpetic ulcer. (Courtesy James W. Reagan, Cleveland.)

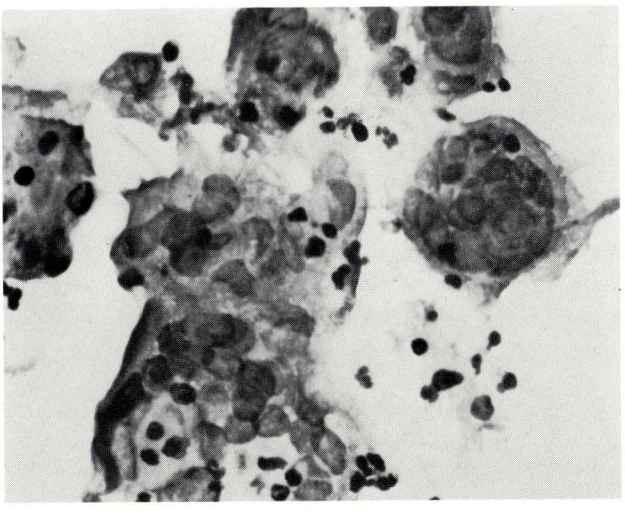

Fig. 16-17. Herpes genitalis. Cervicovaginal smear containing multinucleated giant cells. (Papanicolaou × 450)

and on HeLa cultures, producing typical plaques. The herpes zoster virus does not grow in these media. Various other in vitro culture techniques are in use for the isolation of this virus.

Smear techniques. The herpes virus is seldom observed in direct smears examined under the electron microscope. Biengeleison, Scott, and Lewis have described a rapid diagnostic method involving the use of a specific fluorescent antibody technique.

Serologic methods. A rise in neutralizing antibodies may be demonstrated using serologic methods. Yen found complement fixation tests by the method of Fulton and Dumbell satisfactory for demonstrating titer changes following suspected infection; a rise in titer during convalescence was accepted as evidence of primary herpetic infection. They considered a high antibody titer in the acute phase, which is sustained at essentially the same level in the convalescent phase, an indication of recurrent infection.

Differential diagnosis. The rapid course of herpes genitalis helps to distinguish it from most of the vesiculoulcerative diseases of the vulva. Herpes zoster rarely is a confusing diagnostic problem because of its unilateral distribution, its failure to recur in the same site, its longer duration, and its larger and more persistent lesions. Laboratory methods for distinguishing these conditions are seldom necessary.

Herpes genitalis may easily be confused with multiple chancres of syphilis, condylomata lata, and the lesions of Behçet's syndrome and vaccinia. When secondarily infected, the ulcers of herpes may be mistaken for chancroid. Excoriations from any cause, such as may be present in candidiasis, may be suggestive of herpes. The grayish-white base of coalesced ulcers of herpes may resemble a diphtheritic membrane.

Treatment

No prophylactic treatment is yet available for the prevention of recurrent herpes genitalis, and no specific method is available for blocking virus replication to cut short an acute episode. The experiences of Kaufman, Martola, and Dohlman have been encouraging; they successfully treated patients with herpes simplex keratitis by frequent instillations of aqueous 5-iodo-2'-deoxyuridine (IDU) into the eye. This chemotherapeutic agent is an antimetabolite that reportedly prevents multiplication of the virus. In view of the conflicting reports concerning the efficacy of both the aqueous preparation and the ointment (Stoxil ointment, 0.5%) on herpes genitalis, neither is recommended for the purpose at this time.

Lacking a specific treatment, palliative measures become necessary. Symptomatic relief is often afforded by hot sitz baths, wet dressings, or shake lotions. Wet dressings are difficult to use because of the frequency with which they must be applied. Nevertheless, such dressings as aluminum subacetate solution diluted 1 to 16 parts of water, Burow's solution diluted 1 to 20 parts of water, or a saturated solution of boric acid afford some relief of symptoms. Antibiotic ointments, with or without corticosteroids, seem to relieve symptoms and expedite healing in some cases, presumably by preventing secondary infection.

Recurrent herpes genitalis is distressing to the patient and must be taken seriously by the physician. Every effort should be made to discover and control the precipitating factors. An understanding of the patient's emotional problems might be helpful, as might the use of tranquilizers or sedatives at appropriate times. Aspirin, 5 gr. q.i.d. for several days before menstrual periods, has been reported effective in some patients.

On the assumption that the viruses of smallpox and herpes are related immunologically, repeated inoculations with smallpox vaccine have been advocated for the prevention of recurrences of herpes genitalis. The efficacy of such treatment has been disputed repeatedly, recently by Kern and Schiff. Should the method be used, however, the vaccine should be given between recurrences and should be repeated every 7 to 10 days until six to ten inoculations have been given. If any of the vaccinations "take," the next should be delayed until the site has healed.

Kern and Schiff conducted a well-controlled study to evaluate a specific vaccine prepared from inactivated herpes simplex virus. The results from the control material and the vaccine were essentially identical. Numerous investigators have oberved that over 50 percent of patients who receive repeated inoculations of a vaccine or "control substance" had fewer or no recurrences thereafter. This being true, such methods might be worthy of trial, regardless of the reason for the therapeutic response, whether it is improved immunity or power of suggestion.

Herpes genitalis during pregnancy

The effects of herpes viral infection on the newborn was first reported by Haas, in 1935. The chief danger from herpes genitalis during pregnancy lies in the fact that it can be transmitted to the child during delivery. It then may become widely disseminated, often proving fatal to the newborn infant within 12 days or leadnig to irreversible tragic effects. The more serious disease processes that develop in the infant include pneumonia, hepatic necrosis, necrosis of the adrenal glands, and meningioencephalitis.

Transplacental infection of the newborn, until recently, had not been proved in human beings. Gagnon recently published evidence that such infection had occurred in two of his cases. Nahmias and others feel that this route of transfer is rare. Infants of mothers with active herpes are rarely, if ever, born with signs of the infection. Instead, clinical signs, with or without cutaneous lesions, usually appear 4 to 7 days after birth. Apparently, infants most often acquire the infection during vaginal delivery or in utero after premature rupture of the membranes. Premature infants are more susceptible than term infants. It is believed that infants born of mothers with the recurrent disease, in contrast to the primary type, are much less likely to be affected. This is explained by a passive immunity acquired by the infant in utero from the mother who has an established circulating antibody titer. Whether or not an unborn infant can acquire full protection by passive immunity against direct vaginal contact has not been determined. The evidence is, however, that many infants born of mothers with the recurrent disease escape without contracting the disease or develop only mild infection with insignificant lesions.

Maternal herpes genitalis is of no serious concern during the first and second trimesters; should it develop as term approaches, however, apprehensions are justified. Until more is known of this disease, the logical method of delivery of a patient in labor who has active herpetic lesions of the vulva, either primary or recurrent, is by cesarean section. Also, immediate cesarean section may be indicated should the membranes rupture prematurely near term, although in such an event one cannot be certain that the infant will escape infection. Several reports, in fact, indicate that protection is largely lost after the membranes rupture.

All babies born of infected mothers should be placed in strict isolation, and the baby delivered by cesarean section should be isolated from the mother until she has a complete remission. Hospital personnel suspected of having herpes on any site of the body should be excluded from hospital nurseries. Gamma globulin given to the mother antenatally or to the infant after birth apparently provides little protection to the newborn. A few babies have survived herpes infections after massive doses of gamma globulin, but the mental and physical qualities of babies so salvaged may remain in doubt for some time.

Herpes genitalis and cervical cancer

Considerable evidence has been recently published suggesting an etiologic relationship between herpesvirus type II and cervical anaplasia. Nahmias and others, in Atlanta, found cytologic evidence of herpes genitalis in only 0.5 percent of 44,909 women screened. In contrast, they found that 21.7 percent of patients with cytologically detected genital herpes had cervical dysplasia or carcinoma. Their findings suggested a tenfold difference in incidence of carcinoma in patients with herpes as compared to the overall incidence of cervical anaplasia in patients screened. These workers concluded that herpesvirus type 2 must be regarded as a prime suspect for a cervical carcinogen, and they urge long-term follow-up of patients known to have acquired genital herpes.

The findings of Rawls, Tompkins, Figueroa, and Melnick, working independently, revealed that 88 percent of women with invasive cervical carcinoma yielded herpesvirus type 2 antibodies; in a group of control patients, only 16 percent yielded the antibodies.

Molluscum contagiosum

Molluscum contagiosum is a proliferative process of the skin resembling a localized neoplasm. The disease has a predilection for the vulva and its prevalence is greater than most gynecologists realize. The cases illustrated in Figs. 16-18 and 16-19 were not associated with lesions elsewhere on the body.

Etiology

A mildly contagious growth-stimulating virus, limited in its effect to the epithelium, is responsible for molluscum contagiosum. Although Bateman gave an accurate description of the eruption in 1814, Juliusberg is credited with establishing its viral nature in 1905. Growth of the virus is not supported by chorioallantoic membrane of the chick embryo. Neva, in attempting to propagate the virus in vitro from suspensions of the lesions, demonstrated its cytopathic effect on certain human cells in culture. Epstein and others recently demonstrated circulating antibodies to the virus. The infection is transmissible by both direct and indirect contact. It may be transferred at the time of coitus, yet this is only one of the many routes of transmission. Gudgel reported the finding of many examples of molluscum contagiosum on the external genitalia of men who had repeated intercourse with Korean prostitutes. Lynch and Minkin observed fifty-five patients with molluscum contagiosum confined to the external genitalia, 96 percent of whom admitted extramarital relations during the preceding 6 months. Snell and Fox suggest the name *molluscum contagiosum venereum* for the proven sexually transmitted cases. Autoinoculation of the skin of an infected person is common.

Clinical features

The lesions are usually multiple, the size of the individual growths varying from that of a pinhead to 1 cm. in diameter. The typical lesion is a dome shaped papule (Fig. 16-18). Beginning as a seedling 1 or 2 mm. in diameter, it grows slowly for weeks or months.

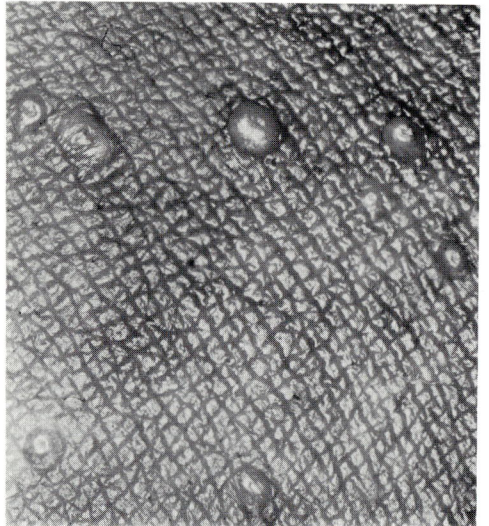

Fig. 16-18. Molluscum contagiosum of vulva. Dome shaped, umbilicated papules. (×3)

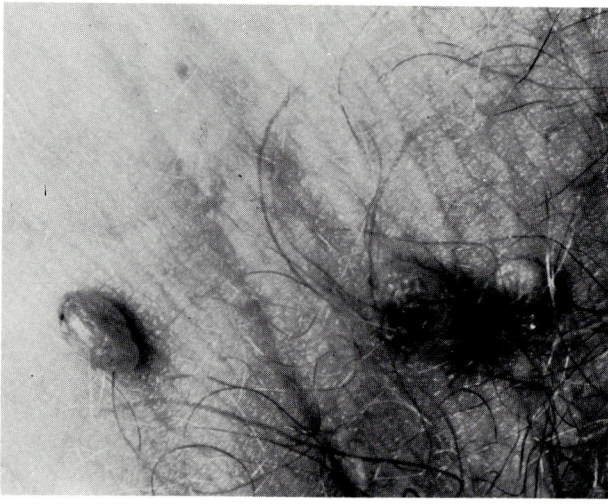

Fig. 16-19. Molluscum contagiosum of vulva, often exhibited by pedunculated growths.

Lesions can remain dormant for months or even years, with no appreciable change in size or gross characteristics being apparent during this period. During growth, the color of the overlying skin appears essentially normal, though later it may appear pearly. We have observed that lesions of molluscum contagiosum of the vulva are often pedunculated (Fig. 16-19); the majority, however, are attached by a sessile base. Necrosis and infection of the overlying skin may produce umbilication with an opening in the center. A curdy or grit-like material composed of dead epithelial cells and keratin frequently can be expressed through the umbilications. Aside from the rare case with associated infection, these lesions do not provoke symptoms.

Histopathology

Basically, the papule is a circumscribed mass of proliferating, acanthotic epithelium with hyperkeratosis. During proliferation, downward growth of the epithelium compresses the connective tissue of the corium to form a capsule. Many of the epidermal cells undergo degeneration as they advance from the basal layer to the surface. As these degenerated cells are desquamated, a central cavity forms at the surface. This degeneration of the epithelial cells is caused by the formation of cytoplasmic inclusion bodies, referred to as *molluscum bodies* (Fig. 16-20). The molluscum body contains numerous elementary bodies representing the virus; this is analogous to the Guarnieri's body of smallpox. Affected cells enlarge as they move toward the surface; the molluscum body ultimately exceeds the original size of the affected cells. The molluscum body compresses the nucleus of the individual cell, displacing it to the periphery of the cell and giving it a crescent appearance. The molluscum bodies near the basal layer are eosinophilic, whereas those in the granular layer become basophilic. Many large basophilic molluscum bodies are found within the horny layer on the surface of the lesions.

Diagnosis

The diagnosis is usually suspected by the characteristic appearance of the lesion, especially if umbilication is present. It can be confirmed by histologic sections. The vulvar lesions may be confused with pyogenic granulomata, nevi, epidermal cysts, acrochordons, neurofibromata, and even with syringomata.

Treatment

Manual expression of the contents from each lesion, followed by the application of carbolic acid to the cavity, is a simple method of treatment. Desiccation of the lesion or freezing with liquid nitrogen or carbon dioxide may also be employed. Another favorite method of therapy consists of removal of the contents with a small dermatologist's curette; following curettage, the bases of the lesions may be lightly desiccated or simply painted with Monsel's solution.

Herpes zoster

Herpes zoster, commonly known as shingles, is an infectious disease similar to herpes genitalis in that it is caused by a virus and is manifested by vesiculoulcerative eruptions. Although the disease is not uncommon, the vulva is seldom affected. During the period of 1953 to 1967, we observed only three patients with herpes zoster of the vulva.

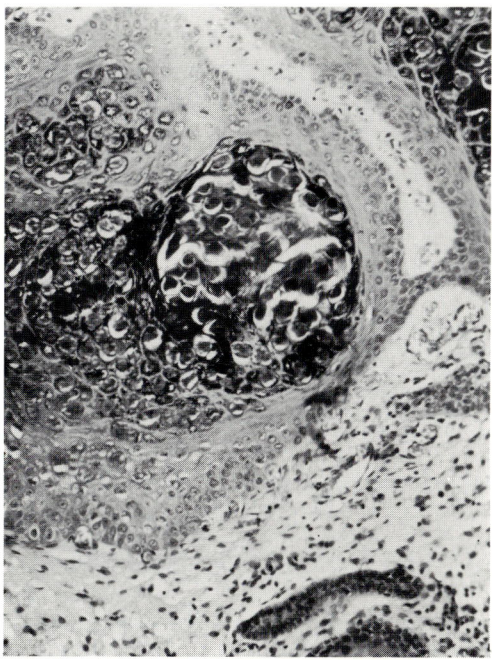

Fig. 16-20. Molluscum contagiosum. Numerous epithelial cells containing cytoplasmic inclusion bodies (molluscum bodies). (H & E × 100)

Etiology

The virus of herpes zoster is believed to be identical to that of varicella (chickenpox). Serological studies have revealed no antigenic differences. Varicella, however, develops in a nonimmune person and is widely disseminated, whereas herpes zoster is a localized infection of a cutaneous nerve segment in an individual with at least partial immunity from a primary varicella infection. The virus apparently first localizes in the dorsal root ganglion, from which it travels along the peripheral nerves to the skin. It is debatable whether herpes zoster is attributable to activation of a virus that has persisted in a latent stage or to a recent exposure.

Clinical features

Symptoms. Herpes zoster is a more serious disease and produces more distressing symptoms than herpes genitalis. At times, a low grade fever and malaise may be associated. A severe neuritic type of pain and hyperesthesia precede the eruption and may persist for weeks after the gross lesion has disappeared. The symptoms are usually more severe and intractable in older patients.

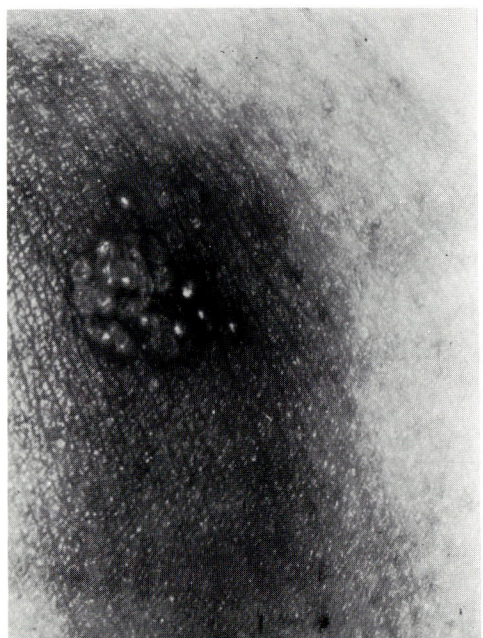

Fig. 16-21. Herpes zoster in genitocrural fold. Numerous vesicles on an erythematous base.

Objective signs. The early cutaneous lesion consists of clusters of discrete vesicles on an erythematous base (Fig. 16-21), and it is accompanied by enlargement and tenderness of the regional lymph nodes. Within 2 or 3 days, the individual vesicular lesions often coalesce, forming a maculopapular plaque of varying diameter (from a few millimeters to several inches). The lesions may appear only in patches where the cutaneous nerves branch to the skin. As a rule, they persist for 3 or 4 weeks. Although they rupture less often than those found in herpes genitalis, they do so at times, occasionally leading to deep ulceration and suppuration. The latter complication usually leaves a scar, with either hyperpigmentation or hypopigmentation of the involved skin. Since herpes zoster starts as a nerve root infection, lesions do not ordinarily cross the midline—a point of diagnostic significance.

Histopathology

Microscopically, the cutaneous lesions are indistinguishable from those of herpes genitalis and varicella. Histologic characteristics common to all include intradermal vesiculation from severe degeneration of the ballooning and reticular types. Intranuclear inclusion bodies in the degenerated epidermal cells are also often observed.

In addition to the cutaneous changes, herpes zoster involves the neural segments supplying the affected skin. The dorsal root ganglion and posterior nerve roots are severely inflamed, and segmental poliomyelitis is observed in the posterior column of the spinal cord.

Diagnosis

Unlike herpes genitalis, recurrences of herpes zoster rarely develop in previously affected sites. Since the two lesions differ in their gross appearance, symptoms, and clinical course, a distinction should be easily established. Any vesicular eruption of the skin could be confused with herpes zoster, yet the location of the lesions along nerve pathways, failure to cross the midline, and severe symptoms should simplify the distinction of herpes zoster. The laboratory distinction between herpes genitalis and herpes zoster is discussed elsewhere in this chapter.

Treatment

No specific cure for this condition is known. The chief objectives are the relief of pain and prevention of bacterial infection and scarring at the site of the lesions. An antibiotic ointment may be applied with the intent of preventing or eradicating secondary infection. Corticosteroids, given locally or systemically, are of questionable value; however, Knox has found that 40 mg. of triamcinolone acetonide (Kenalog) intramuscularly minimizes symptoms and decreases posttherapeutic pain. Since this is a true virus infection, systemic antibiotics do not materially affect its clinical course, unless, perhaps, secondary bacterial cellulitis and lymphadenitis are present. The relief of pain, which is often the chief object of treatment, can usually be accomplished with such agents as codeine or propoxyphene hydrochloride (Darvon). A cooling topical lotion, such as calamine with 0.25% menthol, affords some relief, particularly in the early stages of the disease. Ointments may be required, particularly during the dry and crusted stage of the lesion.

Vaccinia of the vulva

As a rule, vaccinia of the vulva is induced by accidental inoculation of the vulvar tissues with lymph from the vesicopustule that forms after successful smallpox vaccination. Because of the immunity that develops soon after vaccination, the interval between the date of vaccination and the appearance of the secondary vulvar lesions in the autoinoculated patient rarely exceeds 10 days. Cases of primary vulvar vaccinia have followed intercourse with men recently vaccinated and following accidental inoculation with commercial vaccine. According to Humphrey, autoinoculation is most common in children, whereas heteroinoculation is usually responsible for the infection in adults.

The incidence of this complication of vaccination would be exceedingly difficult to determine. It is considered to be extremely rare, although it is probably more prevalent than is supposed, since the majority of cases are either unrecognized or unrecorded. Humphrey, in reviewing the world literature in 1963, found only seventy recorded cases, which were almost equally divided between adults and children.

Clinical features

Heteroinoculation of an unvaccinated person from a vesicopustule of a recently vaccinated person, or autoinoculation from fingers contaminated with material used for routine vaccination, may produce primary lesions and consequent scarring such as follows any initial vaccination. Autoinoculation from the primary vaccination site several days after vaccination is followed by rapidly developing lesions and, usually, subsequent healing without scarring. Most lesions that develop in the previously vaccinated individuals are mild and of the vaccinoid type. Depending upon the degree of immunity, therefore, the severity of a vulvar vaccinia varies from a short-lived immune response to an extensive vulvitis exhibiting all the signs of acute inflammation, including redness, edema, vesiculation, and pustule formation.

The characteristic vesicopustule of the vulva, particularly in the nonimmune patient, is umbilicated. The number of vesicular lesions varies from one to many. They tend to become confluent within a short time and, because of the moisture of the area, ulcerate rapidly. Varying degrees of inguinal lymphadenitis are always present, and a mild elevation of temperature is not unusual. Secondary bacterial infection often develops.

The symptoms include one or more of the following: pain, itching, burning, and dysuria. Pronounced involvement of the meatal area may lead to urinary retention. Constitutional symptoms are not uncommon.

Histopathology

According to Lever, in the center of the vesicles or pustules the epidermis is usually necrotic, while at the periphery reticular and ballooning degeneration may be observed. In view of the innumerable inflammatory cells, the demonstration of inclusion bodies in the cytoplasm is often difficult.

Diagnosis

The nature of vulvar vaccinia should be suspected whenever multiple vesicular lesions appear within 10 days after a successful primary vaccination. Central umbilication of the vesicopustules should also suggest the presence of this disease.

The diagnosis may be confirmed by laboratory tests, including isolation of the vaccinia virus on chorioallantoic membrane of the chick embryo or in tissue culture. In addition, inoculation of material from a suspected lesion into the scarified cornea of a rabbit (Paul's test) will produce characteristic lesions.

The conditions for which vaccinia of the vulva may be mistaken have been considered rather completely by Weary and others. In a large percentage of cases, primary vaccinia of the vulva is confused with a venereal disease; a falsely positive serologic test for syphilis may be caused by vaccination. Primary herpes genitalis is especially likely to be confusing; here, however, the vesicles are not umbilicated, as are those of vaccinia. A change in specific antibody titers in patients with these two conditions will point to the diagnosis. While the viruses of both vaccinia and herpes genitalis produce lesions of the cornea of a rabbit, in vaccinia cytoplastic inclusion bodies are present, and in herpes the inclusion bodies are intranuclear. The vesicular serum in vaccinia contains elementary bodies, whereas the serum in herpes genitalis is likely to contain epithelial giant cells.

Treatment

Since, in the absence of secondary bacterial infection, the vesicular lesions rapidly resolve, the application of cooling lotions is generally adequate. Antibiotics, applied locally or administered systemically, might be useful for controlling or preventing bacterial infection. Bjornberg, Hellgren, and Seebert, in a double blind study, showed that idoxuridine (IDU) does not significantly affect the course of cutaneous vaccinia.

Behçet's syndrome

The "triple symptom complex" of Behçet is observed primarily in the Mediterranean area; it is found only rarely in the United States, especially by gynecologists. Although the disease complex is characterized chiefly by genital and oral ulcerations and ocular inflammation, other clinical manifestations are occasionally associated. These include disorders of the skin resembling erythema nodosum and erythema multiforme, disturbances of the central nervous system, arthritic disease, and thrombophlebitis. Behçet's name was given the entity following the publication of several of his papers on the subject. Ephraim considered the lesion to be similar to ulcus vulvae acutum (Lipschütz ulcer), whereas Phillips and Scott pointedly state that ulcus vulvae acutum are identical with the genital and oral lesions of Behçet's syndrome. The medical literature on the subject was well reviewed by Ayers in 1965.

Etiology

Behçet's descriptions included elementary bodies in cells. The entity has since been generally accepted as being of a viral nature, although there is no unanimity of opinion on this point. Sezer claimed the isolation of a specific virus which, when injected into animals, produced disease of the nature of Behçet's syndrome. Sezer also reported positive antibody titers in convalescent serum. Other workers, including Mortata and Imam, claimed isolation of the virus as well as the discovery of inclusions in scrapings. Phillips and Scott believe that the syndrome may eventually fall into place among collagen diseases. Dudgeon, on the basis of its natural history, pathogenesis, and pathology, does not consider the disease to be of viral origin.

Clinical features

The ulcers begin as small vesicles or papules (Figs. 16-22 and 16-23), ulcerate, become craterous, and are usually covered by a gray slough. They vary in diameter from a few millimeters to several centimeters, tend to heal and recur at intervals, and may last for only a short time or persist for weeks. Those on the mouth, eyes, and genitals may appear on separate occasions. The genital lesions may involve the vulva, vagina, and cervix, and healing may be followed by fibrosis, scarring, and labial perforation. Pain and dyspareunia are the outstanding symptoms, often preceding the visible lesions by several days; incapacitating pain may persist even after the ulcers have healed.

The oral and genital lesions are similar, though the former tend to be smaller and heal more rapidly and without scarring. Ocular lesions begin as a superficial inflammation, at times proceeding to iridocyclitis and even blindness. Lesions involving the joints are of the nature of an arthritis, are monoarticular, and recur in the same joint.

Neural symptoms vary from headache and dizziness to major seizures and death. The joints and nervous system are affected in only the most severe cases.

Histopathology

Most reports of the microscopic appearance of the lesions describe no distinguishing features. The tissues exhibit a chronic inflammatory reaction with granulation.

Diagnosis

The diagnosis may be suspected if the characteristic ulcerative lesions persist beyond 10 to 12 days and involve either the genitalia alone or both the mouth and genitalia at the same time or on separate occasions. This is especially true if a history of exacerbations and remissions of the lesions in both sites is reported. Months or years may separate the appearance of the lesions in the various structures. The patient in Fig. 16-22 had only vulvar, vaginal, and cervical lesions. Subsequent involvement of the eyes is confirmatory evidence of the nature of the condition.

A distinction between herpes genitalis and Behçet's syndrome should be possible from the different clinical course and gross features of the lesions. In Behçet's syndrome, the ulcers are larger and deeper and tend to be more persistent. Laboratory tests are useful for excluding other ulcerative lesions, such as those caused by chancroid, venereal granulomata, and syphilis.

Treatment

Despite its alleged viral nature, systemic corticosteroids are the most consistently successful treatment for this syndrome. The response to other forms of therapy, including antibiotics, has been variable. Since the disease tends to be cyclic, the efficacy of any type of treatment may be falsely interpreted.

TRIC virus genitourinary infection

For many years, pediatricians and ophthalmologists have been aware of a bacteria-free ophthalmia neonatorum, termed *inclusion blennorrhea*, which is now known to be

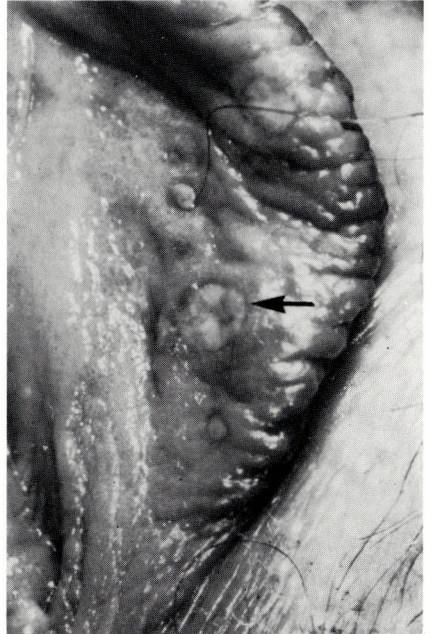

Fig. 16-22. Behçet's syndrome. Lesions are usually larger and more persistent than lesions of herpes genitalis. These lesions had been present for 3 weeks.

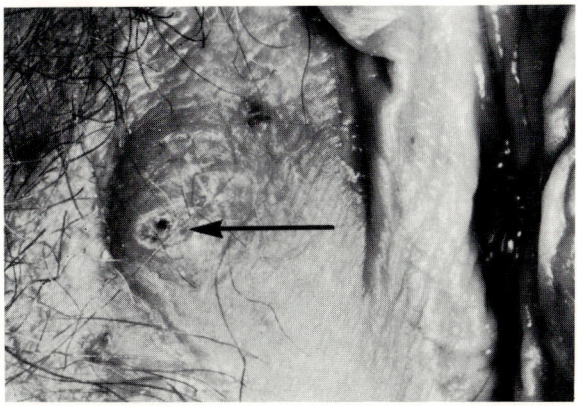

Fig. 16-23. Behçet's syndrome. These lesions, which are almost healed, had been present 6 weeks.

induced by a virus. In 1909, Halberstaedter and Prowazek reported finding similar cytoplasmic inclusions in scrapings from the genitourinary tracts of mothers in whose babies this condition developed. It has since been found that such inclusions are often present in the vaginal smears of mothers of affected babies. From this, it has been assumed that the birth canal of the mother is the most common source of the infection.

Inclusion blennorrhea is an acute papillary mucopurulent conjunctivitis that runs a relatively benign and self-limiting course over a period of several weeks and usually heals without scarring. The same virus is believed to be responsible for inclusion conjunctivitis (swimming pool conjunctivitis) in the adult and, according to Jones, probably for trachoma as well. The causative organism in both the genital and ocular infections has recently been designated as the TRIC virus: TR from trachoma and IC from inclusion conjunctivitis.

Dunlop, Jones, and Al-Hussaini, following colposcopies of the cervices of women from whom the TRIC virus had been isolated, claimed that all the cervices exhibited lesions resembling those produced in the conjunctiva by the TRIC virus. It was their opinion that, in certain cases, so-called nonspecific genital infection may be induced by the TRIC virus. Chiang and others reported "papillary necrotizing cervicitis" in two of five patients from whom the virus was isolated. They considered "distinctive" microscopic findings to be diffuse infiltration of inflammatory cells in the squamocolumnar transitional zone, focal areas of epithelial and subepithelial necrosis, and areas of epithelial cell desquamation. They were unable to demonstrate inclusion bodies in histologic sections resembling inclusions seen in cytologic smears. Kotcher and others discovered inclusion bodies similar to those in inclusion conjunctivitis in the cervical smears of 2.8 percent of approximately 8,000 women examined in a cancer cytology clinic. Despite such observations, we believe that the relationship of the TRIC virus to yet undefined nonspecific genital infections remains to be established.

Vulvar manifestations of systemic viral diseases

Manifestations on the skin and mucosa of the vulva and vagina are usually only one of the many signs of the internal viral diseases. Vulvovaginitis as a part of a systemic viral infection is more commonly observed in children, although it is occasionally found in adults. In view of the seriousness of systemic viral diseases, however, a vaginal discharge and eruptions of the external genitala are most often relatively insignificant and thus are overlooked.

The lesions of varicella (chickenpox), which involve both the vulva and vagina, are manifested initially as small vesicles and later as superficial ulcers. The vesicopustules of smallpox appear on the vulva and occasionally in the vagina; reportedly, the vaginal lesions are diffuse and are associated with leukorrhea. The genital lesions appear simultaneously with those elsewhere on the body, being grossly and histologically similar.

Measles is exhibited by redness of the vulvovaginal tissues and increased vaginal discharge. These signs are rather nonspecific; as is true of other viral lesions, they subside with the systemic disease.

Treatment

As a rule, the vulvovaginal portion of the systemic viral infections requires no special treatment. The prevention of scratching by the use of cooling lotions may be required as a safeguard against secondary infection. Occasionally, broad spectrum antibiotics may be beneficial.

REFERENCES

Ayers, M. A.: Behcet's syndrome, Obstet. Gynec. 26:575, 1965.

Baker, R. L.: OB-GYN collected letters of the International Correspondence Society of Obstetricians and Gynecologists, Series VII, p. 180, Dec. 1, 1966.

Baker, R. L.: Treatment of condyloma acuminatum, Obstet. Gynec. 10:611, 1957.

Barclay, D. L.: Discussion: Symposium on benign diseases of the vulva and vagina, American College of Obstetricians and Gynecologists, District VII, Houston, Tex., 1966.

Bateman, T.: A practical synopsis of cutaneous diseases, ed. 3, London, 1814.

Biegeleison, J. Z., Jr., Scott, L. V., and Lewis, V., Jr.: Rapid diagnosis of herpes simplex virus infections with fluorescent antibody, Science **129**:640, 1959.

Bjornberg, A., Hellgren, L., and Seebert, G.: Treatment of cutaneous vaccinia with idoxuridine, Arch. Derm. **90**:581, 1964.

Chiang, W. T., Alexander, E. R., Wei, P. Y., and Fresh, J. W.: Genital infection with TRIC agents in Taiwan, Amer. J. Obstet. Gynec. **100:** 422, 1968.

Christian, R. T., Ludovici, P. P., Miller, N. F., and Riley, G. M.: Viral studies of the female reproductive tract, Amer. J. Obstet. Gynec. **91:** 430, 1965.

Dudgeon, J. A.: Virological aspects of Behçet's disease, Proc. Roy. Soc. Med. **54:**104, 1961.

Dunlop, E. M. C., Jones, B. R., and Al-Hussaini, M. K.: Genital infection in association with TRIC virus infection of the eye, Brit. J. Vener. Dis. **40:**33, 1964.

Embrey, M. P.: Vulval carcinoma complicating condylomata acuminata, J. Obstet. Gynaec. Brit. Comm. **68:**503, 1961.

Ephraim, H.: Triple symptom complex of Behçet; report of a case, Arch. Derm. Syph. **50:**37, 1944.

Epstein, W. L., Senecal, I., Krasnobrod, H., and Massing, A. M.: Viral antigens in human epidermal tumors, J. Invest. Derm. **40:**51, 1963.

Gagnon, R. A.: Transplacental inoculation of fatal herpes simplex in the newborn, Obstet. Gynec. **31:**682, 1968.

Gorthy, R. L., and Krembs, M. A.: Vulvar condylomata acuminata complicating labor, Obstet. Gynec. **4:**67, 1954.

Graber, E. A., Barber, H. R. K., and O'Rourke, J. J.: Simple surgical treatment for condyloma acuminatum of the vulva, Obstet. Gynec. **29:**247, 1967.

Gudgel, E. F.: Can molluscum contagiosum be a venereal disease?, U. S. Armed Forces Med. J. **5:**1207, 1954.

Haas, G. M.: Hepato-adrenal necrosis with intranuclear inclusion bodies, Amer. J. Path. **11:** 127, 1935.

Halberstaedter, L., and Prowazek, S.: Ueber Chlamydozoen Refunde bei Blenorrhoe neonatorum non gonorrhoica, Klin. Wschr. **46:** 1839, 1909.

Humphrey, D. C.: Localized accidental vaccinia of the vulva, Amer. J. Obstet. Gynec. **86:**460, 1963.

Hunt, E.: Diseases affecting the vulva, ed. 4, St. Louis, 1954, The C. V. Mosby Co.

Jones, B. R.: Ocular syndromes of TRIC virus infection and their possible genital significance, Brit. J. Vener. Dis. **40:**3, 1964.

Josey, W. E., Nahmias, A. J., and Naib, Z. M.: Genital infection with Type 2 herpesvirus hominis: Present knowledge and possible relation to cervical cancer, Amer. J. Obstet. Gynec. **101:**718, 1968.

Josey, W. E., Nahmias, A. J., Naib, Z. M., Utley, P. M., McKenzie, W. J., and Coleman, M. T.: Genital herpes simplex infection in the female, Amer. J. Obstet. Gynec. **96:**493, 1966.

Juliusberg, M.: Zur Kenntnis des Virus der Molluscum contagiosum des Menschen, Deutsch Med. Wschr. **31:**1598, 1905.

Kaplan, I. W.: Condylomata acuminata, New Orleans Med. Surg. J. **94:**388, 1942.

Kaufman, H. E., Martola, E. L., and Dohlman, C. H.: Use of 5-iodo-2′-deoxyuridine (IDU) in treatment of herpes simplex keratitis, Arch. Ophthal. **68:**235, 1962.

Kern, A. B., and Schiff, B. L.: Vaccine therapy in recurrent herpes simplex, Arch. Derm. **89:** 844, 1964.

Knox, J. M.: Personal communication, 1967.

Kotcher, E., Gray, L. A., James, Q. C., Frick, C. A., and Bottorff, D. W.: Cervical cell inclusion bodies and viral infections of the cervix, Ann. N. Y. Acad. Sci. **97:**571, 1962.

Lazar, M. P.: Primary herpetic vulvovaginitis, Arch. Derm. **72:**272, 1955.

Lever, W. F.: Histopathology of the skin, ed. 3, Philadelphia, 1961, J. B. Lippincott Co.

Lynch, P. J., and Minkin, W.: Molluscum contagiosum of the adult: Probable venereal transmission, Arch. Derm. **98:**141, 1968.

Mortata, A., and Imam, I. Z. E.: Virus etiology of Behçet's syndrome, Brit. J. Ophthal. **48:** 250, 1964.

Nahmias, A. J., and Dowdle, W. R.: Prog. Med. Virol. In press.

Nahmias, A. J., Naib, Z. M., Josey, W. E., and Clepper, A. C.: Genital herpes simplex infection, virologic and cytologic studies, Obstet. Gynec. **29:**395, 1967.

Nahmias, A. J., Josey, W. E., and Naib, Z. M.: Neonatal herpes simplex infection, J.A.M.A. **199:**132, 1967.

Neva, F. A.: Studies on molluscum contagiosum, Arch. Intern. Med. **110:**720, 1962.

Phillips, D. L., and Scott, J. S.: Recurrent genital and oral ulceration with associated eye lesions—Behçet's syndrome, Lancet **1:**366, 1955.

Pommerening, R. A., Hill, L. D., and Hammer, C. J.: Perianal verruca acuminata with mucosal lesions, Northwest Med. **62:**348, 1963.

Powell, L. C., Jr., Pollard, M., and Jenkins, J. L., Sr.: Treatment of condyloma acuminatum by autogenous vaccine. In press, 1969.

Rawls, W. E., Laurel, D., Melnick, J. L., Glicksman, G. M., and Kaufman, R. H.: A search for virus in smegma, premalignant and early malignant cervical tissue: The isolation of Herpes virus with distinct antigenic properties, Amer. J. Epidem. **87:**647, 1968.

Rawls, W. E., Thompkins, W. A. F., Figueroa, M. E., and Melnick, J. L.: Herpesvirus Type 2: Association with carcinoma of the cervix, Science **161:**1255, 1966.

Reagan, J. W.: Herpes infections of the female genital tract seen as grave neonatal threat in final trimester, OB-GYN Observer, **7:**2, 1968.

Sezer, F. N.: Isolation of virus as cause of

Behçet's disease, Amer. J. Ophthal. 36:301, 1953.

Sherman, A. L.: Discussion: Symposium on benign diseases of the vulva and vagina, American College of Obstetricians & Gynecologists, District VII, Houston, Tex., 1966.

Slavin, H. B., and Gavett, E.: Primary herpetic vulvovaginitis, Proc. Soc. Exper. Biol. Med. 63:343, 1946.

Snell, E., and Fox, J. G.: Molluscum contagiosum venereum, Canad. Med. Ass. J. 85:1152, 1961.

Unna, P. G.: On herpes progenitalis especially in women, J. Cutan. Ven. Dis. 1:321, 1883.

Weary, P. E., Wheeler, C. E., Lingamfelter, C. S., Jr., and Cawley, E. P.: Localized accidental vaccinia, Arch. Derm. 82:804, 1960.

Wheeler, C. E., and Huffines, W. D.: Primary disseminated herpes simplex of the newborn, J.A.M.A. 191:111, 1965.

Yen, S. S. C., Reagan, J. W., and Rosenthal, M. S.: Herpes simplex infection in female genital tract, Obstet. Gynec. 25:479, 1965.

Chapter 17

Miscellaneous vulvovaginitides

"Nonspecific" vaginitis

Traditionally, any vaginitis or unusual vaginal discharge not explained by readily identifiable agents, particularly trichomonads, *Candida,* or gonococci, has been termed "nonspecific." It has long been generally believed that such conditions are induced by "mixed" bacterial infection. Although vaginal infections are occasionally attributable to bacterial organisms other than *Haemophilus vaginalis,* we have pointed out with considerable care (p. 208) that the isolation of a predominant bacterial agent does not necessarily prove a relationship of that agent to the condition present. In view of the broadened concepts of infectious diseases, the classification of any vulvovaginitis as a "nonspecific" infection becomes increasingly unacceptable. Also, it is hardly tenable that a variety of vaginitides having, perhaps, uniform clinical and laboratory patterns is ascribable to a large and unrelated group of bacteria. Gardner and Dukes, in several reports, have presented evidence that over 90 percent of vaginitides previously classified as "nonspecific" were in reality caused by a short, gram-negative bacillus belonging to the genus *Haemophilus,* for which they suggested the name *Haemophilus vaginalis.* Upon universal acceptance of this premise, the number of unexplained (nonspecific) vaginitides or unusual discharges will have become relatively insignificant.

Medical literature includes frequent references to "nonspecific" vaginitis, yet only a few significant bacteriologic investigations of the problem have been conducted, and even more rarely have investigators attempted to define a clear-cut clinical pattern for such disease. Never have independent investigators agreed upon the physical and microscopic characteristics of the vaginitides or discharges that they term "nonspecific."

Hite, Hesseltine, and Goldstein, in 1947, significantly stated: "Reported results are variable and difficult to correlate, undoubtedly owing, in part, to differences in material and in part, to differences in cultural methods and criteria for identification of the isolated organisms." In 1949, Blinick, Steinberg, and Merendino reported an extensive study of the bacterial flora of the vagina and cervix of patients who complained of nonspecific leukorrhea—a discharge in the absence of trichomonads, *Candida,* and gonococci. These authors isolated twenty-seven microorganisms, the *Staphylococcus albus,* the alpha, beta, and gamma streptococci, the diphtheroids, and colon bacilli being the most prevalent. They also isolated from three to twelve varieties of organisms in the individual patients, the average number of varieties being seven. Weaver, Scott, and Williams, in 1950, reported a study of nonspecific vaginal discharges from which they concluded: "It hardly appears suggestive that any one or more types of bacteria have a cause and effect relationship to nonspecific vaginal discharges." Bernstine and Rakoff have significantly stated: "Indeed, in many instances, the term 'nonspecific vaginitis' is a misnomer, used glibly to conceal ignorance of the true underlying cause."

These opinions and observations illustrate the changing attitude toward the term "nonspecific" vaginitis during the past two decades. We are convinced that the riddle of so-called nonspecific vaginitis was largely solved with the description of *H. vaginalis* vaginitis. Since a specific cause, microbial or otherwise, can be demonstrated in practically every case of vaginitis or leukorrhea, we feel that the term "nonspecific" should be rarely used, if not discarded entirely.

Difficulty occasionally arises in determining whether or not a patient actually has vaginitis. The term *vaginitis* today has a broad interpretation, including conditions unaccompanied by irritative symptoms and gross tissue changes. Perhaps any woman in the childbearing age who has vaginal secretions that are abnormal in color, odor, consistency, volume, and pH should be considered as having vaginitis or leukorrhea. Only when the secretions yield no trichomonads, candidal species, gonococci, *H. vaginalis,* or other pathogenic agent and when other causes are not demonstrable would the diagnosis of "nonspecific" vaginitis ever be acceptable.

Perhaps some leukorrheas or vaginitides without obvious etiology are induced by allergic states, an altered physiology, or chemical irritants. Others may be the result of sexual overindulgence, cervicitis, dietary deficiency, or one of a host of other causes. The overly fastidious woman may interpret perfectly normal physiologic secretions as infection or leukorrhea.

Obviously, as knowledge of infections and altered physiologic processes increases and more reliable laboratory methods become available, the term "nonspecific" vaginitis or leukorrhea should be used with declining frequency. We hasten to admit that, regardless of one's diagnostic capacities, not all such cases can be assigned a specific cause, either microbial, physiologic, irritative, or physical. Nevertheless, the too frequent use of the term "nonspecific" might imply carelessness, indifference, or a failure to employ the available laboratory methods for differential diagnosis.

Vaginitis emphysematosa

Vaginitis emphysematosa is characterized by multiple, discrete, gas-filled, cystoid cavities of the vaginal and cervical mucosa. Although until recently it was considered a distinct entity unrelated to other gynecologic diseases, the findings in a retrospective study strongly suggest that it is a manifestation of trichomoniasis and, occasionally, perhaps, of *H. vaginalis* vaginitis. Aside from a vaginal discharge from these associated infections, most patients are without symptoms, the lesions usually being discovered incidentally during routine examination, investigation of leukorrhea, or at necropsy. In view of the fact that symptoms are few and mild and the condition self-limited, vaginitis emphysematosa is more of a clinicopathologic curiosity than a therapeutic problem; nevertheless, it has been the subject of many reports, most of which are contradictory and inconclusive.

The first description of this condition is usually credited to Hugier. According to the definition of vaginitis emphysematosa, however, he did not include such cases in his account. In 1861, Braun published what is now believed to be the first case report. Although many hypotheses as to the etiology, pathogenesis, and the evolution and chemical nature of the gas have been published, none has been generally accepted.

The designation *vaginitis emphysematosa* was proposed by Zweifel in 1877. It has been given twenty or more other titles, including colpohyperplasia cystica, pneumatosis cystoides vaginae, emphysematous colpitis, and cervicocolpitis emphysematosa. For various reasons, many investigators have objected to the term *vaginitis emphysematosa,* yet it is the one most widely employed, and is our preference.

Etiology

Literature is replete with controversial theories concerning the origin of this disease. These theories include decomposition of cellular debris within tissues or between agglutinated folds of mucosa; entrapment of gas between folds of mucosa; production of gas by bacteria in secreting vaginal glands; bacterial infection in dilated lymph spaces; extravasation of blood into interstitial tissues, with liquefaction and gas formation; decomposition of serous content of lymph follicles; and the forcing of atmospheric air through breaks in the vaginal mucosa and into interstitial spaces.

Wilbanks and Carter, after observing that three of four patients with vaginitis emphysematosa also had trichomoniasis, theorized that *T. vaginalis* is possibly the etiologic agent. At the same time, Gardner and Fernet observed vaginitis emphysematosa in ten living patients, of whom seven had trichomoniasis and three had *H. vaginalis* vaginitis. The finding of a persistent, specific vaginal pathogen in ten consecutive patients with vaginitis emphysematosa would seem to be strong evidence of an etiologic relationship. Even more significant was the disappearance of the vaginitis emphysematosa upon eradication of trichomoniasis.

Gas within living tissues is continuously absorbed; thus, for maintenance or increase in the size of individual cystoid cavities, a continuous source of gas within the tissues is presumed to be essential. It may be concluded that the source of the gas is endogenous, and, hence, the gas is a fermentation product of such microorganisms as *T. vaginalis* and *H. vaginalis*. In support of this view, Newton, Reardon, and DeLera demonstrated that bacteria-free *T. vaginalis* can produce gas in subcutaneous tissues of guinea pigs.

In origin, cardiovascular and pulmonary diseases were, for a long time, assumed to be related to this disease. Undoubtedly, this opinion was based upon the fact that many of the reported cases were found at postmortem examination. That a high percentage of cases of vaginitis emphysematosa was found at autopsy following death from one or the other of these diseases should not be surprising, since a high percentage of all patients die of such disorders. In our opinion, no etiologic relationship exists. Not one of the ten patients with vaginitis emphysematosa reported by Gardner and Fernet had any type of cardiovascular or chronic respiratory disease.

The exact chemical nature of the gas in the lesions has not been determined to the satisfaction of all investigators. Many analyses have disclosed several types of gas, including trimethylamine, carbonic acid, ammonia, hydrogen sulfide, nitrogen, oxygen, and air. Analyses by Hoffman and Grundfest, Gardner and Fernet, and others offer strong evidence that the gas has a high carbon dioxide content.

Incidence

The exact incidence of vaginitis emphysematosa is unknown. In a review by Gardner and Fernet in 1964, a total of 160 reported cases was found. The usual statement that the condition is exceedingly rare could be more presumptive than factual. Abell found eight examples in the material from the Pathology Department of the University of Michigan Hospital during a 17-year period. Ingraham and Hall observed three cases in 1 year. Nagashima reported six cases from surgical material and three cases in 3,804 autopsies during a 9-year period. Gardner and Fernet observed ten cases during 17 years in a private office practice, representing an incidence of one in every 765 pregnant women and one in every 2,400 exclusively gynecologic patients.

The disease apparently develops only after the menarche. It has usually been stated that most patients with the disease are pregnant; an extensive review of the medical literature disclosed that, of patients whose status was known, seventy-three were pregnant and sixty-two were nonpregnant. Gardner and Fernet estimated that among every seventy patients who were both pregnant and infected with *T. vaginalis,* one would develop vaginitis emphysematosa, whereas one nonpregnant patient of every 367 with trichomoniasis would have the disease. From these figures, the incidence of vaginitis emphysematosa is approximately five times higher in pregnant women.

Clinical features

Symptoms. The signs and symptoms of vaginitis emphysematosa center around the classical lesion and associated vaginal infection.

The majority of patients are unaware of

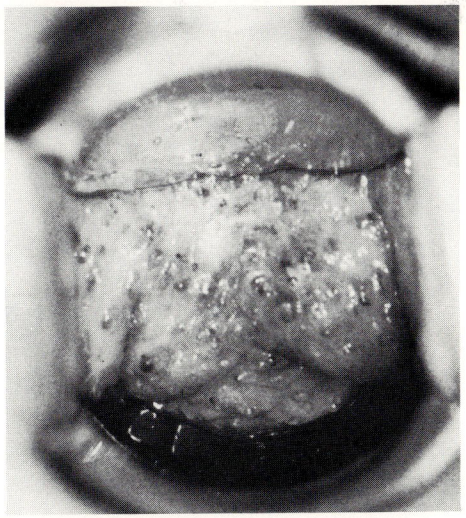

Fig. 17-1. Vaginitis emphysematosa. Multiple gas-filled cystoid cavities of vaginal mucosa.

256 Benign diseases of the vulva and vagina

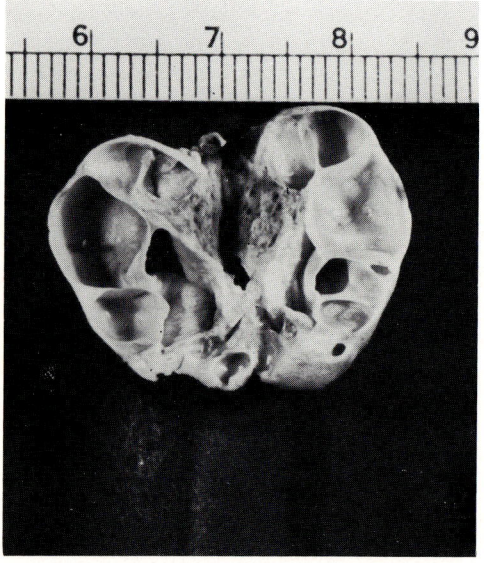

Fig. 17-2. Vaginitis emphysematosa. Cervical tissue removed at time of delivery. Large cystoid cavities. (Gardner, H. L.: Amer. J. Obstet. Gynec. 36:123, 1948.)

the disease per se, although many have a vaginal discharge that usually appears to be attributable to either trichomoniasis or *H. vaginalis* vaginitis. A bloody discharge is sometimes observed after intercourse. Pruritus is a symptom if the associated trichomoniasis is sufficiently active. Some patients are aware of an occasional popping sound from the vaginal area; this is caused by rupture of tense, gas-filled cystoid cavities. The sound may also be elicited by intercourse, douching, vaginal examination, or exercise.

Objective signs. The pathognomonic lesion is a gas-filled, cystoid cavity of the mucosa or submucosa of the vagina or cervix, or both (Figs. 17-1 and 17-2). Many of the gas-filled cavities project slightly above the mucosa. They may be microscopic or of any size up to 2 cm. in diameter. As a rule, these cavities involve the entire length of the vagina and the ectocervix, being most pronounced in the upper two-thirds of the vagina and the ectocervix. One patient, observed by Gardner (1948), had gas-filled cavities is large as 1.5 cm. in diameter in the cervix (Fig. 17-2), yet none in the vagina. Ordinarily, the lesions are uniformly dis-

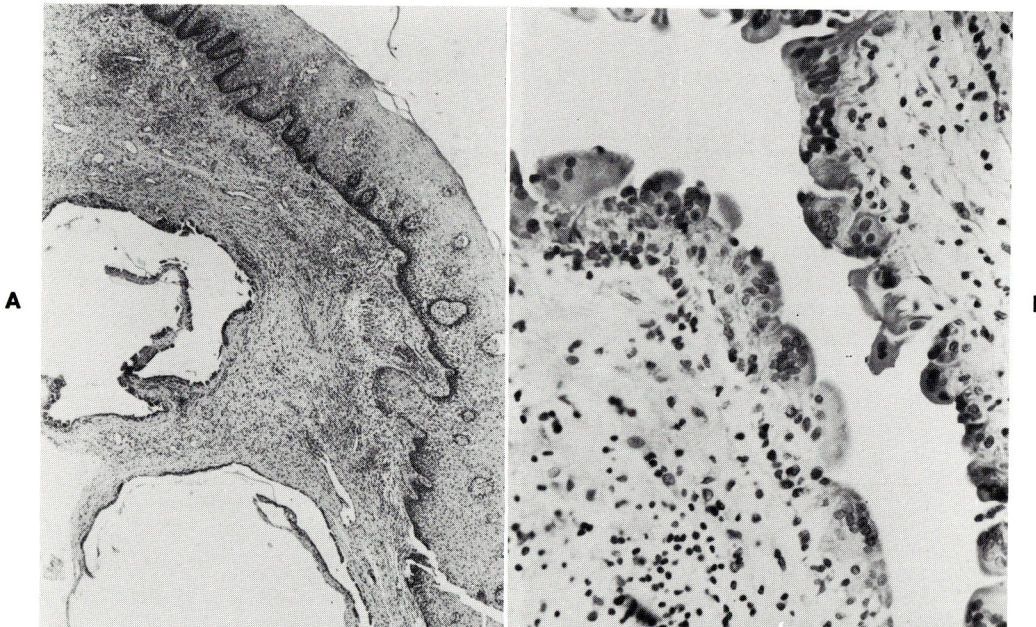

Fig. 17-3. Vaginitis emphysematosa. A, Cystoid spaces beneath intact squamous epithelial lining. B, Vaginitis emphysematosa. Syncytial type giant cells lining a cavity. (Gardner, H. L., and Fernet, P.: Amer. J. Obstet. Gynec. 88:680, 1964.)

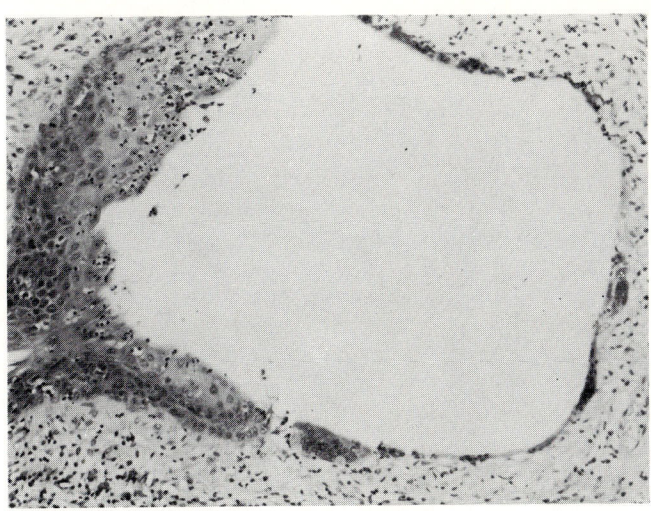

Fig. 17-4. Vaginitis emphysematosa. Cystoid cavity lined partially with squamous epithelium and partially with giant cells. (Gardner, H. L., and Fernet, P.: Amer. J. Obstet. Gynec. **88:** 680, 1964.)

tributed, though they may appear in groups or clusters, constituting an appreciable mass. Individual lesions are tense and smooth; in the aggregate, however, they may produce an effect of roughening or granulation (Fig. 17-1). The affected vaginal wall has been described as honeycombed, pebbled, or seeded with "blebs." The epithelial covering of large vesicles is thin and translucent. There is no crepitation of tissues, as in true emphysema. The number of patients with "granular vaginitis" who would be found to have such lesions on biopsy is a matter of speculation.

Digital examination, insertion of a speculum, and brisk wiping with a cotton-tipped applicator will often rupture a few of the cavities. Usually, rupture is followed by oozing of blood. A few investigators have reported finding fluid as well as gas in the cavities, though we have never observed fluid in a typical lesion. The fact that puncture of a cavity does not cause others in the area to lose gas and contour demonstrates the discrete nature of individual lesions. When involved tissue is excised and submerged in water, it floats rapidly to the surface.

Histopathology

The microscopic picture varies, although the vagina generally exhibits intact squamous epithelium, cystoid spaces in the lamina propria (Fig. 17-3, *A*), acute and chronic in-

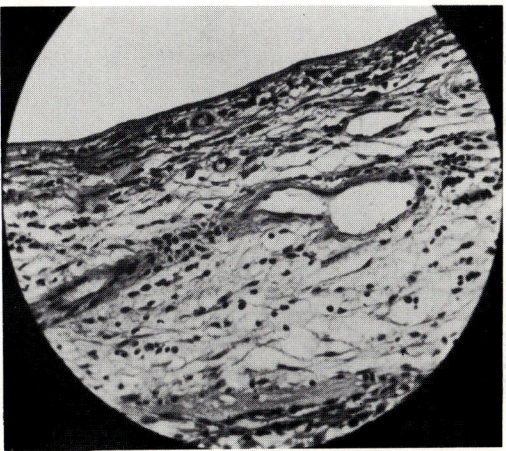

Fig. 17-5. Vaginitis emphysematosa. Large cystoid cavity without identifiable lining. (Gardner, H. L., and Fernet, P.: Amer. J. Obstet. Gynec. **88:** 680, 1964.)

flammatory cells with degrees of reactive fibrosis surrounding the spaces, and syncytial type giant cells lining or partially lining the smaller cavities (Fig. 17-3, *B*). The squamous epithelium is often acanthotic and hyperkeratotic, with invagination and solid downgrowth of epithelial folds. The smaller cystoid lesions are sometimes partially lined with squamous epithelium (Fig. 17-4). In a few cases, PAS stain discloses a glandular epithelial lining. Large cavities may have no identifiable lining (Fig. 17-5).

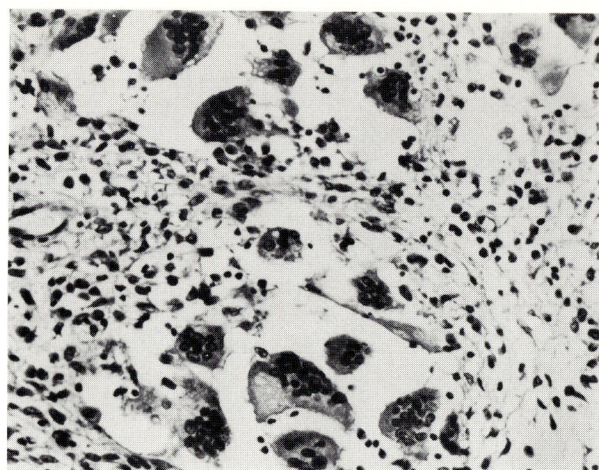

Fig. 17-6. Vaginitis emphysematosa. Clusters of giant cells in early cavities. (Gardner, H. L., and Fernet, P.: Amer. J. Obstet. Gynec. 88:680, 1964.)

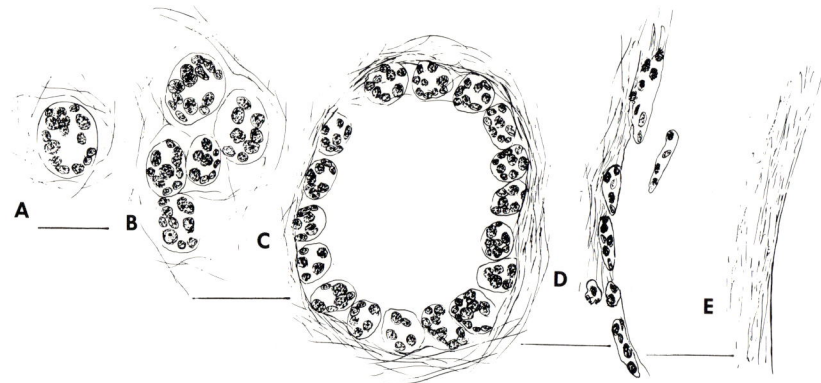

Fig. 17-7. Vaginitis emphysematosa. Diagram of possible stages of pathogenesis. **A,** Giant cell. **B,** Group of giant cells. **C,** Small gas-filled cystoid lesion lined with undistorted giant cells. **D,** Larger lesion with lining giant cells flattened from intracystic pressure. **E,** Largest lesions lined chiefly by stretched-out stroma. (Gardner, H. L.: Amer. J. Obstet. Gynec. 56:123, 1948.)

In patients with trichomoniasis, polymorphonuclear leukocytes or eosinophils are apparent within the squamous epithelium, and the superficial lamina propria often contains masses of acute inflammatory cells (Fig. 17-3, *A*). Chronic inflammatory cells, although often few in number, are consistently present.

The smallest cystoid cavities arise in clusters, chiefly in the superficial stroma. Large cavities are clear, indicating a lack of liquid or cellular content. Usually, reactive fibrosis around the recently developed small cavities is lacking, whereas the converse is true of larger cavities. Almost every cavity contains one or more giant cells, and they are invariably found in small lesions (Figs. 17-3, *B* and 17-6). The giant cells usually have from two to twelve nuclei. The cytoplasm stains pink and exhibits no evidence of PAS-positive vacuoles, bacteria, or fungi. Superficial capillaries and venules are usually dilated, as well as the large veins and lymphatic spaces in deeper portions of the vaginal wall. Special stains do not reveal bacteria, fungi, acid-fast bacilli, fat, or mucicarminophilic material in cells, connective tissue, or vessels.

Some possible stages in pathogenesis are demonstrated in Fig. 17-7.

Diagnosis

Any patient with palpatory evidence of severe "granular" vaginitis should be suspected of having vaginitis emphysematosa. The escape of gas from punctured cystoid cavities is pathognomonic. Specimens of tissue are easily obtained from the vaginal wall by a punch biopsy instrument, without anesthesia, and histologic examination of excised vaginal tissue will confirm the diagnosis.

Treatment

If the theory that vaginitis emphysematosa is caused by vaginal infection is correct, it is only necessary to direct attention to the eradication of the associated specific vaginal pathogens—usually trichomonads or *H. vaginalis*. Although the condition is most interesting, the symptoms are so mild that treatment is not obligatory.

Desquamative inflammatory vaginitis

The condition herein designated as *desquamative inflammatory vaginitis* displays some of the clinical and microscopic features of postmenopausal atrophic vaginitis, yet it develops in women with high estrogen levels. Its peculiar distribution, persistence, poor response to treatment, and tendency to recrudescence after treatment is discontinued are also striking features. In view of these characteristics, the disease should be regarded as a specific entity. Apparently, it is unique among the vaginitides. Gardner (1968) has found this type in only eight of more than 3,000 patients with vaginitis observed in private office practice during the period 1952 through 1967. The clinical and microscopic features closely resembled those observed in six cases reported by Gray and Barnes in 1965. To quote their description: "The vaginas were thin, quite reddened, with numerous pus cells and with oval and round parabasal cells in the secretion." They called the condition "desquamative inflammatory vaginitis."

The clinical and laboratory findings in some of Gardner's eight cases differed in minor respects; also, the clinical picture of the group as a whole differed somewhat from that observed by Gray and Barnes. Nevertheless, most of the affections in the two groups apparently were sufficiently similar to warrant the same designation. With the possible exception of a report by Scheffey, Rakoff, and Lang in 1956 of an unusual case to which they ascribed the term "exudative vaginitis," we are unaware of other reports of a disease that conforms to the condition exhibited in these two groups of cases.

Etiology

Neither Gray and Barnes nor Gardner (1968) could detect a specific causative bacterium in this unusual vaginitis. Of the patients of Gray and Barnes, two initially harbored *Trichomonas vaginalis;* four, *Haemophilus vaginalis;* and three, *Candida albicans.* Presumably, however, these pathogens were subsequently ruled out as causative agents. They were not found in the smears of Gardner's patients. Rather, the bacteria isolated in appreciable numbers were chiefly streptococci of other than the Group A variety (seven), *Staphylococcus aureus* (one), *Escherichia coli* (one), and *Staphylococcus epidermidis* (one). No relationship between the isolated bacteria and development of the lesions was demonstrable. Since the clinical courses of patients are remarkably similar and the predominant bacterial agents isolated remarkably dissimilar, they apparently play no more than a secondary role. That response to antibacterial agents is uniformly poor further suggests that bacterial infection is not primarily responsible for the disease. The essential absence of lactobacilli indicates that the predominant bacteria may become established only as opportunistic organisms, a not uncommon result of vaginal microbial change.

An unidentified chronic viral infection has not been excluded as the primary cause. The cytologic and histologic studies of the vaginitis in two patients disclosed some inconclusive evidence of a viral infection. Theoretically, a dystrophic process involving vaginal metabolism is another etiologic possibility. No patients have displayed a dietary deficiency or obvious allergenic or primary irritant reaction. Biopsy material from the vagina of one patient contained small islands of glandular epithelium of the cervical type; this, perhaps, justified the diagnosis of minimal vaginal adenosis. Any assumption of a relationship between this lesion and desquamative inflammatory vaginitis, however, would be purely speculative.

The pathogenesis of the atrophic status of the vaginal mucosa remains obscure. Gray and Barnes suggested that infection dissolves the superficial cells of the vagina or prevents their maturity. One might presume that basal and parabasal cells in vaginal secretions of women with high estrogen levels are the result of failure of mucosal proliferation, failure of cellular maturation, accelerated desquamation produced by the effects of unknown agents, or other processes.

Cytology and histopathology

As in vaginal atrophy from estrogen deficiency, cytologic smears from the vaginal secretions of these patients exhibit a high percentage of basal and parabasal vaginal epithelial cells (Fig. 17-8), as well as many pus cells, and usually, small numbers of intermediate and superficial cells. Relatively few bacteria are present, and lactobacilli are essentially lacking. A few fragmented nuclei were found in the smears of two of Gardner's patients.

Histologically (Fig. 17-9), acute and chronic inflammatory reactions involve both mucosal and submucosal tissues. Some areas of the epithelium are thin or superficially ulcerated. Vacuolation of a few epithelial cells is sometimes observed. In one case, scattered Russell bodies were discovered, and in another a few small islands of glandular epithelium of the cervical type lay beneath the lining squamous epithelium. Focal areas of stromal hemorrhage are commonly present.

Clinical features

The mucosa of all or part of the upper half of the vagina, especially the opposed surfaces of the posterior fornix and the ectocervix, is acutely inflamed (Fig. 17-10). The margins of the affected areas usually are well delineated. At times, they have serpiginous configurations. Trauma of the lesions frequently leads to superficial ulceration and

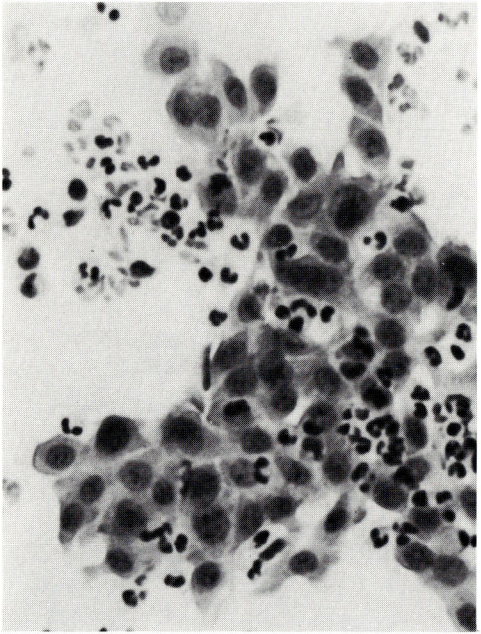

Fig. 17-8. Desquamative inflammatory vaginitis. Vaginal smear containing parabasal squamous epithelial cells and pus cells. (Papanicolaou × 600) (Gardner, H. L.: Amer. J. Obstet. Gynec. **102**: 1102, 1968.)

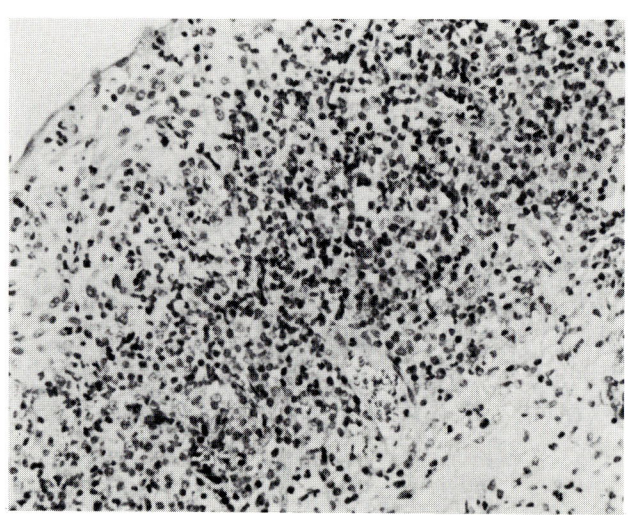

Fig. 17-9. Desquamative inflammatory vaginitis. Numerous acute and chronic inflammatory cells deep to and infiltrating squamous epithelial lining. Vacuolation of cells of squamous epithelium. (H & E × 260) (Gardner, H. L.: Amer. J. Obstet. Gynec. **102**:1102, 1968.)

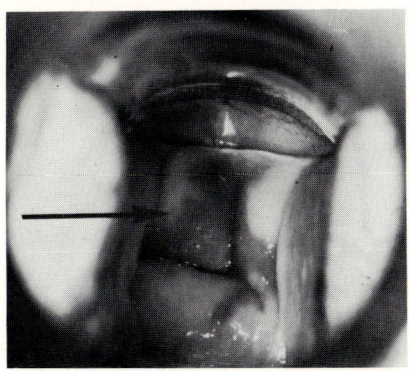

Fig. 17-10. Desquamative inflammatory vaginitis. Localized, well-delineated, erythematous areas of vaginitis (arrow). (Gardner, H. L.: Amer. J. Obstet. Gynec. 102:1102, 1968.)

ecchymotic bleeding points and streaks. Some areas of epithelium may be covered by a grayish pseudomembrane; this peels off when the vagina is wiped, as though it had been parboiled, exposing the inflamed surfaces. The sites of the inflammatory reaction remain unchanged indefinitely.

Most patients complain of a moderate to copious discharge, usually homogeneous and purulent, although it may be seromucoid or bloody. Malodor is not a feature, as it is of the discharge of trichomoniasis or *H. vaginalis* vaginitis. Mild burning and pruritus, reported by the majority of the patients, are the only irritative symptoms. Vaginal acidity is diminished to pH 5.0 to 6.8. Gardner observed a minor stenosis of the vaginal vault in two patients, apparently incident to scar tissue contraction in the affected areas.

Diagnosis

A patient who has normal ovarian activity, a persistent localized vaginitis (especially of the vaginal vault), and an abnormal discharge containing a high percentage of immature epithelial cells and many pus cells not attributable to known specific causes should perhaps be given a diagnosis of desquamative inflammatory vaginitis. Other diseases associated with unusual numbers of immature vaginal epithelial cells in women with normal estrogen levels include trichomoniasis, primary irritant (chemical) vaginitis, and, occasionally, certain bacterial infections. Since the latter two are usually transitory and involve the entire vagina, they should cause little confusion. The discovery of trichomonads often explains the cytologic features of atrophic vaginitis in a patient with normal ovarian activity. Trichomonal vaginitis involves the full length of the vagina rather uniformly, however, whereas desquamative inflammatory vaginitis is patchy in distribution and generally is localized in the upper half of the vagina.

Treatment

With or without treatment, the course of this disease is protracted. None of the lesions in Gardner's group of patients healed spontaneously, and whether any healed completely with treatment was conjectural.

On the basis of the cytologic evidence of vaginal immaturity, four of these eight patients were repeatedly given estrogens, both intravaginally and orally. Little or no beneficial effect upon either the clinical or microscopic patterns of the disease was observed. Actually, this would be expected, since a prerequisite to the diagnosis of desquamative inflammatory vaginitis is active ovarian function. The response to antibacterial agents, including the sulfonamides and antibiotics administered systemically or locally, was also discouraging. These agents may be worthwhile as adjunctive treatment; any rapid therapeutic response, however, would be suggestive of bacterial vaginitis, rather than the desquamative type.

Scheffey, Rakoff, and Lang reported that their patient with an unusual vaginitis, resembling in some respects the type under consideration, was cured by the use of vaginal corticosteroid suppositories (Cortef) for several months. Of five of Gardner's patients who were treated by intravaginal applications of corticosteroids alone or combined with antibacterial agents, four were benefitted. The response was slow, covering a period of months, and even after improvement or apparent cure the vaginitis tended to recur. Nevertheless, intravaginal applications of preparations containing a corticosteroid have thus far proved to be the most effective treatment.

Amebiasis

The prevalence of intestinal amebiasis in the United States is reported to be between 5 and 10 percent. The causative agent *Entamoeba histolytica,* although affecting primarily the colon, is also capable of secondarily infecting practically any organ of the body, including the vulva, vagina, and cer-

vix. It is generally agreed that practically all genital infections are the result of vaginal contamination with fecal material, although Mylius and Ten Seldam reported a case in which sexual contact was the mode of transmission.

Incidence

Probably, few gynecologists in the United States have recognized a case of amebic infection of the vulva, vagina, or cervix. Perhaps discovery of such an infection would not be exceptional, however, if wet mounts were prepared from every leukorrheal discharge and genital ulcer and examined for *E. histolytica* by technologists thoroughly familiar with the organism.

Weinstein and Weed found only ten cases of amebic vaginitis reported in the world's medical literature before 1946, to which they added four cases of their own collected in New Orleans during a period of 9 months. While Bickers, in Virginia, discovered one case in 200 patients with leukorrhea, Bhaduri of Calcutta observed fourteen cases in 123 patients who were examined for leukorrhea. Munguia, Franco, and Valenzuela of Mexico City identified the organism in twenty-four of 100,000 Papanicolaou smears during a 5 year period. It is now recognized that genital amebiasis is not uncommon in tropical countries, where poor hygienic conditions often prevail.

Clinical features

The most characteristic finding in vaginal amebiasis is a malodorous, serosanguineous, or frankly bloody discharge, often containing fragments of necrotic tissue. Ulcerations are usually apparent on both the cervix and upper vagina, yet only rarely is the vulva affected. In diameter, the ulcers vary from a few millimeters to several centimeters and exhibit varying degrees of undermining. The bases of the ulcers are often red, friable, and vascular and frequently are covered by a necrotic slough. An unusual case reported by van Coeverden de Groot was that of a patient who had a necrotic slough of the entire vagina; after her cure with systemic agents, vaginal stenosis developed. Localized vaginal scarring is often a result of this infection.

Patients with amebic vaginitis often experience considerable discomfort in the vaginal and cervical areas, including dyspareunia. Pruritus is seldom a complaint. Since the majority of patients also have amebiasis of the colon, a recent or past history of dysentery would be expected.

Diagnosis

Laboratory findings. Trophozoites of *E. histolytica* with typical motile pseudopodia and ingested red blood cells are usually demonstrable in wet mount preparations of material from affected sites. The examination should be made immediately upon removal of the specimens, with warm slides and physiologic saline being used. Cystic forms are sometimes observed. Munguia, Franco, and Valenzuela readily recognized the organism on Papanicolaou smears (Fig. 17-11); they expressed the opinion that cytologists who keep in mind the morphology of the parasite should be able to detect the protozoan. Cultures are of only limited diagnostic value. Since the intestinal tract is usually affected, stool studies made after the administration of a saline cathartic will frequently yield the organism. They may also be detected in smears taken directly from lesions of the rectosigmoid through the sigmoidoscope.

Histologically, the lesions of amebiasis most often exhibit a chronic inflammatory response, although acute inflammation is not uncommon. Tissue necrosis, ulceration, and autolysis are diagnostic features. *E. histolytica* can often be found within areas of inflammation (Fig. 17-12). These are small, round, pale staining eosinophilic bodies that are strongly PAS-positive.

Differential diagnosis. Since amebic vaginitis is primarily manifested by ulcerations, it must be distinguished from all conditions associated with ulcers—carcinoma, the granulomatous diseases, chancroid, tuberculous ulcers, herpes genitalis, Behçet's syndrome, syphilis, and others. The differential diagnosis of ulcerative lesions of the genitalia frequently requires exhaustive laboratory investigation. Of all the conditions mentioned, carcinoma is most immediately confusing, although it is the easiest to distinguish histologically. Munguia, Franco, and Valenzuela reported that cancer had been suspected in nineteen of their twenty-four cases. Punch biopsy should be taken from any lesion suspected of being a carcinoma. This procedure is also helpful in the

Miscellaneous vulvovaginitides 263

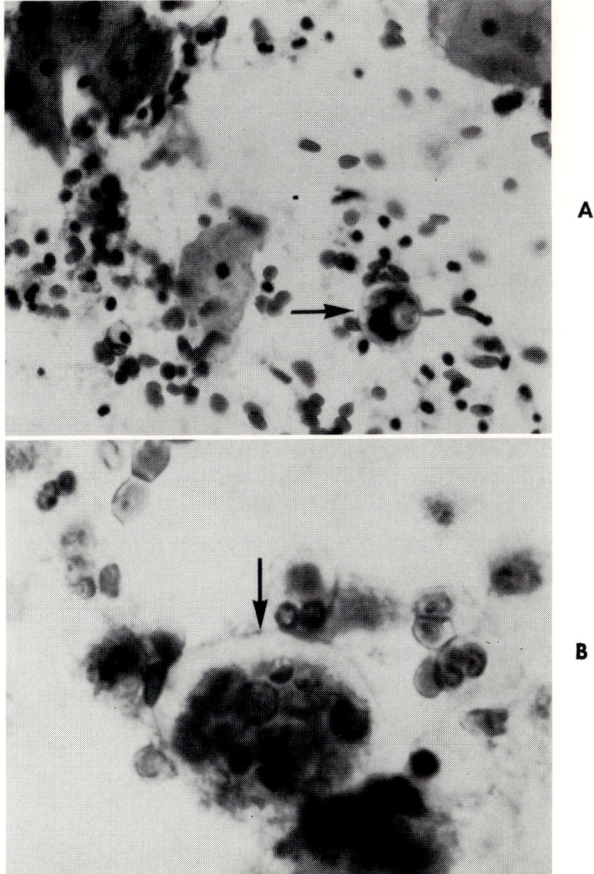

Fig. 17-11. **A,** Amebic vulvovaginitis. Cervicovaginal smear with *Entamoeba histolytica* (arrow). Pap smear. **B,** Amebic vulvovaginitis. Cervicovaginal smear containing *Entamoeba histolytica* with ingested red blood cells (arrow). Pap smear. (Courtesy Patricia Alonzo, Mexico City.)

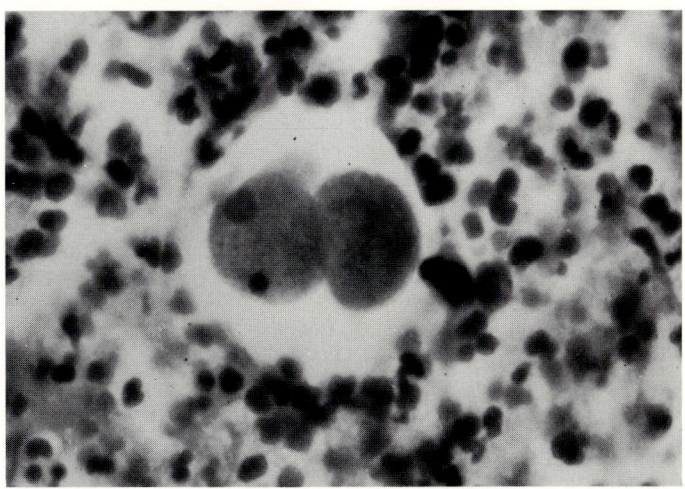

Fig. 17-12. Amebic vulvovaginitis. *Entamoeba histolytica* within an area of inflammation in vaginal biopsy. (Courtesy Conrad G. Collins and David L. Barclay, New Orleans.)

diagnosis of the granulomatous diseases, tuberculosis, and herpes simplex. A dark-field examination is of value in establishing or ruling out the presence of syphilis.

Treatment

Since most patients with vaginal amebiasis are likely to have an intestinal infection as well, their treatment should be left to a physician who is thoroughly familiar with the disease, particularly since eradication of the organisms depends upon the administration of effective systemic amebacides, such as emetine hydrochloride and chloroquine diphosphate (Aralen). Vaginal suppositories that contain carbarsone or chloroquine diphosphate may provide prompt local relief, although they are not curative.

Schistosomiasis (bilharziasis)

Schistosomiasis, while extremely rare in temperate climates, is in reality a world health problem of considerable magnitude. It is primarily a disease of the intestinal tract or urinary bladder and is caused by one of three species of schistosomes or blood flukes. Although practically nonexistent in the United States, it affects approximately 40 percent of the population of Egypt and is endemic in most parts of Africa, the northern part of South America, the West Indies, and the Orient. In North America, schistosomiasis is usually found in persons who have traveled in endemic regions.

Genital schistosomiasis is not uncommon in endemic areas. It is generally caused by *Schistosoma haematobium,* the species that most often inhabits the venules of the bladder and pelvic plexuses. Youssef, Fayad, and Shafeek found 120 cases of genital schistosomiasis among approximately 31,000 gynecologic patients admitted to hospitals in Cairo. Friedberg and Schneider found the cervix the most frequently involved genital site.

Pathogenesis

Man is infected by wading or swimming in, or drinking, water contaminated with the organisms. The life cycle of the parasite is complex, passing through many stages. The blood flukes deposit their eggs in the venules, and the larvae within the eggs supposedly elaborate lytic ferments that weaken the walls of the venules, thus permitting the discharge of eggs into the perivascular tissues. The eggs, by some mechanism, apparently effect a passage to the epithelium to provoke the genital lesions. Commonly, small nodules are discernible beneath the squamous epithelium; these precede the formation of papillomatous lesions.

Clinical features

Charlewood, Shippel, and Renton report that bilharzial lesions of the vulva are well-known in South Africa. Vulvar lesions appear as papillomatous masses similar to those of condyloma acuminatum or carcinoma or as granulomatous ulcerative lesions. The cervical or vaginal disease is represented by visible papillomatous growths, ulcerations, or hard nodules (Fig. 17-13). The lesions of the cervix and vagina are usually friable and tend to bleed on contact. A malodorous discharge is usually present. Since the bladder is also usually involved in these cases, dysuria and hematuria are often associated.

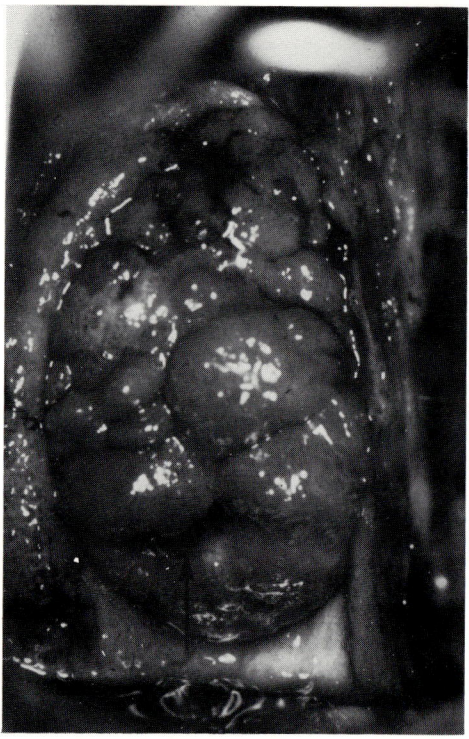

Fig. 17-13. Schistosomiasis. Papillomatous lesion of cervix and vaginal vault. The lesion was friable and bled easily. Arrow points to external os of cervix. (Friedberg, D., and Schneider, J.: Med. Proc. 13:187, 1967.)

Dyspareunia and postcoital bleeding are complained of by some patients.

Histopathology

Charlewood, Shippel, and Renton observed that the degree and type of reaction of the tissues to the ova of schistosomes in different patients and in contiguous tissues in the same patient is highly variable. Squamous epithelium tends to become hypertrophied (Fig. 17-14), whereas connective tissue tends to exhibit a chronic inflammatory reaction. Some degree of fibrous tissue reaction is usually associated. Beneath ulcerated areas, stromal infiltration is pronounced. In most cases, fresh and calcified ova are scattered throughout the affected tissues (Fig. 17-14) and are often accompanied by a foreign body type of giant cell. The cervical and vaginal mucosa may be denuded, atrophic, or hyperplastic. At times, granulomas or pseudotubercles are prominent. Squamous epithelium, particularly of the vulva, commonly has papillomatous projections, the stroma of which is loose and edematous and contains eggs in varying stages of calcification.

Diagnosis

Genital schistosomiasis should be considered in patients who, after being in endemic areas, are found to have ulcerations and papillomatous lesions of the vulva, vagina, or cervix that are otherwise inexplicable. The condition is particularly to be suspected if dysuria and hematuria are present. The papillomatous form of the disease is said to be easily confused with carcinoma and condyloma acuminatum. According to Youssef, Fayad, and Shafeek, the diagnosis of schistosomiasis of the lower genital tract can be established only by the discovery of the eggs in Papanicolaou smears or in histologic sections of tissue. They found eggs in smears from some patients who had no gross evidence of the disease. Reportedly, the ova are readily detected if ulceration or papillomatosis has developed.

Treatment

The systemic use of antimony compounds, such as antimony sodium tartrate, is probably the most effective treatment for this disease.

Erythrasma

Erythrasma, a superficial skin infection, was first described clinically by Burchardt in 1859. The disease is more prevalent in tropical climates and in men; however, it does develop in temperate zones and in women. Knox has found the disease to be extremely common in the Houston area, but many of the patients are asymptomatic. Until Lagana, in 1960, and Sarkany, Taplin, and Blank, in 1961, assigned a bacterial cause for the infection, it was believed to be attributable to a fungus, the *Nocardia minutissima*, an aerobic actinomycete. It has now been established that the disease is caused by a pleomorphic bacillus of the genus *Corynebacterium*. *Corynebacterium minutissimum* has been accepted as the official name for the causative organism. Montes and others have demonstrated, with the use of electron micro-

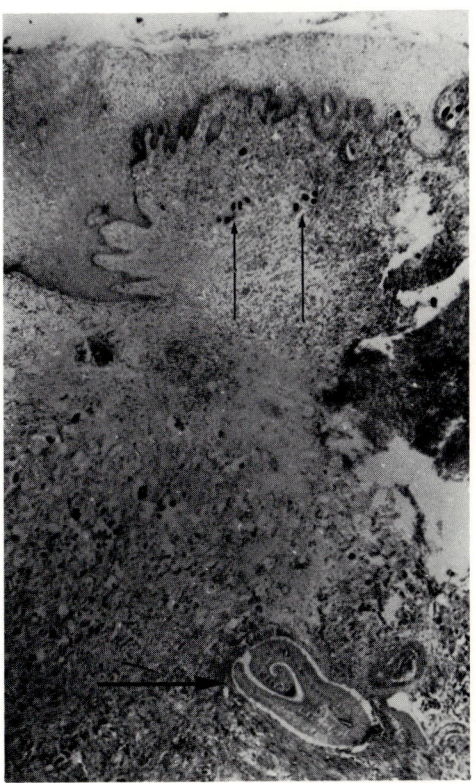

Fig. 17-14. Schistosomiasis. Vaginal papilloma; a schistosome worm (large arrow) in subcutaneous tissue and numerous ova within subepithelial tissue (small arrows). Epithelial hyperplasia also apparent. (Courtesy D. Friedberg, Johannesburg, South Africa.)

graphs, that the bacteria penetrate as deeply as one-half the thickness of the stratum corneum.

Clinical features

The disease affects chiefly intertriginous sites, particularly the groin, toe webs, axillae, and submammary skin. Genitocrural erythrasma (Fig. 17-15) resembles tinea cruris in that both involve the upper thighs, perineum, groin, and gluteal regions and in that both infections give rise to macular, well-defined and confluent lesions. The two diseases differ mainly in that the borders of erythrasma are not appreciably elevated and are without vesiculation. The lesions of erythrasma, as the name suggests, are usually dark red or brown and often are barely visible by daylight. Fine scaling of the involved surfaces of the skin may be present, especially in those lesions distant from the moist vulva. The patients are essentially without symptoms, although minimal pruritus is occasionally experienced.

Diagnosis

Scrapings from suspected lesions will reveal *C. minutissimum* in a potassium hydroxide preparation or when stained with methylene blue (Fig. 17-16), Gram's stain, or Giemsa's stain. The stained smears are the more informative. Gram-positive rod-like organisms or coccobacillary forms are demonstrable. No branching filaments are ob-

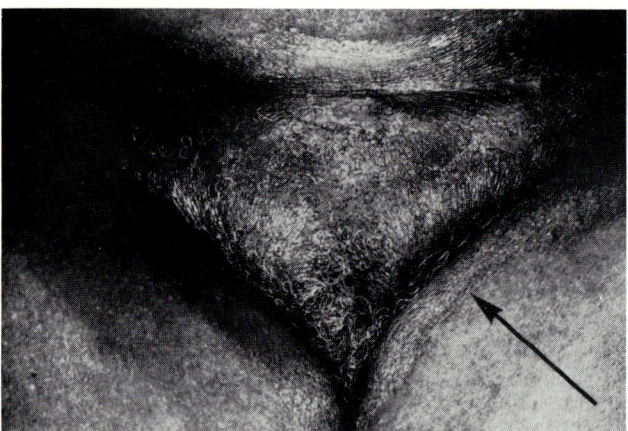

Fig. 17-15. Erythrasma. A flat, sharply demarcated lesion. Arrow points to edge of lesion in left groin. (Courtesy John M. Knox, Houston.)

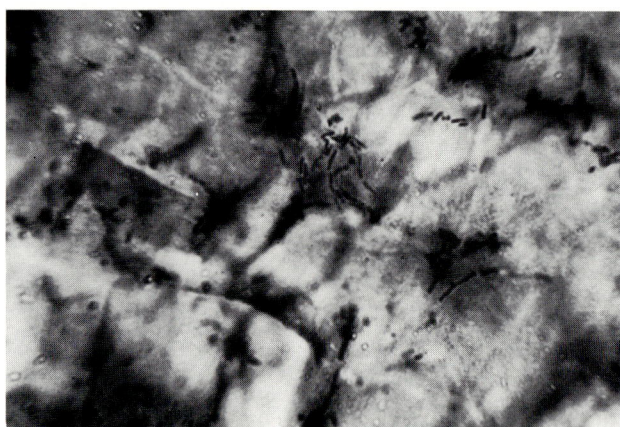

Fig. 17-16. *Corynebacterium minutissimum* in scrapings from vulva of patient with erythrasma. (Methylene blue stain) (Courtesy Robert G. Freeman, Houston.)

served, as in fungal infections and conidia are lacking.

Sarkany, Taplin, and Blank (1962) cultured the scales from patients on a medium containing 20% fetal bovine serum, 2% agar, and 78% tissue culture medium 199 (Morgan, Morgan, and Parker) and incorporating phenol red as an indicator. The pH of the medium was adjusted to between 6.8 and 7.2, with 0.05% tris-(hydroxymethyl)-aminomethane (Tris). Within 12 to 24 hours small (1 to 2 mm.) shiny, translucent, slightly convex colonies appeared; under Wood's light, these produced varying degrees of red to orange fluorescence.

Involved sites, when exposed to Wood's light (ultraviolet lamp with a nickel cobalt filter) in a darkened room, will present a coral-red or pink fluorescence. This is clinically diagnostic of the infection. The fluorescence has been attributed to a bacterial coproporphyrin.

Treatment

Erythrasma, being a mild and superficial infection, responds to such keratolytic agents as ointments of salicylic acid or resorcinol. After the use of these agents for several days, the application of 20% to 25% aqueous solution of sodium hyposulfite is beneficial. The infection also responds to oral antibiotics, especially erythromycin. Simple procedures such as scrubbing the affected area twice daily using an antibacterial soap such as Dial will give a cure in most cases. Griseofulvin, which is of value for the tineas, is ineffective in this condition.

REFERENCES

Abell, M. R.: Cervicocolpitis (vaginitis) emphysematosa, Surg. Gynec. Obstet. **107:**631, 1958.

Arean, V. M.: Manson's schistosomiasis of the female genital tract, Amer. J. Obstet. Gynec. **72:**1038, 1956.

Bernstine, J. B., and Rakoff, A. E.: Vaginal infections, infestations and discharges, New York, 1953, McGraw-Hill Book Co.

Bhaduri, K. P.: Endamoeba histolytica in leukorrhea and salpingitis, Amer. J. Obstet. Gynec. **74:**434, 1957.

Bickers, W.: Leukorrhea, new classification and new approach to treatment, Virginia Med. Monthly **70:**135, 1943.

Blinick, G., Steinberg, P., and Merendino, J. V.: Effect of sulfonamide cream on the bacterial flora of the infected vagina and cervix, Amer. J. Obstet. Gynec. **58:**176, 1949.

Braga, C. A., and Teoh, T. B.: Amoebiasis of the cervix and vagina, J. Obstet. Gynaec. Brit. Comm. **71:**299, 1964.

Braun, C.: Ztschr. Ges. Wiener Aertze **2:**182, 1861; cited by Chiari, H.: Ueber die Gascysten der menschlichen Schiede, Ztschr. Heilk. **6:** 81, 1885.

Burchardt, M.: Ueber eine bei chloasma verkommende Pilzform, Med. Ztschr. **2:**141, 1859.

Carpenter, C. B., Mozley, P. D., and Lewis, N. G.: Schistosomiasis Japonica involvement of the female genital tract, J.A.M.A. **188:**647, 1964.

Charlewood, G. P., Shippel, S., and Renton, H.: Schistosomiasis in gynaecology, J. Obstet. Gynaec. Brit. Comm. **56:**367, 1949.

Chaves, E., and Palitot, P.: Pelvic schistosomiasis, Amer. J. Obstet. Gynec. **89:**1000, 1964.

Chiari, H.: Ueber die Gascysten der menschlichen Schiede, Ztschr. Heilk. **6:**81, 1885.

Friedberg, D., and Schneider, J.: Bilharziasis, Med. Proc. **13:**187, 307, 1967.

Gardner, H. L.: Desquamative inflammatory vaginitis; a newly defined entity, Amer. J. Obstet. Gynec. **102:**1102, 1968.

Gardner, H. L.: Vaginitis emphysematosa, Amer. J. Obstet. Gynec. **56:**123, 1948.

Gardner, H. L., and Dukes, C. D.: Haemophilus vaginalis vaginitis, Amer. J. Obstet. Gynec. **69:**962, 1955.

Gardner, H. L., and Fernet, P.: Etiology of vaginitis emphysematosa, Amer. J. Obstet. Gynec. **88:**680, 1964.

Gray, L. A., and Barnes, M. L.: Vaginitis in women, diagnosis and treatment, Amer. J. Obstet. Gynec. **92:**125, 1965.

Halprin, K. M.: Diagnosis with Wood's light, J.A.M.A. **199:**841, 1967.

Hite, K. E., Hesseltine, H. C., and Goldstein, L.: A study of the bacterial flora of the normal and pathologic vagina and uterus, Amer. J. Obstet. Gynec. **53:**233, 1947.

Hoffman, D. B., and Grundfest, P.: Vaginitis emphysematosa, Amer. J. Obstet. Gynec. **78:** 428, 1959.

Hugier, P. C.: Mémoire sur les kystes de la matrice et sur les kystes folliculaires du vagin, Bull. Soc. Chir. Paris **1:**241, 1847.

Ingraham, C. B., and Hall, I. C.: Emphysematous vaginitis, Amer. J. Obstet. Gynec. **28:** 772, 1934.

Knox, J. M.: Personal communication, 1967.

Lagana, I.: Contribution to the study of the pathogenic agent of erythrasma and its therapy, Acta Microbiol. Hellen **5:**69, 1960.

Montes, L. F., and Black, S. H.: The fine structure of diphtheroids of erythrasma, J. Invest. Derm. **48:**342, 1967.

Montes, L. F., McBride, M. E., Johnson, W. P.,

Owens, D. W., and Knox, J. M.: Ultrastructural study of the host-bacterium relationship in erythrasma, J. Bact. **90:**1489, 1965.

Munguia, H., Franco, E., and Valenzuela, P.: Diagnosis of genital amebiasis in women by the standard Papanicolaou technique, Amer. J. Obstet. Gynec. **94:**181, 1966.

Mylius, R. E., and Ten Seldam, R. E. J.: Venereal infection by Entamoeba Histolytica in a New Guinea native couple, Trop. Geogr. Med. **14:**20, 1962.

Nagashima, Y.: Zur Histologie und Pathogenese der coepitis emphysematosa, Virchows Arch. Path. Anat. **249:**471, 1924.

Newton, W. L., Reardon, L. V., and DeLeva, A. M.: A comparative study of the subcutaneous inoculation of germfree and conventional guinea pigs with two strains of *Trichomonas vaginalis,* Amer. J. Trop. Med. **9:**56, 1960.

Sarkany, I., Taplin, D., and Blank, H.: Erythrasma—common bacterial infection of the skin, J.A.M.A. **177:**130, 1961.

Sarkany, I., Taplin, D., and Blank, H.: Erythrasma, a bacterial disease, Proceedings XII International Congress Dermatology, Washington, D. C., September, 1962.

Sarkany, I., Taplin, D., and Blank, H.: Incidence of bacteriology of erythrasma, Arch. Derm. **85:**578, 1962b.

Scheffey, L. C., Rakoff, A. E., and Lang, W. R.: An unusual case of exudative vaginitis (hydrorrhea vaginalis) treated with local hydrocortisone, Amer. J. Obstet. Gynec. **72:**208, 1956.

van Coeverden de Groot, H. D.: Amoebic vaginitis, South African Med. J. **37:**246, 1963.

Weaver, J. D., Scott, S., and Williams, O. B.: The bacterial flora found in nonspecific vaginal discharge, Amer. J. Obstet. Gynec. **60:**880, 1950.

Weinstein, B. B., and Weed, J. C.: Amebic vaginitis, Amer. J. Obstet. Gynec. **56:**180, 1948.

Wilbanks, G. D., and Carter, B.: Vaginitis emphysematosa, Obstet. Gynec. **22:**301, 1963.

Williams, A. O.: Pathology of schistosomiasis of the uterine cervix due to S. haematobium, Amer. J. Obstet. Gynec. **98:**784, 1967.

Youssef, A. F., Fayad, M. M., and Shafeek, M. A.: The diagnosis of genital bilharziasis by vaginal cytology, Amer. J. Obstet. Gynec. **83:**710, 1962.

Zweifel, P.: Die Vaginitis emphysematosa, oder Colpohyperplasia cystica nach Winkel, Arch. Gynaek. **12:**39, 1877.

Chapter 18

Miscellaneous mycoses

For practical usage, fungal infections are classified as superficial or deep. The superficial types involve only the skin and mucosa, particularly the superficial epithelial layers. The deep fungal infections affect deep organs, though the skin may also be involved. The following simple classification of both types of fungal diseases may be useful to the gynecologist:

A. Superficial mycoses
  1. Candidiasis (Chapter 11)
  2. Torulopsis glabrata vulvovaginitis
  3. Dermatophytoses
     a. Tinea cruris
     b. Tinea versicolor (pityriasis versicolor)
     c. Tinea circinata (tinea corporis)
B. Deep mycoses
  1. Actinomycosis
  2. Blastomycosis
  3. Sporotrichosis
  4. Coccidioidomycosis

SUPERFICIAL MYCOSES
Torulopsis glabrata vulvovaginitis

So little is known about *Torulopsis glabrata* that it receives no mention in most textbooks of medical mycology. Only sketchy information is available regarding the frequency with which the fungus can be isolated or its relationship to clinical disease. Wickerham described it as a marginal pathogen. Guze and Haley pointed out that cases of bronchial pneumonia, urinary tract infection, and septicemia had been attributed to *T. glabrata;* they believed that the factors that predispose to candidiasis are also operative in predisposing to *T. glabrata* infection. These authors also reported that inoculation of the organism into rabbits, guinea pigs, rats, and white mice produced disease in many different organs.

DeSousa and Van Uden found *T. glabrata* in thirty-nine (8.1 percent) of 481 vaginal cultures. The patients who harbored the organism presented no clear-cut evidence of vulvovaginitis; however, those whose vaginal cultures were positive had a much higher incidence of positive stool cultures than a control group of subjects. Smith, Taubert, and Martin reported that *T. glabrata* was the only discernible fungus in the vaginal cultures of six (9.7 percent) of sixty-two pregnant women believed to have "vulvovaginal mycosis." Since no other vaginal pathogens were found in the cultures of these six patients, *T. glabrata* was considered responsible for the clinical disease. Kearns and Gray, in a study of eighty-two patients with symptoms of vaginal mycosis, found *T. glabrata* alone in six (7.3 percent). Four had definite evidence of vulvovaginitis, as indicated by mild itching, erythema, and discharge. The discharge was described as homogeneous and creamy, without curds, and with a pH of 4.5 to 5.0. The signs and symptoms disappeared upon eradication of *T. glabrata.*

Perju, Filip, and Sanda reported sixteen cases of vulvovaginitis that they attributed to *T. glabrata.* They unhesitatingly labeled the organism a pathogen, and their description of the clinical manifestations agrees with that of others. Timonen, Salo, and Haapoja isolated the organism from the vaginas of seventy patients, twenty-one of whom had "inflammation of the vagina."

Since 1963, new interest has been aroused in *T. glabrata.* In our experience since that time, the fungus has been discovered in many patients with mild pruritus and an increased discharge from which no other fungus or known vaginal pathogen could be isolated.

After analyzing and correlating all the

270 Benign diseases of the vulva and vagina

available reports, it seems that *T. glabrata* must be considered a weak pathogen that is capable of producing mild vulvovaginitis in susceptible patients. Actually, it is rather like *Candida*, in that it is often in evidence without inciting clinical disease.

Clinical features

Our observations correspond closely with those of Kearns and Gray and of Perju, Filip, and Sanda. The most common clinical feature is an increase in the vaginal discharge, its gross characteristics being only slightly different from those of normal secretions. No malodor is present; the color is white or slate; the consistency is less curdy than normal; thrush patches do not form; and the acidity is usually about pH 4.5, in contrast to a pH 3.8 to 4.2 in normal subjects. Erythema is only slight, if present. Discharge, mild itching, and a burning sensation are manifestations most often mentioned by the patient.

Diagnosis

The patient with mild symptoms of vulvovaginitis who is found to harbor none of the usual vaginal pathogens might be suspected of having *T. glabrata* infection. As a rule, a wet mount of secretions in physiologic saline, when viewed under high power magnification, contains a tremendous number of spores similar to those of *Candida*, though much smaller and highly variable in size (Fig. 18-1). No hyphae are present and pus cells are relatively few. Vaginal secretions treated with 20% potassium hydroxide, as well as stained smears, also show numerous small spores but no hyphae.

As for cultures, Wickerham reported that *T. glabrata* produced smooth colonies without hyphal tips and caused gaseous fermentation of glucose and trehalose. He pointed out that no other species of yeast is known that ferments these sugars and does not assimilate maltose, sucrose, and cellobiose. In his opinion, *T. glabrata* is readily differentiated from other fungi by its carbon assimilation reactions and by its ability to assimilate nitrate.

Treatment

From limited experience we have found that *T. glabrata* infections respond to most fungicidal agents employed for candidiasis, though preparations containing gentian violet seem superior. Timonen reported a high recurrence rate and a resistance to treatment.

Dermatophytoses (Tineas)

Dermatophytoses are those superficial fungal infections that involve only the skin and its appendages. Involvement of skin appendages of the vulva is rarely, if ever, a problem. The same fungi that invade the superficial layers of the skin are often present

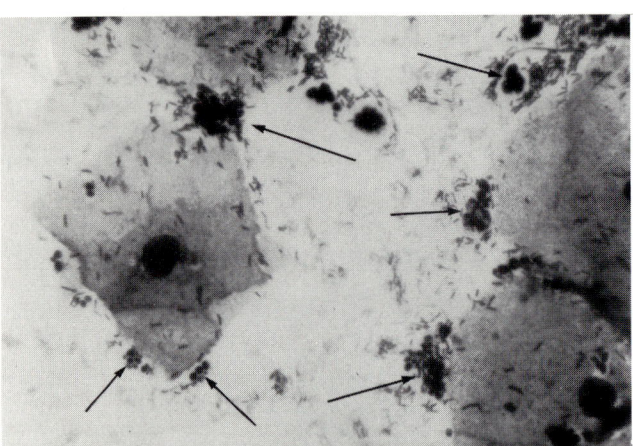

Fig. 18-1. *Torulopsis glabrata*. Direct smear of vaginal secretions containing numerous conidia (arrows). No hyphae present. (Gram's stain) (High power)

as saprophytes on the skin of healthy persons. Their pathogenicity varies widely in different individuals. These fungi thrive best on softened skin such as is found in intertriginous areas, where opposed sweating surfaces are subjected to constant contact and trauma. This environment, which is particularly likely to be found in hot and humid climates, frequently allows fungi to invade the corneum and become pathogenic. If the environment is not particularly favorable or if the pathogenicity of the organism is weak, only a low-grade chronic infection develops. This type of infection may persist for years without causing pruritus and may go unnoticed by the patient.

All of the dermatophytoses (clinical tineas) have a strong tendency to recurrence. The fungi are keratolytic, and thus they are able to digest keratin in the dead horny layer of the skin and to multiply. They neither live nor propagate in viable tissues. Inflammatory reactions apparently are induced by diffusible substances of an allergenic and exotoxic nature, which are excreted by the fungi.

Tinea cruris

Tinea cruris, originally called eczema marginatum, is a fungal infection of the genitocrural areas. It is much more prevalent in men, in whom it is frequently called jockey strap itch. The most common etiologic agents are *Epidermophyton floccosum*, *Trichophyton mentagrophytes*, and *Trichophyton rubrum*. Identification of the exact fungus is of little practical value since the signs and symptoms are essentially identical. *T. rubrum*, however, produces the most resistant infection. Since the causative organisms do not invade living tissues, the lesions remain superficial and limited to the stratum corneum of the epidermis.

Clinical features. The infection begins as a small erythematous patch with vesiculation and crusting or scale formation. The lesions spread peripherally and coalesce as they enlarge, sometimes healing at the center during this process. Ordinarily they are bilateral, although they may be unilateral. They develop most often on the upper inner thighs, usually spreading to the groin, perineum, and buttocks. Generally, the lesions are well-circumscribed and have margins that are erythematous, slightly elevated, and vesiculated (Fig. 18-2). Scaling is minimal on the moist vulvar tissues; in drier areas it can be conspicious. The color varies from almost normal or only slightly pigmented to red. Maceration and "weeping" sometimes follow scratching, especially during the summer months or may result from hypersensitivity to inappropriate therapeutic drugs. Continuous scratching gives rise to lichenification and, occasionally, thickened patches that resemble neurodermatitis in every respect. Mild to intense pruritus is the chief symptom. Transmission from person to per-

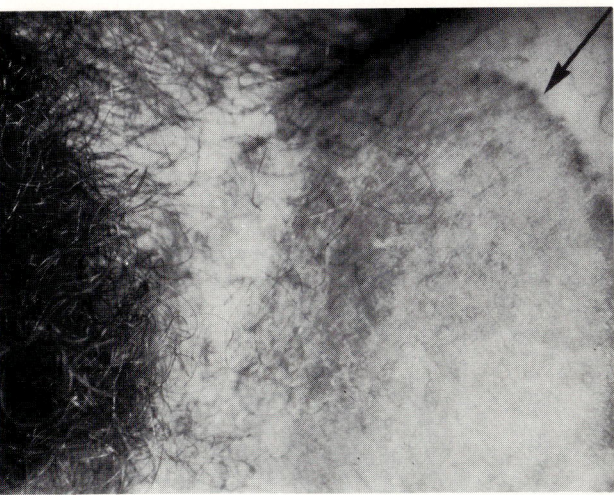

Fig. 18-2. Tinea cruris. Well-circumscribed lesion with active vesiculated margins.

son at the time of coitus is possible, although the infection is not classified as a venereal disease.

Histopathology. The PAS stain of Hotchkiss-McManus demonstrates fungi in the corneum. Since the cell wall is rich in polysaccharides, the fungi stain a deep red. Other structures stain pale pink.

Diagnosis. The presence of a typical lesion strongly suggests the diagnosis, although proof depends upon the laboratory findings. The hyphae of the fungus can be found in marginal scrapings suspended in 20% potassium hydroxide solution (Fig. 18-3). On gentle heating over a flame for 15 to 20 seconds without boiling, the keratinized cellular debris will rapidly dissolve and the organisms will then be easier to find. The fungi can be cultured on Sabouraud's medium, and from this medium a mycologist can make subcultures for identification of the types. It should be remembered that demonstration of fungi is difficult for several days after the use of any topical agent.

In some respects, erythrasma is grossly similar to tinea cruris, yet it lacks an active border, is associated with minimal or no itching, and is fluorescent under Wood's light. Seborrheic dermatitis should rarely be confusing; usually typical lesions are found elsewhere, and oiliness and scaliness are pronounced. Cutaneous moniliasis is a more acute process, and unless the lesions of tinea have become eczematoid incident to trauma or medications, the distinction should not be difficult. The fungi of tinea cruris and moniliasis differ morphologically. As a rule, the former yield only hyphae, whereas in candidal lesions both hyphae and spores can be detected. In psoriasis, lesions are practically always present on other parts of the body, coarse desquamation is apparent, and fungi should not be demonstrable.

Treatment. If the lesions are in an eczematoid stage, the acute inflammatory process should first be alleviated by the use of calamine lotion, frequent applications of wet compresses of Burow's solution 1:20, or compresses prepared from aluminum sulfate (Domeboro) powder (1 tablet or packet in 8 oz. of tap water). Vioform = Hydrocortisone Cream or Lotion (3% iodochlorohydroxyquin and 1% hydrocortisone) is also effective. After the acute inflammatory reaction has been controlled, keratolytic agents such as ointments of salicylic acid (half-strength Whitfield's or Pragmatar), as well as those containing resorcinol, may be used. Salicylic acid is not only keratolytic; it is also fungicidal. Undecylenic acid ointment 5% (Desenex Ointment) is an effective fungicide.

In recent years, griseofulvin, given orally, has been accepted with varying degrees of enthusiasm. Reactions have been reported. The average dose varies from 0.5 to 1.0 gm. per day in divided doses of 250 mg. After the infection has been controlled, the dosage can be reduced to 0.5 gm. daily. Four to six weeks are required for treatment. Improved results have been obtained by the use of micronized griseofulvin, 250 mg. twice daily.

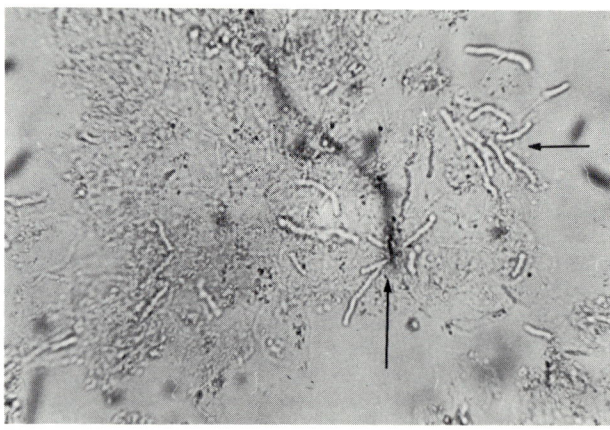

Fig. 18-3. Trichophyton organisms from patient with tinea cruris. Smear contains hyphae only. (Potassium hydroxide preparation)

This agent is not water soluble, and absorption is improved if it is taken with a meal containing some fat. Probably, it should be reserved for patients who are hypersensitive to locally applied agents or those with widespread disease that does not respond to local therapy. The administration of both topical agents and oral griseofulvin might expedite cure, especially of obstinate infections by *T. rubrum*.

Tinea versicolor

This fungal infection, sometimes called *pityriasis versicolor,* usually involves the skin of the trunk; only rarely does it involve the vulva. The causative fungus is *Malassezia furfur,* formerly called *Microsporon furfur.* Intimate contact by a susceptible subject who sweats profusely may be necessary for establishment of the infection.

Clinical features. Tinea versicolor of the vulva is often somewhat symmetrical and may spread over wide areas, including the inner thighs. The lesions are usually multiple, round or discoid, and have a finely scaling, yellowish appearance. Increased moisture, as from sweating, may produce a reddish-brown color that makes the lesions more distinct. As a rule, the edges are not infiltrated or vesiculated as in tinea cruris. The presence of typical lesions on the trunk may give a clue to the nature of the vulvar infection. In light-complexioned patients, an old infection may produce hyperpigmentation, whereas in dark-skinned persons or Negroes, some hypopigmentation may develop and persist long after the active infection has been controlled.

The only symptom is a mild pruritus and this is not always associated.

Histopathology. Histologic sections of involved skin prepared with PAS stain reveal numerous spores and hyphae typical of *Malassezia furfur* in the stratum corneum, particularly the middle layers. Mild inflammatory infiltration is often apparent in the prickle and basal cell layers.

Diagnosis. A definite diagnosis of tinea versicolor can rarely be made by inspection alone; rather, it must depend upon the discovery of the characteristic organism in the scales (Fig. 18-4). They are easily demonstrated by treatment of the scrapings with 20% potassium hydroxide. The hyphae are short, rod-like, and angular, and groups of spores resembling clusters of grapes are usually present.

The differential diagnosis might include vitiligo or postinflammatory pigmentation from any cause. This infection is sometimes grossly indistinguishable from erythrasma. Any disease which exhibits fine scales must be considered.

Treatment. A thorough scrubbing of the area with soap and water followed by careful drying and the application of an ointment containing 2% salicylic acid and 5% sulfur twice daily for several weeks is sufficient to eradicate the infection. The depigmentation may persist for months.

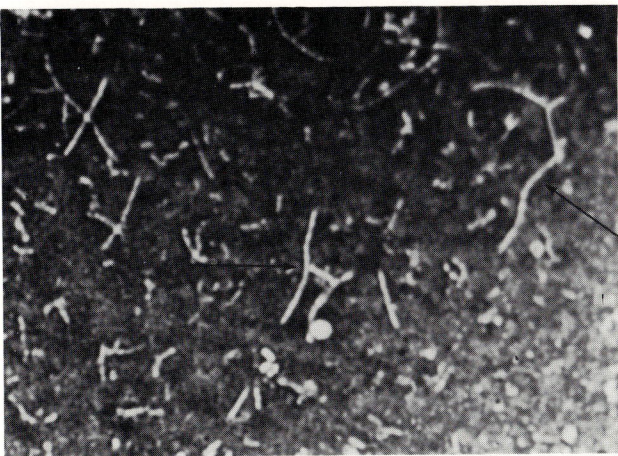

Fig. 18-4. *Malassezia furfur* organisms in scrapings from patient with tinea versicolor. The hyphae are short and angular. (Methylene blue stain)

Tinea circinata (tinea corporis)

Tinea circinata is a lesion of the nonhairy or glabrous skin, although it is occasionally observed in the genitocrural, inguinal, and perianal areas. Actually, this disease is of only slight importance to the gynecologist in the United States.

Several varieties of fungi give rise to morphologically similar lesions that justify the designation tinea circinata. These include *Epidermyphyton floccosum*, *Trichophyton*, and *Microsporum* of animal origin.

Clinical features. The lesions may be single or multiple. As a rule, they begin as papules or vesicopapules, become scaly, and eventually form circumscribed oval or round plaques ranging in size from several millimeters to several centimeters. The larger lesions may be formed by coalescence of small plaques. They tend to heal centrally, which causes the formation of rings with a clearing within the ring. The margins are usually active with minute vesicopapules and scales. The cleared surface between the margins is smooth or, at times, slightly scaly.

Usually, the only subjective symptom is pruritus, which is dependent on the degree of inflammation and the extent of the eruption.

Histopathology. The PAS stain is most helpful in identifying fungi, since the cell walls are rich in polysaccharides. Fungi stain deep red, while most other structures stain pale pink. Microscopic examination of the affected skin will usually reveal only a few hyphae and no spores. Without demonstrable fungi, the histologic picture is not characteristic. Depending upon the acuteness of the infection, varying degrees of dermatitis are observed.

Diagnosis. The diagnosis depends upon demonstration of the fungus in the scales or in the tops of the vesicles. Treatment of scrapings with 20% potassium hydroxide is helpful. Culture methods are necessary for species identification.

Treatment. The majority of these infections yield rapidly to local applications of tincture of iodine, undecylenic acid preparations, half-strength Whitfield's ointment, and Vioform cream. An adequate dosage of oral griseofulvin is usually curative and is sometimes indicated if eruptions are extensive and resistant to treatment.

DEEP MYCOSES

Deep mycoses are those that affect deeper tissues or internal organs, though they may also involve the skin. Usually, they are chronic and their effects are serious. Deep mycoses of the vulvovaginal tissues are so extremely rare that their mention hardly warrants space in a book of this nature. It seems improbable that the average gynecologist will ever observe a single example; nevertheless, if a slowly progressive, chronic granulomatous or suppurative lesion appears on the vulva, the possibility of a deep mycosis deserves consideration. Such a lesion would be unlikely unless all laboratory tests had ruled out the usual venereal granulomata, tuberculosis, and chronic pyogenic suppurative diseases. Consultation with dermatologists, internists, and mycologists may be necessary for a definitive diagnosis. Therapy is difficult and not the responsibility of gynecologists.

Actinomycosis

Although actinomycosis of the genital tract is reported from time to time, primary infections of the external genitalia are extremely rare. The disease is caused by *Actinomyces bovis*, a primary pathogenic fungus of cattle (lumpy jaw). Entry is usually through an abrasion by contact with fungus-harboring material such as hay, straw, or packing material.

Reportedly, the initial lesion is a solid papular nodule of bluish-red color, with firm, deep, inflammatory infiltration. Subsequently, the infiltrate tends to soften, suppurate, and form multiple sinuses. The sinus discharge may contain sulfur yellow granules containing masses of the fungus. The infection spreads into various sites, such as to the perineum, perianal tissues, and vagina.

Blastomycosis

According to Furcolow and others, primary cutaneous blastomycosis is probably more prevalent in this country than is generally supposed. From their investigations within the United States, the disease is most often encountered in persons who live in the Mississippi and Ohio River basins. It has been presumed that virtually all cases are caused by primary inhalation of infective spores into the lungs. This primary infection in the lungs, however, is disseminated systemically via the bloodstream and commonly localizes in the skin, including that of the vulva. The North American form is attributable to *Blastomyces dermatiditis*. *Blastomyces brasiliensis* is found exclusively in South America.

The cutaneous manifestations reportedly are of several clinical types. Lever stated that granulomatous and suppurative lesions develop in any organ, including the skin. In his opinion, the cutaneous disease most often consists of verrucous plaques with an active border and a large number of underlying pustules.

Sporotrichosis

The causative agent of sporotrichosis is *Sporotrichum schenckii*, which usually enters injured skin. The source of infection may be soil, wood, or plants.

The primary lesion may be an inconspicuous red papule or pustular nodule (sporotrichotic chancre) at the inoculation site. This may persist for months or years before the patient seeks treatment. Later manifestations are highly variable; they may include papules, pustules, acneform efflorescences, or ecthyma. Verrucus changes are sometimes observed; skin ulceration is often associated. Frequently, the organisms invade underlying muscles and fascial layers. Since the disease tends to spread through the lymphatics, a cord-like induration along the path of lymphatic drainage may be present, together with subcutaneous nodules, suppuration, and overlying ulceration.

Coccidioidomycosis

The causative organism of coccidioidomycosis is the *Coccidioides immitis*, the lung being the usual portal of entry and the major site of infection. As a rule, infection of the skin follows systemic dissemination. Although primary cutaneous coccidioidomycosis may develop, distinction between primary and secondary varieties is difficult. The incidence of vulvar lesions is so low that few gynecologists will ever observe a single example.

The skin lesions, as in the other deep mycoses, are variable; they may appear as erythema nodosum–like nodules, papules, pustules, verrucose growths, and fungating ulcers.

REFERENCES

DeSousa, H. M., and Van Uden, N.: The mode of infection and reinfection in yeast vulvovaginitis, Amer. J. Obstet. Gynec. 80:1096, 1960.

Furcolow, M. L., Balows, A., Menges, R. W., Picker, D., McClellan, J. T., and Saliba, A.: Blastomycosis, J.A.M.A. 198:529, 1966.

Guze, L. B., and Haley, L. D.: Fungus infections of the urinary tract, Yale J. Biol. Med. 30:292, 1958.

Kearns, P. R., and Gray, J. E.: Mycotic vulvovaginitis, Obstet. Gynec. 22:621, 1963.

Lever, W. F.: Histopathology of the skin, ed. 3, Philadelphia, 1961, J. B. Lippincott Co.

Perju, A., Filip, E., and Sanda, G.: Un champignon peu connu des organes génitaux: La torulopsis glabrata, Arch. l'Union Med. Balkanique, Vol. 1, 1963.

Smith, A. G., Taubert, H. D., and Martin, C. W.: The use of Trichomycin in the treatment of vulvovaginal mycosis in pregnant women, Amer. J. Obstet. Gynec. 87:455, 1963.

Timonen, S., Salo, O. P., and Haapoja, H.: Vaginal mycoses, Acta Obstet. Gynec. 45:232, 1966.

Wickerham, L. J.: Apparent increase in frequency of infections involving Torulopsis glabrata, J.A.M.A. 165:47, 1957.

Chapter 19

Pediatric vulvovaginitis

"Pediatric vulvovaginitis" is applied herein to all cases of leukorrhea and vulvovaginal infection or inflammation in children from birth until the effects of ovarian estrogens have become manifest. In view of the differences in the ages of girls at the menarche and the variable physiologic changes that take place in the vagina at this time, the term cannot be applied to all cases in patients up to any specified age. Most children with vulvovaginitis are between the ages of 2 and 9 years. The incidence falls rapidly after initiation of ovarian activity and epithelial proliferation. Vulvovaginitis is the most common gynecologic disorder among children; even so, a distinction between disease and normality is sometimes difficult.

Although to many clinicians the gonococcus is still the principal cause of vaginitis in childhood, it is today seldom responsible, particularly in patients observed in the private practice of medicine; nevertheless, the necessity for eliminating the gonococcus as the offending agent remains. The vaginitides commonly observed in women (trichomoniasis, candidiasis, and *Haemophilus vaginalis* vaginitis) seldom affect children.

With few exceptions, the etiology of pediatric vulvovaginitis cannot be determined from clinical findings alone. For example, the clinical picture of gonorrhea varies widely in different patients and in the same patient at different stages of infection. Actually, most cases of pediatric vulvovaginitis cannot be directly attributed to specific microbial agents, and thus they must be classified as nonspecific. Hypoestrogenic vaginal atrophy is the most important predisposing factor.

AGE GROUP VARIATIONS IN VAGINAL PHYSIOLOGY AND BACTERIOLOGY

Before birth and for several days after birth, an infant has high estrogen levels acquired from the mother during intrauterine life. The estrogens stimulate a thick, well-cornified vaginal epithelium resembling that of the adult. The vaginal pH at birth is high (essentially that of the amniotic fluid), though it soon becomes acid (pH 4.0 to 4.5) and remains so for 2 to 4 weeks. The glycogen content is also high at birth, gradually diminishing during the next several weeks. For 2 or 3 days following birth the flora is mixed, but lactobacilli soon become the predominant organism.

After birth, the blood estrogen levels of the infant slowly and continuously decrease and the vaginal epithelial cells soon begin a rapid exfoliation. Since cellular regeneration proceeds more slowly than epithelial shedding, the vaginal epithelium becomes thinner and within 3 to 6 weeks regresses to a thickness of two to six layers of cells. At this stage, the epithelial cells in the cytologic smear are primarily of the parabasal type. Cellular glycogen is soon lost, and the vaginal acidity decreases, usually to pH 6.0 to 7.5. The lactobacilli are replaced by a flora that varies in different children and in the same child from day to day. Diphtheroids are usually the predominant organism, although species of staphylococci, streptococci, and coliform bacteria, including *Escherichia coli*, are often present. The characteristics of hypoestrogenism persist until puberty approaches.

Prepubescence, which usually starts when the child reaches the age of 9 to 11 years, is a period of gradually increasing ovarian estrogenic activity. The vaginal epithelium begins to thicken, glycogen increases, lactobacilli become reestablished, and acidity approaches the level of the normal adult. Once vaginal maturity is attained, the child is more susceptible to the common pathogens of adults and less susceptible to the causes of pediatric vulvovaginitis.

DIAGNOSTIC METHODS IN PEDIATRIC VULVOVAGINITIS

Special problems are involved in examining children. Friendliness toward the child and the development of rapport before examination is important, as is gentleness during the examination. Anesthesia is rarely required; however, local application of a topical anesthetic, such as Xylocaine jelly (2% lidocaine), to the vestibule before introduction of an applicator or instrument is sometimes advisable.

Since the epithelium of the introitus is thin and lies over a vascular stroma, the tissues are normally somewhat red and might be considered inflamed. The severity of infection is usually indicated by the degree of inflammation of the vulvar tissues; these changes, however, are often too nonspecific for differential diagnosis. Frequently, even gonorrheal infections are clinically indistinguishable from nonspecific types.

Vaginoscopy is extremely useful in differential diagnosis. Through an appropriate instrument, the entire vagina and cervix can be observed. Satisfactory instruments for visualization of the vaginal canal include the Kelly air cystoscope, Boehm female urethroscope, veterinary otoscope, and, for older children, the Huffman or Peterson bivalve speculum. Smears and material for cultures can also be taken through these instruments. Nasal specula do not permit proper visualization, nor does the human otoscope, both being too short.

Rectal examination with a finger can be helpful in the detection and removal of foreign bodies in the vagina. By this means, discharge also can be expressed from the vagina for laboratory study. In some patients, the need for vaginal instrumentation might thus be obviated. If the patient is an infant or small child, the little finger, thoroughly lubricated, should be used.

Other methods may be used to obtain vaginal material. The vestibule should first be wiped clean. A small glass catheter that has been dipped in physiologic saline may be inserted the full length of the vagina without causing pain or bleeding. Through the small openings, the tip will attract enough material for stained smears, wet mount preparations, and cultures. Another method consists of the injection and aspiration of physiologic saline through a small medicine dropper. Capraro aspirates material through a dry sterile plastic disposable aspirator, from which he makes eight laboratory examinations. A small, sterile, tightly wound, cotton-tipped applicator is also satisfactory for obtaining vaginal material, although this technique may cause slight bleeding from the vagina and make the child uncomfortable.

pH determination of secretions in the immature vagina is of little value in making a differential diagnosis of vulvovaginitis. Whether the vagina is infected or not, the pH approaches neutrality, whereas the normal mature vagina usually has a pH of 3.8 to 4.2.

Wet mount preparations are of less diagnostic value in the child than in the adult; they are useful chiefly for the detection of trichomonads, spores, and filaments of *Candida,* and the clue cells of *H. vaginalis,* none of which is ordinarily found in children. Wet mount preparations show the maturity of the epithelial cells and the number of pus and red blood cells. Pus cells are present in all immature vaginas, yet a high ratio of pus cells to epithelial cells is suggestive of infection. Frequently, red blood cells are attributable to the mechanical trauma of examination. Since parabasal epithelial cells are uniformly found in young children, their presence is without diagnostic significance.

The *gram-stained smear* is of particular value for determining the relative percentage of various types of bacteria, particularly after they have been identified by culture techniques. Some workers find that the gram-stained smear affords a more accurate quantitation of vaginal bacteria than a count of the colonies on solid culture media. The material must be obtained directly from the vagina; smears taken from secretions within the vestibule are essentially worthless. No special attempt to take urethral and cervical smears in a child is necessary, since these structures are seldom independently infected; rather, they would reflect only the bacteriologic status of the vagina. Moreover, endocervical smears are extremely difficult to obtain. The gram-stained smear is especially useful in the diagnosis of acute gonorrhea, although it is unreliable and frequently falsely negative in the chronic stage, after secondary infections have developed. From a medicolegal standpoint, the gram-stained smear is unacceptable as a definitive test. Other gram-negative diplococci, such as *Micrococcus catarrhalis, Neisseria sicca,* the meningococcus, and the pneumococcus, may be confused with the gonococcus. With the use of differential culture techniques, Weaver demonstrated that smears from twelve of sixteen patients that yielded gram-negative intracellular diplococci contained *Neisseria sicca* rather than *Neisseria gonorrhoeae.* The spores and filaments of *Candida* are easily identified on the gram-stained smear. This is not true of trichomonads.

The *immunofluorescent method* of positive identification of the gonococcus was developed by Deacon and others in 1959. An immediate direct fluorescent antibody (FA) method and a delayed FA technique are employed. The former affords a fairly accurate answer within an hour. The delayed FA test is more accurate in chronic cases, although 16 to 20 hours is necessary for cultivation of the vaginal exudate.

Culture techniques offer the most reliable method for accurate recognition of vaginal bacteria. As already mentioned, however, aside from the gonococcus, isolation and identification of a predominant bacterial organism does not prove its etiologic relationship to the apparent vulvovaginitis problem. Except for the gonococcus, thioglycollate broth is an excellent transport medium. Direct cultures on chocolate agar and fermentation reactions are necessary for positive identification of the gonococcus. According to Wende and others, the Thayer-Martin medium is particularly useful in the isolation of gonococci. Subcultures from thioglycollate broth can be made on Nickerson's or Sabouraud's medium for species of *Candida,* STS medium for trichomonads, Casman's blood agar for *Haemophilus vaginalis,* and others according to indications.

A Scotch tape swab of the anal margin permits detection of the ova of pinworms. Frequently, pinworm infestation must be eliminated as a cause of nonspecific vulvovaginitis in children, particularly in those who have unexplained chronic or recurrent pruritus and vulvitis.

LEUKORRHEA AND VARIETIES OF VULVOVAGINITIS
Physiologic leukorrheas
Neonatal leukorrhea

During intrauterine life, the vaginal epithelium and cervical mucosa are under the influence of maternal estrogens. As a result, not uncommonly, a large volume of desquamated epithelial cells (and perhaps some mucus) collects in the vagina, to be expelled gradually or suddenly soon after birth. This is a nonirritating and transient physiologic discharge. Having been acted upon by maternal estrogens, the endometrium sometimes partially sheds after estrogen withdrawal, as exhibited by a scant bloody discharge within a few days after birth.

Premenarchal leukorrhea

With the increased production of unopposed estrogens in the months or years immediately before the menarche, a physiologic type of leukorrhea may develop. Since its true nature is not understood by the child and mother, and not always by the physician, it may be interpreted as indicative of vaginal infection. The increased secretions result from proliferation and desquamation of vaginal epithelium and from increased production of mucus by the cervical glands. Ordinarily, the discharge first appears during the development of secondary sexual characteristics, being particularly prevalent in girls with congenital erosion. Since odor and irritative signs and symptoms are not associated, a distinction from infection is relatively easy. The only treatment usually required is reassurance of the patient and parent and instructions regarding vulvar hygiene. An occasional patient has a large congenital erosion and a profuse discharge, for which cauterization of the cervix may be necessary. As a rule, this is best deferred until the child has reached full sexual and anatomic development.

Leukorrhea from developmental anomalies

Developmental anomalies that may cause discharge or vulvovaginitis include ectopic ureteral openings into the vagina, a short anomalous urethra that permits partial emptying of the bladder into the vagina, and anomalous openings of the anus into the vestibule (anus vestibularis) or posterior vagina (see Chapter 3).

Nonspecific pediatric vulvovaginitis

The term "nonspecific" reflects our ignorance of the specific etiology of most cases of pediatric vulvovaginitis; however, in view of our inability to assign definite causes to these cases, be they real or imaginary, its use must be retained for the present. Thus, little girls who have abnormal vulvovaginal secretions and perhaps irritative signs and symptoms, without specific demonstrable cause, must be considered to have nonspecific vulvovaginitis. Although the term is still acceptable as applied to the disease in children, it is hardly acceptable for infections in the adult, since they are almost always attributable to a demonstrable etiologic agent.

Etiology

The vaginal flora in children with nonspecific vulvovaginitis is usually highly mixed, so there is little likelihood of incriminating a single bacterium as the causative factor. In fact, the range of bacterial organisms is similar to that recovered from any child with or without evidence of infection. As is true of senile vaginitis, nonspecific vulvovaginitis in children is directly related to the effects of extreme hypoestrogenism. Schauffler concluded that this was actually the explanation for most cases of nonspecific vaginitis in children.

The role of pinworms in the transference of bacteria from the rectum to the vagina is unknown, although it is probable that nonspecific infections develop more often in children with pinworm infestation. Because of the proximity of the anus and vagina, fecal contamination or filth of the vulva from neglect may also play a part. Other factors may consist of trauma from masturbation, the wearing of tight-fitting, nonabsorbent underclothing, and too vigorous cleansing by the mother. Many cases of supposed discharge or vulvovaginitis in children are explained solely by the imagination of an overly solicitous parent.

Clinical features

Nonspecific vulvovaginitis has no characteristic manifestations. The discharge may be thin and watery or purulent; it may irritate the vulva, leading to erythema, excoriations (Fig. 19-1), and edema. Irritation may cause the child to scratch and further manipulate the parts; as a result, the exudation may become more profuse, and dried secretions may appear on the underclothing. Urinary symptoms such as burning, frequency, and dysuria may also develop. Occasionally, a bloody discharge and enuresis are associated.

Treatment

Any disease of unknown etiology can present therapeutic problems. Frequently, nonspecific pediatric vulvovaginitis clears following the institution of hygienic measures alone. Local cleanliness with a mild soap and an abundance of water is helpful; strong soaps and overzealous scrubbing must be avoided. Medicated soaps, although useful in some cases, may be harmful in others. After a soapy water soaking and rinsing, the vulva should be gently dried, preferably by a blotting action instead of rubbing. The child should be taught to wipe from front to back after defecation to prevent fecal contamination of the vulva. The wearing of loose-fitting cotton panties instead of tight ones made of synthetic materials will help to prevent the accumulation of moisture. Topi-

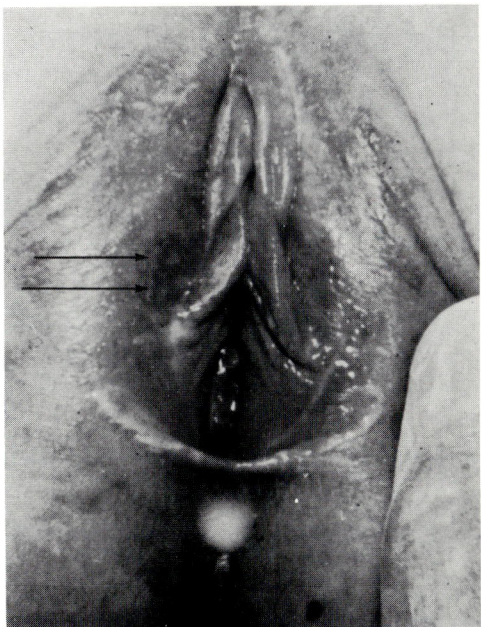

Fig. 19-1. Nonspecific vulvovaginitis in 10-year-old child. A wide area of erythema is present. Arrows indicate excoriations. These are not consistent findings. (Courtesy V. J. Capraro, Buffalo, N. Y.)

Table 9. Varieties of pediatric vulvovaginitis found by four investigators

	Macey-Barclay (1963)	Lang (1962)	Capraro (1965)	Tudor (1963)
Nonspecific (mixed)	31	67	42	0
Gonorrhea	2	4	6	0
Trichomoniasis	0	7	9	21
Candidiasis	2	5	8	2
Specific bacterial (streptococci, staphylococci, E. coli)	0	21	15	43
Pinworms	5	3	2	1
Foreign body	15	3	17	0
Physiologic	0	20	10	0
Congenital anomalies	0	0	4	0
Diphtheria	0	0	0	0
Miscellaneous	0	0	1	1

cal applications of antiseptics and germicides are essentially useless and might aggravate the disease.

The introduction, by Robert Lewis in 1933, of hypodermic injections of estrogens for pediatric vulvovaginitis was a significant milestone in gynecology. TeLinde and Brawner (1935) were the first to describe the topical use of estrogens for vaginitis. These agents continue as a mainstay in the treatment of patients with vulvovaginitis and estrogen deficiency, whether they are children or postmenopausal women. For pediatric patients with clinical evidence of vulvovaginitis without demonstrable cause, and particularly if the condition has not responded to hygienic measures, estrogens are not only warranted but indicated to compensate for the lack of the hormone. Estrogens, either applied locally or given systemically, produce thickening of the epithelium, an increase of vaginal acidity, and more abundant lactobacilli in the flora, all of which are inimical to many bacteria.

Gray and Kotcher (1961) and Capraro report excellent physiologic and therapeutic responses to the application of estrogenic creams (Premarin and dienestrol) to the vulvar tissues alone. Gray and Kotcher recommended the application of Premarin cream at bedtime for 2 to 3 weeks, and thereafter two or three times weekly for an additional 2 or 3 months. They found that the vaginal epithelium became well cornified within 2 weeks.

Intravaginal application of estrogenic creams and suppositories is effective, though actually it is unnecessary and often is emotionally traumatic to the child. If the intravaginal route is to be used, Premarin vaginal cream (0.625 mg. of equine conjugated estrogens per gram) and dienestrol cream (0.01%) are probably equally effective. If the patient is an infant or young child, the cream is best instilled through a glass or rubber catheter. A satisfactory regimen consists of 1 gm. of cream instilled nightly for 2 weeks and thereafter every three to four nights for an additional 6 weeks. Estrogenic suppositories containing 0.1 mg. of stilbestrol or any of several others designed for children may be used. A lubricating jelly will facilitate insertion. The mother must be taught how to insert suppositories with a forcep.

Estrogens, given systemically, are preferable to the intravaginal preparations for reasons already mentioned. Cornification of the vagina can be effected and maintained by the oral use of 0.1 mg. of stilbestrol daily for 2 weeks, and then 0.1 mg. twice weekly. Equine conjugated estrogens (Premarin 0.3 mg.) may be given in a similar manner. Usually, the treatment is continued for 6 to 12 weeks. Gray and Kotcher reported twenty-four cures in twenty-seven patients by means of these oral agents. In view of the possibility of premature development of secondary sexual characteristics and the remotely possible effects upon the epiphyses, estrogens should not be used indefinitely in the dosage recommended, even though the danger of significant adverse effects is slight.

Occasionally, antibiotics and chemotherapeutic agents, applied locally or given systemically, are indicated when the response to hygienic measures and estrogens proves disappointing. In general, the response of nonspecific vulvovaginitis to antibiotics and sulfonamides is poor, since most vaginal bacteria are resistant to these agents. Broad spectrum antibiotics, such as the tetracyclines, are more likely to elicit a response than penicillin. Such intravaginal sulfonamides as Sultrin cream (containing three sulfonamides) probably are as effective as intravaginal antibiotics. Rapid response to any of these medications points to a specific bacterial agent, such as a streptococcus, as the cause of the vaginitis. Another reportedly successful preparation is intravaginal Furacin (nitrofurazone) in cream or suppository form. Furacin-E urethral inserts (0.2% nitrofurazone and 0.1 mg. stilbestrol) are easily applied and are effective in some cases. Intravaginal use of Gynben cream (containing stilbestrol and sulfadiazine) might also be curative. Ointments and creams containing a corticosteroid (antiinflammatory) and an antibacterial agent, such as neomycin, frequently bring excellent results.

Gonorrheal vulvovaginitis

The diagnosis of gonorrhea in a child carries with it serious responsibilities for the physician and can stigmatize the patient. It should always be confirmed by cultures or by immunofluorescent methods. The rigors to which a child can be subjected by an apprehensive and distrustful parent can seriously and adversely influence sexual and other emotional behavior in later life.

Incidence

As an epidemic problem, infection with *Neisseria gonorrhoeae* has virtually disappeared in this country. Whether, because of questionable laboratory methods, gonorrhea was formerly too often regarded as responsible for vaginitis is debatable. The current low incidence (Table 9) is probably related to the availability of specific therapeutic agents and to a better appreciation of epidemiologic factors, as well as to improved diagnostic methods. Whatever the reason, relatively few children with gonorrhea are observed today. Gray and Kotcher (1961), in a study of 192 girls with vulvovaginitis who had anestrogenic vaginas, found gonococci in eighteen (9.3 percent). Most of their patients were from public clinics. Grossi and Buchman found no gonorrhea in thirty-five patients with vulvovaginitis. Table 9 presents a summary of the findings of several other investigators. Discrepancies in the reported incidence are easily explained by differences in patient material and perhaps occasionally by different diagnostic criteria. The incidence among institutionalized children of low social strata is higher than that in children from prosperous homes. According to a recent poll, the majority of gynecologists in the Houston area had never observed a child with gonorrhea in private practice.

Route of transmission

The most common route of transmission is unknown. Schauffler believed that it was most often transmitted from one child to another and that this was the most likely explanation for institutional epidemics. Most isolated cases probably are attributable to contact with infected individuals. The incidence of genital contact with infected adults is unknown.

If the assumption that the rectum sometimes harbors the organisms is correct, then rectal thermometers could be a source in poorly run institutions, as could communal fomites. Over a period of 1 year, Strauss found no secondary infections in a group of uninfected children who lived in close contact with a group of children with proved gonorrheal vaginitis in the wards of a large city hospital. From this observation, it seems unlikely that toilet seats are a source of infection. He found, however, that in 90 percent of the homes of children with gonorrhea, some other member of the family was also infected. In his opinion, sex play in older children is an important factor in transmission.

Clinical features

The thin, atrophic vaginal mucosa in childhood is susceptible to invasion by the gonococcus. The infection is superficial, diffuse, and limited primarily to the mucosa and submucosa. The vulvar tissues become reddened, edematous, and occasionally excoriated. Bartholin's glands, the cervix, and urethra are rarely involved. Ascending infection to the endocervix, uterus, tubes, and peritoneum is exceptional, usually being observed in children only after estrogenic activity has begun. As a rule, the discharge is creamy and yellowish or greenish; it may be profuse or scant. Signs and symptoms may include itching, burning, vulvar dysuria, and chafing. Untreated children with chronic disease frequently have relapses and remissions, with predictable variations in clinical signs.

Treatment

Antibiotics have replaced estrogens as the treatment of choice. Practically all cases of gonorrhea respond to penicillin. Although the dosage may be varied according to the age of the patient, as a rule, 600,000 U. of procaine penicillin intramuscularly given daily for 3 days should be more than adequate to effect a cure. For several reasons, injectable penicillin is more reliable than oral preparations. The tetracyclines may be employed for a penicillin-resistant strain of gonococcus. Although the sulfonamides have been used successfully, they are less effective than penicillin.

In addition, the usual hygienic measures should be carried out. Shake lotions or a powder, such as zinc stearate, might be beneficial in patients with dermatitis of the vulva. Vaginal douches, irrigations, antiseptics, and germicides are probably contraindicated.

Before specific therapeutic agents were available, the production of vaginal cornification by the use of estrogens was the most effective method of treatment. Estrogens cannot, however, be relied upon for microbiologic cures of gonorrhea with anything approaching the reliability of antibiotics. Occasionally, estrogens are valuable for combating secondary bacteria that may persist and cause a discharge after eradication of the gonococcus.

Nongonococcal specific bacterial infections

The bacteria in the normal and infected immature vagina are often remarkably similar. Except in gonorrhea or diphtheria, a predominant bacterium in the vagina of a child with vulvovaginitis is not necessarily proof of an etiologic relationship. Gray and Kotcher (1961) stated that, statistically, the various organisms isolated can rarely be incriminated as etiologic agents and that patients in control groups yield microbiologic populations similar to those of patients with vulvovaginitis. Nevertheless, we have found the *Streptococcus* a not uncommon exception. Several types of streptococci have been observed in pure cultures from children with vulvovaginitis. Capraro reported eight cases of streptococcal vaginitis, and Hedlund found vulvovaginitis from hemolytic streptococci in 105 of 758 patients with scarlet fever. That hemolytic streptococci can cause pronounced inflammatory reactions seems well-established. Usually, the tissues are erythematous and edematous; the discharge varies from a thin, watery type during the early stages of disease to one which is more purulent later. Such systemic reactions as fever and malaise may be associated.

Among other possible bacterial pathogens are different types of staphylococci, *Neisseria catarrhalis,* pneumococci, proteus, *Escherichia coli,* and various other coliform bacilli. No generally acceptable clinical patterns of infection from these organisms have been defined. Seemingly, no bacterial agent should be incriminated as the etiologic agent unless it is highly predominant and persistent, and unless its eradication brings about a complete cure of the patient. Even then, absolute proof of its causative role is not assured.

Treatment

When a predominant bacterium is suspected as being responsible for vulvovaginitis in a child, treatment should be delayed until sensitivity tests have been made. Most antibiotics are available for local application, including the tetracyclines, penicillin, and Mycitracin (polymyxin-neomycin-bactracin mixture). Furacin (nitrofurazone) cream and suppositories are also effective against many bacteria. Estrogens may bring about a cure, even though a particular bacterial agent is believed to be the cause of the infection. The administration of antibiotics systemically is only rarely indicated.

Diphtheritic vulvovaginitis

Diphtheritic vulvovaginitis is caused by *Corynebacterium diphtheriae* (the Klebs-Loeffler bacillus). After susceptibility testing and immunization became available, diphtheria in any form all but disappeared in this country. Few physicians will ever encounter a single case of diphtheritic vaginal infection. The majority of reported cases have been primary infections, although many have been associated with diphtheritic respiratory infections.

Clinical features

According to published reports, the area most often affected is the vestibule of the vulva, yet all vulvar and vaginal surfaces may be involved. The characteristic lesion is an adherent, grayish or yellowish pseudomembrane of varying thickness. Separation of the membrane from the underlying tissues leaves a bleeding surface. Vulvar excoriations and inguinal adenopathy may be observed. The discharge is usually profuse and serous, although it may be sanguinopurulent and malodorous. The systemic effects are identical to those of the respiratory form of disease.

Diagnosis

During an epidemic or when a history of contact is given, diphtheritic vulvovaginitis should be suspected if a child has the typical adherent pseudomembrane, and especially if the usual systemic reactions associated with the disease are apparent. Laboratory diagnosis depends upon isolation of the Klebs-Loeffler bacillus, Loeffler's being a suitable culture medium for this purpose. Because of the similarity of the Klebs-Loeffler bacillus to the diphtheroids that inhabit most vaginas, a diagnosis from smears in unreliable. The organisms can be easily isolated from vaginal secretions, though cultures may be falsely negative if the patient is taking antibiotics.

Treatment

The services of a physician who is familiar with all aspects of diphtheria is required. If the presence of the disease is suspected, specific antitoxin should be administered immediately. Penicillin or erythromycin, or both, should also be given. Aside from ordinary hygienic care, local treatment is contraindicated. Vaginal adhesions between ulcerated surfaces can be prevented by the insertion of strips of gauze impregnated with an antibiotic ointment.

Trichomoniasis, candidiasis, and *Haemophilus vaginalis* vaginitis

These infections are unimportant in the overall problem of pediatric vulvovaginitis, especially in infants and young girls, since the immature vagina does not provide a suitable environment for growth of the causative organisms. Binder found it worthwhile to publish a report of a single case of trichomoniasis in a 2-month-old girl. We have never observed trichomoniasis in a patient under the age of 8 years. The trichomonal infection is usually traceable to an infected person in the family. *H. vaginalis* has been isolated in a young patient only by de la Fuente, Rico, and Soria, who discovered the organism in a child 3 years old. We have never found *H. vaginalis* in a premenarchal patient, nor has Lang (1959) or Gray and Kotcher (1961) reported such a finding. Candidiasis is also rare in children less than 8 years old. This infection in a child before natural estrogenic activity begins suggests the recent administration of an antibiotic or estrogen or the presence of diabetes.

Treatment

In children, these infections require the use of the same therapeutic agents that are employed in adults—metronidazole for trichomoniasis, topical applications of nystatin for candidiasis, and a tetracycline given systemically for *H. vaginalis* vaginitis.

Worm infestations

Pinworms *(Oxyuris vermicularis* [Fig. 19-2], also called *Enterobius vermicularis)* are not uncommon in children with vulvovaginitis, although the worms are seldom found in the vagina. Roundworms *(Ascaris lumbricoides)* and whipworms *(Trichuris trichiura)* have been reported in the vagina of a few children. In the transport of bacterial agents to the vagina, the role of migrating worms in nonspecific infections is unknown. Their presence, like that of the gonococcus and foreign bodies, should be excluded in every case of pediatric vulvovaginitis.

Pinworms are thin, thread-like organisms varying in length from 3 to 12 mm. They are commonly found in the feces and around the anus, and occasionally between the labia. The ova are usually deposited on the perianal skin, where they are picked up on the fingers of children and ingested, thus starting another life cycle.

Pruritus and vulvovaginitis in children may be more often attributable to pinworms than is generally appreciated, even though Capraro found only two cases among 114 children with vulvovaginitis. Macey and Barclay found five cases among fifty-five children. Gray and Kotcher (1960), however, consider pinworms of little importance in the etiology of vaginitis in children. Whether those found between the labia produce a chemical irritative effect upon the tissues is not clear. Their presence is sufficient to cause pruritus, and the resultant trauma from scratching must explain some cases of vulvovaginitis.

Clinical features

Pruritus ani and vulvae is the chief manifestation of pinworm infestation. Changes in the tissues of the perianal and vulvar regions are most conspicuous, while the vaginal reaction is minimal. Pinworm infestation should be suspected if fingernail excoriations are visible in the perianal skin.

Treatment

Treatment consists of the administration of some piperazine preparation, such as Antepar or of pyrvinium pamoate (Povan). Antepar is given orally once daily before breakfast for 7 consecutive days. The recommended daily dosage, according to weight, is as follows: under 15 pounds, 250 mg.; 15 to 30 pounds, 500 mg.; 30 to 60 pounds, 1 gm.; and over 60 pounds, 2 gm. Povan is given as a single oral dose, equivalent to 5 mg. per kilogram of body weight. No laxatives, enemas, or special diets are necessary.

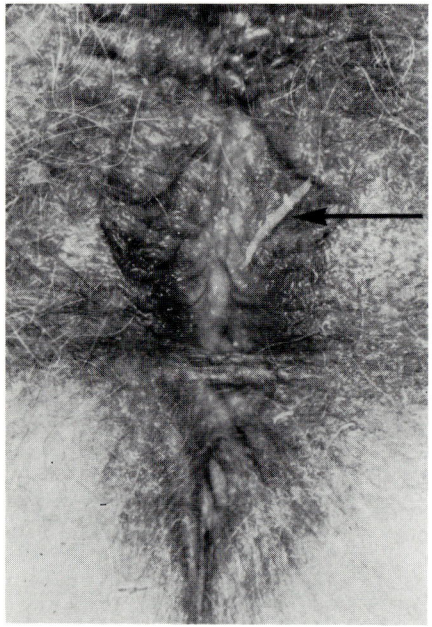

Fig. 19-2. Pinworms. Arrow demonstrates *Oxyuris vermicularis* (female) lying on vulva, a finding rarely observed.

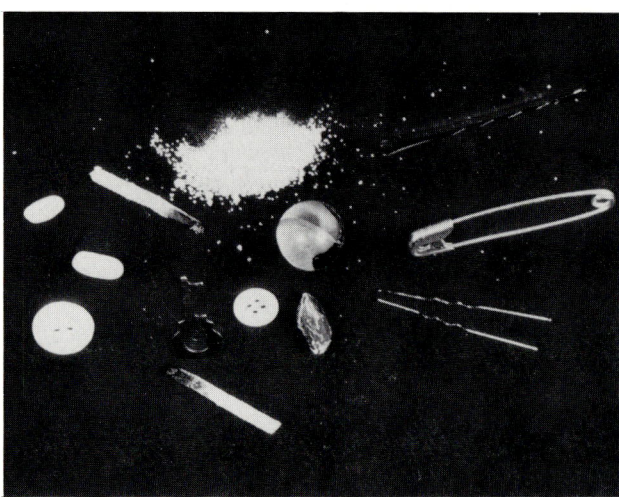

Fig. 19-3. Foreign bodies removed from vaginas of children. (Altchek, A.: GP **34:**85, 1966.)

Foreign bodies

The objects (Fig. 19-3) most often recovered from the vagina include wax crayons, pencils, safety pins, hairpins, wads of paper, marbles, twigs, chewing gum, erasers, and dried beans. Taylor has mentioned "sandbox" vaginitis, which is caused by particles of sand or grit in the vagina. Henderson and Scott described eleven cases of "toilet tissue" vaginitis, which appeared to be accidental rather than a result of exploratory curiosity (Fig. 19-4). Usually, the introduction of foreign bodies into the vagina has no more sexual basis than the introduction of objects into the ears and nose.

Incidence

The finding of objects in the vagina of children is considerably less common than is generally supposed. For example, Schauffler found only nine foreign bodies in 302 children with a vaginal discharge; Lang found only three in 110 patients with premenarchal vaginitis; and Tudor, in sixty-two cases of pediatric vulvovaginitis, found none.

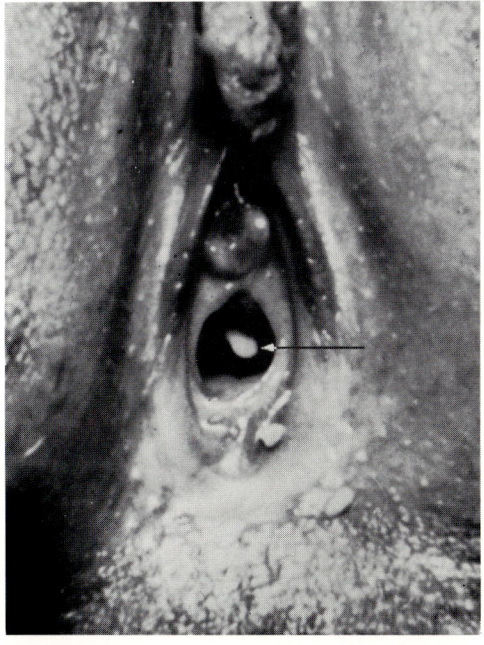

Fig. 19-4. Toilet paper within the vagina of a 6-year-old child. (Courtesy V. J. Capraro, Buffalo, N. Y.)

Clinical features

The symptoms produced by foreign bodies depend upon the shape, consistency, and chemical constituents of the objects. Those made of organic materials (erasers, chewing gum, beans, and paper) may provoke an acute chemical irritation. Such objects as pencils and hairpins occasionally cause lacerations, punctures, pain, and bleeding. Smooth and totally inert objects may remain in the vagina indefinitely without giving rise to much irritation; nevertheless, in general, foreign bodies ultimately produce a profuse, blood-tinged, malodorous vaginal discharge. The combination of persistent slight bleeding, discharge, and malodor should perhaps be called "Schauffler's syndrome," since Schauffler most actively publicized the importance of this symptom complex. Thus any child with this syndrome should be suspected of having a foreign body in the vagina, even though no history can be obtained of the introduction of an object. Also to be considered, however, is the possibility of a severe infection or a neoplasm.

The diagnosis is best established by vaginoscopic examination. A metal or glass object can be detected by probing the vagina with a metal instrument. If necessary, a radiogram will disclose a metal object. Rectal examination may afford additional information.

Treatment

Foreign bodies in the vagina must, of course, be removed. As a rule, this can be accomplished without the administration of a general anesthetic. Topical anesthesia with the use of such agents as Xylocaine jelly (2% lidocaine) is frequently advisable. The method of removal depends upon the shape, size, and consistency of the object. Its manipulation toward the introitus with a finger in the rectum is often possible. A grasping instrument, such as those used by the urologist, may be operated through a Kelly air cystoscope. Removal of such objects as safety pins or any hard substance that has become imbedded in the vaginal wall may require general anesthesia and, rarely, a short midline episiotomy.

REFERENCES

Altcheck, A.: Vulvovaginitis in children, GP **34:** 85, 1966.

Binder, S. S.: Vaginal trichomoniasis in a 2-month-old child, Obstet. Gynec. **21**:354, 1963.

Capraro, V. J.: Pediatric vulvovaginitis, J. Newark City Hosp. **2**:15, 1965.

Deacon, W. E., Peacock, W. L., Jr., Freeman, E. M., and Harris, A.: Indentification of *Neisseria gonorhoeae* by means of fluorescent antibodies, Proc. Soc. Exp. Biol. **101**:322, 1959.

de la Fuente, F., Rico, L. R., and Soria, F.: Hemofilasis urogenital—affeccion venereal, Rev. Esp. Obstet. Ginec. **18**:252, 1959.

Gray, L. A., and Kotcher, E.: Vaginitis in childhood, Amer. J. Obstet. Gynec. **82**:530, 1961.

Gray, L. A., and Kotcher, E.: Vulvovaginitis in childhood, Clin. Obstet. Gynec. **3**:165, 1960.

Grossi, M. T., and Buchman, M. I.: Vaginitis in children, Amer. J. Dis. Child. **97**:613, 1959.

Hedlund, P.: Acute vulvovaginitis in streptococcal infections, Acta. Paediat. **42**:388, 1953.

Henderson, P. A., and Scott, R. B.: Foreign body vaginitis caused by toilet tissue, Amer. J. Dis. Child. **111**:529, 1966.

Lang, W. R.: Pediatric vaginitis exhibit, American College of Obstetricians & Gynecologists, Chicago, April 1-4, 1962.

Lewis, R. M.: A study of effects of theelin on gonorrheal vaginitis in children, Am. J. Obstet. Gynec. **26**:593, 1933.

Macey, H. B., Jr., and Barclay, D. L.: Gynecologic problems of children, Bull. Tulane Univ. Med. Fac. **23**:95, 1964.

Schauffler, G. C.: Pediatric gynecology, ed. 4, Chicago, 1958, The Year Book Publishers, Inc.

Strauss, H.: Gynecology and obstetrics (Davis and Carter), Hagerstown, Md., 1964, W. F. Prior Co., Inc.

Taylor, E. S.: Essentials of gynecology, ed. 3, Philadelphia, 1965, Lea and Febiger.

TeLinde, R. W., and Brawner, J. N., Jr.: Experiences with amniotin in the treatment of gonococcal vaginitis in children, Amer. J. Obstet. Gynec. **30**:512, 1935.

Tudor, R. B.: Vulvovaginitis in children, Lancet **83**:401, 1963.

Weaver, J. D.: Nongonorrheal vulvovaginitis due to gram-negative intracellular diplococci, Amer. J. Obstet. Gynec. **60**:257, 1950.

Wende, R. D., Forshner, J. G., and Knox, J. M.: Field evaluation of the Thyer-Martin selective medium in the detection of *Neisseria gonorrheae*, Public Health Lab. **22**:104, 1964.

Chapter 20
Contact vulvovaginitis
Primary irritant and allergic reactions

Contact dermatitis is an inflammatory reaction of the skin to a primary irritant or allergenic substance. Eruptions from either cause are often clinically indistinguishable, and each may mimic many other types of skin disorder. The vaginal mucosa and the skin frequently respond in a similar manner. Reactions to contactants involve primarily the epithelium, although the dermis and submucosa usually undergo secondary changes. The majority of contact vulvovaginal reactions are induced by agents intentionally applied for therapeutic or hygienic purposes. Individuals susceptible to a topical agent are often considered to be "allergic" to that substance; however, most such individuals are merely hypersensitive rather than truly allergic to the particular agent.

Primary irritant reactions

A primary irritant is a substance that will produce an irritative response in the majority of persons upon first exposure. The corrosive chemicals, such as concentrated acids applied to the skin and potassium permanganate tablets applied to the vagina, are examples of strong primary irritants that affect tissues of all persons. Some primary irritants produce a response only after repeated contacts or in the presence of moisture or occlusiveness. An irritative response that develops only after prolonged exposure has been designated a *cumulative primary irritation*. The latter is not uncommonly associated with prolonged use of intravaginal medicaments for vulvovaginitis.

Allergic reactions

Allergic contact dermatitis, sometimes called allergenic contact dermatitis, eczematous dermatitis, or allergic eczema, is an eruption arising from contact with allergenic substances in susceptible individuals. An allergic reaction indicates that the subject has been sensitized through previous exposure to the allergenic substance. Subsequent reactions may follow either systemic administration of the allergen or contact of the skin with the substance. Usually, allergic reactions do not provoke clinical changes until several days or weeks after contact; this fact often is of value in the distinction between the two general varieties of contact reactions.

Clinical features

The following descriptions do not apply to the lesions of dermatitis medicamentosa.

Primary irritant reactions and allergic responses are so similar that the most expert dermatologist, much less the gynecologist, is frequently unable to make a clinical distinction between the two. The contactant in most vulvovaginal reactions probably is a primary irritant. With the exception of lesions caused by a strong corrosive substance, such as potassium permanganate, the clinical features of the acute responses to the two general varieties of contactants are essentially identical, both often consisting of erythema, edema, vesicles or bullae, and weeping (Fig. 20-1). Although crusting may develop in the drier areas of the body, it is less likely in the environment of the vulva. Vulvovaginal reactions, however, are highly variable; the majority do not exhibit the classical eczematoid response. Usually, erythema and edema of the vulva are the earliest signs and are frequently the only ones observed. Vesiculation and ulceration are more often induced by primary irritants used in strong concentrations or over a prolonged period of time or by allergenic substances. The severity of a reaction is also influenced by the sensitivity of the affected person, as well as by the environmental conditions at the site of contact. The intertriginous areas of the skin such as the intralabial and genitocrural folds and the groins, which are subject to moisture and rubbing, are also particularly susceptible to reactions from offending agents.

The features of contact dermatitis of long duration may include lichenification, scaling, thickening of the skin, and even white plaques. Perhaps some of the lesions interpreted as a dystrophy or "leukoplakia" represent, in reality, examples of chronic contact dermatitis, the histologic features of which might also be remarkably similar.

The symptoms of contact vulvovaginitis usually consist of varying degrees of tenderness, pain, burning, and pruritus, the last being the principal symptom. Complete disability and insomnia are possible. Urinary retention is not unusual in cases of severe reaction. Occasionally, painful adenitis is also experienced.

Histopathology

Mild reactions, with erythema, may be exhibited by only microscopic epithelial edema and hyperemia, whereas the more advanced reactions present evidence of vesiculation incident to intracellular and intercellular edema (spongiosis) and burst-

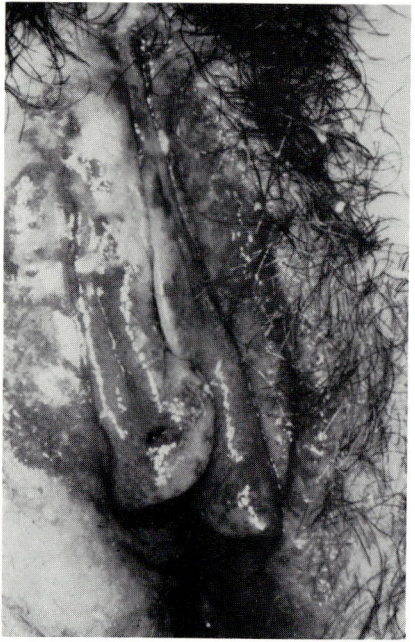

Fig. 20-1. Severe contact vulvitis following use of several topical medicaments. Eczematoid reaction.

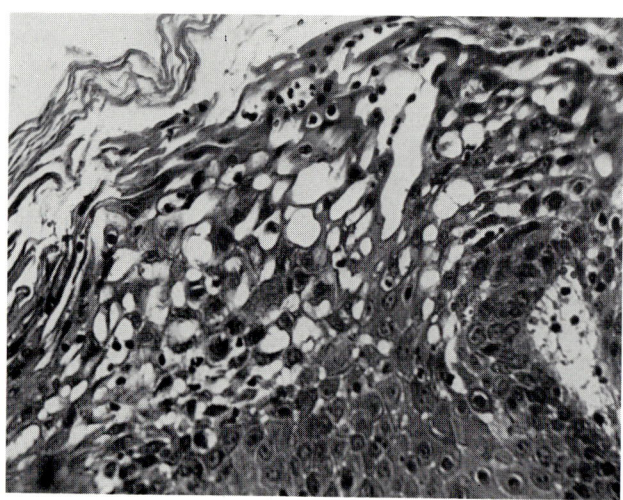

Fig. 20-2. Contact vulvitis. Advanced intracellular edema and early vesicle formation. A few inflammatory cells are present in the epidermis. (H & E × 200)

ing of cells (Fig. 20-2). Usually, the blood vessels in the upper cutis are dilated. In most cases, some edema and infiltration with lymphocytes and histiocytes are associated. Eosinophils may or may not be observed. Primary irritant and allergic reactions are often histologically indistinguishable. The chief difference lies in the nature of the cellular infiltrate in the early stages. In the allergic response, the infiltration is mainly monocytic, with the granulocytes appearing late, whereas, in the primary irritant response, granulocytes are present from the onset. A severe necrotizing irritant type of vulvitis is likely to be manifested by an abundance of neutrophilic leukocytes, necrosis of the epithelium, and an acute inflammatory reaction in the cutis.

Diagnosis

The clinical features of contact vulvovaginitis may be of little value in the detection of the responsible agent. A careful inquiry regarding possible contactants should elicit information on this point. Reactions to primary irritants are often easily recognized, since the patient is usually aware of the medicinal preparations used. Allergic vulvovaginitis, however, may require a more extensive investigation, true allergens being sometimes difficult to trace.

Patch test. Patch tests may offer information as to whether a patient is sensitive or allergic to suspected agents. The suspected substance is placed on the skin surface and covered with an adhesive band or a patch test dressing. The substance should be left in contact with the skin for 48 to 72 hours. The immediate appearance of redness or vesiculation beneath the applied agent is suggestive of a primary irritant type of reaction, whereas a delayed response is highly suggestive of an allergic sensitivity. A positive reaction, especially to primary irritants, may not appear at test sites such as the back or forearm, since the environment in these areas is entirely different from that of the vulva.

The performance and interpretation of patch tests are perhaps more complex than is generally realized; neither is to be considered lightly. For valid interpretation, experience in their performance seems essential.

Contact dermatitis of the vulva must be differentiated from a large variety of eruptions. Some of the conditions with which it is likely to be confused are acute candidiasis, trichomoniasis, tinea cruris, seborrheic dermatitis, herpes genitalis, psoriasis, and neurodermatitis.

Treatment

Practically all vulvovaginal reactions respond rapidly after the causative agent is withdrawn; if so, active therapy is obviously unnecessary. For a severe reaction, immediate institution of external treatment is usually indicated, regardless of whether or not the responsible agent has been discovered. This, of course, is only after the diagnosis of contact vulvovaginitis is made or is highly suspected and after infectious diseases have been eliminated as causes of the lesions. The use of remedies that may further aggravate the eruption—for example, antibiotics for lesions induced by candidal species—should be avoided. Properly applied wet compresses, such as Burow's solution (diluted 1:20) or concentrated boric acid solution, may afford considerable immediate relief. Initially, wet compresses are probably more effective as a treatment for eczematoid eruptions than are preparations with a cream base, since the latter do not adhere to moist surfaces. After 24 to 48 hours under wet compresses, a previously weeping, tender lesion may become dry, clean, and less painful and more suitable for the application of therapeutic creams.

Topical applications of an appropriate corticosteroid preparation, such as fluocinolone acetonide (S y n a l a r) cream or ointment, hydrocortisone acetate (Cortef) ointment, or triamcinolone acetonide (Aristocort) cream, often promptly relieve the patient's symptoms and bring about an objective improvement in the lesions.

Whereas acute inflammatory reactions may respond rapidly to corticosteroid preparations, several weeks of treatment with these agents may be necessary for lichenified plaques of chronic contact dermatitis. True allergic reactions respond more rapidly to corticosteroids than to any other therapeutic agent. Primary irritant reactions may not require the use of corticosteroids; if severe or persistent, however, they may also be benefited by the use of these agents.

Systemic corticosteroids, taken daily, are

particularly beneficial as a treatment for severe allergic reactions, such as those produced by the oleoresins of poison ivy or poison oak. They are best administered in diminishing doses over about 3 weeks, the gradual decrease serving to prevent a "rebound" of the allergic reaction.

Antihistamines, such as diphenhydramine (Benadryl), although widely employed in contact dermatitis, leave much to be desired in effectiveness. Allegedly, they are moderately effective in certain types of reactions, such as those that might develop from treatment with penicillin. Their topical use involves considerable risk of inducing an allergic reaction to the agents themselves. For this reason, antihistamines should rarely, if ever, be applied locally to the vulvar tissues.

Prophylactic measures such as desensitization are not within the scope of this book.

Specific contactants

Essentially every organic and inorganic chemical agent, whether a component of a vaginal contraceptive agent, a vaginal medicament, a vaginal douche preparation, or an accidental contaminant, has caused vulvovaginitis. We have observed vulvovaginal reactions to almost all the vaginal medicaments, those purchased across the counter as well as prescription preparations. In view of the many preparations currently in use, an attempt to discuss each one is impractical, as is also an attempt to classify the constituent agents, individually or in combinations, as primary irritants or allergenic substances. In fact, some chemicals appear to act as a primary irritant in one person and as an allergenic substance in another.

Reactions to douches

The pharmaceutical industry has been most successful in formulating combinations of medicinal agents for use as douche

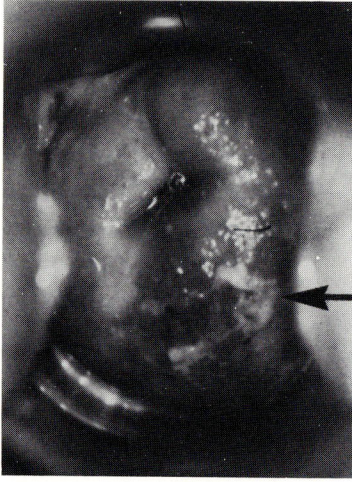

Fig. 20-3. Chemical vaginitis incident to introduction of a proprietary douche power directly into vagina. Patient had an eczematoid reaction of the vulva.

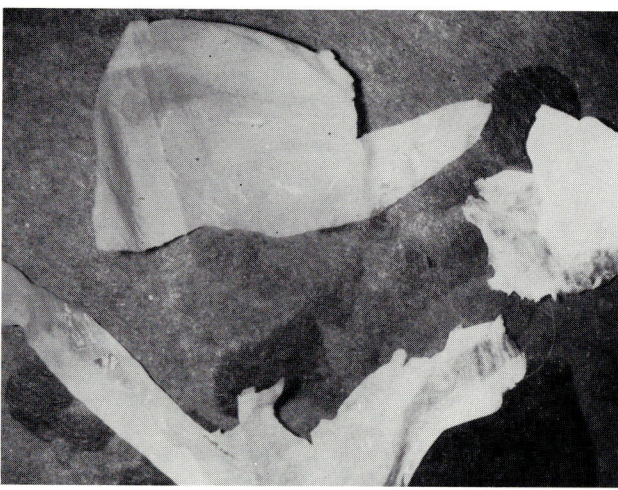

Fig. 20-4. Pseudomembrane passed from the vagina as a thin cast after a strong vinegar douche.

preparations. Every proprietary preparation and any one of its constituents have a potential for inciting reactions in a small percentage of women. The reactions that develop are often ascribable to the patient's failure to follow appended instructions—for example, douching with a solution containing undissolved aggregates of medicinal douche powder or undissolved particles of corrosive agents such as potassium permanganate or mercuric chloride. Fortunately, vulvovaginitis from douche preparations is rare, usually transient, and of only minor consequence. We have observed severe, acute eczematous vulvovaginitis following the purposeful introduction of popularly used proprietary douche powders directly into the vagina (Fig. 20-3). The instructions on the containers of douche preparations generally warn against their use in this manner.

Other proprietary preparations that may cause reactions when used in too strong a concentration or by highly susceptible women include Lysol, chlorinated solutions, and detergents. The formation of a pseudomembrane is often observed in the vaginas of patients who have recently douched with vinegar solutions. Presumably, the concentration of acetic acid is sometimes sufficient to precipitate the glycoproteins and mucus of the vagina, or possibly it causes the superficial epithelial cells to desquamate in a sheet (Fig. 20-4). Such a reaction appears to be clinically insignificant.

Reactions to vaginal contraceptives

The chemical agents in vaginal contraceptives have been wisely chosen for their safety; nevertheless, they occasionally act as either a primary irritant or allergenic substance to the patient or her coital partner. Many women are unable to use one or another brand of contraceptive jelly or cream because of consequent burning and pruritus. On inspection, these patients rarely have more than slight degrees of erythema and labial edema. We have never observed a serious eczematoid reaction to vaginal contraceptives. Following the introduction of some contraceptives, a white adherent film resembling a pseudomembrane commonly forms over the vaginal mucosa. This, likewise, is transitory and presumably insignificant.

Reactions to therapeutic vaginal agents

Varying degrees of reactions may appear as a result of treatment for vulvovaginitis with medicinal agents. The majority of reactions are of short duration and consist only of erythema, mild edema, pruritus, and burning. Practically every vaginal medicament is capable of inciting an eczematoid rash in the susceptible patient, especially when used injudiciously.

Chlordantoin (Sporastacin), widely employed as a candidacidal agent, has caused moderately severe reactions in several of our patients (Fig. 20-5). Epstein (1966a) reported two cases of vulvovaginitis that he attributed to an allergic response to chlordantoin. His claim was supported by positive patch tests.

Candicidin (Candeptin), a candidacidal agent, only rarely gives rise to a contact type of vulvovaginitis. We have observed reactions to this agent (Fig. 20-6).

Nystatin (Mycostatin) vaginal suppositories have seldom, if ever, produced a clinically apparent irritative response in any patient personally observed, although the agent has been extensively used.

Proprionic acids (Proprion) have been

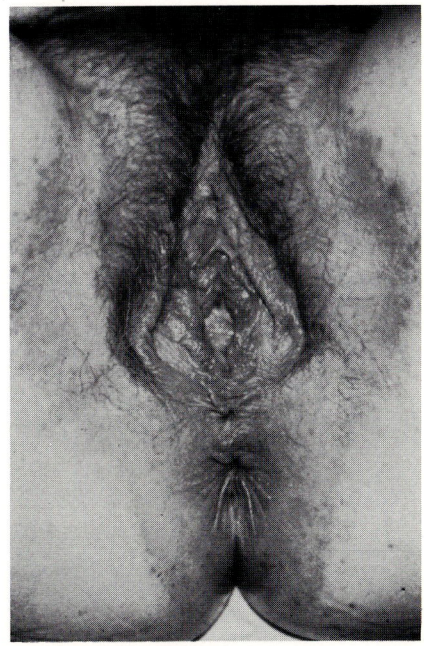

Fig. 20-5. Widespread contact vulvitis following applications of chlordantoin (Sporastacin) cream.

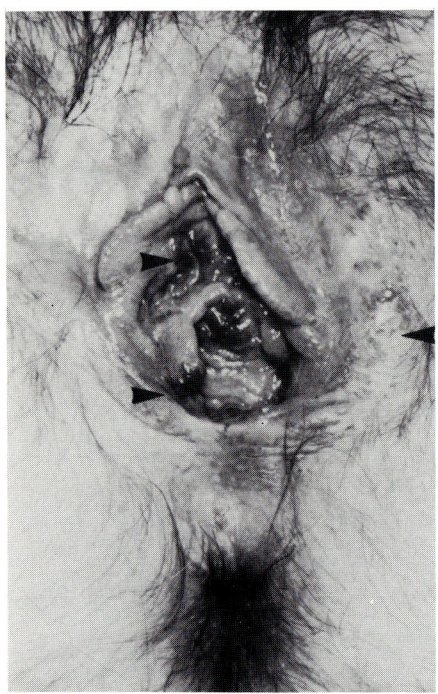

Fig. 20-6. Vulvovaginitis secondary to the use of candicidin (Candeptin). Superficial hemorrhagic ulcerations of vestibule are apparent (arrow, left), as well as dermatitis of labia majora (arrow, right).

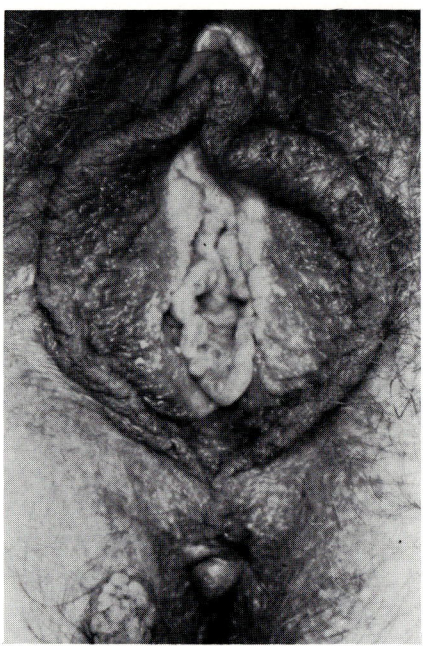

Fig. 20-7. Reaction following injudicious use of proprionic acids (Propion Gel) over several months. The mucosa of the vagina and vestibule of this patient was thickened and leathery.

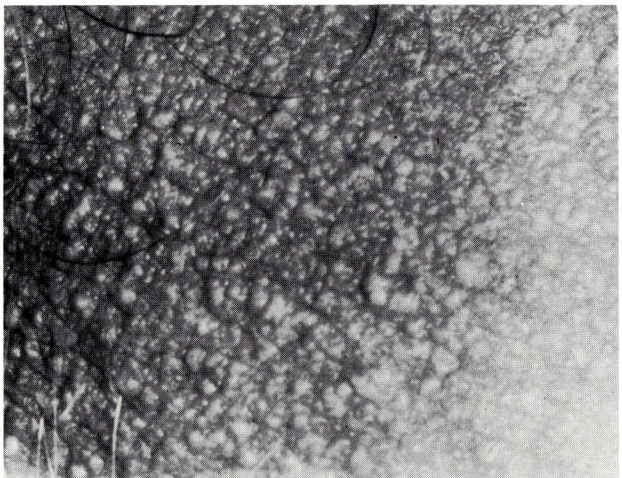

Fig. 20-8. Reaction of vulvar skin to topical use of triple sulfa cream. (×3)

observed to produce an occasional reaction after prolonged use. Such response, however, is probably rare (Fig. 20-7).

Sulfonamide creams and tablets such as Sultrin, sometimes inserted into the vagina preoperatively and postoperatively as well as in treatment for bacterial vaginitis, are followed by irritative responses in a limited number of patients (Fig. 20-8). Such reactions are surprisingly infrequent and are rarely of more than minor consequence.

Tricofuron suppositories, containing furazolidone and nifuroxime, which are allegedly effective against each of the three common varieties of infectious vaginitis, induce reactions in a definite but disputed percentage of patients.

Nitrofurazone (Furacin), a preparation widely employed for bacterial vaginitis as well as preoperatively and postoperatively for the prevention of bacterial infection, is associated with reactions in up to 1 percent of patients. We have knowledge of several patients who received treatment with nitrofurazone presurgically whose operations were necessarily delayed because of eczematoid reactions.

Silver picrate (Fig. 20-9) and arsenic preparations, which until recently were commonly used as trichomonicidal agents, are often associated with some degree of contact vulvovaginitis. Some of these agents seem to produce reactions only after prolonged use; thus, the reactions may be of the cumulative primary irritant type or a true allergic reaction.

Gentian violet is recognized as one of the most effective candidacidal agents. It is, however, capable of inciting eczematoid

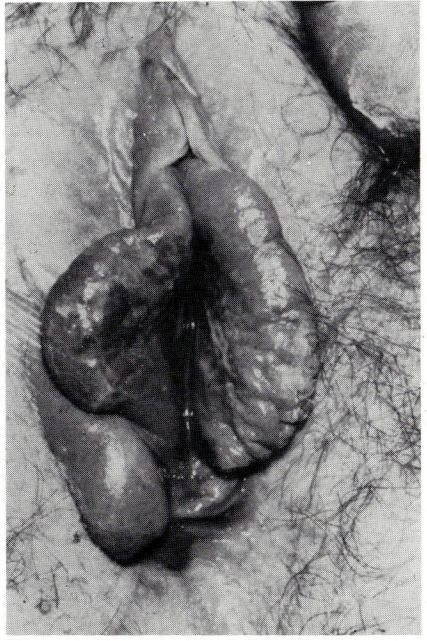

Fig. 20-9. Severe reaction to silver picrate preparation, exhibited by edema, erythema, and ulcerations.

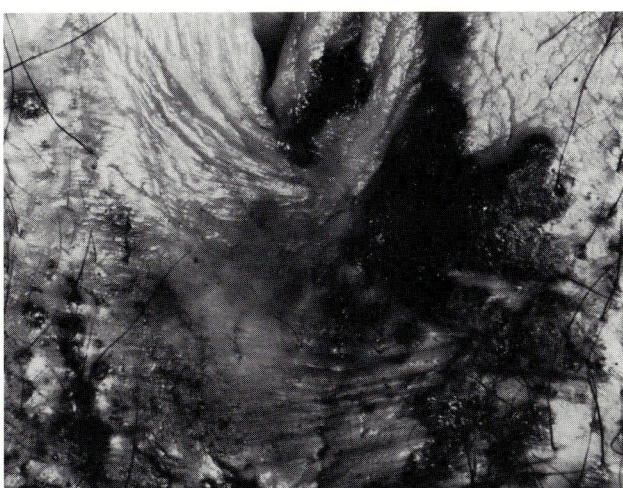

Fig. 20-10. Reaction to applications of 2% gentian violet every other day. Stained superficial ulcerations are present.

reactions in every patient if applied over too long a period of time or if too concentrated. Our experience indicates that if this agent is used as a 2% aqueous solution daily, or even every other day, an eczematoid reaction will ultimately develop, almost without fail (Fig. 20-10). We have observed reactions in patients during the use of any and all of the proprietary vaginal medicaments in which the active principal is gentian violet. Patients should be forewarned of this possibility. The reactions are of the primary irritant type and are easily controlled by lengthening the interval between applications. The typical change caused by the dye is a superficial, incomplete ulceration of the vulvar and vaginal tissues. Severe cases may be classified as eczematoid, although vesicles and bullae are rarely observed. Such reactions to gentian violet serve as a good example of the "over-treatment syndrome."

All antibiotics, including the tetracyclines, penicillin, and the strictly topical agents such as Neomycin, have the potential for producing allergic vulvovaginitis. Their chief relationship to vulvovaginitis, however, is their stimulation to overgrowth of candidal organisms and consequent clinical candidiasis. The physician must often distinguish between a true contact vulvovaginitis and an aggravation of a preexistent candidiasis.

Although the majority of reactions are allergic in nature, irritant reactions to concentrated antibiotic preparations in the vagina is a possibility. Such reactions are highly variable, both as to type and to degree. Existent eruptions from one of several other causes also are sometimes aggravated by the use of topically applied antibiotics.

Topically applied anesthetic preparations are often allergenic, and repeated applications can produce severe eczematoid vulvitis. These agents have been commonly employed for the relief of vulvar pruritus and for pain following episiotomy repair. Also, they are occasionally used by the male during coitus to delay ejaculation and are thus brought into contact with the vulvovaginal tissues. In view of their relative ineffectiveness and their sensitizing nature, we question the wisdom of their application to the vulvovaginal tissues for any purpose.

Reactions to poison oak and posion ivy

Oleoresins produced by these plants are classic models for the study of allergic contact dermatitis. The allergen is generally transmitted to the vulvar tissues by contaminated hands, less often by direct contact with the genital area. The period between contact with the allergen and the eruption varies from only a few hours to several days. Redness and wheals at the point of contact are the initial signs. This is followed within 24 to 48 hours by vesicles (Fig. 20-11) and bullae. The arrangement of the lesions in linear streaks when present,

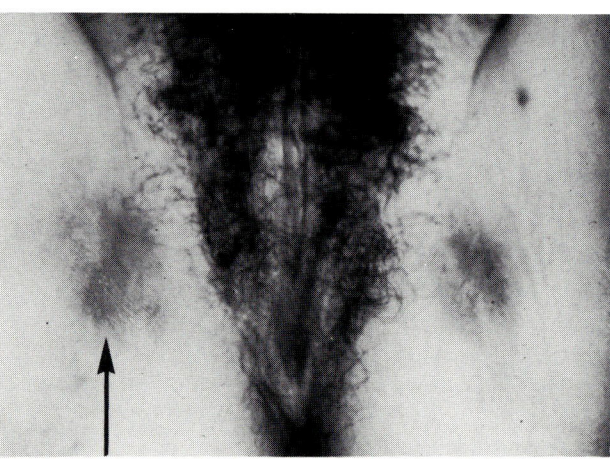

Fig. 20-11. Allergic reaction to poison ivy. Erythema and minute vesiculations were present in area indicated by arrow.

may be a diagnostic feature. Spontaneous healing takes place within 3 to 4 weeks.

Reactions to miscellaneous agents

Allegedly, the dyes of colored toilet tissue and cheap underwear may cause vulvitis. The incidence of such reactions would be difficult to determine. Undoubtedly, the dermatologist is more alert to the possibility of reactions of this nature than is the gynecologist. Perfumes are well known for their potential as allergenic or irritant agents. Such reactions are observed especially about the neck. Those observed in the vulvar skin have been traced to the regular application of perfume to the area.

Dermatitis medicamentosa (drug eruption)

Dermatitis medicamentosa is a cutaneous reaction secondary to allergenic substances circulating throughout the body, rather than the result of contact of the skin with the offending agent. In other words, it is an external manifestation of a generalized reaction taking place in the body. The etiologic agents usually gain entry into the body by ingestion, inhalation, or inoculation. Lesions of dermatitis medicamentosa may be manifested on the vulva and even the vagina, although such manifestations are usually only an incidental part of the total clinical picture and may often be unnoticed. The lesions of this type of reaction are highly variable; they do not resemble the usual eczematoid changes induced by surface contactants. Since dermatitis medicamentosa is hardly within the scope of this book, it will not be discussed beyond the citing of two patients we have observed who developed different types of reactions. One patient developed deep-seated, tender maculopapules of the vulva as a part of a generalized rash several days after taking a systemic trichomonicide, 2-acetylamino-5-nitrothiazole (Tritheon). In the other case, a localized reaction of the vulvovaginal tissues followed the systemic use of penicillin, the patient having developed a localized sensitivity incident to previous topical use of penicillin on the vulvovaginal tissues. This is an extremely rare reaction, called a *fixed drug eruption,* which recurs precisely in the same area whenever the incriminating drug is administered.

Reactions to corrosive chemicals

Corrosive agents, as mercuric chloride (Fig. 20-12) and potassium permanganate (Fig. 20-13), as well as strong solutions of alkali, are members of a group of chemicals that affect the tissues of practically all exposed persons.

Strong alkali solutions deeply penetrate

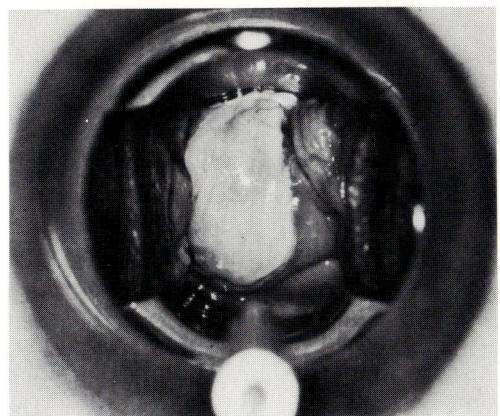

Fig. 20-12. Necrotic ulceration covered by pseudomembrane (blue in the original) subsequent to insertion of a bichloride of mercury tablet into vaginal vault.

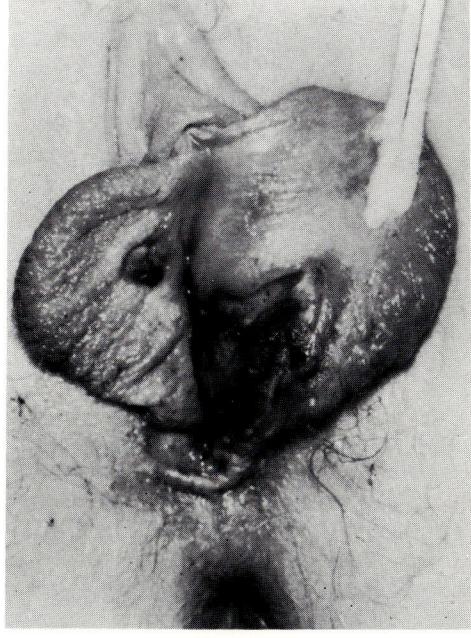

Fig. 20-13. Deep necrotic ulceration of vulva, secondary to contact with a potassium permanganate tablet.

and destroy the tissues by dissolution. Concentrated chlorinated solutions can cause serious injuries; even in relatively dilute solutions, they may produce eczematous eruptions. The chemical basis of chlorinated disinfectants is believed to be the liberation of HOCl and nascent oxygen. The vaginal mucosa is particularly susceptible, ulceration and necrosis sometimes following application of only moderate concentrations of the agent.

Potassium permanganate burns. Potassium permanganate in dilute solution was once frequently used as a medicament or douche for vulvovaginitis. During the middle 1930's, the belief that the insertion of a potassium permanganate tablet into the vagina would induce abortion became widespread among the laity. Shull, in 1941, was the first to call attention to the complications arising from its usage for this purpose.

Although the exact incidence of complications resulting from the vaginal insertion of potassium permanganate tablets is unknown, every county hospital in which clinic patients are treated has had a significant number of these cases. Many reports of fifty or more such complications have been published. For example, in 1945, McDonough reported sixty-five cases from the Boston City Hospital, and in 1961, Hill and Thomas reported eighty-three cases from the San Francisco General Hospital. In view of the increasing number of women who incurred their injury as a result of the practice, the U. S. Food and Drug Administration has now ruled that potassium permanganate, except in weak solution, may not be sold without a prescription.

Jetter and Hunter have described the pharmacology of potassium permanganate salt as follows. When the substance comes in contact with the vaginal tissues, it is reduced to potassium hydroxide and manganese dioxide with the liberation of nascent oxygen. The reaction has been expressed in the equation: $4 KMnO_4 + 2 H_2O = 4 KOH + 4 MnO_2 + 3 O_2$. The nascent oxygen supposedly causes superficial necrosis, and the corrosive action of the resulting potassium hydroxide produces necrosis of the underlying tissues. Since potassium permanganate tablets dissolve slowly in water, requiring probably from 20 to 30 minutes for complete dissolution, minor burns may result from potassium permanganate douches containing particles of the drug.

Clinical features. Profuse, painless vaginal bleeding is practically always the chief presenting symptom. Usually, the bleeding begins within 24 hours, although it may not begin until as late as 2 weeks after insertion of the tablet. Hill and Thomas reported that of fifty-six patients who acknowledged the insertion of the agent, fifty-five experienced vaginal bleeding within 24 hours. Twenty-three of the patients were in clinical shock at the time of their admission to the hospital, and twenty-nine others required blood transfusions.

Vandergriff and Diddle have emphasized the likelihood of error in the initial diagnosis and the importance of speculum examination of every pregnant patient with painless vaginal bleeding. Error in diagnosis is understandable, since the majority of these patients are pregnant and logically are assumed to be bleeding from the uterine cavity. These authors also point out the inadequacy of potassium permanganate as an abortifacient. Their experience suggested that abortion was seldom induced by this means. Other investigators, however, have reported a higher incidence of abortion and premature labor from its use.

The necrotic process is initiated immediately following the insertion of one or more potassium permanganate tablets (usually gr. v) into the vagina. The lesions are generally described as multiple, sharply demarcated, deep, punched-out ulcers, with a characteristic brownish-black eschar over the base and the immediately surrounding mucosa. The vulva may be similarly involved (Fig. 20-13). This characteristic eschar has been attributed to insoluble manganese dioxide. The ulcerations vary in size from only a few millimeters to several centimeters. The upper third of the vagina is most seriously affected. The cervix may also be involved, occasionally to an extensive degree. Active arterial bleeding is frequently observed, the vagina being full of bright red and clotted blood.

Several authors have described severe sequelae of the ulcerations. Necrosis of the posterior vaginal fornix with perforation into the cul-de-sac has been reported. Jetter and Hunter observed a patient with intestinal obstruction following penetration of the cul-de-sac. Also, necrosis of the vagina and overlying bladder has led to vesicovaginal fistulas. Lin and Davis reported the cases of five patients with cicatricial tissue formation that caused cervical dystocia or vaginal stenosis sufficient to require cesarean section.

Treatment. Many of these patients are in shock at their initial observation and thus must promptly be given transfusions. All residual corrosive agents should be removed by thorough irrigation of the vagina with water. Bleeding may be controlled by the use of sutures or accurate placement of dry gauze packs; if multiple bleeding points are present, both sutures and packs may be necessary. Since the patients often have swelling and tenderness, as well as much apprehension, general anesthesia is usually required. The patient should be forewarned that further bleeding at a later date is a distinct possibility.

REFERENCES

Andrews, G. C., and Domonkos, A. N.: Diseases of the skin, ed. 5, Philadelphia, 1963, W. B. Saunders Co.
Baer, R. L., and Harris, H.: Types of cutaneous reactions to drugs, J.A.M.A. **202**:120, 1967.
Beam, L. R.: Principles of adverse drug reactions, Southern Med. J. **59**:142, 1966.
Berman, B. A.: Seasonal allergic vulvovaginitis caused by pollen, Ann. Allergy **22**:594, 1964.
Burckhardt, W., and Epstein, S.: Atlas and manual of dermatology and venereology, ed. 2, Zurich, 1963, The Williams & Wilkins Co.
Caillouette, J. C., and Chambers, C. B.: Potassium permanganate burns of the vagina, another cause of third trimester bleeding, Western J. Surg. **66**:225, 1958.
Criep, L. H.: Dermatologic allergy: Immunology, diagnosis, management, Philadelphia, 1967, W. B. Saunders Co.
Epstein, E.: Allergic dermatitis from chlordantoin vaginal cream, Obstet. Gynec. **27**:369, 1966a.
Epstein, E.: Allergy to dermatologic agents, J.A.M.A. **198**:103, 1966b.
Grater, W. C., and Grover, F. W.: Evolution of a topical corticosteroid (flumethasone pivalate) in allergic dermatoses, Southern Med. J. **60**: 1153, 1967.
Hill, E. C., and Thomas, J. M.: Potassium permanganate ulcers of the vagina, Obstet. Gynec. **18**:747, 1961.
Jetter, W. W., and Hunter, F. T.: Death from attempted abortion with a potassium permanganate douche, New Eng. J. Med. **240**:794, 1949.
Kobak, A. F., and Wishnick, S.: Potassium permanganate burn of vagina followed by bowel obstructions, Amer. J. Obstet. Gynec. **70**:409, 1955.
Lin, T. J., and Davis, S. S., Jr.: Obstetric hazards following the application of corrosive substances to the vagina and cervix, Obstet. Gynec. **12**:333, 1958.
Lockey, S. D.: Reactions to drugs, Med. Sci. **18**:: 43, 1967.
Lubin, S., and Waltman, R.: Vaginal hemorrhage due to potassium permanganate, Amer. J. Surg. **82**:227, 1951.
McDonough, J. F.: Vaginal bleeding from potassium permanganate as an abortifacient, New Eng. J. Med. **232**:189, 1945.
O'Donnell, R. P.: Vesico-vaginal fistula produced by potassium permanganate, Obstet. Gynec. **4**: 122, 1954.
Perlman, H. H.: Contact dermatitis caused by poison ivy, poison sumac and poison oak, Med. Sci. **15**:31, 1964.
Perlman, H. H.:: Highlights in diagnosis: vesiculobullous eruptions, Med. Sci. **18**:49, 1967.
Rees, R. B.: Dermatoses due to environmental and physical factors, Springfield, Ill., 1962, Charles C Thomas, Publisher.
Shull, J. C.: Vaginal bleeding from potassium permanganate burns, Amer. J. Obstet. Gynec. **41**:161, 1941.
Sulzberger, M. B., Wolf, J., Witten, V. H., and Kopf, A. W.: Dermatology—diagnosis and treatment, ed. 2, Chicago, 1961, The Year Book Publishers.
Vandergriff, W., and Diddle, A. W.: Intravaginal use of potassium permanganate as an abortifacient: The error in diagnosis, Obstet. Gynec. **28**:155, 1966.
Von Oettingen, W. F.: Poisoning, New York, 1954, Harper & Row, Publishers.

Chapter 21

Pyodermas of the vulva

Pyodermas are skin infections in which the responsible organism is usually a coagulase-positive staphylococcus or hemolytic streptococcus. In a smaller number of cases, the causative bacteria are transient contaminants of the skin that produce infection mainly because of lowered resistance of the subject or because of precipitating factors. The following classification of the pyodermas, although incomplete from the viewpoint of a dermatologist, includes the infections likely to affect the vulva.

- A. Infections of hair follicles
    1. Folliculitis
    2. Furuncle
    3. Carbuncle
- B. Infection of apocrine glands: hidradenitis suppurativa
- C. Pyogenic ulcers
    1. Impetigo
    2. Ecthyma
- D. Infections of the cellular planes
    1. Erysipelas
    2. Cellulitis

Follicular pyodermas

Infections arising within hair follicles, known as follicular pyodermas, are the most important and prevalent of all the pyodermas. They consist of folliculitis, furuncle, and carbuncle.

Etiology and pathogenesis

Since the infectious agent, usually a staphylococcus such as *Micrococcus pyogenes*, produces infection by entering the opening of a hair follicle, the follicular infections are considered to be "infections from without." Conditions that predispose to these infections include obesity, sweating, maceration, malnutrition, diabetes, seborrhea, poor hygiene, scabies, and pediculosis.

The role of foci of infection in the teeth and tonsils is unknown. An occasional patient with chronic folliculitis or furunculosis relates the initial infection to shaving of the vulva in connection with childbirth, a surgical procedure, or other reasons. Most often, however, no apparent predisposing or precipitating factor can be detected.

Apparently, follicular pyodermas follow inoculation of pilosebaceous ducts and hair follicles of susceptible subjects with a staphylococcus. Whether or not a resultant infection persists as a folliculitis or progresses to a furuncle or carbuncle is dependent upon many factors, including susceptibility of the individual and virulence of the infectious agent. The infection may be limited to the upper part of the pilosebaceous duct and thus may be considered a *superficial folliculitis;* or it may involve the entire follicle and the sebaceous glands and be appropriately called *deep folliculitis*. Should infection spread into the perifollicular tissues, producing localized cellulitis, the lesion may then be called a *furuncle*. The infection may retrogress at any of these stages and eventually absorb, or it may progress to suppuration and subsequent formation of an abscess with a core of necrotic follicular tissue and purulent material. Suppurative folliculitis or furuncles usually drain spontaneously and heal within a few days. Closely associated multiple furuncles with intervening communications and multiple areas of drainage to the skin are known as *carbuncles*.

Clinical features

Pain and tenderness are common features of the follicular pyodermas, the pain increasing commensurately with the depth and extent of the lesion. Painful lymphadenitis may be associated.

The majority of lesions of superficial folliculitis (Fig. 21-1) are represented by a small erythematous papule or pustule in the orifice of the follicle, in the center of which a hair is sometimes visible. Often, the hair is only a small lanugo hair and may be difficult to detect. The amount of purulent material present is hardly more than a droplet. Frequently, deep folliculitis is clinically indistinguishable from a furuncle. Many lesions of deep folliculitis are palpable as tender, red nodules. They may resolve without suppuration, although the nodules may persist for several weeks. Folliculitis is subject to exacerbations, and it may recur without apparent provocation.

A furuncle (Fig. 21-2), sometimes called a boil, is similar to deep folliculitis; usually, however, it is a more extensive infection, involving tissues beyond the hair follicle. In the early stage, the lesion consists of a hard, tender, erythematous nodule. After several days, a small pustule forms at the apex of the nodule; this may eventually rupture and drain a small amount of bloody, purulent material. Healing follows expulsion of the core of necrotic tissue. Few patients escape with only a single furuncle. New lesions may appear continuously or intermittently for months or years; in this event, the condition is called *furunculosis*.

When several adjoining hair follicles become infected, intercommunicate with each other, and have multiple openings onto the surface of the skin, the lesion is called a carbuncle (Fig. 21-3). If the overlying skin is thick and resistant to spontaneous rupture of the lesions, the process may spread laterally in the tissue planes. This spreading process may lead to a deep lesion involving a large area of tissue. Unlike furunculosis and folliculitis, recurrence of a carbuncle is exceptional. None of several carbuncles we have observed have recurred.

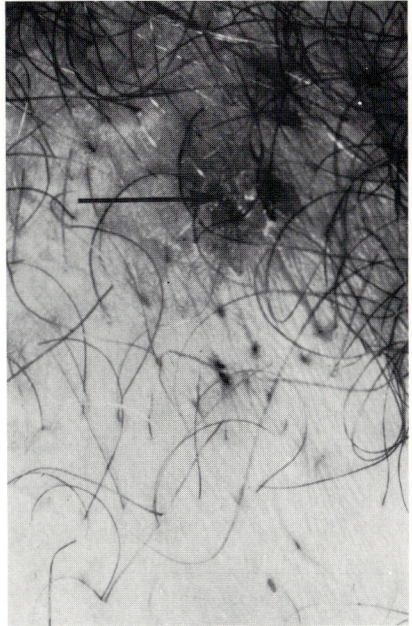

Fig. 21-1. Folliculitis. Erythematous papule at orifice of hair follicle.

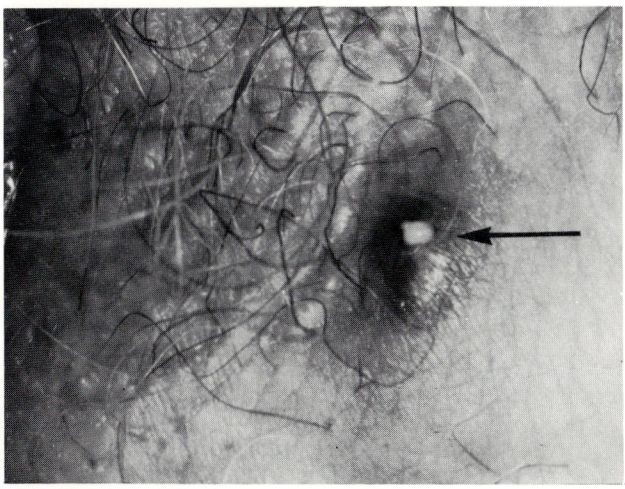

Fig. 21-2. Furuncle. A red, tender nodule, with purulent material exuding through an orifice.

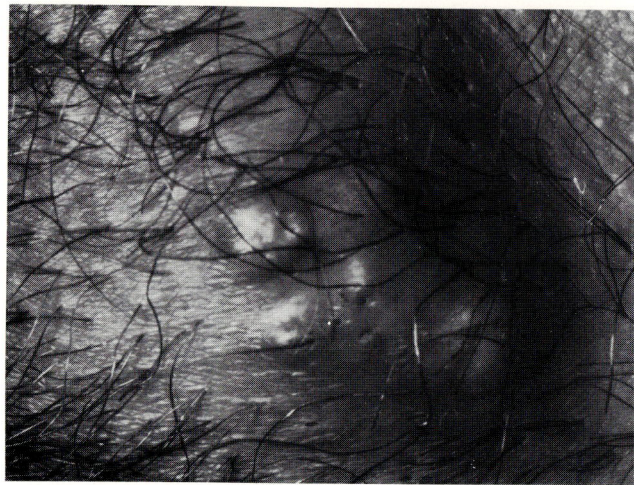

Fig. 21-3. Early carbuncle. Multiple intercommunicating, infected hair follicles. These lesions subsequently drained from several orifices.

Histopathology

The pathologic changes in the follicular pyodermas include folliculitis, perifolliculitis, and abscess formation. In the acute stage, neutrophils are predominant. In the abscess stage, a core of necrotic tissue and purulent material is present. Older lesions consist of chronic granulation tissue containing numerous lymphocytes and plasma cells. Foreign body giant cells are often present. Eventually, a deep pyoderma is accompanied by proliferation of connective tissue; this is often followed by microscopically (and grossly) visible scar tissue.

Treatment

Superficial folliculitis often responds well to the application of an antibiotic lotion. Treatment for the deeper follicular pyodermas is more vigorous but is essentially identical for the several varieties. The application of hot packs accelerates pointing; once this takes place, the lesions should be incised, though not squeezed. For extensive furunculosis and carbuncles, systemic antibiotics have proved invaluable, both for their immediate effects upon established lesions and for the prevention of new lesions. Bacterial sensitivity tests are recommended for the selection of the appropriate agent. The penicillins and the tetracyclines (250 mg. every 6 hours) have proved curative for most lesions. Ampicillin, which can be given orally, has been highly successful in some cases. Obstinate or recurrent lesions may require administration of these agents over a period of weeks or even months. After the development of new lesions has been arrested, the dosage of the drug may be reduced. The sulfonamides, 1 gm. every 6 hours, have also been found effective in some cases; they may be indicated in patients who do not tolerate antibiotics. If identifiable, predisposing conditions should be given appropriate attention.

Since it appears that the entry of bacteria into follicles through the pilosebaceous ducts is the cause of new lesions, an adjunctive measure might be antisepsis of the surrounding skin. This may be accomplished by frequent bathing with antiseptic soaps, such as Dial, and perhaps by repeated local applications of antibiotic lotions or creams. Preparations such as Neosporin G cream, containing polymyxin B-neomycin-gramicidin, are particularly useful.

Hidradenitis suppurativa

Hidradenitis suppurativa is a resistant infection of the apocrine glands. The vulva and the axillae, the areas in which apocrine glands are most abundant, are the sites of predilection. Since activity of these glands is dependent upon endocrine function, hidradenitis is rarely, if ever, observed before puberty. The infection appears to originate in occluded apocrine glands. The pathogenesis may be partially attributable to inflammatory reactions to the materials that accumulate in the resultant cystic lesions. One or more species of staphylococci or streptococci is usually the infectious agent. The conditions discussed on p. 298 may also predispose patients to hidradenitis, although some patients with the disease do not clearly display any of these conditions.

Clinicial features

The disease is exhibited by nodules, usually multiple, deep in the skin. Eventually, most of the nodules develop into abscesses. Some of the abscesses rupture spontaneously, whereas others may remain as indurated, inflammatory masses. Usually, the disease is characterized by the continual development of new lesions; this ultimately leads to a chronic, widespread, deep infectious process, frequently involving the entire vulva (Fig. 21-4). Multiple chronic draining sinuses are often present. Widespread scarring, pitting, and induration (Fig. 21-5) of the apocrine gland areas, being features of the disease, help to distinguish it from the follicular pyodermas; the latter are associated with minimal or no scarring. Occasionally, the condition may be confused with the granulomatous diseases or even with tuberculous adenitis.

Histopathology

Reportedly, the earliest infiltration with inflammatory cells is apparent within the lumina of apocrine glands and in the adjacent periglandular tissues. From this, it has been assumed that infection enters through the hair follicles. According to Montgomery,

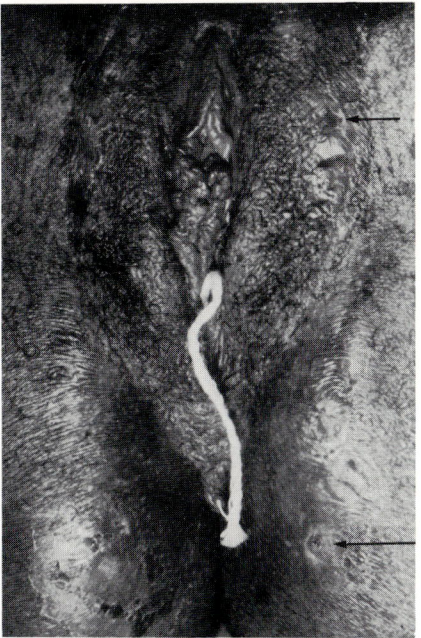

Fig. 21-4. Hydradenitis suppurativa. Pitting, demonstrated by arrows, is a distinguishing feature from folliculitis.

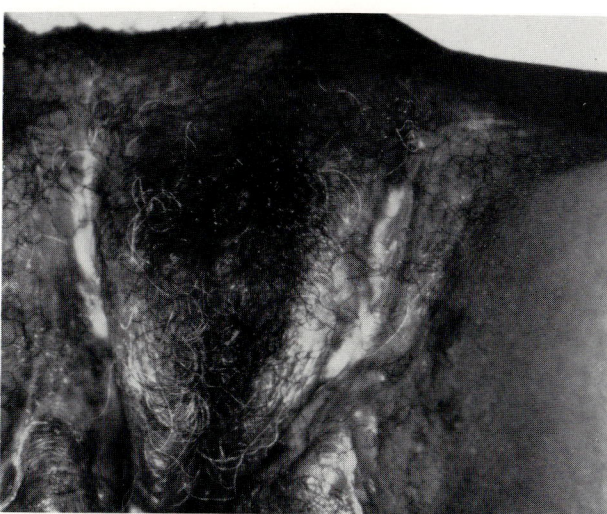

Fig. 21-5. Hydradenitis suppurativa of many years' duration. Scarring and induration are widespread.

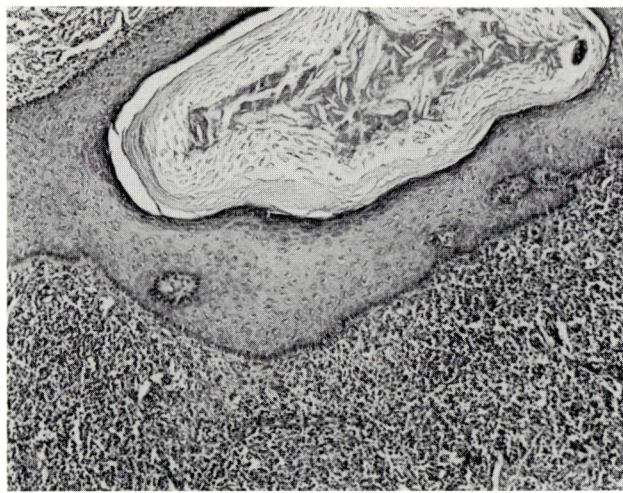

Fig. 21-6. Hydradenitis suppurativa. Sinus tract lined by squamous epithelium filled with keratinized material and surrounded by chronic inflammatory infiltrate. Such a tract is often present in the healing stage. (H & E × 100)

the histopathologic changes in the early stages of hidradenitis are diagnostic. He found that the condition is characterized by inflammation within the apocrine glands and, often, by the presence of many cocci. The inflammatory infiltrate consists chiefly of neutrophils; subsequently, lymphocytes and plasma cells predominate, and foreign body giant cells may be observed. The infection eventually spreads throughout the subcutaneous tissues. The latter phases are exhibited by extensive abscesses and destruction of tissue. Pseudoepitheliomatous hyperplasia of the epithelium is sometimes present, perhaps causing confusion of the lesion with squamous cell carcinoma. During the process of healing, sinus tracts, lined with squamous epithelium, frequently develop (Fig. 21-6).

Treatment

The same therapeutic measures apply in the treatment for this condition as for the follicular pyodermas—namely, incision and drainage, antibiotics and skin antisepsis. The most appropriate antibiotic should be selected, as indicated by sensitivity tests. Systemic corticosteroids reportedly are beneficial in some cases. Patients resistant to all forms of conservative treatment may eventually require partial or complete vulvectomy; this effects a cure by removal of the apocrine glands. We recently performed a vulvectomy on a young Negro woman. Although her infection improved to a pronounced degree under prolonged antibiotic therapy, it became acutely exacerbated when the antibiotics were discontinued. If the disease is limited, partial vulvectomy may be curative. Before vulvectomy is undertaken, a period of relative quiescence should be induced with antibiotics, and following the operation, the antibiotics should be continued for 2 to 3 weeks.

Impetigo contagiosa

Impetigo is an infectious and contagious disease caused by staphylococci or streptococci, or both, and involving the superficial layers of the epidermis. Since the disease is autoinoculable, the lesions are practically always multiple; they may spread rapidly to remote parts of the body, including the vulva. It is almost exclusively a disease of children, being rarely observed in the adult. Even in children, impetigo of the vulva is usually only a part of the widespread disease.

Clinically, the lesion appears initially as a vesicle. A pustule soon develops and readily ruptures, leaving a superficial ulcer. A crust, usually brown or yellow, then forms. Removal of the crust discloses a superficial ulcer with thin, overhanging edges of epidermis. As a rule, a zone of erythema is present. Since the infection is superficial and limited to the epidermis, scarring does not follow. The absence of significant inguinal adenopathy in the uncomplicated case helps to distinguish impetigo from other ulcerative conditions and the deeper pyodermas.

Treatment

Because of the superficial nature of the infection, local measures—removal of crusts with soap and water, hydrogen peroxide, or boric acid soaks—followed by the application of a cream containing antibiotics (such as Neosporin G) three or four times daily usually bring about a rapid response of the lesions. Bathing with an antibacterial soap is recommended for skin antisepsis and the prevention of new vesicles.

Ecthyma

Ecthyma is a pustular infection of the skin similar to impetigo, although it involves the full thickness of the epidermis and the superficial layers of the corium. In the majority of cases, the causative agent is a streptococcus; less often, a staphylococcus is responsible. The infection may be a complication of scabies or other skin diseases associated with pruritus. Unlike impetigo, healing is usually followed by scarring. Like impetigo, it is primarily a disease of children, is contagious, and autoinoculable. Occasionally debilitated patients are affected.

The lesions most often develop on the lower legs, although the posterior aspects of the buttocks and, occasionally, the vulva are involved. The primary lesion is a pustule; this ruptures and becomes crusted and deeply ulcerated. The ulcer tends to spread peripherally and to heal slowly.

Treatment

In addition to local measures, treatment often must be directed to improvement of the general condition of the patient. The same therapy as that employed for the treatment of impetigo is effective—removal of the crusts and local applications of antibiotics. The use of systemic antibiotics is sometimes indicated.

Erysipelas

Erysipelas is a rapidly spreading acute infection of the skin caused by invasion of the superficial lymphatics by a beta hemolytic streptococcus. It is usually the result of bacterial inoculation incident to trauma, especially in patients with a streptococcal sore throat or an associated pyoderma. Erysipelas of the vulva is exceedingly rare.

The chief symptoms are constitutional; these include chills, fever, and malaise, all of which should lead one to suspect the presence of erysipelas, rather than other types of erythematous vulvitis. The infection is characterized by a raised, indurated area of erythema having a rapidly spreading, well-defined border. Tenderness is usually acute. Vesiculations and bullae may appear over the glazed surface of the affected skin. Erythematous streaks leading to the inguinal nodes may or may not be apparent.

Microscopically, according to Lever, the dermis exhibits pronounced edema and dilation of the lymphatics and capillaries. A diffuse infiltrate, composed of polymorphonuclear leukocytes and some lymphocytes, involves the dermis and occasionally extends into the subcutaneous tissues. Bacterial stains may reveal streptococci in the tissues.

Treatment

Treatment for this condition consists of bed rest and the administration of large doses of penicillin or a tetracycline.

Cellulitis

Cellulitis is inflammation of cellular tissue, especially inflammation of the loose subcutaneous tissue. The majority of cases of cellulitis of the vulva follow inoculation of bacterial organisms incident to episiotomy and such surgical procedures as bartholinectomy and plastic repair. Every obstetrician has observed cellulitis in the tissues of an episiotomy repair. The offending bacteria are usually of low virulence and generally are of several types, such as staphylococci, streptococci, and coliform organisms. Since vulvar cellulitis is most often incident to episiotomies, the present discussion will concern itself chiefly with this variety.

Clinical features

Following episiotomy, most patients experience some degree of pain, though the patient with a low grade fever, a distressed look, and tears in her eyes from severe perineal pain, often has cellulitis about the repair.

Some of these patients are not relieved by the usual analgesics used postpartally.

The objective signs include swelling, tenderness, and erythema about the episiotomy site. Because of edema, the suture line may be slightly separated. The process, with or without treatment of the patient with antibiotics, will sometimes progress to suppuration and spontaneous drainage. This type of infection has often been erroneously attributed to "catgut reaction." Although cases of catgut reaction have been documented, the majority of such affections represent confluent low grade cellulitis.

Treatment

Without appropriate treatment, semi-invalidism may afflict the patient for a matter of weeks, especially if early spontaneous drainage does not occur. The treatment for cellulitis incident to episiotomy and surgical procedures, therefore, often becomes of major importance. Hot packs afford considerable relief of pain and perhaps facilitate localization of the inflammatory process. Drainage of the deeper structures by means of a mosquito forcep inserted between sutures is often highly effective in relieving pain. This should be carried out within 4 to 7 days after the repair. Quite remarkable in the majority of patients is the immediate relief of pain following infiltration of both sides of the episiotomy line with 2% lidocaine; this is especially true following infiltration in the area of the posterior fourchette, where so-called stitch pain is often maximal. Another procedure that we have found of value at the time of infiltration is gentle stretching of the perineum, particularly over the stitches of the episiotomy at the fourchette. Relief of pain from the latter procedure is perhaps explained by the relief of tension on certain tissues in the affected area. Regardless of the explanation, practically all patients can be relieved of the distressing pain that sometimes follows repair of episiotomy or colpoperineorrhaphy by adequate local infiltration with such agents as lidocaine, by probing to the depth of the incision to release any purulent, sanguineous, or serous fluid that may have accumulated, and by gentle stretching of the perineum under local anesthesia.

The systemic use of antibiotics, while being theoretically highly effective, is often of minimal value. Nevertheless, the administration of the tetracyclines to some patients appears to alleviate the degree of inflammatory reaction, which in turn partially relieves pain. The patient should perhaps be given the benefit of the doubt, yet we do not consider antibiotics an essential part of the treatment for cellulitis caused by perineal repair unless the patient is running more than a low grade fever.

As a final statement, we should like to stress that remarkable results are obtainable with appropriate treatment for cellulitis incident to episiotomy, and the approximated tissues, almost without exception, can be preserved intact. Infiltration of infectious cellulitis may be contrary to good surgical principles; however, the results of infiltration for uncontrollable pain justify the risk. We have never observed an unfavorable response to its use.

Although the treatment for vulvar cellulitis incident to surgical procedures and trauma is essentially identical with that following episiotomy, we are reluctant to infiltrate extensively the affected tissues. In these cases, the clinical features often resemble those of a localized erysipelas, in which such treatment would not be recommended.

REFERENCES

Burckhardt, W., and Epstein, S.: Atlas and manual of dermatology and venereology, ed. 2, Baltimore, 1963, The Williams & Wilkins Co.
Burns, R. E.: Hidradenitis suppurativa. In Conn, H. F., editor: Current therapy, Philadelphia, 1967, W. B. Saunders Co.
Chernosky, M. E.: Personal communication, 1968.
Knox, J. M.: Personal communication, 1968.
Montgomery, H.: Dermatopathology, New York, 1967, Harper & Row, Publishers.
Percival, G. H., and Dodds, T. C.: An atlas of regional dermatology, London, 1955, E. & S. Livingstone, Ltd.
Sauer, G. C.: Manual of skin diseases, ed. 2, Philadelphia, 1966, J. B. Lippincott Co.

Chapter 22

Venereal diseases

A venereal disease is an infection that usually arises from sexual intercourse with an infected person. In the exceptional case, however, it is transmitted by other means. Such infections as herpes genitalis and condyloma acuminatum are occasionally transmitted by sexual contact, yet their classification as venereal diseases is hardly acceptable. We regard the following infections as incontestable members of the family of venereal diseases:

Gonorrhea
Syphilis
Chancroid
Lymphogranuloma venereum
Granuloma inguinale
Trichomoniasis (Chapter 12)
Haemophilus vaginalis vaginitis (Chapter 13)

Gonorrhea

Gonorrhea, without reference to affected body structures, is usually interpreted as an infection of the lower genitalia—the structures below the internal cervical os. The os is believed to be a significant barrier to the upward spread of the disease. The features of salpingo-oophoro-peritonitis and their results are outside the sphere of this book.

Infections of the lower tract—the urethra, Skene's ducts, paraurethral glands, Bartholin's glands, vagina, and cervix—are symptomatically so dissimilar from infections of the upper genitalia that the two could actually be considered separate clinical entities caused by a common etiologic agent. The term "specific infection" was once used synonymously for gonorrhea; since the etiologic agents of practically all genital infections are now identifiable, the term is outmoded.

Etiology

Gonorrhea is caused by the diplococcus *Neisseria gonorrhoeae,* which was first described by Neisser in 1879. With few exceptions, infections in adults are traceable to sexual contact.

Incidence

Gonorrhea is the most prevalent of the major venereal diseases, the incidence being five to ten times that of syphilis. The incidence in different geographic, racial, and socioeconomic groups differs widely. According to the public health officials, an estimated 1,500,000 persons (male and female) in the United States became infected in 1962. Changed morals, removal of fear of venereal diseases, and reduced usage of prophylactics by men with the increased use of birth control pills by women are only a few of the factors contributing to the rising rate of venereal diseases, including gonorrhea. Harris and others, using modern diagnostic methods, found gonorrhea in forty-four (20.6 percent) of 213 female jail inmates who had no signs or symptoms of the infection.

Clinical features

The majority of gonorrheal infections of women do not conform to the textbook picture of the disease. Shapiro, for example, reported that 85 percent of a group of infected clinic patients in Philadelphia had no symptoms at all. In the lower genital tract, the gonococcus affects mainly the glandular epithelia of the involved structures. More often than not, the infection is mild and fails to produce the classic signs and symptoms. Many patients with mild

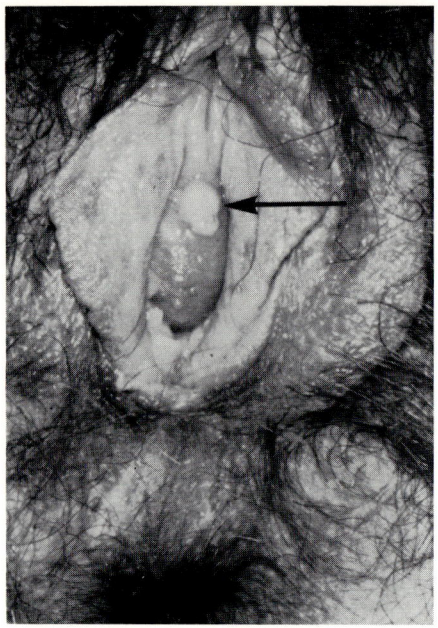

Fig. 22-1. Gonorrhea. Purulent exudate at urethral orifice (only seldom present in such volume).

asymptomatic infections do not seek medical attention and apparently remain in good health. It has been suggested that totally asymptomatic women should be called "gonorrhea Gerties" and their infections "epidemiologic cases." Such patients frequently become chronic carriers without knowledge of ever having been infected.

The incubation period of the disease is 2 to 7 days. Burning and frequency of urination from urethritis are usually the first symptoms to appear. Discomfort may be minimal and brief, or, if the infection spreads to the bladder trigone, extreme dysuria and tenesmus may be experienced. Many patients complain of a discharge. Although the amount, color, and consistency of the discharge are highly variable, characteristically it is frankly purulent. Exudate can often be expressed from the urethra and Skene's ducts (Fig. 22-1). Redness, edema, and "pouting" of the urethral meatus are sometimes observed. Abscesses in paraurethral glands are rare; when present, however, they may be distressingly painful and give rise to urethral obstruction and urinary retention. Most such abscesses are small and rupture spontaneously into the urethral lumen. The relationship of gonorrhea to urethral diverticula is still undetermined. If the patient receives no treatment, chronic foci of infection may persist indefinitely in Skene's ducts and the urethra.

Gonorrheal bartholinitis is observed, as a rule, only in patients who also have gonorrheal urethritis. The main duct is affected initially, and pus may be expressed so long as the ducts remain patent. If they do not become occluded, the acute process may subside without abscess formation, although the gland may remain tender and indurated for some time. Ductal occlusion is almost invariably followed by a Bartholin's abscess. Glandular swelling increases; the overlying skin becomes edematous, red, and tender; the involved labium majus enlarges, leading to flattening of the labium minus of the involved side; and a fluctuant abscess is soon palpable. The majority of such abscesses rupture spontaneously within a few days, whereas others may require incision and drainage. Pain and acute tenderness are the most prominent symptoms of Bartholin's abscess.

Although *N. gonorrhoeae* may be implicated, it should be remembered that abscesses of Bartholin's ducts are generally unrelated to neisserian infection. Routine culture of pus from the abscesses most often yields such organisms as staphylococci, streptococci, and *E. coli*. These bacteria may predominate, even though gonococci are recoverable from the urethra and cervix.

Although the cervix is involved in practically every case of gonorrhea, its gross appearance is not diagnostic. Any purulent cervical discharge should, however, lead one to suspect the presence of gonorrhea, as should erythema about the external os. Aside from leukorrhea, gonorrheal cervicitis is essentially asymptomatic.

Vulvitis and vaginitis are often transitory signs of acute gonorrhea in the adult. The stratified squamous epithelium of the vagina is said to be highly resistant to invasion by the gonococcus and most authors believe that the organism has no role in the inflammatory process. Nevertheless, in the early phase of the acute disease, obvious gross changes are predictable. The vulvar skin may also undergo visible inflammatory changes (Fig. 22-2). These transitory changes in the vulvovaginal tissues may represent an allergic-irritant phenomenon from the inflammatory exudates arising in the

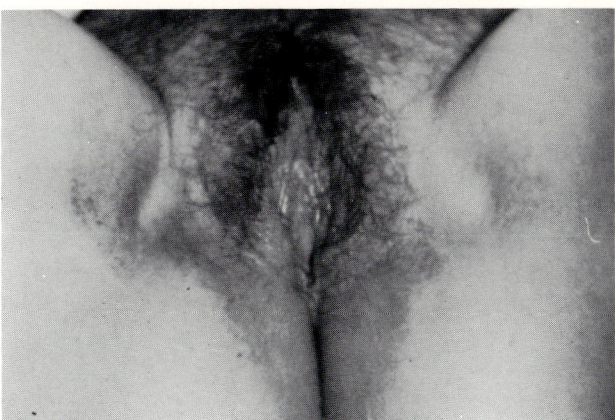

Fig. 22-2. Gonorrheal vulvitis (occasionally observed). Possible transitory allergic-irritant phenomenon.

glandular tissues of the other lower genital structures. Inflammation of vulvar skin and vaginal mucosa is not a part of chronic gonorrheal infections.

The results of gonorrhea in the lower genitalia include Bartholin's cyst, recurrent Bartholin's abscess, cyst of Skene's duct, urethral stricture (rare), chronic urethritis, and chronic cervicitis. Condylomata acuminata are at times associated with gonorrhea, yet they are induced by a virus rather than by *N. gonorrhoeae*. Their association with gonorrhea serves as another example of the simultaneous presence of different genital infections.

Histopathology

The gonococcus affects chiefly the glandular mucosa of the involved structures. In the acute infection, the histologic picture is one of hyperemia, edema, and polymorphonuclear leukocytic infiltration of both mucosa and submucosa. Varying degrees of mucosal destruction are commonly observed; this explains how opposed surfaces of the ducts may heal together, producing occlusion. Circumferential fibrosis and stricture may also explain ductal occlusion.

In acute gonorrheal bartholinitis, a nonspecific inflammatory reaction with hyperemia, edema, and pronounced inflammatory infiltration is noted. Chronic inflammatory changes develop later.

Diagnosis

Although the typical acute clinical features, if present, are highly suggestive of gonorrhea, final proof must be based upon laboratory evidence. Of the several affected structures, the cervix is the most reliable source of secreted material for laboratory examination; urethral secretions, however, should also be examined. Before material is obtained for laboratory tests, the structures should be cleansed of external secretions by swabbing. Bartholin's glands may be squeezed between the thumb and forefinger to obtain secretions from infected ducts, the urethra may be milked, and the cervix may be compressed between the blades of a speculum.

Direct smears. In the acute disease, gonococci appear on Gram-stained smears (Fig. 22-3) as kidney shaped, gram-negative diplococci, 1.25 to 1.6 μ long and approximately 0.8 μ wide, within polymorphonuclear leukocytes. Characteristically, several paired organisms are present in a single leukocyte. In view of the serious implications of the diagnosis of gonorrhea and the fact that information afforded by smears can be equivocal, the ultimate diagnosis should depend upon confirmation by culture. On smears, other organisms such as *Neisseria catarrhalis* and species of *Mima* may be difficult to distinguish from the gonococcus. Gonococci are also often difficult to demonstrate on smears from patients with chronic infections; thus, negative smears are of little value. In the chronic disease, organisms are often found only outside leukocytes. Numerous morphologically characteristic gram-negative intracellular diplococci in smears from patients suspected of having gonorrhea make

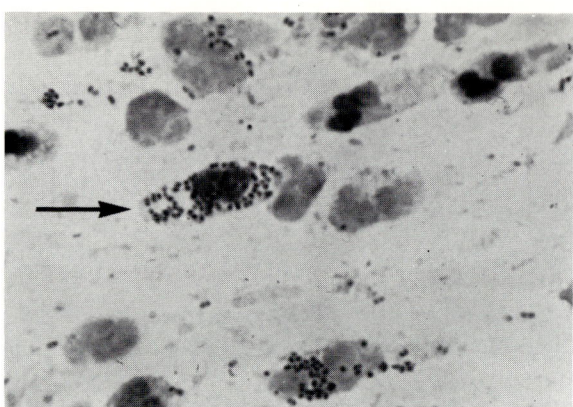

Fig. 22-3. Gonorrhea. Gram-negative intracellular diplococci.

the diagnosis highly probable and positively indicate treatment when more reliable diagnostic methods are unavailable.

Cultures. At present, differential cultures are the most reliable test for gonorrhea, particularly of the chronic type, in which the organisms are few, mixed with other bacteria, and chiefly extracellular. Culture techniques for identification of the gonococcus are slow, costly, difficult to perform, and not always as accurate as would be desirable. Chocolate blood agar, particularly when used in an environment of 3 to 10 percent carbon dioxide at 35° to 36° C. is one of the better media for cultivation of the organism. A distinction from N. catarrhalis and Neisseria intracellularis (meningococcus) in cultures depends upon sugar fermentation reactions. N. catarrhalis does not ferment sugar, the gonococcus ferments only dextrose, and the meningococcus ferments dextrose and maltose. Wende, Forshner, and Knox found that, if compared in duplicate with routine media, the Thayer-Martin selective medium affords a considerably higher percentage of isolations of N. gonorrhoeae. This medium inhibits many diagnostically confusing bacteria that often appear on most culture materials.

Fluorescent antibody techniques. The development of fluorescent antibody techniques by Deacon and others (1959) for identification of the gonococcus was accepted with considerable enthusiasm, though some recent reports bring their diagnostic accuracy into question. Wende, for example, found a lack of specificity, since strains of staphylococci, streptococci, and Mima herellea, as well as some saprophytes, occasionally were stained by the supposedly specific fluorescein-tagged antibody. Either direct smears or smears from culture (delayed technique) may be employed. The smear is stained with fluorescein-labeled N. gonorrhoeae antiserum, then examined through the microscope under ultraviolet illumination. Since many direct smears from patients with chronic disease contain few gonococci, only the indirect or delayed technique is acceptably reliable following negative reports.

Delayed fluorescent antibody technique. For this test, the material is cultured on chocolate agar and the fluorescent antibody technique is used to examine suspected colonies. The delayed method has proved more accurate, particularly for the diagnosis of gonorrhea in the asymptomatic patient.

Complement fixation test. This test has proved to be practically worthless in the diagnosis of gonorrhea.

Treatment

Local methods of treatment such as douching, suppositories, irrigations, and instrumentation are contraindicated for acute gonorrhea. Sulfonamides, penicillin, and, later, broad spectrum antibiotics have revolutionized the treatment for this disease. Before these agents were introduced, treatment often required hospitalization of the patient; now it can be effectively carried out on an out-patient basis. Although the sulfonamides were once highly effective, the organism rapidly developed resistance to these agents. Currently, penicillin is considered the most effective drug available; however, strains of gonococci resistant to penicillin are being reported with increasing frequency. Most resistant strains observed by us have come from the Mexican border towns, where prostitutes often receive small doses of long-acting penicillin semimonthly, mainly for the control of syphilis. Unquestionably, penicillin-resistant strains have evolved, yet the majority of patients will respond to an increased dosage and prolonged treatment. Whereas, originally, 300,000 U. of penicillin was usually effective, today such dosage is totally undependable. We have recently observed a patient who, despite the administration of 6,600,000 U. of benzathine penicillin G (Bicillin) during a 4 day period, continued to manifest the classic signs of the disease and the smears and cultures remained positive. According to Shapiro, the evidence indicates that women require a higher dosage than men. It is his further opinion that most treatment schedules currently in use are inadequate. Many failures are attributable to inadequate blood levels obtained with the sole use of long-acting penicillin, such as benzathine penicillin G (Bicillin). The simultaneous treatment of all sexual partners is important. Schedules of antibiotic therapy that have been found effective include:

1. Aqueous procaine penicillin G, 2,400,000 U., into each buttock, for a total dosage of 4,800,000 U.
2. Shapiro and Lentz found that the highest cure rate (94.2 percent) was obtained with the use of a combination of aqueous procaine penicillin G, 2,400,000 U., in one buttock, and procaine penicillin G in oil, 2,400,000 U., in the other buttock.
3. Amies recommended soluble penicillin in a single dose of as much as 8,000,000 U. for resistant infections.
4. Tetracycline antibiotics, given orally, 250 to 500 mg. every 6 hr. for 3 to 5 days, have been followed by good results in penicillin resistant infections and in penicillin sensitive patients.

Dosages smaller than the foregoing will probably be ineffective in more patients and will contribute to increasing resistance of the organism. Retreatment is indicated if signs or symptoms persist 3 or more days after treatment or if laboratory tests remain positive. Retreatment demands an increase of the original dosage, whether given in single or divided injections. If a patient fails to respond initially to adequate penicillin, change to a tetracycline should be seriously considered.

A laboratory follow-up of patients who are treated for gonorrhea should include Gram-stained smears and cultures. Material from both the cervix and urethra should be examined at weekly intervals for 3 or more weeks before the patient is pronounced cured.

As in every other venereal disease, the epidemiologic aspects of gonorrhea should be considered. To be remembered is the fact that a high percentage of infected women are asymptomatic and that apparent failures of treatment can frequently be traced to untreated or inadequately treated consorts. Every individual with a known exposure to gonorrhea should be treated prophylactically with a full therapeutic dosage of an appropriate antibiotic.

Special therapeutic considerations

Bartholin's abscess is best incised and drained. Drainage may be facilitated and premature closure of the opening prevented by use of an iodoform wick for a few days. We do not advocate the marsupialization of a Bartholin's abscess associated with acute gonorrheal infection. The field is surgically unsuitable and the ultimate condition of the duct cannot be foretold. Should a cyst subsequently develop, marsupialization is then indicated (Chapter 5).

Abscess of Skene's duct, although relatively uncommon, may require incision and drainage. Should a Skene's duct cyst subsequently form, its removal may be indicated (Chapter 5). Chronic skenitis is seldom observed today, since most infections of the duct respond completely to specific therapeutic agents. A chronic discharge from Skene's ducts is more often a manifestation of trichomoniasis than gonorrhea. Destruction by cautery of Skene's ducts, because of chronic infection, is seldom indicated now that specific therapeutic agents are available.

Urethral stricture may develop late, although it is a rare result of gonorrhea in the female and is seldom severe. It usually consists of a uniform narrowing, unlike the multiple scar tissue contractions that develop in men. The stricture is manifested by varying degrees of urinary retention, frequency, and dribbling. Recurrent cystitis may result. The extent of urethral narrowing can be determined with graduated dilators. Office dilations, performed after urethral application of 2% lidocaine (Xylocaine), are usually adequate treatment.

Chronic cervicitis is too often mentioned in connection with gonorrhea. It is not an inevitable result, and definitely gonorrhea is not the most common cause of chronic cervicitis. The cervicitis that may follow gonorrhea is not distinctive, and treatment is more correctly determined by the gross appearance of the cervix. Cauterization or other destructive procedures for cervicitis in a patient who has had gonorrhea should not be employed until several weeks or months have elapsed subsequent to microbiologic proof of a cure of the gonorrhea.

The following points deserve reiteration:

1. In many women, gonorrhea is asymptomatic and unsuspected.
2. Smears (particularly) and cultures are subject to a high percentage of error, especially when the findings are negative.
3. Penicillin-resistant strains of gonococci are on the increase; to assume cure of all patients who receive a recommended dosage would be erroneous.
4. The patient's sexual partner should be treated simultaneously.

Syphilis

Syphilis is a continuous infectious process that is initiated at the time of contact. It passes through well-known clinical stages: primary, secondary, latent, and late (tertiary). Although syphilis is a systemic disease almost from the moment of transmission, its discussion in this book concerns mainly lesions in the lower genitalia. Here, the primary (chancres) and the secondary lesions (condylomata lata) develop. Tertiary lesions (gummata) are rarely observed.

Etiology

The organism causing syphilis, *Treponema pallidum,* is a motile, anaerobic spirochete that dies quickly if denied moist tissue. Transmission of syphilis involves intimacy, and in the vast majority of cases it is attributable to sexual contact. Spirochetes readily invade intact, moist mucosa; invasion through dry, unbroken skin is unlikely. Ordinarily, no organisms are found in the vaginal tract or on the vulva unless early lesions are present from which organisms are continuously discharged. During the early latent stage of the disease, the menstrual blood often contains the organisms. In the words of Pariser, "Transmission of spirochetes reduced to its simplest terms is a lesion to lesion affair except by means of the blood." In other words, spirochetes survive in the vaginal tract or on the vulva only if discharged from chancres and condylomata lata or when present in menstrual blood. Of epidemiologic importance is the fact that infectious lesions are often painless and inconspicuous to the patient.

Incidence

When penicillin became plentiful after World War II, the incidence of syphilis declined rapidly. The belief that penicillin had all but eradicated the disease apparently resulted in deemphasis of V.D. education. This, combined with the indiscriminate use of antibiotics that often masked the primary and secondary lesions, accounted for an abrupt increase in its incidence after 1958. Although syphilis may never be totally eradicated, it can be effectively controlled by appropriate use of available therapeutic agents, educational programs, and conscientious attention to its epidemiologic aspects.

Clinical features

According to estimates, approximately half the patients with syphilis have either been unaware of its presence or have considered the lesions to be inconsequential until the disease has passed through its early stages. Although the patient is actually infected from the moment of inoculation, the primary lesion usually does not appear for 10 to 90 days, the average being 3 weeks; serologic tests do not become positive (reactive) for an additional week or longer. Approximately 9 weeks (6 weeks to 6 months) after inoculation, the disease may enter the secondary stage. At this time, all the serologic tests should be positive. The signs and symptoms of late syphilis may develop immediately after the secondary stage; usually, however, a latent period intervenes before any signs and symptoms are evident. The use of antibiotics for unrelated diseases frequently alters the clinical pattern and serologic reactions of syphilis.

Primary syphilis. A chancre may develop at any site of entry of the spirochete: the vulva, vagina, cervix, tongue, nipples, or lips. Ordinarily, the lesion is single, yet multiple chancres (Fig. 22-4, *A*) of the vulva are relatively common. The primary lesion often begins as an indurated papule, the surface of which promptly erodes, forming an ulcer. The lesion with the most diagnostic features is the classical hard chancre (Fig. 22-4, *B*), although more often than not lesions of the vulva are not characteristic. The so-called typical hard chancre has a punched-out, indurated base, with firm, rolled edges. The erosive or softer type of chancre of the vulva is an irregularly shaped "sore" that at times resembles a traumatic ulcer or erosion (Fig. 22-4, *A*, top arrow). There may be no induration, and the base may be level with the surrounding skin. In the untreated patient, 3 to 9 weeks are usually required for complete healing of the chancre. Any ulcer of the vulva should be suspect, particularly if it is painless and indurated.

Unfortunately, many chancres develop

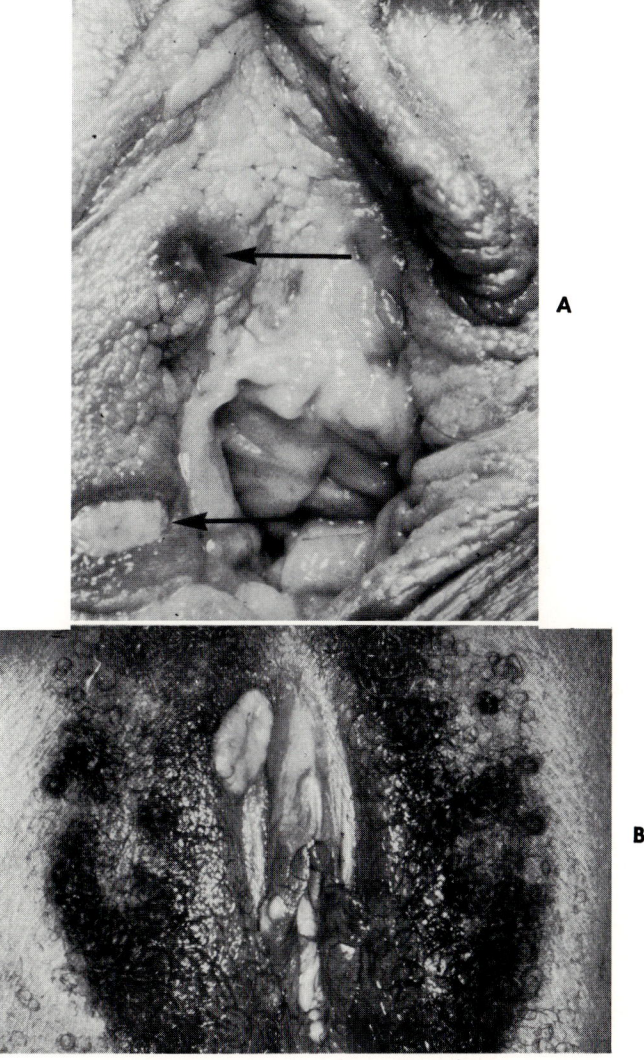

Fig. 22-4. **A,** Syphilis. Multiple chancres of vulva, indicated by arrows. **B,** Typical hard chancre. Although perhaps classical, this type of primary lesion is seldom observed on the vulva.

on the cervix without being detected, and even when found they are frequently unrecognized. Cervical and vaginal chancres are less characteristic than the vulvar lesions. They may appear as well-delineated mucous patches resembling leukoplakic spots, or they may be sharply defined ulcers near the external cervical os or separated from the os by an area of normal squamous epithelium. Any lesion of the cervix that seems to be an ulcer or erosion and is separated from the os by apparently normal epithelium should be suspected of having an infectious origin.

Unless secondarily infected, chancres are essentially painless. Regardless of their location, they are usually associated with enlargement of the regional lymph nodes; in the presence of a vulvar chancre, these would be the nodes in the groin. The deep pelvic lymph nodes draining the upper vagina and cervix are not accessible to palpation. Nodal enlargement does not appear until several days after the chancre has developed. The nodes remain discrete and are not adherent to the skin.

Secondary syphilis. Because of the multiple lesions present, the secondary stage is the most infectious phase of the disease. These lesions may appear before the primary lesions have completely healed. Mild systemic symptoms include malaise, headache, and a low grade fever. The characteristic vulvar lesions of secondary syphilis are the condylomata lata (Fig. 22-5) or syphilitic papules. They are raised, flat-topped, moist, and grayish in color. Many are appreciably ulcerated and indurated. A pseudomembranous exudate may be present on the surface. These excrescences in the moist environment of the vulva are literally teeming with spirochetes, thus accounting for their highly infectious nature. Similar lesions are sometimes found in the mouth and pharnyx, beneath the breasts, and in the axillae. Secondary infection, particularly with Vincent's organisms, frequently causes them to have a foul odor. Generalized adenopathy is suggestive of the disease. Painless inguinal adenopathy is practically always associated.

During the early latent stage (usually the first 2 years), relapses to the secondary lesions are occasionally observed. Supposedly, after this time the patient's resistance prevents relapses in the skin.

Tertiary syphilis. The usual tertiary lesion of the vulva is the gumma, although it is extremely rare. It appears as a nodule that enlarges, and, because of necrosis of the overlying skin, ulcerates and sloughs. Large, multiple ulcerating gummata can destroy practically all of the vulvar tissues.

Histopathology

Chancre. As a rule, the involved epidermis is acanthotic at the margin of the chancre. The epidermis becomes progressively thinner toward the center of the lesion; here, ulceration is usually present. Infiltration of the dermis with neutrophils, lymphocytes, and plasma cells is prominent. Perivascular islands of inflammatory infiltrate are generally apparent at the periphery of the lesion. Arterioles, capillaries, and venules exhibit endothelial proliferation; it is believed that necrosis and ulceration may be the result of a frequently associated vascular thrombosis. Spirochetes are occasionally found in sections stained by Levaditi's method. In most cases, only a nonspecific

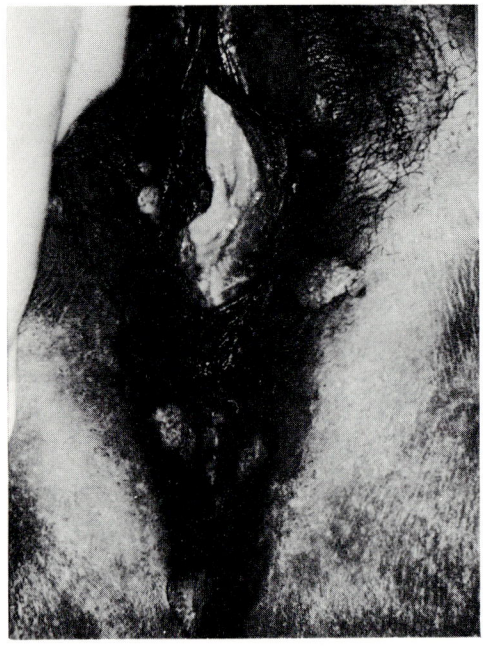

Fig. 22-5. Secondary syphilis. Multiple lesions of condylomata lata on vulva and perineum. Patient also had typical oral lesions. Darkfield was positive.

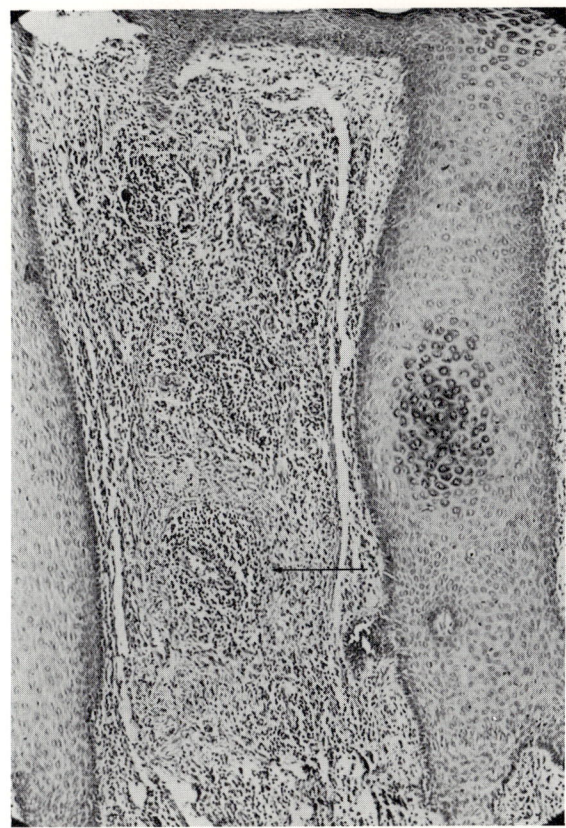

Fig. 22-6. Condyloma latum. Pronounced elongation and broadening of rete pegs. Also, perivascular cuffing with inflammatory cells (arrow). (H & E × 78)

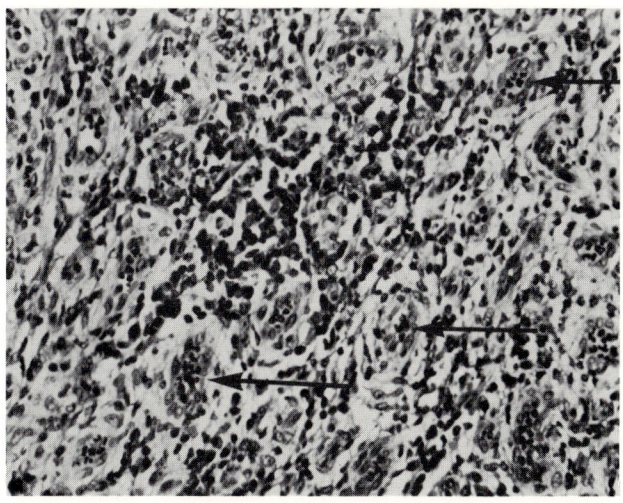

Fig. 22-7. Condyloma latum. Endothelial swelling and chronic inflammatory infiltrate about vessels in coat-sleeve fashion (arrow). (H & E × 273)

inflammatory reaction of the regional lymph nodes is observed.

Condyloma latum. The most diagnostic microscopic findings (Figs. 22-6 and 22-7) consist of pronounced vascular endothelial swelling and a dense coat-sleeve-like inflammatory infiltrate, consisting largely of plasma cells about the vessels in the lower dermis. Acanthosis with elongation and broadening of the rete pegs is frequently apparent. Levaditi's silver stain occasionally reveals the presence of spirochetes.

Gumma. Caseation necrosis in the center of the lesions and numerous epithelioid cells and foreign body type giant cells near the necrotic areas are features of the gumma. Endothelial proliferation and thickening of the vascular walls often lead to narrowing of their lumina. Plasma cell infiltration is conspicuous. The healing stage is exhibited by the presence of fibroblasts and the end-stage by fibrosis.

The chief microscopic findings in syphilis that distinguish it from tuberculosis are the vascular changes and the prevalence of plasma cells.

Diagnosis

Most physicians trained since 1945 have seen, at most, only an occasional case of classic early syphilis. This stage was once readily suspected and usually confirmable by darkfield examinations of the lesions and by serologic tests. Since the use of penicillin and other treponemacidal antibiotics has become widespread, the signs of early syphilis are so frequently modified or eliminated and the serologic activity so weakened that problems in diagnosis often arise. This means that physicians must remain even more vigilant and ever conscious of the existence of the disease; they should always suspect *T. pallidum* as the etiologic agent of every sore or open lesion of the genitalia, as well as every rash of obscure origin.

Darkfield examination. If the serologic test is negative, immediate proof of the presence of syphilis must depend upon the demonstration of *T. pallidum* (Fig. 22-8) from a lesion of the skin or mucosa or from the regional lymph nodes. Since the serum from primary and secondary lesions of syphilis contains *T. pallidum,* darkfield microscopy becomes a valuable and rapid method of laboratory diagnosis. It is particularly valuable in the seronegative primary disease, since specific therapy can be instituted at an early stage.

Proper collection of material for examination is important. The lesion is cleansed and abraded with a gauze square to the point of superficial bleeding. The blood is removed and the serum allowed to ooze from the lesion. Serum is picked up on the surface of a glass slide and a cover slip is applied. Reading of the darkfield is necessary before the slide dries. Drying may be prevented if the serum is collected and

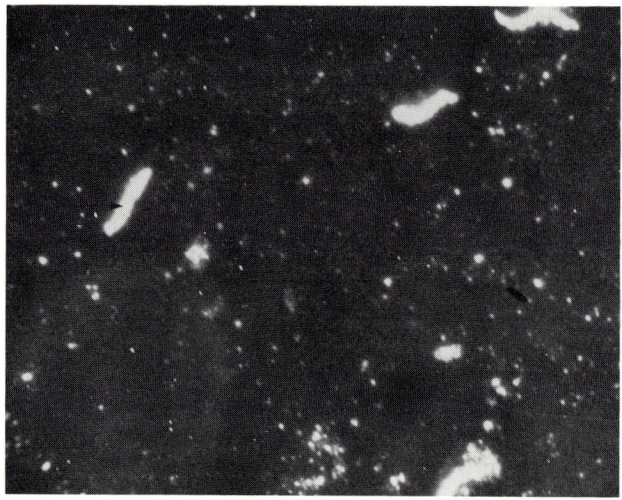

Fig. 22-8. Syphilis. Darkfield shows *Treponema pallidum*.

sealed in a capillary tube or if the edges of the cover slip are coated with petroleum jelly or clear nail polish. Only the technician thoroughly trained in the technique can readily distinguish *T. pallidum* from nonpathogenic spirochetes. The *T. pallidum* may be difficult to find if topical medications have recently been applied, as is often true.

Serologic tests. *T. pallidum* stimulates production of an antibody complex (reagin) that appears in the patient's serum, usually 4 to 6 weeks after infection or 1 to 3 weeks following the appearance of the chancre. Thereafter, titers rapidly rise. The reagin in serum can be measured serologically by the use of nontreponemal antigens prepared from beef heart. The most commonly used flocculation test today is the Venereal Disease Research Laboratories (VDRL) test. The Mazzini, the Kline, and the Kahn tests are still occasionally used. The Kolmer is the most popular complement fixation test. Although these tests with nontreponemal antigens are not 100 percent specific, they are highly indicative of the disease when properly interpreted and correlated with clinical findings. Qualitative results are usually reported as:

1. Reactive, positive, or 4+ or 3+ (synonymous terms); or
2. Weakly reactive, weakly positive, doubtful, or 2+ or 1+ (relatively synonymous terms); or
3. Nonreactive (NR) or negative (synonymous terms)

When nontreponemal antigens are employed, quantitative results are obtained by serologic titration in geometric progression. The results are particularly useful in evaluation of therapeutic response. The titer is generally high in secondary syphilis.

Treponema pallidum immobilization (TPI). Serologic tests in which treponemal antigens are employed are more specific, yet their use has proved difficult and costly, and they should not be considered to be routine screening tests. They are valuable as confirmatory tests if the diagnosis is questionable.

Fluorescent antibody test. Recently, fluorescent antibody techniques, especially the indirect method, have been successful. The fluorescent treponemal antibody (FTA) tests, particularly the FTA-absorption technique (FTA-ABS), have been found to be both sensitive and specific. The direct technique, probably still experimental, involves the use of antibodies labeled with fluorescein as a histochemical stain for identifying *T. pallidum* (the antigen), whereas the antigen *(T. pallidum)* may be used to identify the antibodies in the patient's blood. The latter, known as the indirect method, has proved to be the most practical. Knox and others have written a good description of the technique.

Differential diagnosis. Syphilitic sores on the vulva mimic numerous other ulcers and thus must always be considered in the differential diagnosis of ulcers in this area. Chancres must be distinguished from the diseases listed below, as well as many others associated with vulvovaginal ulceration. Also, the possibility of coexistence is always present. Chancroidal lesions are usually multiple and painful (Fig. 22-9), and *T. pallidum* is not demonstrable in the darkfield, whereas *Haemophilus ducreyi* may be demonstrable in smears or appropriately performed cultures. In granuloma inguinale, the darkfield is negative; Donovan bodies are demonstrable in tissue smears and sometimes in histologic sections. In lymphogranuloma venereum, the darkfield is negative and the Frei test positive unless the disease is in the earliest stages. Ulcers of herpes genitalis are preceded by the development of vesicles. The ulcers are small, multiple, more superficial, and more painful; usually the patient gives a history of their recurrence. Further, in contrast to chancres, they heal within 7 to 10 days. The darkfield is negative. The lesions of syphilis are never vesicular except in the congenital stage. Carcinoma follows a longer clinical course, and the distinction is readily made by a biopsy study. The ulcers of Behçet's syndrome may be highly confusing, though they are darkfield-negative. Condylomata lata must also be distinguished from such lesions as chancroid, granuloma inguinale, lymphogranuloma venereum, and condyloma acuminatum. Tertiary lesions are most likely to be confused with carcinomata, tuberculosis, deep fungal infections, and granulomata from other causes.

The assumption that all eruptions of the vulvovaginal tissues are syphilitic because the patient has a positive serologic test is an error to be avoided. The failure of lesions to heal rapidly with appropriate treatment is suggestive evidence of a concomitant disease.

Treatment

For decades before antibiotics became available, most patients with syphilis were treated by specialists in venereal diseases or in public health clinics. Since the treatment has been simplified by the use of antibiotics, an ever-increasing number of patients is being treated by physicians in private practice.

Antibiotics have replaced arsenicals and bismuth as the treatment for syphilis. Penicillin is the drug of choice. Many preparations and schedules of dosage are in use. The oral method of administration is unacceptable, since absorption of the penicillin is too variable and the cooperation of the patient is too unreliable. Since many patients have been sensitized to penicillin and are thus subject to allergic anaphylactic reactions, careful inquiry regarding this possibility is mandatory before intramuscular injections are given. The patient should be detained for 15 to 20 minutes after the initial injection, and the physician should be fully prepared to cope with an anaphylactic reaction.

An effective penicillin blood level can be easily maintained by intramuscular administration of the drug according to one of the following schedules:

1. Benzathine penicillin G (Bicillin), 4,800,000 U. total dosage—2.4 million U. initially (1.2 million U. into each hip) and repeated in 1 week.
2. Procaine penicillin G in oil, with 2% aluminum monostearate (PAM), 6,000,000 U. total dosage—2.4 million U. initially and 1.2 million U. at each of three subsequent injections 3 days apart.
3. Aqueous procaine penicillin G, 600,000 U. daily for 10 days or a total dosage of 6,000,000 U.

Patients who are sensitive to penicillin may be treated by broad spectrum antibiotics including:

1. Erythromycin estolate (Ilosone), 500 mg. every 6 hours for 10 to 15 days. This agent should not be used in pregnancy because of the placental barrier, as demonstrated by South, Short, and Knox.
2. Tetracyclines, 500 mg. every 4 hours for 10 to 15 days. These agents in such dosage are contraindicated in the third trimester of pregnancy because of possible discoloration of the infant's teeth and retardation of skeletal growth.

With the exceptions mentioned, the treatment schedule of the pregnant and non-pregnant patient is essentially identical. Follow-up examinations should include clinical inspection and quantitative serologic tests monthly for 6 months and at intervals of 3 months for 1 year thereafter. If a patient is adequately treated during the seronegative primary stage of the disease, serologic tests usually remain negative. If treatment is not given until the seropositive stage is reached, tests are likely to be positive for several months, although 90 percent revert within 12 months. Treatment during the secondary stage generally brings about a serologic reversal within 12 to 18 months. Any patient seropositive 12 months after treatment should have a lumbar puncture. If the disease has been present for several years before treatment, the serologic tests may be positive for the life of the patient.

Epidemiologic control

The results of recent research suggest that a protective vaccine against syphilis may some day be available. At present, the private physician holds the key to effective control of the disease. The professional staff members of health departments are usually skillful and are anxious to cooperate with the private physician. The majority of patients will cooperate after the importance of contact-tracing is explained. Contacts should be appropriately investigated and treatment given to the obviously infected.

The majority of patients exposed to early syphilis should be treated prophylactically, even though no evidence of the disease can be found. Prevention is usually provided by a single injection of 2,400,000 U. of benzathine penicillin G. The occasional severe reaction from hypersensitivity to penicillin might be offered as an argument against the routine prophylactic treatment, although it would appear that the benefits to the community and to the innocent would far outweigh the dangers. Patients who are allergic to penicillin may be treated prophylactically with the broad spectrum group of antibiotics—for example, erythromycin estolate or tetracycline—the dosage of these being the same as for the established disease.

Chancroid

Chancroid (soft chancre), first described by Ducrey in 1889, is a highly contagious, localized, acute venereal disease caused by the bacillus *Hemophilus ducreyi*. Although its overall incidence is low, the disease has a world-wide distribution. It is more prevalent in tropical and subtropical countries and in a clinic type of practice; it is seldom observed in private practice.

Clinical features

Unlike vulvar sores from syphilis, a chancroid is always tender and painful. Ordinarily, the ulcers appear on the vulva, particularly the vestibule, and occasionally on the vagina or cervix. The incubation period varies from 3 to 7 days, depending upon virulence of the agent and perhaps upon the hygienic status of the vulvar tissues. Usually, the earliest lesion is visible within 3 days and rapidly changes from papule to intradermal abscess to ulcer.

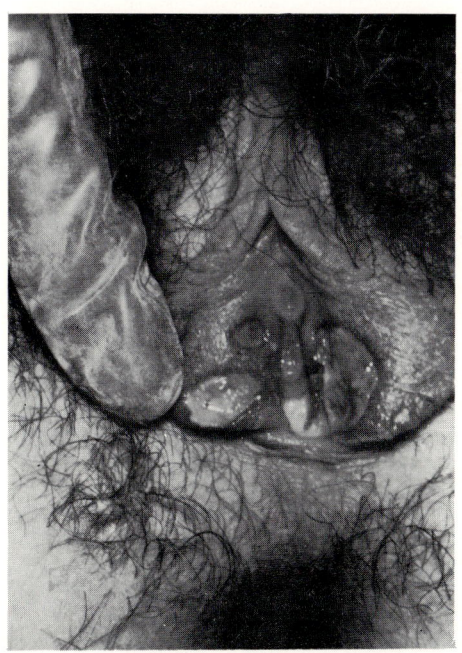

Fig. 22-9. Chancroid. Multiple, irregular, well-defined ulcers with dirty, gray necrotic bases.

Since the disease is autoinoculable, the majority of patients have multiple ulcers (Fig. 22-9) in various stages of development. Most of the lesions are irregular in shape, have well-defined sloping or ragged edges, and are surrounded by an erythematous halo. Some are undermined. Initially, the ulcers are suppurative, their bases appearing to be dirty, grayish, and necrotic. The lesions are softer than the classic syphilitic chancre and often are extremely malodorous incident to secondary infection, particularly with fusospirochetal organisms. In the untreated patient, extensive ulceration, destruction of tissue, and edema at times involve the entire vulva, perineum, and perianal tissues. Chronic, nonhealing ulcerations may spread to the inner thighs and to the groins and persist for years.

One or more inguinal lymph nodes become involved in about half the infected patients, usually within 14 days. If treatment is delayed, the overlying skin often becomes infected and necrotic, and the nodes suppurate and drain. Pain is more often associated with the bubo of chancroid than with other granulomatous diseases.

Histopathology

Although the microscopic changes in chancroid are said to be nonspecific, Heyman, Beeson, and Sheldon found that, in almost every case, the diagnosis can be established with reasonable certainty by microscopic study. According to these authors, unless the lesion is in the earliest stage, sufficient tissue for examination can be removed by a biopsy punch instrument without anesthesia and with little pain. (We have always used a local anesthetic.) They describe the lesion as having three fairly distinct zones:

> The surface zone or base of the ulcer is rather shallow and is made up of polymorphonuclear leukocytes, fibrin, red blood cells and necrotic tissue. Below this is a fairly wide layer of edematous tissue in which endothelial cells in various stages of proliferation outnumber all other cellular components. Newly formed blood vessels are numerous and may show palisading with occasional degeneration of the vessel walls and thrombosis. Finally there is a deep zone in which there is a dense infiltration by plasma cells and lymphocytes. Demonstration of Ducrey bacilli in the tissue is occasionally possible.

Diagnosis

For all practical purposes, the diagnosis of chancroid is based upon the patient's history, the clinical signs and symptoms, and the exclusion of other ulcerative diseases of the genitalia. A variety of laboratory procedures not only provides some confirmatory evidence of the disease but is also helpful in the exclusion of other granulomatous lesions.

Stained smears. A diagnosis by smear, not always successful, is based chiefly upon the morphology, staining characteristics, and arrangement of the bacilli of Ducrey. The organisms are short, plump, and gram-negative. Pappenheim's staining method discloses that they have rounded ends. Although the bacilli are sometimes intracellular, they are more often observed in clusters outside of pus cells, in a "school of fish" arrangement.

The base of a clean, early ulcer is preferable for removal of smear material. Secondary infection often alters the microscopic picture, including a reduction in Ducrey's bacilli. The aspirate of a suppurative bubo sometimes contains the organism. Smears from this source are more diagnostic than smears from ulcers.

Bacteriologic cultures. Properly performed cultures made before secondary infection has developed afford an accurate diagnosis of approximately 75 percent of chancroids. In most cultures, a mixed growth is present; thus, certain identification of *H. ducreyi* is difficult. Aspirate of buboes provides good material for study by culture.

Skin tests. In view of conflicting reports on the use of intradermal reactions to both bubo pus antigen and bacillary vaccine, the value of such tests is debatable. Reactions become positive only after 8 to 25 days following the onset of the disease, and they remain positive for life. False positive reactions are not uncommon. According to Glicksman, skin tests are rarely used in venereal disease clinics.

Biopsy. Heyman, Beeson, and Sheldon reported that histologic examination of excised tissue can be dependable for diagnosis.

Differential diagnosis. The distinction of chancroid from other diseases is mandatory. Darkfield examination and serologic tests for syphilis are necessary in every questionable case of ulceration of the lower genital tract. A positive serologic test for syphilis does not, however, prove that an obvious sore is syphilitic in origin, since positive findings may be incident to latent or late syphilis. The possibility of concomitant lesions of other origin is always present, particularly in persons of the lower social strata. In differential diagnosis, syphilis, lymphogranuloma inguinale, granuloma inguinale, Behçet's syndrome, and ulcers from many other causes must be considered.

Treatment

Immediate subjective relief can be afforded the patient by the local application of soaks, such as diluted Burow's solution. Antibiotic ointments are of questionable value; moreover, they may mask a positive darkfield. For curative treatment, the systemic use of sulfonamides or antibiotics is necessary. Possible schedules of the dosages include:

1. Sulfadiazine or a triple sulfa preparation, 1.0 gm. four times daily for 7 to 10 days, depending upon the response. Sulfonamides are advantageous since they do not suppress syphilis and thus do not alter the clinical and serologic patterns.
2. Tetracycline, aureomycin, or terramycin, 250 mg. orally four times daily for 7 to 10 days, depending upon the response. Because of the danger of their masking associated early syphilis, these drugs should perhaps be reserved for lesions that do not respond to sulfadiazine and streptomycin.

In the presence of inguinal adenitis or if the response is slow, the systemic agents should be administered for longer periods. Fluctuant inguinal buboes may be aspirated with a large needle; incision is not recommended.

For phagedenic chancroids associated with Vincent's organisms, penicillin may be required, despite the fact that penicillin is relatively ineffective against Ducrey's bacilli. An ulcer that fails to heal after the use of known effective medication warrants further investigation.

Lymphogranuloma venereum

Lymphogranuloma venereum (lymphogranuloma inguinale, lymphopathia venereum) is a highly contagious venereal disease caused by a virus-like organism of the psittacosis-lymphogranuloma group, which has an affinity for lymphatic structures. Contact with infectious secretions may be a possible source of infection, particularly in children. Since the virus-like organisms contain both ribonucleic and deoxyribonucleic acids, they cannot be called true viruses.

The disease is most prevalent in tropical and subtropical climates, in patients of low socioeconomic level, and in Negroes (10:1). Approximately 50 percent of the patients are between 21 and 30 years old. The actual prevalence of lymphogranuloma venereum (L.G.V.) in the general population is unknown. De Sousa and Brandao reported positive complement fixation tests on 60 percent of fifty prostitutes, and positive Frei tests on ten of thirty-two prostitutes. Although the significance of such figures is not clear, they are strongly suggestive of a considerable number of subclinical infections. Sigel has stated: "We have at least indirect evidence that L.G.V. may occur in an inapparent form in as many as 90 percent of infected individuals." The disease is perhaps more common than chancroid and, according to Douglas, the ratio of cases of lymphogranuloma venereum to those of granuloma inguinale is approximately 3:1.

Clinical features

After an incubation period of 3 to 21 days, the initial or primary lesion appears as a papule or vesicle, usually single, located in the vicinity of the posterior fourchette. It is evanescent and painless, and generally it is unnoticed by the patient. The earliest lesion is rarely observed by a physician. The subsequent clinical course of lymphogranuloma venereum is highly variable; in some patients it gives rise to only transient, minimal lymphadenitis, while in other it leads to extensive disease with chronic disability.

Within a matter of weeks after the appearance of the first lesion, the disease is manifested by lymphadenitis; this may be the only discernible lesion. Perhaps lymphogranuloma venereum should be suspected when lymphadenitis is present without obvious cause. Systemic symptoms consist principally of fever and headaches. Occasionally, inguinal buboes are the first noticeable sign of L.G.V.; however, they never develop in the vast majority of female patients. The perirectal lymph nodes are more likely to be involved, presumably because of the lymphatic drainage to these nodes from the usual initial sites in the posterior portions of the vulva and vagina. This explanation has not been generally accepted, although it is well known that inguinal buboes rarely precede or are associated with rectal L.G.V. Buboes, when they develop, are unilateral in approximately two-thirds of the patients. They are most often multiple and discrete, yet they are frequently matted together and to the overlying skin by perinodal inflammation (Fig. 22-10). The buboes tend to elongate in the direction of the inguinal ligament. According to their

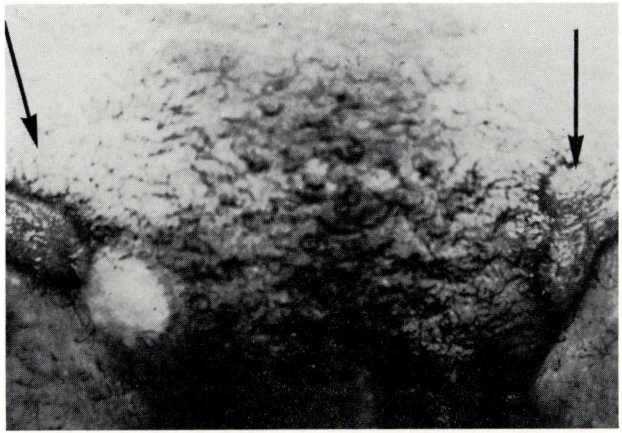

Fig. 22-10. Lymphopathia venereum with inguinal lymphadenopathy. The latter is rarely observed in women. (Courtesy John M. Knox, Houston.)

stage and extent, their consistency varies from hard to soft and fluctuant. In about one-fourth of untreated patients the adenopathy regresses without eruption; in the others, suppurating buboes erupt through the overlying skin forming draining fistulous tracts. The fistulous openings remain relatively clean, with little inflammatory reaction, in contrast to the large, dirty ulcers that follow chancroidal buboes. Slow, though eventual healing leaves irregular inguinal scars. The exuberant granulations of granuloma inguinale do not develop in L.G.V.

Proctocolitis followed by anorectal stricture is the most clinically significant manifestation of this disease in the female. The chief early symptom of proctitis is the passage of mucus, blood, and pus from the rectum. Edematous perianal tags are often associated. On digital examination, the anal and rectal mucosa are roughened and leathery, frequently seeming to be granular or nodular. The subsequent formation of fibrous strictures is possibly attributable to uncontrolled secondary bacterial infection over months or years. The anal and rectal walls become indurated, rigid, and roughened; the examining finger is frequently admitted with difficulty, if at all. Although the strictures may extend as high as the lower sigmoid, the anorectal junction is usually their upper limit. Strictures are chronically progressive and are often complicated by perirectal and ischiorectal abscesses. In the advanced stages, fistulae to the vagina and perineum may develop. Constipation with small stools and, eventually, alternate obstipation and diarrhea are results of such strictures. Even complete obstruction of the lower bowel may ensue. Many patients are troubled with rectal bleeding, pain, and a varying rectal discharge. Frequently, the posterior aspect of the lower half of the vagina also becomes indurated and scarred.

Elephantiasis of the labia and clitoris develops incident to lymphatic obstruction. The degree of swelling is highly variable, and the increased size of the vulva from lymph stasis is augmented by hyperplasia and hypertrophy of the skin and subjacent tissues. The surfaces of the swollen parts may be verrucoid, smooth, or ulcerated, and the tissues may be of a rubbery consistency. These edematous tumefactions can resemble pedunculated neoplasms.

Destructive ulcerative lesions sometimes follow the lymphadenitis. The labia minora and prepuce may be partially or totally destroyed. Fenestrations and tunneling of the vulvar skin are not uncommon results. Progressive destruction of the urethra and adjacent tissues can ultimately lead to complete urinary incontinence.

Since carcinoma of the vulva arises in younger patients with granulomatous infections including L.G.V., the latter are believed to constitute a predisposing factor. This assumption is supported by the observations collected by Sigel, as well as those of Collins and others, Douglas, Saltzstein, Woodruff, and Novak, and Lunin. Levin and others reported that postlymphogranulomatous rectal strictures increase the incidence of carcinoma of the rectum.

Histopathology

The microscopic appearance of lymphogranuloma venereum is not usually specific, yet it may be strongly suggestive of the disease. Although inguinal buboes are rarely available for examination in the female, they exhibit the most diagnostic microscopic feature—stellate abscesses surrounded by epithelioid cells in palisade formation. The typical abscesses soon merge, however, and lose their characteristic stellate appearance. Later, caseation necrosis of the lymph nodes and infiltration with plasma cells take place.

The microscopic picture of the elephantiasic lesion includes peritubular infiltration with plasma cells and lymphocytes, fibroblastic activity, and dilated lymph vessels. Pronounced fibrosis of the involved tissues is a late development. Epithelial thinning may be present at the edge of the ulcers. At times, epithelial hyperplasia with pronounced and irregular elongation of the epithelial folds may be present. This hyperplasia may be so advanced that differentiation from carcinoma may be difficult. The term "pseudoepitheliomatous hyperplasia" is commonly used to refer to these changes.

Diagnosis

The clinical course of the disease and the gross appearance of the lesion offer clues to the diagnosis. Acute inguinal adenitis without an associated vulvar lesion and unexplained fibrotic anorectal stricture are particularly significant. Regardless of the clinical evidence, proof of the disease must depend upon laboratory confirmation.

Frei test. The Frei test is performed by the intradermal injection of virus antigen. Originally, the antigen was prepared from diluted pasteurized aspirate of buboes; the antigen now in common use is Lygranum S.T. (Squibb), prepared from chick embryo yolk sac cultures of the virus. For the test, 0.1 ml of the prepared antigen is injected intradermally into the forearm of the suspect. A positive reaction is indicated by the appearance within 48 to 72 hours of a papule or papulopustule 0.6 to 1.0 cm. in diameter, surrounded by a red areola. The papule is the important part of the reaction, and its diameter should be read with a millimeter scale. An intradermal control, provided with the Frei antigen, should be administered at the same time. Reactions to the control material are rare. A positive response can be elicited between 10 and 40 days after the primary lesion appears. If the presence of the disease is strongly suspected, negative tests should always be repeated. Test findings usually remain positive for life, especially if the patient has not been treated during an early stage of the disease; the findings can be reversed, however, if curative treatment is given in the beginning. Since positive reactions are reportedly obtained in only about 80 percent of infected patients, a negative reaction does not always exclude the presence of the disease. In view of the usual lifetime persistence of a positive reaction, the response cannot be interpreted as proof of active disease. A vesicle in the center of the Frei-antigen-produced papule suggests a high antibody titer. Because of the antigenic relationship between the various viruses of the psittacosis-lymphogranuloma group, false positive reactions may be obtained, especially in association with psittacosis, orinthosis, and certain pneumonias.

Complement fixation test. Lygranum C. F. (Squibb) is prepared from yolk sac membranes infected with the virus of L.G.V. Serologic findings are usually positive before those from the Frei test. A positive reaction in dilutions of 1:40 or higher should be interpreted as strong evidence of active disease, although positive reactions up to 1:40 should be carefully interpreted with a full knowledge of the clinical findings. Low titer findings should always be repeated. A rising titer is of highest significance. The diagnosis should probably be based only upon serial serum testings.

Inverted Frei test. This is performed by doing a Frei test on a subject known to have had lymphogranuloma venereum, using antigen prepared from the aspirate of a bubo from a patient suspected of having the disease. It is of particular value if the reactions to the Frei and complement fixation tests are negative.

Differential diagnosis. Chronic lymphogranuloma venereum with buboes or ulcerations requires differentiation from other granulomatous diseases, such as syphilis, chancroid, granuloma inguinale, and carcinoma. Rectal strictures must be distinguished from other proctologic diseases, including rectal carcinoma. Frequently, all available diagnostic tools—biopsies, smears, cultures, serologic tests, and darkfield examinations—are necessary for exclusion of the various other granulomatous and ulcerative diseases.

Treatment

The large virus causing L.G.V. may succumb to the recommended therapeutic agents, although some observers believe that the responses are attributable to the control of the secondary infections, and, with this accomplished, the viral infection becomes self-limited. The treatment of choice is the broad spectrum antibiotics, especially the tetracyclines. Effective treatment schedules include:

1. Chlortetracycline (aureomycin), oxytetracycline (terramycin), or tetracycline, 500 mg. every 6 hr. for 10 to 15 days. Failure of the lesion to heal, or their recurrence, necessitates a larger dosage, a longer course, or a change in medication.
2. Sulfadizine, 1 gm. every 6 hours for 14 to 21 days.

Special considerations. Buboes should never be incised, although, if fluctuant, they may be aspirated. Usually, they continue to resolve after the therapeutic agents have been discontinued.

For patients with rectal stricture, Packer (1963) suggests that, after the initial 21 day course of sulfadiazine therapy, medication should be continued for several months in the reduced dosage of 0.5 gm. q.i.d. Following chemotherapy, the diameter of the anorectal lumen, with or without digital dilations, may gradually increase. Prolonged antibiotic therapy will probably prove similarly effective.

A "pull through" procedure will afford good results in some patients with severe stricture yet with a good rectal sphincter. Colostomy should be reserved for those patients with strictures that do not respond to prolonged chemotherapy or antibiotics and digital dilations and for patients with an incompetent anal sphincter. An embarrassing or uncomfortable elephantiasis, especially when subject to ulcerations (esthiomene), may best be overcome by vulvectomy. This procedure is also indicated for persistent histologic atypias. Fistulous tracts may heal after prolonged drug therapy and gradual rectal dilatations. Vulvar disease with pronounced destructive changes, particularly of the urethra, offers a real surgical challenge for which serious preoperative planning is required. Regardless of the procedure chosen, sulfadiazine or one of the tetracyclines should be administered before it is undertaken and during convalescence; even under optimal conditions, poor healing can be expected.

Granuloma inguinale

Granuloma inguinale (donovanosis, venereal granuloma) is a mildly contagious disease caused by the unusual bacterial organism *Donovania granulomatis*. McLeod, in 1882, was the first to describe granuloma inguinale, though the causative organism was discovered by Charles Donovan in 1905. When this morphologically characteristic organism is present in tissues, it is referred to as a *Donovan body*. Aside from the determination of the nature of Donovan bodies and discovery of the response of the infection to antibiotics, little knowledge of this disease has been gained since these original descriptions.

In contrast to lymphogranuloma venereum, which is chiefly a disease of the lymphatics, granuloma inguinale primarily involves the skin and subcutaneous tissues. It is a slowly progressive, ulcerative, granulomatous process that most often affects the anogenital and adjacent tissues of patients between 20 and 40 years old. Being only mildly contagious, it remains relatively uncommon. In the United States, granuloma inguinale predominates in Negroes by a ratio of eight cases to one in Caucasians. Whether this is attributable to a racial or socioeconomic factor is unknown.

Etiology

The causative organism *D. granulomatis* is believed to be a bacterium, and it is currently the only known representative of its group. It is oblong and frequently bipolar and is found chiefly in large mononuclear cells. Carter, Jones, and Thomas isolated the bacillus in pure cultures from pseudobuboes, though they were unable to maintain the cultures. In 1943, Anderson, de Monbreun, and Goodpasture reported in vivo culture of the organisms in yolk sacs of chick embryos; they were subsequently able to maintain the organisms in vitro in culture, utilizing egg yolk material. It was they who named the organism *D. granulomatis*. Although Koch's postulates have never been fulfilled, the evidence points to *D. granulomatis* as the true etiologic agent. Dienst, Greenblatt, and Sanderson were able to transmit the disease in human beings by inoculation with aspirate of pseudobuboes. Although granuloma inguinale has always been considered a venereal disease, it is of interest that Packer (1959) found only two cases in the marital partners of over 500 patients with the disease.

Clinical features

The incubation period of granuloma inguinale in 8 days to 12 weeks. The initial lesion, which is a papule, breaks down to form an ulcer. The disease is only rarely observed and recognized in the preulcerative stage. The early ulcer, which commonly appears on the vulva, perianal tissues, vagina, or cervix, is frequently undermined, although it soon displays a red, granulomatous base. The ulcers, usually multiple because of autoinoculation, may be confluent. They slowly spread to adjacent skin and thus may involve tissues well beyond the genitalia, particularly the groins. Most of the lesions are essentially painless; others, however, are tender and painful, especially if secondarily infected. Characteristically, the ulcers ulti-

Venereal diseases

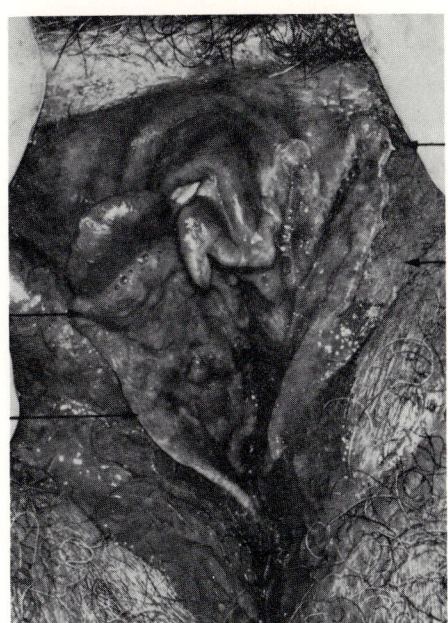

Fig. 22-11. Granuloma inguinale. Large granular, raised ulceration involving extensive areas of vulva. This lesion had been mistaken clinically for carcinoma.

mately form profuse vascular granulations (Fig. 22-11) above the surface of the skin, producing varying degrees of tumefaction. Frequently, the margins are raised and serpiginous. Extensive destruction and mutilation of the vulvar, perianal, and inguinal tissues sometimes follow severe secondary infection, especially if the patient is debilitated and untreated.

After months or years of slow healing, fibrosis is often pronounced, although even in the fibrotic stages small areas of ulceration are usually discernible. After healing, depigmented scars can be expected, and, in Negroes, keloid formation is not uncommon. A massive enlargement of the vulva, resembling elephantiasis, sometimes follows healing; this is believed to be induced by lymphatic obstruction from scar tissue contraction.

Generally, advanced disease may be of either of three clinical types or stages. The *exuberant* type, which appears relatively early, before secondary infection develops, exhibits a notable overgrowth of granulation tissue. The *ulcerative* type, in which the lesions are secondarily infected and necrotic, is less elevated and malodorous.

The latest stage or *cicatricial* type, which is reached after much healing, may be characterized by fibrosis, scarring, depigmentation, keloid formation, elephantiasis, or even stenosis of the vaginal and anal orifices.

Lymphadenitis is not a characteristic of this disease, although it occasionally develops from secondary infection. Subcutaneous inguinal granulomas or pseudobuboes are often observed. These ultimately penetrate the overlying skin, producing typical granulating ulcers. Whether they are the result of lymphatic spread or of autoinfection is not clear. Thus, inguinal lesions may arise from pseudobuboes or by direct extension from the vulva.

Granuloma inguinale of the cervix, which also appears as a granulating ulcer, is easily mistaken for carcinoma. Rarely, vaginal lesions develop, usually being direct extensions from the vulva. Stenosis of the vagina from fibrosis can ensue. Disseminated granuloma inguinale, although extremely uncommon, is sometimes found in pregnant patients with cervical lesions. In such patients, it is extremely dangerous.

Histopathology

Microscopically, the epithelium at the margins of the ulcers exhibits increased activity without keratinization. This proliferation can become pronounced, leading to acanthosis with irregular elongation of the rete pegs, a condition that might justifiably be called *pseudoepitheliomatous hyperplasia* (Fig. 22-12). At this stage, differentiation from carcinoma is sometimes a problem. Microabscesses are often found between the elongated rete pegs. Tissues beneath the denuded areas are densely infiltrated by histiocytes and plasma cells, as well as aggregates of polymorphonuclear cells (Fig. 22-13). In these exuberantly granulating lesions, small hemorrhages are seen, capillary proliferation is conspicuous, and connective tissue scarce.

Donovan bodies in large mononuclear cells (Fig. 22-14) provide the most diagnostic feature, yet they are at times difficult to demonstrate histologically, even with silver stains. Frequently, the cytoplasm of these monocytes has a cystic appearance; it is in these cysts that the encapsulated organisms are most often observed. Al-

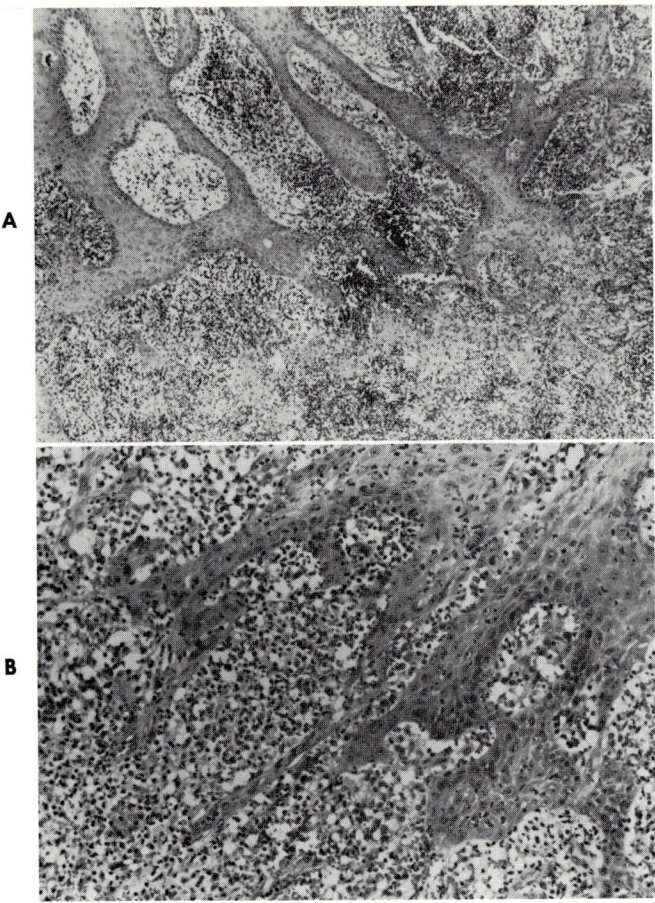

Fig. 22-12. A and B, Granuloma inguinale. Pseudoepitheliomatous hyperplasia with marked elongation and irregularity of rete pegs. (A, H & E × 40; B, H & E × 100)

though Donovan bodies can be detected with hematoxylin-eosin stains, Giemsa's stain, in which the organisms appear brick red, is preferable. Donovan bodies are black in silver stains and, because of intense bipolar staining, resemble a closed safety pin. Extracellular organisms are seldom visible.

Diagnosis

Although this disease may be strongly suspected on the basis of its clinical features, laboratory confirmation is necessary. The diagnosis depends upon the demonstration of Donovan bodies (Fig. 22-14) in scrapings, tissue smears, or histologic sections. Tissue smears are highly satisfactory and are easily made by smearing the cut side of granulation tissue removed without an anesthetic by means of a punch biopsy instrument. The smear is air dried and stained with Giemsa's or Wright's stain. Serologic and skin tests are highly sensitive, though nonspecific, and hence afford only presumptive evidence of the disease. With the use of antigens prepared from strains of *Donovania*, Goldberg, Weaver, and Packer found 136 positive responses to complement fixation tests of 151 sera from infected patients. Only one of 112 controls gave a positive reaction. Thus, when expertly performed, the complement fixation reaction may be valuable in excluding the disease.

Differential diagnosis. The distinction of granuloma inguinale from carcinoma, deep fungal infection, genital amebiasis, and various other diseases such as syphilis, chancroid, and lymphogranuloma venereum can frequently be accomplished only after careful interpretation of serologic tests, skin tests, biopsies, tissue and bacterial smears, and cultures of both ulcers and aspirate of buboes. The administration of antibiotics before the various tests sometimes makes definitive diagnosis difficult, if not impossible.

Treatment

At this time, the tetracycline group of antibiotics appears to be the most effective treatment. This would include chlortetracycline (aureomycin), oxytetracycline (terramycin), and tetracycline, given orally, 500 mg. every 6 hours for 10 to 21 days. None of these agents has been proved superior to the others. Penicillin is of no value unless the lesions are complicated by fusospirochetosis.

The lesions may heal rapidly during treatment, or the response may be slow or delayed for several weeks. For this reason, according to Douglas, failure of the treatment is not to be presumed until after 6 weeks. If healing does not take place or a relapse follows, a change of the antibiotic or a longer course of treatment is indicated.

Vulvectomy is reserved for those lesions that do not heal completely with medical treatment or for the vulva that remains conspicuously swollen. Vulvar swelling does not always give rise to discomfort, although it subjects the patients to ulcerations and possibly emotional reactions. Saltzstein, Woodruff, Novak and Collins (1951), and others reported an increased incidence of carcinoma of the vulva in groups of patients with granulomatous diseases, including granuloma inguinale. Vulvectomy, however, is not warranted as a routine procedure for the sole purpose of prophylaxis against carcinoma.

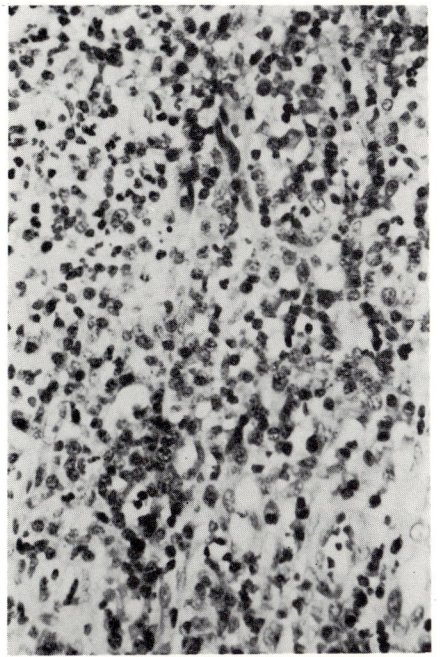

Fig. 22-13. Granuloma inguinale. Intense inflammatory infiltrate consisting primarily of plasma cells. (H & E × 250)

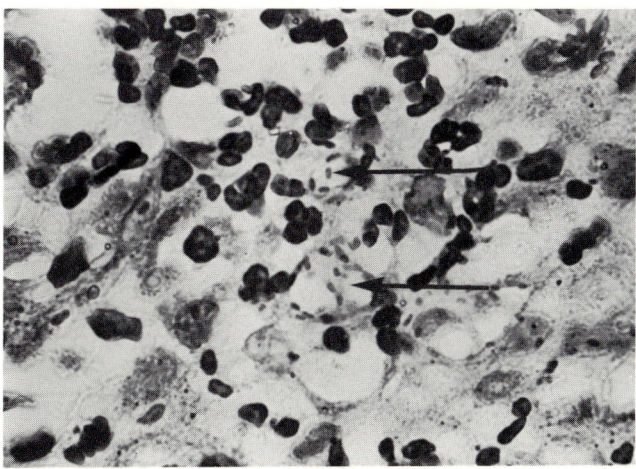

Fig. 22-14. Granuloma inguinale. Donovan bodies (bacteria) in vacuolated histiocytes. (Silver stain × 960)

REFERENCES

Amies, C. R.: Development of resistance of gonococci to penicillin: An eight year study, Canad. Med. Ass. J. **96:**33, 1967.

Anderson, K., de Monbreun, W. A., and Goodpasture, E. W.: Etiologic consideration of *Donovania granulomatis* cultivated from granuloma inguinale (three cases) in embryonic yolk, J. Exper. Med. **81:**25, 1945.

Blinick, G.: Gonorrheal disease in the female, Clin. Obstet. Gynec. **2:**492, 1959.

Brown, L., Copeloff, M. B., and Peacock, W. L., Jr.: Study of gonorrhea in treated and untreated asymptomatic women as determined by fluorescent antibody and culture methods, Amer. J. Obstet. Gynec. **84:**753, 1962.

Brown, W. J.: Primary and secondary syphilis. In Conn, H. F., editor: Current therapy, Philadelphia, 1963, W. B. Saunders Co.

Burckhardt, W., and Epstein, S.: Atlas and manual of dermatology and venereology, ed. 2, Baltimore, 1963, The Williams & Wilkins Co.

Carter, B., Jones, C. P., and Thomas, W. L.: The attempted cultivation of Donovan bodies from granuloma inguinale, J. Infect. Dis. **64:**314, 1939.

Cherny, W. B. V., Jones, C. P., and Peete, C. H.: Disseminated granuloma inguinale and its relationship to granuloma of the cervix and pregnancy, Amer. J. Obstet. Gynec. **74:**597, 1957.

Collins, C. G., Collins, J. H., Nelson, E. W., Smith, R. C., and MacCallum, E. A.: Malignant tumors involving the vulva, Amer. J. Obstet. Gynec. **62:**1198, 1951.

Collins, C. G., Kushner, J., Lewis, G. N., and Lapointe, R.: Noninvasive malignancy of the vulva, Obstet. Gynec. **6:**339, 1955.

Deacon, W. E., Albritton, D. C., Olansky, S., and Kaplan, W.: V.D.R.L. chancroid studies I: A simple procedure for the isolation and identification of *Hemophilus ducreyi*, J. Invest. Derm. **26:**399, 1956.

Deacon, W. E., Peacock, W. L., Jr., Freeman, E. M., and Harris, A.: Identification of *Neisseria gonorrhoeae* by means of fluorescent antibodies II, Proc. Soc. Exp. Biol. Med. **101:**322, 1959.

Deacon, W. E., Peacock, W. L., Jr., Freeman, E. M., Harris, A., and Bunch, W. L., Jr.: Fluorescent antibody tests for detection of the gonococcus in women, Pub. Health Rep. **75:**125, 1960.

De Sousa, C. P., and Brandao, F. N.: Epidemiological aspects of lymphogranuloma venereum, Brit. J. Vener. Dis. **37:**179, 1961.

Dienst, R. B., Greenblatt, R. B., and Sanderson, E. S.: Cultural studies on the "Donovan bodies" of granuloma inguinale, J. Infect. Dis. **62:**112, 1938.

Donovan, C.: Medical cases from the Madras General Hospital, Indian Med. Gaz. **40:**411, 1905.

Douglas, C. P.: Lymphogranuloma venereum and granuloma inguinale of the vulva, J. Obstet. Gynaec. Brit. Comm. **69:**871, 1962.

Ducrey, A.: Le virus dell'ulcera venerea non e state ancora cultivator, Giorn. Internaz. Sci. Med. (Napoli M.S.) **11:**44, 1889.

Dunlop, E. M. C.: Epidemiology of gonorrhoea, Brit. J. Vener. Dis. **39:**109, 1963.

Glicksman, J. M.: Personal communication, 1968.

Goldberg, J.: Studies on granuloma inguinale IV, Brit. J. Vener. Dis. **35:**266, 1959.

Goldberg, J., Weaver, R. H., and Packer, H.: Studies on granuloma inguinale I, Amer. J. Syph. **37:**60, 1953.

Greenblatt, R. B., Baldwin, K. R., and Dienst, R. B.: The minor venereal diseases, Clin. Obstet. Gynec. **2:**549, 1959.

Greenblatt, R. B., Pund, E. R., Sanderson, E. S., Torpin, R., and Dienst, R. B.: Management of chancroid, granuloma inguinale, lymphogranuloma venereum in general practice, Public Health Service Publication No. 255, ed. 2, Washington, 1953.

Harris, A., Deacon, W. E., Tiedemann, J., and Peacock, W. L., Jr.: Fluorescent antibody method of detecting gonorrhea in asymptomatic females, Pub. Health Rep. **76:**93, 1961.

Hellerstrom, S., and Skog, E.: Outcome of penicillin therapy of syphilis, Acta Dermatovener. **42:**179, 1962.

Heyman, A., Beeson, P. B., and Sheldon, W. H.: Diagnosis of chancroid, J.A.M.A. **129:**935, 1945.

Jorgensen, L.: Lymphogranuloma venereum, Acta Path. Microbiol. Scand. **47:**113, 1959.

Kampmeier, R. H.: Responsibility of a physician in a program for eradication of syphilis, J.A.M.A. **183:**1094, 1963.

Knox, J. M., Short, D. H., Wende, R. D., and Glicksman, J. M.: The FTA-ABS test for syphilis: Performance in 11033 patients, Brit. J. Vener. Dis. **42:**16, 1966.

Lever, W. F.: Histopathology of the skin, ed. 3, Philadelphia, 1961, J. B. Lippincott Co.

Levin, I., Romano, S., Steinberg, M., and Welsh, R. A.: Lymphogranuloma venereum: Rectal stricture and carcinoma, Dis. Colon Rectum **7:**129, 1964.

Lunin, A. B.: Carcinoma of the vulva, Amer. J. Obstet. Gynec. **57:**742, 1949.

Management of chancroid, granuloma inguinale, lymphogranuloma inguinale in general practice, U. S. Public Health Service, Pub. 255 (Revised 1964).

McLeod, K.: Precis of operations performed in the wards of the first surgeon Medical College Hospital, during the year 1881, Indian Med. Gaz. **17:**113, 143, 1882.

Moore, M. B., Jr., Price, E. V., Knox, J. M., and Elgin, L. W.: Epidemiologic treatment of contacts to infectious syphilis, Pub. Health Rep. 78:966, 1963.

Neisser, A. L. S.: Ueber eine der Gonorrhoe eigentumliche Micrococcusform, Zbl. Med. Wiss. 17:497, 1879.

Packer, N., Lymphogranuloma venereum. In Conn, H. F., editor: Current therapy, Philadelphia, 1963, W. B. Saunders Co.

Packer, N., quoted by Goldberg, J.: Studies on granuloma inguinale IV, Brit. J. Vener. Dis. 35:266, 1959.

Pariser, H.: Infectious syphilis, Med. Clin. N. Amer. 48:625, 1964.

Pund, E. R., Greenblatt, R. B., and Huie, G. B.: The role of biopsy in diagnosis of venereal diseases, Amer. J. Syph. Gonor. Vener. Dis. 22:495, 1938.

Saltzstein, S. L., Woodruff, J. D., and Novak, E. R.: Postgranulomatous carcinoma of the vulva, Obstet. Gynec. 7:80, 1956.

Shapiro, L. H.: Gonorrhea in females, G.P. 28:78, 1963.

Shapiro, L. H., and Lentz, J. W.: Clinical evaluation of treatment of gonorrhea in the female, Amer J. Obstet. Gynec. 97:968, 1967.

Shapiro, L. H., Lentz, J. W., and MacVicar, D. N.: Large doses of penicillin for treatment of gonorrhea in women, Obstet. Gynec. 30:89, 1967.

Sheldon, W. H., and Heyman, A.: Studies on chancroid, Amer. J. Path. 22:415, 1946.

Sigel, M. M., editor: Lymphogranuloma venereum, Coral Gables, Fla., 1962, The University of Miami Press.

South, M. A., Short, D. H., and Knox, J. M.: Failure of erythromycinestolate therapy in in utero syphilis, J.A.M.A. 190:70, 1964.

Syphilis, modern diagnosis and management, U. S. Public Health Service Pub. 743, Washington, D. C., 1961.

Thambiah, A. S.: Venereal granuloma, Trans. St. John Hosp. Derm. Soc. 43:44, 1959.

Thayer, J. D., Field, F. W., Perry, M. I., Martin, J. E., Jr., and Garson, W.: Surveillance studies of *Neisseria gonorrhoeae*, sensitivity to penicillin and nine other antibiotics, Bull. W.H.O. 24:327, 1961.

Wende, R. D.: Personal communication, October, 1967.

Wende, R. D., Forshner, J. G., and Knox, J. M.: Field evaluation of the Thayer-Martin selective medium in the detection of *Neisseria gonorrhea*, Public Health Lab. 22:104, 1964.

Willcox, R. R.: Factors leading to a failure of control of gonorrhea, Brit. J. Prev. Soc. Med. 16:113, 1962.

Willcox, R. R.: The treatment of chancroid, Brit. J. Clin. Pract. 17:455, 1963.

Chapter 23

Traumatic lesions of the vulva and vagina

This discussion of traumatic lesions involving the vulva and vagina does not include obstetric and surgical injuries. Lesions such as endometriosis, inclusion cysts (which are often incident to trauma), and chemical burns are discussed elsewhere.

ACCIDENTAL INJURIES

Because of their protected location, the vulva and vagina are seldom injured accidentally. These areas are, however, subject to almost any form of accidental injury. These injuries are most commonly seen in prepubertal girls as a result of traumatic straddling of such objects as fence rails, gymnasium equipment, bicycle frames, edges of chairs, baths, toilet seats, and even occasionally as a result of splinters acquired from boards on which they slide. Occasionally, the insertion of various objects by the patient is responsible. Injuries are manifested by the development of hematomata and lacerations.

Hematomata

Hematomata are seldom serious, though ecchymosis may be extremely alarming. They are manifested by swelling and tenderness, and, if the hematoma is large, often by pain. Usually, the hematomata are small and localized, although they may be extensive, extending from the vulva through the paravaginal tissues and into the broad ligament. The skin over large hamatomata is frequently black, shiny, edematous, and susceptible to surface trauma. On rare occasions, the blood loss into tissue spaces may be sufficiently severe to produce shock. In the adult, considerable edema may develop in the vulvar area following severe trauma, due to the dependent location of the lesion and the loose structure of the tissues.

Treatment

Small hematomata require merely the use of analgesics and careful observation for evidence of continued enlargement. A large, fluctuant collection of blood usually should be aspirated or incised and evacuated; in most cases, the latter method is preferable. In our own experience, most significant hematomata usually rupture and drain spontaneously. A significant number of infections occurs in these patients. Recovery is often more rapid if the hematoma is evacuated by a physician. If an obvious bleeding vessel is found, this should be ligated. Extensive exploration for obscure bleeding vessels, however, is inadvisable. In the presence of considerable generalized oozing, the cavity of the hematoma should be carefully packed, or, if it appears dry, a drain should be inserted and left in place for at least 24 hours.

Wilson reported ten labial hematomata observed over a period of 10 years, all of which followed astride injuries. Eight patients were treated by analgesics alone and two by evacuation of the hematoma and suturing. In Wilson's opinion, conservative treatment is best for labial hematomata unless a break in the skin surface gives rise to bleeding. Williams recommends aspiration or incision and evacuation of fluctuant collections of blood.

The application of cold compresses immediately following trauma and, subsequently, of local heat are helpful. If extravasation of blood into the tissue is extensive, the oral administration of the proteolytic enzymes may possibly facilitate absorption of the blood, although their value is debatable.

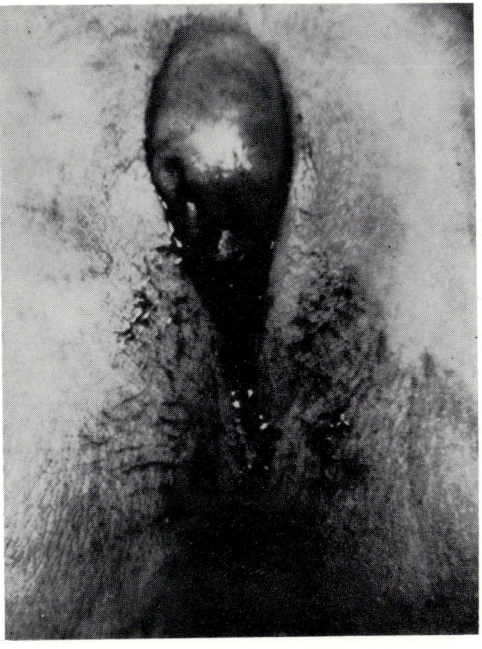

Fig. 23-1. Lacerations of perineum and periclitoral hematoma in 7-year-old child following a bicycle injury. (Courtesy V. J. Capraro, Buffalo, N. Y.)

Lacerations

Laceration of the vulva and vagina is especially likely to be received by a violent fall upon a slender object, such as a stake or picket fence (Fig. 23-1). Occasionally, this injury may extend through the vagina into an adjacent organ, such as the rectum, bladder, urethra, or even through the cul-de-sac into the peritoneal cavity. Under these circumstances, hemorrhage may be severe. The patient in Figs. 23-2 and 23-3 sustained her injuries in a motorcycle accident. Extensive deep lacerations of the labia majora were received, as well as vaginal lacerations extending through the posterior vaginal wall into the rectum and severing the anal sphincter.

When multiple severe lacerations are found in the vagina, a foreign body should be suspected as the cause; one should carefully search for remnants of foreign bodies such as glass, metal, or plastic. Anteroposterior and lateral radiograms, including the vaginal area, should be taken to locate metallic objects. Lacerations of this type may also result in profuse hemorrhage and severe pain.

Treatment

Treatment for vulvar and vaginal lacerations should be directed toward the restoration of normal anatomic relationships. Bleed-

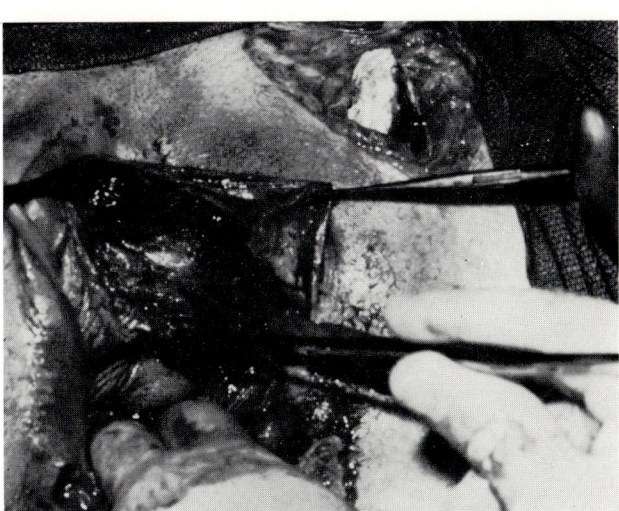

Fig. 23-2. Extensive injuries incident to a motorcycle accident. Fingers in vagina. Laceration extended through anal sphincter and also into retropubic space. (Courtesy James A. Friedman, Houston.)

330 Benign diseases of the vulva and vagina

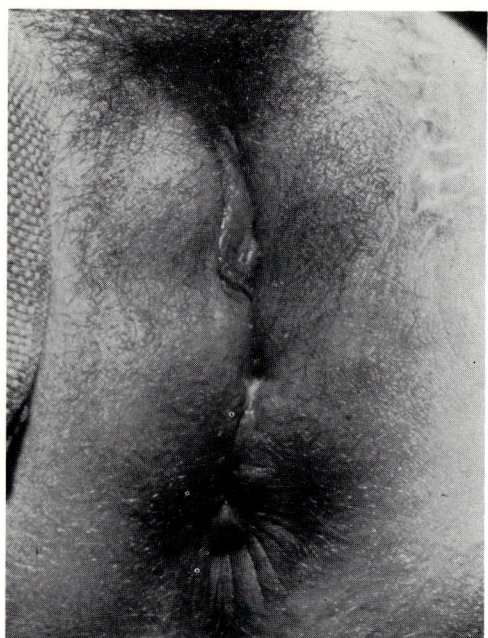

Fig. 23-3. Same patient as in Fig. 23-2, 3 months after accident and repair of defects. (Courtesy James A. Friedman, Houston.)

ing vessels should be ligated and the tissue edges carefully approximated. Large traumatic areas should be thoroughly irrigated with sterile saline, and necrotic tissue debrided. Adjacent organs such as the bladder and rectum should be examined for evidence of damage; if any is found, it should be repaired. If the peritoneal cavity has been penetrated, it should be explored for evidence of visceral lacerations and intraabdominal bleeding.

Forcible examination of a child should not be attempted. In the presence of considerable pain, bleeding, or evidence of laceration, she should be examined under anesthesia. Lacerations should be repaired by careful approximation of the tissue edges with small instruments, with small bites of tissue being taken.

As already mentioned, a meticulous examination should be carried out to determine whether adjacent organs have been injured. If they have, their anatomic structure must be restored. If loss of blood has been significant, it should be replaced. Reassurance of the patient and, if she is a child, of the parents that the injury will not impair her ability to have children normally, if this is true, is of extreme importance after the injury has been repaired.

SEXUAL INJURIES

Another major source of injuries to the vagina and vulva is sexual in nature. Such injuries are received during the process of defloration, rape, or insertion of foreign bodies into the vagina.

Wilson, in a review of traumas of the lower genital tract over a period of 10 years, found that sixty-three of seventy-three were secondary to coital trauma. Twenty of these sixty-three involved the introitus alone, and forty-three involved the vagina at varying sites. Seventeen of the twenty introital injuries were associated with first coitus, and three of the seventeen patients required transfusions. Of forty-three vaginal lacerations incident to coitus, ten followed the initial coitus, eight followed coitus in the postpartum period, five were in postmenopausal women, and five followed hysterectomy. Over half of the forty-three patients were parous. The lateral vaginal wall was most often lacerated, this area being involved in twenty-four patients. Twelve patients had lacerations of the posterior fornix, and five, lacerations of the posterior vaginal wall and the vaginal vault, post-hysterectomy. In one patient, the rent extended into the posterior broad ligament with no breech in the vaginal wall. Another patient had a complete perineal, posterior vaginal wall, and rectal tear extending up into the pouch of Douglas and peritoneal cavity. Twenty of the forty-three patients required transfusions.

The majority of introital injuries associated with first coitus are of rather minor degree and are accompanied by minimal bleeding. These can be managed by simple compression. Occasionally, however, the injury may involve an extensive laceration of the hymeneal ring and extend into the vagina, giving rise to profuse bleeding. In this event, suturing of the laceration is indicated after obviously bleeding vessels have been ligated.

Lacerations caused by rape are usually much more extensive than defloration injuries, especially in the virgin or young child. Frequently, trauma to the vulvar region, the hymeneal ring, and vagina is severe and is accompanied by considerable hemorrhage, hematoma, and laceration of the hymen

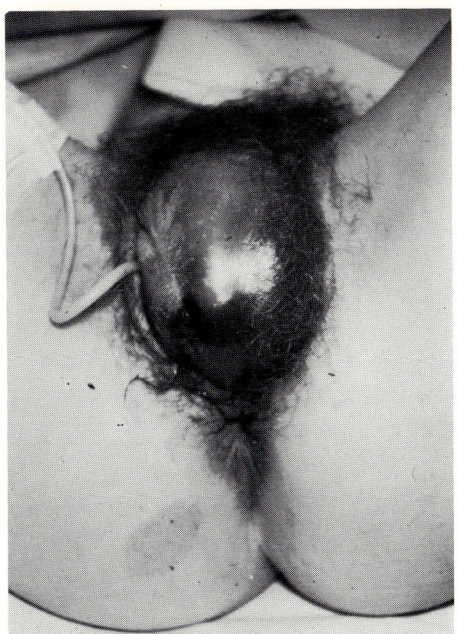

Fig. 23-4. Massive hematoma in a 14-year-old girl following rape.

(Fig. 23-4). Especially in a child, these lacerations may be quite deep, extending into the rectum or even the bladder. Rarely, the cul-de-sac may be ripped through and the peritoneal cavity penetrated. If bleeding is extensive, the patient should usually be given an anesthetic before hemostasis and repair of the lacerated tissue are undertaken.

Since the gynecologist is frequently the initial physician to examine the alleged victim of rape, it is essential that he obtain an accurate history and carefully document his findings, since he may be called upon to give testimony in a court of law. Not only must the examining physician note any evidence that will substantiate the individual's claim of rape, but he must also look for any information that may indicate a false claim of rape. Rape is defined as unlawful sexual intercourse with a woman by force and against her will. In Texas and several other states, in the case of a minor under the age of 18, even consent for intercourse is considered statutory rape. Obviously, there are various legal exceptions to this, which we will not go into in detail.

Before a charge of rape can be substantiated, medical evidence of signs of lack of consent and proof of intercourse must be present. The passage of the penis between the labia minora constitutes intercourse. It is well for the examining physician to follow a fixed routine in each case, making a note of all statements and findings. The following procedures are suggested:

1. Before the alleged victim is examined, consent for this must be obtained, preferably in the presence of a witness. If she is a child or is mentally deficient, the consent of the parents or guardian is necessary.

2. The time and place of the examination should be recorded. Also, the length of time since the alleged assault took place. The emotional status of the patient should be noted.

3. The age, marital status, parity, and last menstrual period of the patient should be obtained. If she was not a virgin, the date of last coitus should be recorded. Also, she should be questioned as to whether she has taken a douche or a bath since the alleged rape. The patient's clothing should be examined for missing buttons, tears, and stains and should be saved for examination by the police.

4. Physical examination of the patient should include a search for signs of violence, not only to the genital area, where lacerations and hematomata may be found, but also the entire body. Bruises and scratches on the face, extremities, and trunk should be recorded. Matted pubic hair should be noted, as well as the presence of foreign hairs on the patient; if found, the latter should be saved and labeled. If the pubic hair appears matted, some of this should be obtained for laboratory examination for the presence of semen. The presence or absence of the hymen should be noted, as well as whether laceration and bleeding of this tissue is present. In addition, the vagina should be examined for lacerations.

5. Laboratory studies should be made. It is preferable that all material obtained for laboratory examination be given directly to the clinical pathologist who will examine the specimens. If this is not feasible, a signed receipt should be given for each specimen delivered to the laboratory by the technologist who will make the tests.

   a. A wet mount of secretions should be obtained from the vaginal fornices to determine the presence of sperm. If the vagina is dry, it may be irrigated with saline and the preparation made from the solution. Motile sperm should be looked for. These may be found in the vagina for 30 minutes to 6 hours after intercourse, the average time being 3 hours. Nonmotile sperm may be found for 7 to 12 hours, and, at times, for 18 to 24 hours. A dry smear, stained with methylene blue or Wright's or Gram's stain, should also be studied for spermatozoa.

b. The absence of sperm does not preclude intercourse, since the assailant may have been azospermic or may have withdrawn. Dried stains on the clothing or the pubic hair may be examined for the presence of seminal fluid. Ultraviolet light produces a bluish fluorescence on seminal fluid stains, quite unlike that observed on material from the bladder or rectum. A vaginal aspirate and dried stains may be studied for acid phosphatase, which presumes the presence of seminal fluid. The finding of a positive fluorescence, together with a high acid phosphatase (for an immediate answer, Phosphatabs-Acid, Warner-Chilcott, may be used) or high creatinine phosphokinase level, or both, provides good presumptive evidence of seminal fluid.

c. Secretors of A and B substances will have these in their seminal fluid. If they are present, A or B blood group can be determined and compared with the blood group of the alleged assailant.

d. Dried stains of blood on the victim should be typed and compared with the blood of the suspected assailant as well as that of the victim.

e. Foreign hairs found on the clothing or body of the victim should be saved for comparison with the hair of the alleged assailant.

f. Smears, cultures, and serology studies should be made as indicated.

6. If possible, photographs should be taken of any bruise marks on the body of the patient, and of lacerations and bruises of the genital area.

7. The use of large doses of stilbestrol for several days following the assault may prevent a resultant pregnancy.

Special attention must be afforded the child who has been sexually assaulted. The immediate physical and emotional needs of the child must be met, as well as the emotional needs of the parents. The response of the parents to this tragic event may affect the psychosexual development of the child.

INJURIES BY FOREIGN BODIES

Occasionally, one observes lacerations of the vulvovaginal tissues incident to the insertion of foreign bodies by either a child or an adult. The subject of intravaginal foreign bodies in children has already been discussed in the section on pediatric vulvovaginitis. In most cases, the insertion of a foreign body into a nonvirginal or parous woman will not result in significant injury. When this is attempted in a virginal female, however, it may cause laceration of the hymeneal tissue as well as of the perineum. We have seen several unusual molded "phalluses" that have been used in homosexual activity, and, occasionally, they have rather severely lacerated the vagina. Glass objects, such as soda bottles or drinking glasses, may be introduced into the vagina; if they should happen to break, the vulvovaginal tissues can be severely damaged. Following laceration from these causes, the tissues must be carefully inspected for the presence of residual foreign bodies. If it is known that a glass object was broken in the vagina, a careful search must be made for glass fragments before repair of the lacerated tissue is undertaken. All bleeding points should be ligated and any necrotic tissue removed. The tissues should be approximated surgically.

Not uncommonly, a patient will leave a tampon in the vagina and then forget its presence. Practically always, the patient will notice a foul, copious, brownish discharge. In most cases, examination will readily indicate the source of the discharge. It is corrected by simple removal of the tampon.

The use of various vaginal pessaries and supports for uterine prolapse and large cystocele is less popular today than formerly. Not uncommonly, however, these devices are still employed in older women in the hope of deferring vaginal surgery. When left in place for a prolonged period of time, especially if the device is made of hard plastic or has sharp edges, the cervical portio and vaginal walls may become ulcerated (Fig. 23-5, *A*). On rare occasions, the pessaries become embedded in the paravaginal tissues, giving rise

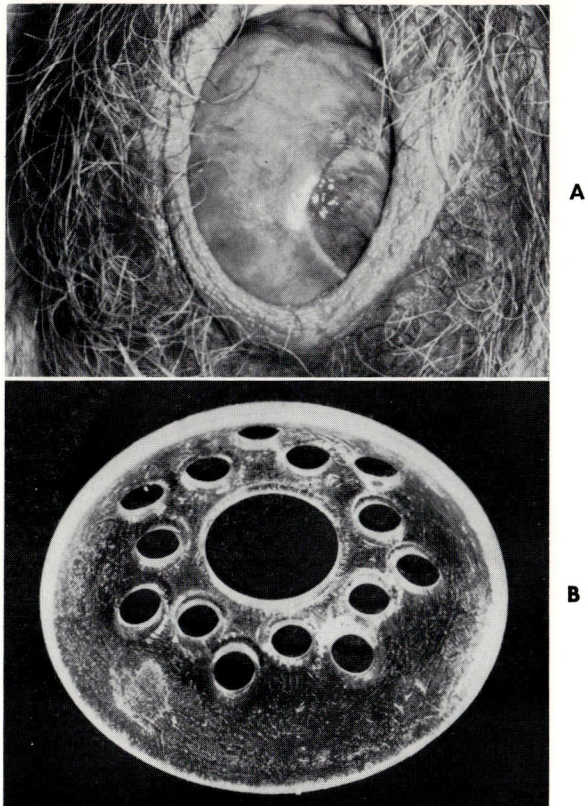

Fig. 23-5. **A,** Ulceration of vagina incident to pressure necrosis from plastic pessary. **B,** Pessary removed from patient shown in **A.**

to a bloody discharge and, rarely, to rather severe vaginal infection and parametritis. The pessary pictured in Fig. 23-5, *B* had been present in the vagina of a 70-year-old woman for approximately 1 year. For 2 months prior to its removal, she had a copious, bloody discharge. The pessary was tightly wedged into the vagina, pressing tightly upon both lateral vaginal walls. Following its removal, two deep, granulomatous appearing ulcerations were observed on each lateral wall. Russell has reported a case in which a vaginal pessary ulcerated into the bladder and rectum, producing large fistulae. He suggested that prolonged chronic irritation from a pessary may be a factor in the development of some vaginal carcinomata.

The treatment for injuries secondary to intravaginal pessaries consists first of removal of the pessary and, then, of application of topical antibiotic creams or suppositories, as well as topical estrogen cream, to stimulate reparative growth of the vaginal epithelium.

If a patient with procidentia has a severe ulceration, her confinement to bed while the ulceration is healing may be necessary. The use of lamb's wool tampons soaked in borogylcerin is also of value in promoting healing, as well as in keeping the vaginal contents in place.

The use of a vaginal pessary as a treatment for genital prolapse has little place in the modern gynecologist's armamentarium. For severe prolapse in elderly sick women, the LeForte operation offers good results, with few serious complications. Rarely, pessaries such as the Gellhorn type or inflatable rubber doughnuts afford temporary relief from the symptoms of severe genital prolapse.

INTERTRIGO

Intertrigo is essentially a chronic dermatitis induced by friction between moist, opposed surfaces of the skin, particularly of the genitocrural folds and the upper inner thighs. The inguinal folds and the intergluteal regions also may be affected. The condition is more prevalent in the obese patient, especially during the warm months of the year. Vaginal infections such as trichomoniasis and candidiasis aggravate the lesion.

Clinical features

Initially, the surfaces of the opposed affected areas become erythematous. If no treatment is administered, maceration, exudation, and fissuring of the skin may ensue, and ultimately verrucose changes and increased pigmentation may appear (Fig. 23-6).

Chafing, itching, and burning are the chief symptoms.

Differential diagnosis

Intertrigo is sometimes differentiated from infectious conditions with considerable difficulty. It may also be confused with dermatitis, neurodermatitis, erythrasma, tinea cruris, and a host of other affections. Severe intertrigo may resemble acanthosis nigricans. Involvement of the axillary and inframammary regions assist one in establishing the diagnosis, although some conditions, such as erythrasma, also affect the axillary skin. The discovery of nonpathogenic fungi in the scrapings may further confuse the differential diagnosis, such fungi perhaps suggesting the presence of candidiasis or tinea cruris.

Treatment

Since moisture predisposes to the development of intertrigo, the control of vaginal discharges, regardless of their etiology, will facilitate treatment. The vulva and inner thighs should be kept as clean and dry as possible. The wearing of cotton panties, rather than those made of synthetic mate-

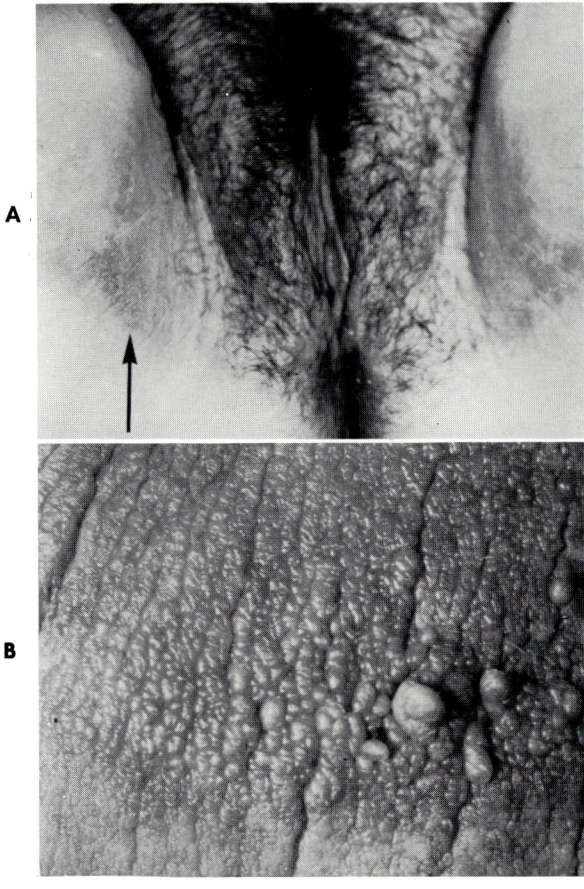

Fig. 23-6. **A**, Intertrigo of inner thighs. **B**, Verrucose changes from area indicated by arrow in **A**.

rials, is helpful in that they permit better aeration and evaporation of moisture. After the area is cleansed and dried, the application of dusting powders containing zinc stearate and talc is often helpful. Also, lotions with 5% zinc oxide are usually effective. Local applications of antiinflammatory agents, such as corticosteroids, or the use of antibacterial or fungicidal agents are occasionally beneficial, especially if a secondary infection has developed.

REFERENCES

Ashton, W. E.: A textbook on the practice of gynecology, Philadelphia, 1907, W. B. Saunders Co.

Barnes, J.: Rape and other sexual offences, Brit. Med. J. 2:293, 1967.

Capraro, V. J.: Sexual assault of female children, Ann. N. Y. Acad. Sci. 142:817, 1967.

Cook, W. R.: Essentials of gynecology, Philadelphia, 1943, Philadelphia, 1943, J. B. Lippincott Co.

Frachtman, K. G.: Foreign body in the vagina, Obstet. Gynec. 21:257, 1963.

Graves, L. R., and Francisco, J. T.: A clinical and laboratory evaluation of rape, J. Tenn. Med. Ass. 55:389, 1962.

Griffiths, P. D., and Lehmann, H.: Estimation of creatinine phosphokinase as an additional method for identification of seminal stains, Med. Sci. Law 4:32, 1964.

Hakanson, E. Y.: Genital injuries, Ob-Gyn News 2:1, 1967.

Parrott, M. H., and Millder, N. F.: Diseases of the vulva, In Davis, C. H., editor: Davis' gynecology and obstetrics, Hagerstown, Md., 1953, W. F. Prior Co.

Polson, C. J.: The essentials of forensic medicine, Springfield, Ill., 1965, Charles C Thomas, Publisher.

Russell, J. K.: The dangerous vaginal pessary, Brit. Med. J. 2:195, 1961.

Sharpe, N.: The significance of spermatozoa in victims of sexual offences, Canad. Med. Ass. J. 89:513, 1963.

Simpson, K.: Forensic medicine, London, 1964, Edward Arnold (Publishers) Ltd.

Simpson, K.: Taylor's principles and practice of medical jurisprudence, ed. 12, London, 1965, J. & A. Churchill Ltd.

Williams, G. A.: Postsurgical and post-traumatic tumors, Clin. Obstet. Gynec. 8:1020, 1965.

Wilson, K. F. G.: Lower genital tract trauma, Aust. New Zeal. J. Obstet. Gynaec. 6:291, 1966.

Chapter 24

Miscellaneous conditions

SYSTEMIC DISEASES

A number of systemic diseases may produce manifestations of the vulva and vagina. Among these, several—varicella, smallpox, diphtheria, diabetes, and the dermatoses—have already been discussed. The lesions discussed in this section are seldom encountered, yet they are mentioned for completeness. Obviously, not every systemic disease that might conceivably affect the lower genitalia will be reviewed.

Childhood diseases

On occasion, vulvovaginitis may develop in association with chickenpox and measles in their prodromal phase. This is also true with diphtheria and scarlet fever. Not uncommonly, the vulva becomes inflamed and irritated. Once the full-blown clinical picture of these disease entities is recognized, their relation to the vulvovaginal changes becomes apparent.

Blood disorders

Hunt discusses the association of an iron deficiency anemia of the microcytic type with vulvar symptoms and changes. Patients with this condition occasionally seek advice because of an intractable vulvar pruritus. On examination, the vulvar tissues, especially the mucosa, may appear dry and pale, and the mucosa may be fissured. Fissures may also be present at the angles of the mouth. The diagnosis should be suspected upon discovery of an iron deficiency anemia of the microcytic type. Treatment for the vulvar lesion alone will afford only temporary relief; the symptoms will return once the local therapy is discontinued. Upon treatment for the anemia, the vulvar discomfort will usually subside. While this is being carried out, the local application of hydrocortisone creams will afford the patient relief.

Hunt also reports a case of a 60-year-old woman who complained of irritation associated with an edematous, purpuric appearance of the vulva. The patient was given a diagnosis of acute myeloid leukemia. We have encountered one patient with malignant lymphoma who had multiple nodules of the vulva and vagina (Fig. 24-1); biopsy of the lesions established the diagnosis of malignant lymphoma (Fig. 24-2). Review of this patient's history revealed that 6 months prior to the detection of the vulvar and vaginal lesions, she had had a pneumonectomy because of a similar nodule in the lung.

Vitamin deficiency

At present, patients with vitamin deficiencies are rarely encountered in private clinical practice. Occasionally, however, they are observed in the out-patient clinics of hospitals. Deficiencies of vitamin A and B are most often associated with vulvar changes, although vitamin C deficiency can also give rise to changes in this area. Of course, most patients suffering from avitaminosis have multiple vitamin deficiencies.

Vitamin A deficiency

Vitamin A deficiency is usually associated with changes in the mucosal surfaces of the entire body, as well as of the vulva. The mucosa becomes fissured and ulcerated, and small papules appear in the vicinity of the hair follicles of the vulva. Patients complain of pruritus, and frequently the fissures become painful. Gastrointestinal symptoms, achlorhydria, night blindness, and subsequent keratomalacia may also be present.

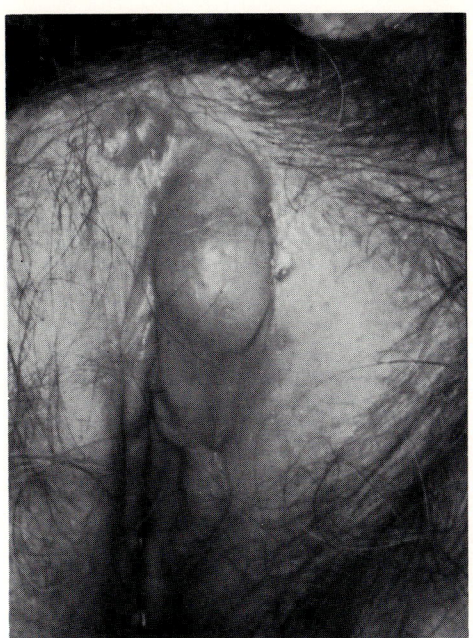

Fig. 24-1. Malignant lymphoma involving the vulva.

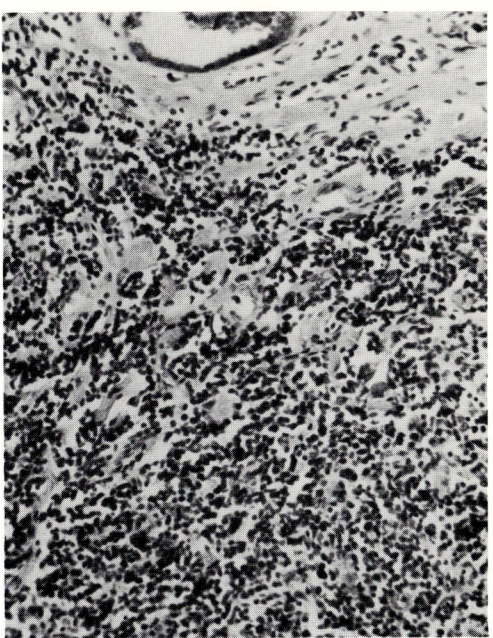

Fig. 24-2. Malignant lymphoma. Biopsy taken from lesion in Fig. 24-1. (H & E × 260)

Microscopic examination of the vulvar tissues will reveal hyperkeratosis and considerable edema of the connective tissue of the corium. Treatment consists of correction of the vitamin A deficiency by means of large doses of vitamin A by mouth (250,000 to 500,000 U. daily). If achlorhydria is associated, dilute hydrochloric acid should be given. The pruritus is usually relieved by the local application of hydrocortisone cream. Secondary infection within fissures can be controlled by the use of local antibiotics.

Vitamin B deficiency

Most authorities agree that the vitamin B factor plays the most important role in the deficiency diseases. Riboflavin, niacin, and thiamine chloride are essential agents in the process of cellular nutrition and respiration. As demonstrated by Parks and Martin, the vulvar skin and mucosa respond to prolonged deficiency of vitamin B. They found that riboflavin deficiency will predispose to a candidal infection.

Pellagra. The relation of pellagra to deficiency of vitamin B_2 (nicotinic acid) is well recognized. The vulvar lesions associated with this disease are usually erythematous and symmetrical, with sharp borders. The skin is hyperkeratotic and thickened. Finally, atrophic changes develop. As a rule, patients with pellagra complain of anorexia, vomiting, and diarrhea; the lesions on the skin develop later. As is true with most of the other diseases discussed in this section, evidence of vitamin deficiency elsewhere in the body is usually apparent. Treatment consists of an adequate diet, together with supplements of vitamin B complex and the other vitamins.

Vitamin C deficiency

Hemorrhagic ulcers of the vulvar and vaginal mucosa, similar to those of the oral, tonsillar, and pharyngeal regions, may accompany vitamin C deficiency. Such ulcers easily become infected. Submucosal hemorrhages of the vaginal mucosa may also develop, being exhibited by indistinct, painful swellings and usually associated with petechiae and ecchymoses of other parts of the skin surface. The diagnosis is based upon other symptoms of scurvy, such as swelling of the gums, oral hemorrhages, painful joints, anemia, and radiographic evidence of changes in the bones. Treatment consists of an adequate diet and large amounts of vitamin C and other vitamins.

Pemphigus vulgaris

Pemphigus vulgaris is characterized by the development of bullae on apparently normal skin and mucosa. The eruption usually involves the scalp, inguinocrural, perianal, umbilical, and inframammary regions, although ultimately it becomes disseminated over the entire body. Because of the frequent involvement of mucous membrane surfaces, the vagina and vulva are frequently affected. Despite this, there is little mention in the medical literature of genital involvement with pemphigus vulgaris.

The bullae usually develop rapidly. They vary in size from a few millimeters to several centimeters, are filled with a clear, straw-colored fluid, and have an apparently normal base. Eventually, the base may become erythematous and the contents of the cyst, turbid. The bullae on mucosal surfaces usu-

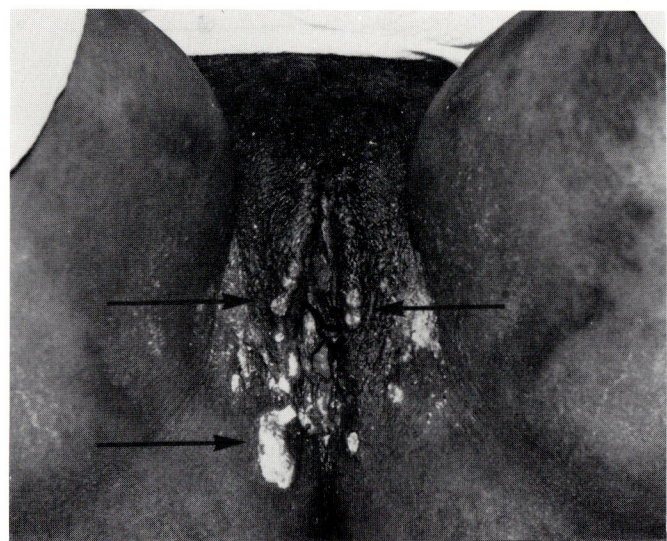

Fig. 24-3. Pemphigus vulgaris with crusted ulcers. (Kaufman, R. H., Watts, J. M., and Gardner, H. L.: Obstet. Gynec. 33:264, 1969.)

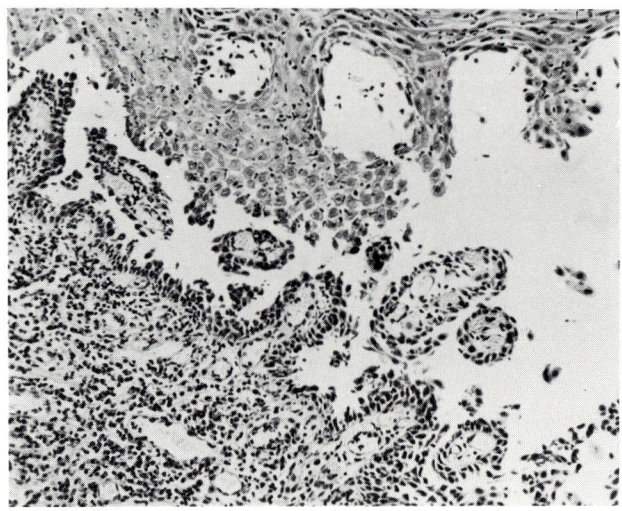

Fig. 24-4. Pemphigus vulgaris. Same patient as in Fig. 24-3, showing intraepidermal bullus. Epidermal cells and so-called villi are apparent within the bullus. (H & E × 160) (Kaufman, R. H., Watts, J. M., and Gardner, H. L.: Obstet. Gynec. 33:264, 1969.)

ally rupture early, leaving red, shallow ulcers. These become crusted, with the crusts eventually being shed (Fig. 24-3). Pemphigus may possibly be limited to a mucosal surface before the cutaneous lesions develop.

As a rule, the gynecologist is unlikely to consider a diagnosis of pemphigus unless the systemic disease is associated. In this case it is then wise to refer the patient to a dermatologist for confirmation of the diagnosis and treatment. If, perchance, only vulvar and vaginal lesions are present, the diagnosis may be suggested by the demonstration of acantholytic cells in a Tzanck smear or biopsy specimen (Fig. 24-4).

Before the discovery of ACTH and the corticosteroids, the course of pemphigus was progressive, resulting in death. With the use of these medications, the disease can now be fairly well controlled.

VARICOSE VEINS

Varicose veins commonly develop on the vulva during pregnancy, disappearing thereafter. As a significant clinical entity, they are rare in the nonpregnant woman, even one whose legs are severely affected.

Clinical features

The varicose veins may present as small, isolated protrusions, particularly on the labia majora (Fig. 24-5), or as large, sac-like, undulant masses covering extensive areas of the vulva (Fig. 24-6). Occasionally, the vari-

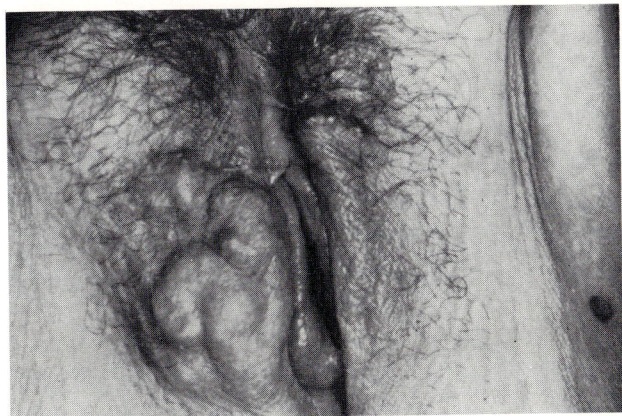

Fig. 24-5. Classical varicosities of right labium majus.

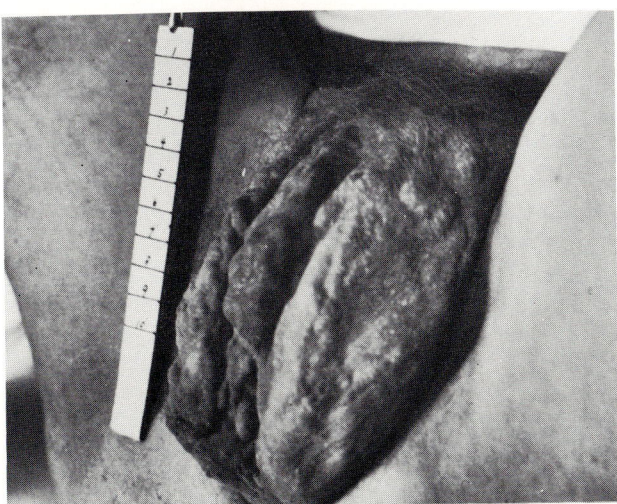

Fig. 24-6. Varicose veins of vulva, unusually massive, in patient with twin pregnancy at term.

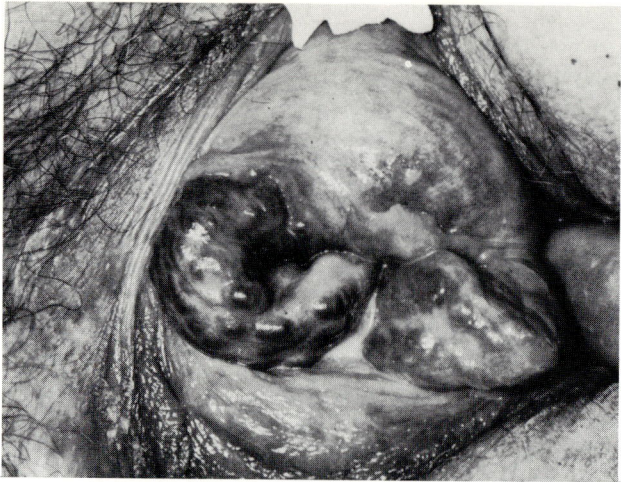

Fig. 24-7. Varicosities of lower vagina and introitus.

cosities involve the vagina and vestibule (Fig. 24-7).

The prominent symptoms of large varicose veins are heaviness and pressure in the vulvar area. Many women also complain of pruritus. Trauma may lead to large ecchymoses or hematomata. Rupture of a varix may give rise to severe or, rarely, even fatal hemorrhage.

Treatment

Opinion regarding the treatment for symptomatic varicose veins in the pregnant woman is divided. For large and progressive varicosities, Betson recommends ligation of the veins before the end of the seventh month of gestation. At delivery, he suggested a midline episiotomy to avoid cutting into the varicosities. Nabatoff recommended vulvar support for compression of the veins. Since most vulvar varicosities may regress to a pronounced degree following the termination of pregnancy, our approach has been conservative, consisting of the use of special support by pads and underwear. If repeated hemorrhage occurs, ligation of the veins may be necessary. Ligation may also be necessary for symptomatic vulvar varicosities in the nonpregnant woman. When ligation is required, Foote recommends high resection of the internal saphenous vein. He then opens the foramen ovale, locates the femoral vein, and ligates the deep internal pudendal vein. In the presence of repeated hemorrhage, the individual vulvar varicosities may be ligated. This is especially true during pregnancy, since regression of the remaining varicosities is to be anticipated following delivery. Practically speaking, the necessity for venous ligation for vulvar varicosities is extremely rare. On the few occasions when we have had to resort to this treatment, the uppermost and lowermost ends of the varicose veins were simply ligated. The use of sclerosing solutions has proved unsatisfactory; according to Foote, this method of treatment is difficult, painful, and only temporarily beneficial.

INSECT BITES

The skin, including that of the vulva, may be attacked by animal parasites such as the itch mite and the crab louse, which habitually inhabit the human skin; by those such as the bed bug, which live in the human environment but attack only for nourishment; and those such as ticks, which accidentally come in contact with human beings. A discussion of parasitic bites, other than perhaps pediculosis pubis, may seem superfluous in a book of this nature, yet we have observed one or more examples of each of those described herein. Since any classification of parasitic bites or any histologic description of the resultant lesions could be of only academic interest, they are not included, nor are the many systemic diseases that may be transmitted by parasites.

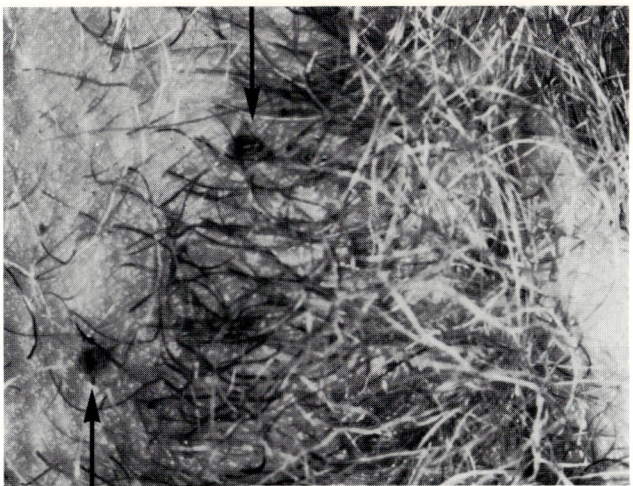

Fig. 24-8. Pediculosis pubis. Small, inflamed maculopapules.

Pediculosis pubis

Pediculosis pubis is an infestation of the hair-bearing area of the vulva by the crab louse *Phthirus pubis (Pediculus pubis),* an insect about 1.5 mm. long and usually dark gray in appearance. Occasionally, the same organism may be found in the axillae, the eyebrows, and hairy areas of the sternum of heavily infested persons. The pubic louse bites the skin of the hairy portion of the vulva and lives on the blood. The female deposits her eggs (nits) at the bases of the hairs. The organisms are usually transmitted through sexual relations, although they may be acquired by contact with bedding and toilet seats.

Itching is a constant symptom. Scratching may induce secondary lesions of the skin, such as lichenification, pigmentation, small excoriations, and pyodermas.

Careful examination will reveal nits and parasites at the bases of the hairs. The finding of ova and parasites is facilitated by the use of a magnifying glass; for certain identification, they may be caught with a forceps and placed on white paper. If present, lesions of the skin consist mainly of minute, inflamed maculopapules (Fig. 24-8). If the papules are excoriated, crusts may form.

Pediculosis may be confused with scabies. Lesions of the latter, however, are usually widespread over the body, including non-hairy areas; also, scabies lesions exhibit small burrows and are not accompanied by nits.

Topocide lotion and Kwell lotion are effective medicaments for the treatment of pediculosis pubis. The vulva should be thoroughly shampooed and dried before the preparation is applied. The treatment should be repeated after 3 days.

Scabies

Scabies of the vulva, which is caused by the itch mite *Sarcoptes scabiei,* is usually a part of widespread disease. It is transmitted from one person to another by close contact. The female of the species burrows into and deposits her ova and feces in the epidermis, producing a minute papule or vesicle. Itching, essentially the only symptom, is particularly severe in the warmth of the bed, where the mite is more active.

Treatment consists of the application of appropriate mite-killing substances such as Topocide (benzyl benzoate, D.D.T., and benzocaine) to all body surfaces other than the head and neck. The medication is applied on 2 consecutive days after a thorough cleansing of the skin.

Chigger bites

Chigger bites are acquired during the summer months, particularly in the southern parts of the United States and especially during berry picking season. The common chigger of the United States, *Eutrombicula alfreddugesi,* is a six-legged red mite barely discernible to the naked eye. Its favorite habitat is grassy lawns and pastures.

The bite of this organism gives rise to intense pruritus. The typical lesion is a minute papule. Some persons are unusually sensitive and develop allergic papulovesicular eruptions or papular urticaria. Excoriations, commonly present, may lead to follicular pyodermas.

Preventive measures are highly important to individuals exposed to infested areas. Flowers of sulphur powder applied to the stockings before exposure, as well as Six-Twelve (containing ethahexanediol in a light mineral oil base) applied to the legs and thighs, are effective repellants. A shake lotion is helpful in controlling pruritus, and the addition of sulphur (3%) to the lotion will kill the chiggers.

Bed bug bites

The common bed bug *Cimex lectularius* is a wingless, blood-sucking insect, about 5 mm. long and yellowish-brown in color. The insect inhabits beds and upholstered furniture, and also lives behind wallpaper and in the cracks of woodwork. From these locations, it makes nocturnal excursions, biting human beings, its favorite source of sustenance, during their sleep. Soon after the bite, the victim experiences a burning or stinging sensation at the site.

Depending upon the susceptibility of the subject, the lesion produced by a bed bug bite may be a wheal, papule, or blister. The lesions, which usually are found in groups or in a straight line, probably result from the mechanical effects of the bite as well as from the injection of a secretion. The fact that patients exhibit an increasing reaction to successive bites suggests that the reactions are primarily allergenic rather than caused by an irritant.

Treatment consists of the eradication of bed bugs from the household. The subject of insect extermination is not within the sphere of this book.

Tick bites

Ticks depend upon blood-sucking for sustenance. Several varieties, most of which are referred to as wood ticks, feed upon human beings as well as upon animals. The skin lesion is usually a minor inflammatory reaction around the tick bite; if the tick carries certain bacterial agents, however, a localized erysipelas-like eruption may develop. When the head of a tick is left imbedded in the skin, as often happens if mechanical removal of the tick is attempted, its presence gives rise to a longstanding (several months to a year or more) pruritic papule.

Any attempt at mechanical removal of an attached tick should be avoided, since the implanted head will usually break off and remain imbedded. The tick may be partially smothered and induced to drop off by the application of an oily substance, such as petrolatum. If the imbedded head cannot be extracted, the affected site may be excised.

Flea bites

Flea bites are all but nonexistent in the Houston area, and it would be particularly unusual for the gynecologist to be called upon to detect lesions arising from this source. According to Ayers, flea bites by the human flea *Pulex irritans* are not unusual in the California area, particularly around San Francisco. Fleas that normally inhabit cats and dogs also occasionally infest human beings.

As a rule, a flea bite gives rise to a small wheal in which a minute, hemorrhagic point is present. These small lesions are often typically grouped. In the hypersensitive patient, more impressive lesions, such as giant wheals or blisters, may develop. When an obscure papular skin eruption of the vulva exhibits a hemorrhagic pinpoint puncta, flea bites may be suspected. Preparations containing D.D.T. are highly effective against this insect.

Mosquito bites

Mosquito bites of the vulva could hardly be of much importance to the gynecologist. The resultant lesion is usually a pruritic papule, although the degree of reaction is highly variable in different persons. Secondary infection may lead to pyodermas.

REFERENCES

Ayers, S., III, quoted by Sauer, G. C.: Manual of skin diseases, ed. 2, Philadelphia, 1966, J. B. Lippincott Co.

Betson, J. R., Jr.: Varicosities of the pelvirectal area and the lower extremity in gravid women: Current therapy, J. Int. Coll. Surg. 42:50, 1964.

Burckhardt, W., and Epstein, S.: Atlas and manual of dermatology and venereology, ed. 2, Baltimore, 1963, The Williams & Wilkins Co.

Callomon, F. T., and Wilson, J. F.: The nonvenereal disease of the genitals, Springfield, Ill., 1956, Charles C Thomas, Publisher.

Dodd, H., and Wright, H. P.: Vulvar varicose veins in pregnancy, Brit. Med. J. **1**:831, 1959.

Foote, R. R.: Varicose veins, Bristol, England, 1960, John Wright & Sons Ltd.

Hunt, E.: Diseases affecting the vulva, London, 1954, Henry Kimpton Co.

Kaufman, R. H., Watts, J. M., and Gardner, H. L.: Pemphigus vulgaris: Genital involvement, Obstet. Gynec. **33**:264, 1969.

Kreek, M. J., Raziano, J. V., Hardy, R. E., and Jeffries, G. H.: Portal hypertension with bleeding vaginal varices, Ann. Int. Med. **66**:756, 1967.

Montgomery, H.: Dermatopathology, New York, 1967, Harper & Row.

Nabatoff, R. A.: Vulvar varicose veins during pregnancy, J.A.M.A. **173**:1932, 1960.

Parks, J., and Martin, S.: Reactions of the vulva to systemic diseases, Amer. J. Obstet. Gynec. **55**:117, 1948.

Sauer, G. C.: Manual of skin diseases, ed. 2, Philadelphia, J. B. Lippincott Co.

Simpson, G. W., and Mason, K. E.: Vitamin A deficiency vaginitis, Amer. J. Obstet. Gynec. **32**:125, 1936.

Sulzberger, M. B., Wolf, J., Witten, V. H., and Kopf, A. W.: Dermatology. Diagnosis and treatment, Chicago, 1961, Year Book Medical Publishers, Inc.

Tzanck, A.: Le cytodiagnostic immédiat en dermatologie, Ann. Derm. Syph. **8**:205, 1948.

Glossary

abscess A circumscribed collection of pus. Includes collections of pus in a cavity with an identifiable epithelial lining, the latter being at times referred to as *pseudoabscess*.

acantholysis Loss of coherence and sometimes polarity between epidermal cells incident to degeneration of the intercellular bridges, which may lead to the formation of vesicles within the epidermis.

acanthosis An increase in thickness of squamous epithelium through hyperplasia of the malpighian layers of cells.

acuminate With narrow point.

antibody A substance formed in the blood or tissues in response to the presence of an antigen.

antigen A substance which, when introduced into the body of an animal, promotes the formation of antibodies.

atypical clue cell Certain vaginal epithelial cells resembling, though not precisely identical to, clue cells.

ballooning degeneration Degeneration of epidermal cells characterized by intracytoplasmic edema and vacuolation and loss of intercellular bridges found in virus diseases. Also frequently present is amitotic division of the nucleus to form multinucleated giant cells.

basal cell layer of mucosa The deepest layer of cells of mucosa composed of squamous epithelium.

basal cell layer of skin (stratum germinativum) The deepest layer of the epidermis, being one layer of cells in thickness. The cells are columnar in shape. Interposed between some of the columnar basal cells are melanocytes, which, when stained with hematoxylin and eosin, appear as clear cells with small dark nuclei. These cells are capable of forming melanin.

bulla Same as vesicle, except they are greater than 1 cm. in diameter.

chromatophores Large cells in the dermis that ingest and carry pigment.

clue cell Vaginal epithelial cell with a granular or stippled appearance, incident to the adherence and uniform spacing of *H. vaginalis* upon its surface.

collagen Normal fibrillar connective tissue in the corium.

conidia Spores borne externally by fungi, sometimes called yeast cells or buds.

crust A dried layer of serum, blood, sebum, or pus on the surface of the skin, usually overlying a disrupted, eroded, or ulcerated epidermis.

cyst A sac containing a liquid or semisolid material.

dyskeratosis Faulty keratinization of epidermal cells, usually signifying premature keratin formation.

dysplasia Abnormality of development. This term has been used synonymously with the term "atypical epithelial hyperplasia" to designate nuclear pleomorphism and loss of normal cell polarity within the squamous epithelium. The changes are less pronounced than those exhibited by in situ carcinoma.

dystrophy A disorder arising from defective or faulty nutrition.

ecchymosis Same as petechia, but larger.

erosion A moist, well-defined, usually depressed lesion resulting from the loss of the epidermis above the basal cell layer. An example is excoriation from scratch marks.

excoriation A scratch mark or linear break in the skin surface; loss of superficial layers of skin, usually produced by trauma.

fissure A linear excoriation of the skin extending into the dermis, usually at mucocutaneous junctions and frequently in natural skin folds.

foreign body giant cells Multinucleated macrophages in which the nuclei are irregularly distributed in the cytoplasm.

glabrous skin Smooth, hairless skin.

granular layer of skin (stratum granulosum) The layer of skin, usually one to three cells in thickness, between the horny (keratinized) layer and the prickle cell layer. Individual cells are diamond shaped and filled with basophilic granules. The thickness of this layer frequently increases in proportion to the degree of keratinization, although it can be absent in the presence of parakeratosis. The chemical nature of the granules from which the layer derives its name is unknown.

histiocytes Cells from the reticuloendothelial system, having phagocytic properties.

homogeneous Of uniform structure or composition.

horny layer of skin (stratum corneum) The outermost layer of the epidermis. Its thickness is highly variable, depending somewhat upon external trauma. No intercellular bridges are visible between the horny cells, and, normally, they have no nuclei.

hyalin degeneration A condition in which the connective tissue layer has become homogeneous and takes a deep eosin stain.

hyperkeratosis An increase in thickness of the keratinized (horny) layer of the skin, caused by formation of excessive keratin in some conditions and by abnormal retention of the horny layer in others.

hyperplasia An increase in size incident to an increase in cellular elements.

hypertrophy An increase in size of individual cells, usually resulting in an increase in size of the involved organ.

hypha (hyphae) One of the tubular, usually branching and septate cells which make up the vegetative portion or mycelium of fungi. Sometimes called a filament.

intermediate cell layer of mucosa Cells of squamous epithelium lying between parabasal and superficial cells. The cells are polygonal, the cytoplasm is thin, and the nuclei are vesicular.

intertriginous Between folds of skin, as between the labia and upper thigh.

karyorrhexis Fragmentation or dissolution of nuclei.

Langhans' giant cells Multinucleated giant cells, the nuclei usually being arranged at the periphery of the cells.

lichenification Thickening of the skin and gross exaggeration of normal skin markings, usually induced by chronic trauma such as rubbing, and frequently associated with increased pigment.

macrophages Histiocytes that have ingested particulate matter or microorganisms.

macule A discolored area of the skin without depression or elevation.

maculopapule A macule with slight elevation.

metaplasia Transformation of one type of tissue into another.

microabscess Small abscess. An example is a microabscess of Munro in psoriasis.

Munro's abscess Microscopic abscess found in the stratum corneum in psoriasis.

mycelium (mycelia) The mass of hyphae composing the colony of a fungus.

nodule Similar to a papule, although the term is usually applied to solid lesions larger than 1 cm. in diameter that project above the surface of the skin and involve the dermis or subcutaneous tissues.

papilloma A circumscribed overgrowth or proliferation of the papillae of mucous membranes or skin; actually, an epithelial tumor in which the cells cover projections of stroma.

papule A solid, circumscribed elevation on the skin, generally used when elevations are 1 cm. or less in diameter.

parabasal layer of mucosa The layer of cells lying above the basal layer of cells of lining squamous epithelium. The cells are usually oval, have vesicular nuclei and thick cytoplasm.

parakeratosis Incomplete keratinization resulting in retention of nuclei in the cells of the stratum corneum. The granular layer is usually absent.

petechia A discrete deposit of blood or blood pigments, less than 5 mm. in diameter, in extravascular tissues that is visible through the surface of the skin or mucous membrane.

phagedenic Rapidly spreading and eroding: like phagedena, a rapidly spreading and sloughing ulceration.

pleomorphic Having two or more forms.

prickle cell layer of skin (stratum malpighii) The layer immediately superficial to the basal cell layer which is several cells in thickness. The individual cells, called squamous or prickle cells, are polygonal in shape and appear as a mosaic. The more superficial cells of this layer become flattened. Intercellular bridges are prominent.

prosoplasia Abnormal differentiation of tissue; development into a higher state of organization.

pseudoepitheliomatous hyperplasia Pronounced acanthosis with extensive downward extension of the rete malpighii. It frequently appears at the periphery of an ulcer and overlying certain tumors and may be mistaken for carcinoma.

pseudohypha A fragile chain of cells with characteristics intermediate between a chain of budding cells and a hypha.

pustule Small, circumscribed elevation on the skin, containing pus; also, vesicle containing pus.

pyknosis Shrinkage of the nuclei of cells.

rete pegs The elongated epithelial folds of squamous epithelium that extend down into the dermis.

recticular degeneration of epidermal cells Advanced intracellular edema with bursting of the cells and formation of multilocular bulla. The septa in the bulla represent cellular walls that have not undergone degeneration.

scale A thin plate of cornified epithelial cells resulting from decreased shedding or increased keratinization.

scaling Desquamation or shedding of a thin plate of horny epithelium.

scar Replacement by scar tissue of injured dermis or subcutaneous tissues; a replacement fibrosis.

spongiosis Intercellular edema of the epidermis giving rise to increase in the width of the spaces between the cells.

stratum malpighii The stratum between the basal and granular layers of the skin, also referred to as prickle cell layer.

superficial cell layers of mucosa Mature cells of outer layers of squamous epithelium. The cells are polygonal in shape, have thin cytoplasm, and pyknotic nuclei (6 μ or less).

telangiectasis A spot formed on the skin or mucosa by a dilated capillary or terminal artery.

ulcer A depressed lesion of the skin or mucous membrane resulting from the loss of all layers of the epidermis, thus extending into the dermis.

vegetation A growth or excrescence of any type; usually multiple.

vesicle A well-delineated elevation of the epidermis containing serum, plasma, or blood. This term is reserved for elevations less than 1 cm. in diameter.

virulence Degree of pathogenicity.

wheal An acute, transitory area of edema of the skin, usually rather sharply circumscribed, that appears and disappears rapidly, without leaving permanent changes.

Index

A

Acanthosis nigricans
 benign, 118
 clinical features, 118
 etiology, 118
 histopathology, 119
 malignant, 118
 pseudoacanthosis nigricans, 118, 119
 treatment, 119
Acrochordon
 clinical features, 43
 histopathology, 43
 treatment, 43-44
Actinomycosis, 274
Adenofibroma of Bartholin's gland, 64
Adenoma, sebaceous; see Sebaceous adenoma
Adenosis, vaginal, 107-110
 clinical features, 108-109
 histogenesis, 107
 histopathology, 108, 109
 objective signs, 109
 symptoms, 109
 treatment, 109
 types
  adenomatous, 108
  cystic, 108
  effluent, 108
  occult, 108
Adrenogenital syndrome, 15-16; see also Anomalies, developmental
Agenesis, vaginal, 27-28
Agonadism, primary, 15
Allergic reactions caused by contact vulvovaginitis; see Vulvovaginitis, contact
Amebiasis, 261-264
 clinical features, 262
 diagnosis, 262, 263
  differential, 262
  laboratory, 262, 263
 incidence, 262
 treatment, 264

Anaerobic bacterial vaginitis, 212-213
Angiokeratoma (Fordyce type), 60-61
 clinical features, 60, 61
 histopathology, 60, 61
 treatment, 60
Anomalies
 developmental, of external genitalia
  adrenogenital syndrome, 15
  agonadism, primary, 15
  classification, 24
  of clitoris, 25
   hypoplasia, 25
   hypertrophy, 25
  genetic and hormonal factors in, 15-23
  genetic-chromosomal, 33-35
  hermaphroditism, 16, 33, 34
  hormonal factors and intersex, 16-17
  mosaicism, 15
  pseudohermaphroditism
   female, 15, 29-32
   male, 34-35
  testicular feminization, 17, 34-35
  Turner's syndrome, 15
  urogenital sinus, variations in, 25
 diagnostic approach, 36-38
 female, 15-23; see also specific sites
  histogenic process, 18-23
  hormonal factors, 16-17
  intersex syndromes, 15-16
  morphogenetic processes, 17-18
 treatment, 38-39
 of the urinary tract, 35-36
  ectopic anus, 36
  ectopic ureteral orifice, 35
  epispadias, 35
  exstrophy of bladder, 35
 of the vagina, 27-29; see also Vagina
  congenital absence (agenesis), 27-28
  duplication, 28-29
  Gartner's duct cyst, 78
  imperforate hymen, 27
  prolapse of urethral mucosa, 67

Anomalies—cont'd
  of the vagina—cont'd
    transverse septa, 29
    vulvovaginitis from, in children, 279
  of the vulva, 25-27; see also Vulva
    fusion of the labia majora, 25-26, 29-31
    hypertrophy of the labia minora, 26-27
    hypoplasia, 25
Anus, ectopic, 36
Atrophic dystrophy; see Lichen sclerosus et atrophicus
Atrophic vulvovaginitis; see Vulvovaginitis, atrophic
Atypical epithelial hyperplasia; see Dysplasia

B

Bacterial vulvovaginitis; see Vulvovaginitis, bacterial, nonvenereal
Bartholin's abscess, 91-92, 306
  clinical features, 91
  objective signs, 91
  symptoms, 91
  treatment, 91-92
Bartholin's duct
  anatomy, 7, 8
  cyst; see Cysts, Bartholin's duct
Bartholin's gland
  anatomy, 7-8
  cyst; see Cysts, Bartholin's gland
  solid tumors, 64
Basal cell epithelioma, 48-50
  clinical features, 48-49
  histogenesis, 48
  histopathology, 49, 50
  treatment, 50
Bed bug bites; see Insect bites
Behçet's syndrome, 248-249
  clinical features, 248-249
  diagnosis, 249
  etiology, 248
  histopathology, 249
  treatment, 249
Bilharziasis; see Schistosomiasis
Bites, insect; see Insect bites
Blastomycosis, 274-275
Blood disorders, vulvovaginal manifestations, 336
Bowen's disease
  clinical features, 139-141
  general features, 146-147
  histopathology, 141
  treatment, 147
Burns, potassium permanganate, 295, 296-297
  clinical features, 296-297
  treatment, 297

C

Canal of Nuck, cyst; see Cysts of embryonic origin
Candidiasis
  primary cutaneous
    clinical features, 162-163
    diagnosis, 163
    treatment, 163

Candidiasis—cont'd
  vulvovaginal
    bacteriology, 153-154
    in children, treatment, 283
    chronic, treatment, 160
    clinical features, 154-156
    diabetic vulvitis; see Diabetic vulvitis
    diagnosis
      clinical, 157-158
      laboratory, 158-159
    etiology, 149-152
    histopathology, 156-157
    incidence, 152-153
    objective signs, 154-156
    predisposing factors, 150
    recurrent, treatment, 160
    sources of infection, 150
    symptoms, 154
    treatment, 158-162
      chronic and recurrent types, 160-162
    vestibular, 156
Carbuncle; see Follicular pyodermas
Carcinoma
  cervical, with herpes genitalis, 243
  intraepithelial, 139
    Bowen's disease; see Bowen's disease
    erythroplasia of Queyrat; see Erythroplasia of Queyrat
    general characteristics, 146-147
    Paget's disease; see Paget's disease
    squamous cell in situ; see Squamous cell carcinoma in situ
    treatment, 147
  related to dystrophies, 133-135
Caruncle, urethral
  clinical features, 65-66
  histopathology, 66
  treatment, 66-67
Cavernous hemangioma
  clinical features, 58-59
  histopathology, 59
  treatment
    of the adult, 59
    of the child, 59
Cellulitis
  clinical features, 303-304
  treatment, 304
Cervix
  duplication, 28
  endometriosis; see Endometriosis
Chancre, histopathology; see Syphilis, chancre; Syphilis, histopathology
Chancroid
  clinical features, 317
  diagnosis
    differential, 318
    laboratory, 318
  histopathology, 317
  treatment, 318
Chigger bites; see Insect bites

Childhood diseases, vulvovaginal manifestations, 336
Clitoris
  abnormalities
    hypertrophy, 25, 31, 32
    hypoplasia, 25
  anatomy, 5-6
  histology, 6
Coccidioidomycosis, 275
Condyloma latum, histopathology; see Syphilis, condyloma latum; Syphilis, histopathology
Condylomata acuminata
  clinical features, 231-233
  etiology, 230-231
  histopathology, 233
  malignant potential, 233
  objective signs, 232-233
  symptoms, 231-232
  treatment, 233-236
Congenital absence of the vagina; see Anomalies of the vagina
Contact vulvovaginitis; see Vulvovaginitis, contact
Contraceptives, vaginal, vulvovaginal reactions, 291-294
Corynebacterium
  in erythrasma, 265, 266
  in vulvovaginitis, 212
Cystic tumors; see Cysts; specific cysts
Cysts
  Bartholin's duct, 8, 86
    clinical features, 86-87
    etiology and pathogenesis, 86
    histopathology, 87
    marsupialization, 88-90
    objective signs, 87
    symptoms, 86-87
    treatment, 87-91
  Bartholin's gland, 8
  of embryonic origin
    in adenosis, 108
    canal of Nuck
      clinical features, 83-84
      treatment, 84
    dermoid, 85-86
    mesonephric and paramesonephric (Gartner's duct)
      clinical features, 79-82
      histogenesis, 78-79
      histopathology, 82-83
      incidence, 79
      treatment, 83
    supernumerary mammary glands
      clinical features, 84
      treatment, 84
  of epidermal appendage origin
    Fox-Fordyce disease
      clinical features, 76-77
      etiology, 76
      histopathology, 77
      treatment, 77
    hidradenoma; see Hidradenoma

Cysts—cont'd
  of epidermal appendage origin—cont'd
    sebaceous
      clinical features, 73
      histopathology, 73
      treatment, 73
    syringoma; see Syringoma
  of epidermal origin
    pilonidal
      clinical features, 72
      histopathology, 73
      treatment, 73
    traumatic inclusion and epidermal
      clinical features, 70-71
      histopathology, 71-72
      treatment, 72
  of miscellaneous origin
    endometriosis; see Endometriosis
    liquified hematoma; see Hematoma
    lymphangioma; see Lymphangioma
    vaginitis emphysematosa; see Vaginitis emphysematosa
  of urethral and para-urethral origin
    Skene's duct
      clinical features, 92
      treatment, 92
    urethral diverticulum; see Urethral diverticulum

D

Dermatitis
  contact; see Vulvovaginitis, contact
  seborrheic
    clinical features, 115
    etiology, 114
    histopathology, 115-116
    treatment, 116
Dermatitis medicamentosa (drug eruption), 295
Dermatophytoses, 270-274; see also Tinea circinata (tinea corporis); Tinea cruris; Tinea versicolor
Dermatoses of the vulva, 111-119; see also specific dermatoses
  acanthosis nigricans, 118-119
  contact dermatitis; see Vulvovaginitis, contact
  intertrigo, 333-335
  lichen planus, 116-118
  neurodermatitis; see Lichen simplex chronicus
  psoriasis, 111-114
  seborrheic dermatitis, 114-116; see also Dermatitis, seborrheic
Dermoid cyst; see Cysts of embryonic origin
Desquamative inflammatory vaginitis, 258-261
  clinical features, 260-261
  cytology, 260
  diagnosis, 261
  etiology, 259-260
  histopathology, 260
  treatment, 261

Developmental anomalies of the vulva and vagina; *see* Anomalies
Diabetic vulvitis
  clinical features, 165-166
  etiology and pathogenesis, 164-165
  objective signs, 165-166
  symptoms, 165
  treatment, 166
Diphtheritic vulvovaginitis in children; *see* Vulvovaginitis, pediatric
Diverticulum, urethral; *see* Urethral diverticulum
Double cervix, 28
Double uterus, 28
Double vagina, 28
Douches, vulvovaginal reactions, 290-291
Drug eruptions, 295
Dyspareunia in atrophic vulvovaginitis, treatment, 223
Dysplasia, 125-127
  gross and microscopic appearance, 126-127
Dystrophies, vulvar, 121-137
  atrophic (lichen sclerosus et atrophicus); *see* Lichen sclerosus et atrophicus
  classification, 122
  etiology, 132-135
  hyperplastic, 122-127; *see* Hyperplastic dystrophies
  mixed (lichen sclerosus et atrophicus), 131-132; *see also* Lichen sclerosus et atrophicus
  relationship to cancer, 133-135
  symptoms, 135
  treatment, 135-137

E

Ecthyma, 303
  treatment, 303
Ectopic anus, 36
Ectopic ureteral orifice, 35
Embryology
  differentiation of uterine and vaginal portions, 17
  embryonic and early fetal development of internal genital tracts, 12-14
  external structures, development, 14-15
  female sex anomalies; *see* Anomalies, developmental
  genetic and hormonal factors, 15-22
  and intersex, 16-17
  gross morphogenetic processes, 17-18
  histogenetic processes, 18-22
  internal structures, embryonic and early fetal stages, 12, 13, 19
Endometriosis
  of the cervix, 99
    clinical features, 102
    diagnosis of superficial type, 104
    etiology
      primary type, 99-101
      secondary type, 101
    histopathology, 103-104

Endometriosis—cont'd
  of the cervix—cont'd
    incidence, 102
    objective signs, 102-103
    symptoms, 102
    treatment, 104
  of the vagina, 104
    primary type, 104-105
    secondary type, 105
    treatment, 106
  of the vulva, 98
    clinical features, 98-99
    etiology, 98
    histopathology, 99
    incidence, 98
    treatment, 99
Epidermal cyst; *see* Cysts of epidermal origin
Epispadias, 35
Epithelioma, basal cell; *see* Basal cell epithelioma
Erysipelas, 303
  treatment, 303
Erythrasma, 265-267
  clinical features, 266
  diagnosis, 266-267
  treatment, 267
Erythroplasia of Queyrat, 141-142
  general characteristics, 146
  treatment, 147
Escherichia coli infection, 211
Exstrophy of bladder, 35

F

Female pseudohermaphroditism, 29-33
Feminization, testicular, 34-35
Fibroma
  clinical features, 51
  histopathology, 51
  treatment, 51
Flea bites; *see* Insect bites
Follicular pyodermas
  clinical features, 298-299
  etiology and pathogenesis, 298
  histopathology, 300
  treatment, 300
Folliculitis; *see* Follicular pyodermas
Fordyce angiokeratoma; *see* Angiokeratoma
Foreign bodies
  injuries, 332-333
  removed from vaginas of children, 285
    clinical features, 285
    incidence, 285
    treatment, 285
Fox-Fordyce disease, 74-77
  clinical features, 76-77
  etiology, 76
  histopathology, 77
  treatment, 77
Frei test, 321
Furuncle; *see* Follicular pyodermas

Fusion of the labia majora; see Labia majora, fusion
Fusospirochetosis; see Vincent's infection

G

Gartner's duct cyst; see Cysts of embryonic origin, mesonephric and paramesonephric
Genetic-chromosomal abnormalities, 33-35
    testicular feminization, 34-35
    true hermaphroditism, 34
Gonorrhea
    clinical features, 305-307
    diagnosis, 307-308
    etiology, 305
    histopathology, 307
    incidence, 305
    pediatric; see Vulvovaginitis, pediatric
    treatment, 308-310
        special considerations, 309-310
    vulvitis, 307
Granular cell myoblastoma
    clinical features, 55
    histogenesis, 55
    histopathology, 55-56
    treatment, 56-57
Granuloma, pyogenic; see Pyogenic granuloma
Granuloma inguinale
    clinical features, 322-323
    diagnosis, 324-325
        differential, 324
    etiology, 322
    histopathology, 323-324
    treatment, 325
Gumma, 312, 314; see also Syphilis
    in tertiary syphilis, 312

H

Haemophilus vaginalis infection in men, 204-205
    treatment, 205
Haemophilus vaginalis vaginitis
    bacteriology, 196
    causative agent, 191
    in children; see Pediatric vulvovaginitis
    clinical features, 196
    clinical findings, 199
    diagnosis, 199-203
    etiology, 191-193
    histopathology, 199
    laboratory findings, 199-203
    objective signs, 198-199
    pathogenesis, 195-196
    pathogenicity, 193-195
    predisposing factors, 193
    prevalence, 193
    sources of infection, 191-193
    symptoms, 197-198
    treatment
        miscellaneous measures, 204
        prophylaxis, 204

Haemophilus vaginalis vaginitis—cont'd
    treatment—cont'd
        systemic agents, 203
        topical agents, 203-204
Hemangiomas
    angiokeratoma; see Angiokeratoma
    cavernous
        clinical features, 58-59
        histopathology, 59
        treatment
            of the adult, 59
            of the child, 59
    granuloma, pyogenic; see Pyogenic granuloma
    senile, 59-60
        clinical features, 60
        histopathology, 60
        treatment, 60
    strawberry
        clinical features, 57
        histopathology, 57
        treatment, 57-58
Hematocolpos, 27
Hematomata, 328-329, 331
    treatment, 328-329
Hermaphroditism, true, 16, 33, 34; see also Genetic-chromosomal abnormalities
Herpes genitalis
    clinical features, 237-239
    diagnosis, 240-242
        differential, 242
        laboratory, 240-242
    etiology, 236-237
    histopathology, 239-240
    incidence, 237
    objective signs, 238-239
    during pregnancy, 243
    relationship to cervical carcinoma, 243
    symptoms, 237-238
    treatment, 242-243
Herpes zoster, 245-247
    clinical features, 246
    diagnosis, 246
    etiology, 246
    histopathology, 246
    objective signs, 246
    symptoms, 246
    treatment, 247
Hidradenitis suppurativa, 300-302
    clinical features, 301
    histopathology, 301-302
    treatment, 302
Hidradenoma, 47, 73-74
    clinical features, 74
    histogenesis, 73-74
    histopathology, 74
    treatment, 74
Hydrocele; see Cysts of embryonic origin
Hymen
    anatomy, 6-7
    imperforate, 27

Hyperplastic dystrophies
  atypical epithelial; *see* Dysplasia
  benign epithelial, 122-125; *see also* "Leukoplakia"
    gross and microscopic appearance, 122-125
  lichen simplex chronicus (neurodermatitis); *see* Lichen simplex chronicus
  unclassified, 125
Hypertrophy; *see* specific site
Hypoplasia; *see* specific site

I

Imperforate hymen, 27
Impetigo contagiosa, 302-303
  treatment, 303
Inclusion cysts, traumatic; *see* Cysts of epidermal origin
Infections
  bacterial, nonvenereal; *see* Vulvovaginitis, bacterial
  candidiasis; *see* Candidiasis
  Haemophilus vaginalis, in men, 204-205
  Haemophilus vaginalis vaginitis; *see* *Haemophilus vaginalis* vaginitis
  Mycoplasma, 212
  mycoses; *see* Mycoses
  nonspecific; *see* Vaginitis, "nonspecific"
  pediatric; *see* Vulvovaginitis, pediatric
  proteus, 212
  pseudomonas, 212
  pyodermas of the vulva; *see* Pyodermas of the vulva; specific pyodermas
  skin; *see* Pyodermas of the vulva
  trichomoniasis; *see* Trichomoniasis
  venereal; *see* Venereal diseases
  viral; *see also* specific infection
    Behçet's syndrome, 248-249
    condylomata acuminata, 230-236
    herpes genitalis, 236-243
    herpes zoster, 245-247
    molluscum contagiosum, 243-245
    systemic, vulvovaginal manifestations, 250
      treatment, 250
    TRIC virus, 249-250
    vaccinia of vulva, 247-248
Injuries
  accidental
    hematomata; *see* Hematomata
    lacerations; *see* Lacerations
  by foreign bodies, 332-333
  intertrigo; *see* Intertrigo
  sexual, 330-332
Insect bites, 340-342
  bed bug, 342
  chigger, 341-342
  flea, 342
  mosquito, 342
  pediculosis pubis, 341
  scabies, 341
  tick, 342
Intersex syndromes; *see* Anomalies, female

Intertrigo, 333-335
  clinical features, 334
  differential diagnosis, 334
  treatment, 334-335
Intraepithelial carcinoma; *see* Carcinoma, intraepithelial

K

Keratosis, seborrheic; *see* Seborrheic keratosis
Kraurosis vulvae, 127; *see also* Lichen sclerosus et atrophicus

L

Labia majora
  anatomy, 1
  fusion, 25-26, 29-31
  histology, 1-4
Labia minora
  anatomy, 4
  histology, 4-5
  hypertrophy, 26, 27
Labial adhesions, 26
Lacerations, 329-330
  treatment, 329-330
Leiomyoma
  vaginal, 63
    clinical features, 63-64
    histopathology, 64
    treatment, 64
  vulvar
    clinical features, 53
    histopathology, 53, 54
    treatment, 55
Leptothrix vulvovaginitis, 213
"Leukoplakia," 122, 133-134; *see also* Hyperplasia, benign epithelial; Lichen simplex chronicus
  relationship to cancer, 133-134
Leukorrhea
  from developmental anomalies, 279
  neonatal, 278-279
  physiologic, in pediatric vulvovaginitis, 278-279
  premenarchal, 279
Lichen planus, 116-118
  clinical features, 117
  etiology, 117
  histopathology, 117-118
  treatment, 118
Lichen sclerosus et atrophicus, 127-131
  with epithelial hyperplasia, gross and microscopic appearance, 131-132
  gross and microscopic appearance, 128-132
  relationship to cancer, 134-135
Lichen simplex chronicus (neurodermatitis), 122-124; *see also* Hyperplasia, benign epithelial; "Leukoplakia"
  gross and microscopic appearance, 122-124
  symptoms, 135
  treatment, 135

Lipoma
  clinical features, 51, 52
  histopathology, 51
  treatment, 52
Lipschütz ulcer (ulcus vulvae acutum); *see* Ulcer, Lipschütz
Lupus vulgaris, 214
Lymphangioma; *see* specific type
Lymphangioma cavernosum
  clinical features, 63
  histopathology, 63
  treatment, 63
Lymphangioma circumscriptum, 63
Lymphangioma simplex
  clinical features, 62, 63
  histopathology, 62-63
  treatment, 63
Lymphogranuloma venereum, 318-322
  clinical features, 319-320
  diagnosis, 320-321
    differential, 321
    laboratory, 321
  histopathology, 320
  special considerations, 321-322
  tests for, 321
  treatment, 321-322

M

Mammary glands, cysts of; *see* Cysts of embryonic origin
Marsupialization of Bartholin's cyst, 88-90
Mesonephric cysts; *see* Cysts of embryonic origin
Miscellaneous conditions; *see also* specific conditions
  mycoses; *see* Mycoses
  systemic diseases
    blood disorders, 336
    childhood diseases, 336
    insect bites, 340-342
    pemphigus vulgaris, 338-339
    vitamin deficiencies, 336-337
  vaginitides; *see* Vaginitis, nonspecific
  varicose veins, 339-340
Molluscum contagiosum, 243-245
  clinical features, 244-245
  diagnosis, 245
  etiology, 244
  histopathology, 245
  treatment, 245
Moniliasis; *see* Candidiasis
Mosaicism, 15
Mosquito bites; *see* Insect bites
Mycoplasma infections, 212
Mycoses; *see also* specific mycoses
  classification, 269
  deep
    actinomycosis, 274
    blastomycosis, 274-275
    coccidioidomycosis, 275
    sporotrichosis, 275

Mycoses—cont'd
  superficial, 269-274
    candidiasis; *see* Candidiasis
    dermatophytoses (tineas), 270-274
    torulopsis glabrata vulvovaginitis, 269-270

N

Neurodermatitis; *see* Lichen simplex chronicus
Neurofibroma
  clinical features, 52-53
  histopathology, 53
  treatment, 53
Nevus, pigmented, 45-47
  clinical features, 46
  histopathology, 46-47
  treatment, 47
  types, 46
"Nonspecific" vaginitis; *see* Vaginitis, "nonspecific"
Nonvenereal bacterial vulvovaginitides; *see* Vulvovaginitis, bacterial
Nuck, cysts of canal of; *see* Cysts of embryonic origin

P

Paget's disease
  clinical features, 143-144
  general features, 146
  histogenesis, 143
  histopathology, 144-146
Papilloma
  clinical features, 42
  histopathology, 42-43
  treatment, 43
Paramesonephric cysts; *see* Cysts of embryonic origin
Patch test for contact vulvovaginitis, 289
Pediatric vulvovaginitis; *see* Vulvovaginitis, pediatric
Pediculosis pubis, 341
Pellagra, vulvovaginal manifestations, 337
Pemphigus vulgaris, 338-339
Pigmented nevus; *see* Nevus, pigmented
Pilonidal cyst; *see* Cysts of epidermal origin
Pityriasis versicolor; *see* Tinea versicolor
Poison ivy and poison oak vulvovaginitis, 294
Postirradiation vulvovaginitis; *see* Vulvovaginitis, postirradiation
Postmenopausal vaginitis; *see* Vulvovaginitis, atrophic, postmenopausal
Potassium permanganate burns
  clinical features, 296-297
  treatment, 297
Primary cutaneous candidiasis; *see* Candidiasis, primary cutaneous
Primary irritant reactions in contact vulvovaginitis; *see* Vulvovaginitis, contact
Prolapse of urethral mucosa
  clinical features, 67-68
  treatment, 68
Proteus infection, 212

Pseudoacanthosis nigricans, 118, 119; see also Acanthosis nigricans
Pseudohermaphroditism, 15; see also Anomalies, developmental; Female pseudohermaphroditism
Pseudomonas infection, 212
Psoriasis
    clinical features, 111-113
    etiology, 111
    histopathology, 113-114
    treatment, 114
Pyodermas of the vulva; see also specific pyodermas
    carbuncle; see Follicular pyodermas
    cellulitis, 303-304
    classification, 298
    ecthyma, 303
    erysipelas, 303
    folliculitis; see Follicular pyodermas
    furuncle; see Follicular pyodermas
    hydradenitis suppurativa, 300-302
    impetigo contagiosa, 302-303
    infection of the apocrine glands, 298
    pyogenic ulcers, 298, 302-303
Pyogenic granuloma
    clinical features, 61
    histopathology, 61-62
    treatment, 62
Pyogenic skin infections; see Pyodermas of the vulva
Postirradiation vulvovaginitis; see Vulvovaginitis, postirradiation

Q

Queyrat, erythroplasia of; see Erythroplasia of Queyrat

S

Scabies, 341
Schistosomiasis
    clinical features, 264-265
    diagnosis, 265
    histopathology, 265
    pathogenesis, 264
    treatment, 265
Scrofuloderma, 214
Sebaceous adenoma
    clinical features, 47
    histopathology, 48
    treatment, 48
Sebaceous cyst; see Cysts of epidermal appendage origin
Seborrheic dermatitis; see Dermatitis, seborrheič
Seborrheic keratosis
    clinical features, 44-45
    histopathology, 44, 45
    treatment 45
Senile hemangioma; see Hemangiomas, senile
Senile vaginitis; see Vulvovaginitis, atrophic
Sexual injuries, 330-332
Skene's duct cyst; see Cysts of urethral and paraurethral origin

Skin infections; see Pyodermas of the vulva
Solid tumors; see Tumors, solid; specific tumors
Sporotrichosis, 275
Squamous cell carcinoma in situ
    general characteristics, 146
    histopathology, 142-143
    treatment, 147
Staphylococcal vaginitis, 210
Strawberry hemangioma, 57
Streptococcal vaginitis, 209-210
Supernumerary mammary glands, cysts; see Cysts of embryonic origin
Syphilis
    chancre (q.v.), 310, 311, 312, 314, 315, 316
    clinical features, 310-312
        primary, 311-312
        secondary, 312
        tertiary, 312
    condyloma latum (q.v.), 312-314, 316
    diagnosis, 314-316
    epidemiologic control, 316-317
    etiology, 310
    gumma (q.v.), 312, 314
    histopathology
        chancre, 312
        condyloma latum, 314
        gumma, 314
    incidence, 310
    treatment, 316
Syringoma
    clinical features, 77-78
    histopathology, 78
    treatment, 78
Systemic diseases
    blood disorders, 336
    childhood diseases, 336
    pemphigus vulgaris, 338-339
    vitamin deficiencies
        pellagra, 337
        vitamin A, 336-337
        vitamin B, 337
        vitamin C, 337

T

Testicular feminization, 17, 34-35; see also Anomalies, developmental
Testicular feminization syndrome, 17
Tests
    for lymphogranuloma venereum
        complement fixation, 321
        Frei, 321
        inverted Frei, 321
    for contact vulvovaginitis
        patch, 289
Tick bites; see Insect bites
Tinea circinata
    clinical features, 274
    diagnosis, 274
    histopathology, 274
    treatment, 274

Tinea corporis; *see* Tinea circinata
Tinea cruris
   clinical features, 271-272
   diagnosis, 272
   histopathology, 272
   treatment, 272-273
Tinea versicolor
   clinical features, 273
   diagnosis, 273
   histopathology, 273
   treatment, 273
Torulopsis glabrata vulvovaginitis, 269-270
   clinical features, 270
   diagnosis, 270
   treatment, 270
Transverse vaginal septa, 29; *see also* Anomalies of the vagina
Traumatic inclusion cysts; *see* Cysts of epidermal origin
Traumatic lesions; *see* Injuries
TRIC virus genitourinary infection, 249-250
Trichomonas vaginalis
   as a cause of trichomoniasis, 169-170; *see also* Trichomoniasis
   morphology, 169
Trichomonas vaginalis vaginitis, 168; *see also* Trichomoniasis
Trichomoniasis
   acute, 168-170, 173, 176, 179, 180, 181, 183
     objective vaginal signs, 176, 178
   asymptomatic, 168
   bacteriology, 174-175
   causative agent, 169-170
   in children, treatment, 283
   chronic, 168, 181
   classification, 168-169
   clinical features, 176-180
   cytology, 175-176, 178, 182, 183
   diagnosis, 182-184
     clinical, 182
     laboratory, 182-184
   etiology, 169-172
   histopathology, 180-182
   leukorrhea in, 176, 179-180
   of lower urinary tract, 178, 182, 187-188
     symptoms, 188
     treatment, 188
   in men
     diagnosis, 188-189
     treatment, 189
   pathogenesis, 173-174, 182
   predisposing factors, 171-172
   prevalence, 172-173
   relationship to carcinoma, 189
   signs
     objective vaginal, 176, 178
     vulvar, 176, 177-178
   sources of infection, 170-171

Trichomoniasis—cont'd
   symptoms, 176-177
   treatment, 184-187
Tuberculosis of the vulva and vagina, 213-214
Tumors
   classification, 42, 70
   cystic; *see* Cysts
   solid; *see also* specific solid tumors
     Bartholin's gland, adenofibroma, 64-65
     of epidermal appendage origin
       basal cell epithelioma, 48-50
       hidradenoma, 47
       sebaceous adenoma, 47-48
     of epidermal origin
       acrochordon, 43-44
       condyloma acuminatum, 42, 230-236
       nevus, pigmented, 45-47
       papilloma, 42-43
       seborrheic keratosis, 44-45
     of mesodermal origin
       angiokeratoma (Fordyce type), 60-61
       fibroma, 51
       granular cell myoblastoma, 55-57
       hemangioma, 57-60
       leiomyoma, 53, 55, 63-64
       lipoma, 51-52
       lymphangioma, 62-63
       neurofibroma, 52-53
       pyogenic granuloma, 61-62
     of urethral origin
       caruncle, 65-67
       prolapse of urethral mucosa, 67-68
Turner's syndrome, 15

U

Ulcer
   Lipschütz (ulcus vulvae acutum), 214
   tuberculous, 214
Ulcus vulvae acutum; *see* Ulcer, Lipschütz
Urethra
   anatomy, 8-9
   caruncle; *see* Caruncle, urethral
   diverticulum; *see* Urethral diverticulum
   prolapse of mucosa; *see* Prolapse of urethral mucosa
Urethral diverticulum, 93
   clinical features, 93
   diagnosis, 95
   etiology and pathogenesis, 93
   histopathology, 94
   objective signs, 93, 94
   symptoms, 93
   treatment, 95
Urethrocystitis
   atrophic, treatment of, 223
   trichomonal, 187
Urinary tract, anomalies; *see* Anomalies of the urinary tract
Urogenital sinus, variations, 25
Uterus, duplication of, 28

V

Vaccinia of the vulva
  clinical features, 247
  diagnosis, 247-248
  histopathology, 247
  treatment, 248
Vagina
  absence of, congenital; see Anomalies of the vagina
  adenosis, 107
  anatomy, 9-11
  anomalies; see Anomalies of the vagina
  blood supply, 11
  candidiasis; see Candidiasis, vulvovaginal
  duplication of, 28
  embryonic and fetal development, 12-14; see Embryology
  endometriosis; see Endometriosis of the vagina
  infection; see Vulvovaginitis; specific infections
  injuries
    by foreign bodies, 332-333
    sexual, 330-332
  lacerations; see Lacerations
  leiomyoma; see Leiomyoma, vaginal
  lymph supply, 11
  trichomoniasis; see Trichomoniasis
  tumors, cystic; see Cysts
Vaginitides, miscellaneous; see Vaginitis; specific types
Vaginitis; see also Vulvovaginitis; specific types
  amebiasis, 261-264
  candidal (moniliasis); see Candidiasis
  desquamative inflammatory; see Desquamative inflammatory vaginitis
  "nonspecific," 191, 253-254
  pediatric; see Vulvovaginitis, pediatric
  schistosomal (bilharzial); see Schistosomiasis
  staphylococcal, 210-211
  streptococcal, 209-210
  Trichomonas vaginalis; see *Trichomonas vaginalis;* Trichomoniasis
Vaginitis emphysematosa
  clinical features, 255-256
  diagnosis, 258
  etiology, 254-255
  histopathology, 256-258
  incidence, 255
  objective signs, 255-256
  symptoms, 255
  treatment, 258
Varicose veins
  clinical features, 339-340
  treatment, 340
Venereal diseases; see also specific diseases
  chancroid, 317-318
  gonorrhea, 305-310
  granuloma inguinale, 322-325
  Haemophilus vaginalis vaginitis, 191-205
  lymphogranuloma venereum, 318-322

Venereal diseases—cont'd
  syphilis, 310-317
  trichomoniasis, 168-189
Vestibule
  anatomy, 6
  bulb of
    anatomy, 8
  candidiasis of 156
Vincent's infection, 211-212
Viral infections; see Infections, viral; specific infections
Vitamin deficiencies, vulvovaginal manifestations, 336-337
  pellagra, 337
  vitamin A, 336-337
  vitamin B, 337
  vitamin C, 337
Vitiligo, resemblance to lichen sclerosus et atrophicus, 129
Vulva; see also specific diseases of the vulva
  anatomy, 1-9
  anomalies; see Anomalies of the vulva
  basal cell epithelioma, 48-50
  blood supply, 9
  candidiasis; see Candidiasis, vulvovaginal
    primary cutaneous, 154, 162-163
  carcinoma, 133, 134
    intraepithelial, 139-147; see also Carcinoma, intraepithelial
    in situ, squamous cell, 142-143, 146-147
  dermatoses; see Dermatoses of the vulva; specific dermatoses
  dystrophies; see Dystrophies, vulvar; specific dystrophies
  embryonic and fetal development, 12-14
  endometriosis, 98-99; see also Endometriosis of the vulva
  hypoplasia, 25
  infections; see Vulvovaginitis; specific infections
  injuries
    by foreign bodies, 332-333
    sexual, 330-332
  insect bites, 340-342; see also Insect bites
  lacerations; see Lacerations
  leiomyoma; see Leiomyoma, vulvar
  lymph supply, 9
  nerve supply, 9
  pyodermas; see Pyodermas
  tumors, cystic; see Cysts
  vaccinia; see Vaccinia of the vulva
  varicose veins, 339-340
Vulvar manifestations of systemic viral infections, 250
  treatment, 250
Vulvitis; see also Vulvovaginitis
  candidal (moniliasis); see Candidiasis
  diabetic, 163-166
    clinical features, 165-166
    etiology and pathogenesis, 164-165

Vulvitis—cont'd
  diabetic—cont'd
    objective signs, 165-166
    symptoms, 165
    treatment, 166
  gonorrheal, 307
Vulvovaginal candidiasis; see Candidiasis
Vulvovaginitis
  atrophic, 216-229
    postirradiation, 223-229
      clinical features, 226-227
      cytology, 224-226
      histopathology, 227-228
      objective signs, 226-227
      symptoms, 226
      treatment, 228-229
    postmenopausal, 216-223
      bacteriology, 217
      clinical features, 218-220
      cytology, 217-218
      diagnosis
        clinical, 222
        differential, 222
        laboratory, 222
      etiology, 216-217
      histopathology, 220-222
      objective signs, 218-220
      symptoms, 218
      treatment, 222-223
        for atrophic urethrocystitis, 223
        for dyspareunia, 223
  bacterial, nonvenereal, 208-214; see also specific diseases
    anaerobic, 212-213
    Corynebacterium infections, 212
    diagnosis, 208-209
    Escherichia coli infection, 211
    fusospirochetosis, 211
    Leptothrix infection, 213
    Lipschütz ulcer (ulcus vulvae acutum), 214-215
    Mycoplasma infection, 212
    proteus infection, 212
    pseudomonas infection, 212
    staphylococcal, 210-211
    streptococcal, 209-210
    tuberculous origin, 213-214
    Vincent's infection, 211-212
  contact, 287-297
    allergic reactions, 287
    clinical features, 287-288
    diagnosis, 289
    histopathology, 288-289
    patch test for, 289
    potassium permanganate burns; see Potassium permanganate burns
    primary irritant reactions, 287

Vulvovaginitis—cont'd
  contact—cont'd
    specific contactants, reactions, 290-297
      to corrosive chemicals, 295-297
      to douches, 290-291
      to drugs, 295
      to miscellaneous agents, 295
      to poison oak and poison ivy, 294-295
      to therapeutic vaginal agents, 291-294
      to vaginal contraceptives, 291
    treatment, 289-290
  pediatric, 276-285
    age group variations in vaginal physiology and bacteriology, 276-277
    candidal origin, 283
      treatment, 283
    diagnosis, 277-278
    diphtheritic origin, 282-283
      clinical features, 283
      diagnosis, 283
      treatment, 283
    foreign body origin, 284, 285
      clinical features, 285
      incidence, 285
      treatment, 285
    gonorrheal
      clinical features, 281-282
      incidence, 281
      route of transmission, 281
      treatment, 282
    Haemophilus vaginalis origin, 283
      treatment, 283
    leukorrhea
      from developmental anomalies, 279
      neonatal, 278-279
      physiologic, 278-279
      premenarchal, 279
    nongonococcal bacterial infections, 282
      treatment, 282
    nonspecific
      clinical features, 279
      etiology, 279
      treatment, 279-281
    trichomonal origin, 283
      treatment, 283
    types, 277
    vaginal physiology and bacteriology, age group variations, 276-277
    worm infestations, 283-284
      clinical features, 284
      treatment, 284
  torulopsis glabrata; see Torulopsis glabrata vulvovaginitis

W

Worm infestations, vulvovaginitis from, in children, 283-284